About the Editors

Max More, PhD is President and CEO of the Alcor Life Extension Foundation, the world's leading cryonics organization. An internationally acclaimed strategic philosopher and co-founder of the first explicitly transhumanist organization, Extropy Institute, Dr. More is recognized for his thinking on the philosophical and cultural implications of emerging technologies.

Natasha Vita-More, PhD is a leading expert on human enhancement and emerging and speculative technologies and is a Professor at the University of Advancing Technology. Dr. Vita-More's writings have appeared in *Technoetic Arts: A Journal of Speculative Research, Metaverse Creativity,* and *Sistemi Intelligenti*. She has been featured in numerous televised documentaries on media design, culture, and the future.

Classical and Contemporary
Essays on the Science,
Technology, and Philosophy
of the Human Future

THE
TRANSHUMANIST
READER

Edited by Max More and Natasha Vita-More

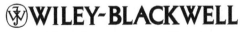
WILEY-BLACKWELL

A John Wiley & Sons, Inc., Publication

This edition first published 2013
© 2013 John Wiley & Sons, Inc

Wiley-Blackwell is an imprint of John Wiley & Sons, formed by the merger of Wiley's global Scientific, Technical and Medical business with Blackwell Publishing.

Registered Office
John Wiley & Sons, Ltd, The Atrium, Southern Gate, Chichester, West Sussex, PO19 8SQ, UK

Editorial Offices
350 Main Street, Malden, MA 02148-5020, USA
9600 Garsington Road, Oxford, OX4 2DQ, UK
The Atrium, Southern Gate, Chichester, West Sussex, PO19 8SQ, UK

For details of our global editorial offices, for customer services, and for information about how to apply for permission to reuse the copyright material in this book please see our website at www.wiley.com/wiley-blackwell.

The right of Max More and Natasha Vita-More to be identified as the authors of the editorial material in this work has been asserted in accordance with the UK Copyright, Designs and Patents Act 1988.

Library of Congress Cataloging-in-Publication Data

The transhumanist reader : classical and contemporary essays on the science, technology, and philosophy of the human future / edited by Max More and Natasha Vita-More.
     pages   cm
   Includes bibliographical references and index.
   ISBN 978-1-118-33431-7 (pbk. : alk. paper) – ISBN 978-1-118-33429-4 (cloth : alk. paper)
1. Medical technology–Social aspects.   2. Humanism–History.   3. Human body (Philosophy)–History.
4. Genetic engineering–Social aspects.   I. More, Max, 1964–   II. Vita-More, Natasha, 1950–
   R855.3.T73 2013
   610.285–dc23

2012050378

A catalogue record for this book is available from the British Library.

Cover designer: www.simonlevyassociates.co.uk
Cover images: Main image © Edvard March/Corbis. Chip © Aldis Kotlers / Shutterstock

Set in 9.5/13pt Minion by SPi Publisher Services, Pondicherry, India

1   2013

Contents

Contributor Biographies

Rachel Armstrong, MD, is a Teaching Fellow, the Bartlett School of Architecture, and a TED Global Fellow. She authored *Living Architecture* (TED Books, 2012); and co-authored with Neill Spiller *Protocell Architecture: Architectural Design* (Wiley-Blackwell, 2011).

Roy Ascott, is President, Planetary Collegium, Visiting Professor, School of the Arts, University of California Los Angeles. He authored "Behaviourist Art and the Cybernetic Vision" (*Cybernetica: Journal of the International Association for Cybernetics*, 1964); and co-authored with Edward A. Shanken *Telematic Embrace: Visionary Theories of Art, Technology, and Consciousness* (University of California Press, 2007).

Ronald Bailey, is Science Correspondent, *Reason Magazine*, and University Lecturer, Harvard University. He authored *Liberation Biology: The Scientific and Moral Case for the Biotech Revolution* (Prometheus Books, 2005); and *Ecoscam: The False Prophets of Ecological Apocalypse* (St. Martin's Press, 1994).

William Sims Bainbridge, PhD, is Co-Director, Human-Centered Computing, at the National Science Foundation. He authored *The Warcraft Civilization: Social Science in a Virtual World* (MIT Press, 2010); *Nanotechnology: Societal Implications* (Springer, 2007); and co-edited with Mihail C. Roco *Converging Technologies for Improving Human Performance* (Kluwer Academic Publishers, 2010).

Laura Beloff, PhD, is Associate Professor, IT University of Copenhagen and a Visiting Lecturer, Aalto University, Helsinki, Finland. She authored "Shared Motifs: Body Attachments in RL; and SL" (*Metaverse Creativity* 1, 2011), and "Wearable Artifacts as Research Vehicles" (*Technoetic Arts: A Journal of Speculative Research* 8.1, 2010).

Russell Blackford, PhD, is Editor-in-Chief, *Journal of Evolution & Technology*. He authored *Freedom of Religion and the Secular State* (Wiley-Blackwell, 2012) and *An Evil Hour* (I Books, 2003); and co-authored with Van Ikin and Sean McMullen *Strange Constellations: A History of Australian Science Fiction* (Praeger, 1999).

Nick Bostrom, PhD, is Director, Future of Humanity Institute, Oxford University. He has written numerous papers and authored *Anthropic Bias* (Routledge, 2010); and co-edited with Julian Savulescu *Human Enhancement* (Oxford University Press, 2011) and *Global Catastrophic Risks* with Milan Cirkovic (Oxford University Press, 2011).

David Brin, PhD, authored *Existence* (Tor Books, 2012); *The Transparent Society: Will Technology Force Us to Choose Between Privacy and Freedom?* (Basic Books, 1999); *The Postman* (Bantam Spectra, 1997); and "Future of Surveillance," in *Changing Minds* (Penguin Academics Series, 2009).

Damien Broderick, PhD, is Senior Fellow, School of Culture and Communication, University of Melbourne. He authored *The Spike: How Our Lives Are Being Transformed by Rapidly Advancing Technologies* (Tor, 2002); co-authored with Paul di Fillippo and David Pringle *Science Fiction: The 101 Best Novels 1985–2010* (Nonstop, 2012); and co-authored with Barbara Lamar *Post Mortal Syndrome* (Wildside, 2011).

Alexander "Sasha" Chislenko (1959–2000) MS, was an AI theorist, former Researcher Society of Mind Group, MIT. He authored "Technology as Extension of Human Functional Architecture," delivered at Extro3 Conference 1999, and "Intelligent Information Filters and Enhanced Reality" (1997). Many of his essays can be found at http://www.lucifer.com/~Sasha/.

Andy Clark, PhD, is Professor and Chair in Logic and Metaphysics, University of Edinburgh. He authored *Supersizing the Mind: Embodiment, Action, and Cognitive Extension* (Oxford University Press, 2010); *Natural Born Cyborgs: Minds, Technologies, and the Future of Human* (2003); and *Intelligence Mindware* (Oxford University Press, 2000).

Aubrey de Grey, PhD, is Chief Science Officer, Strategies for Engineered Negligible Senescence Foundation. He co-authored with Michael Rae *Ending Aging: The Rejuvenation Breakthroughs that Could Reverse Human Aging in Our Lifetime* (St. Martin's Griffin, 2008); and "Combating the Tithonus Error: What Works?" (*Rejuvenation Research* 11, 2008).

Eric Drexler, PhD, is an academic visitor at Oxford University. He authored *Engines of Creation: The Coming Era of Nanotechnology* (Doubleday, 1986); and *Nanosystems: Molecular Machinery, Manufacturing and Computation* (Wiley, 1992).

Robert A. Freitas Jr., JD, is Senior Research Fellow, Institute of Molecular Manufacturing. He has published three books: co-authored with Ralph Merkle, *Kinematic Self-Replicating Machines* (Landes Bioscience, 2004); authored *Nanomedicine*, vol. 1: *Basic Capabilities* (Landes Bioscience, 1999); and *Nanomedicine*, vol. 11a: *Biocompatibility* (Landes Bioscience, 2003).

Ben Goertzel, PhD, is an AGI Researcher, Novamente LLC, Chief Scientist, Aidyia Holdings, and Vice Chair, Humanity+. He authored *The Hidden Pattern: A Patternist Philosophy of Mind* (Brown Walker Press, 2006); *A Cosmist Manifesto: Practical Philosophy for the Posthuman Age* (Humanity+ Press, 2010); and co-edited with Cassio Pennachin *Artificial General Intelligence* (Springer, 2007).

Robin Hanson, PhD, is Associate Professor of Economics, George Mason University. He authored "Meet the New Conflict, Same as the Old Conflict" (*Journal of Consciousness Studies* 19, 2012); "Enhancing our Truth Orientation" (*Human Enhancement*, Oxford University Press, 2009); and "Insider Trading and Prediction Markets" (*Journal of Law, Economics, and Policy* 4, 2008).

Patrick D. Hopkins, PhD, is Associate Professor, Philosophy and Gender Studies, Millsaps College. He authored *Sex/Machine: Readings in Culture, Gender, and Technology* (Indiana University Press, 1999); and co-authored with Larry May et al. *Rethinking Masculinity: Philosophical Explorations in Light of Feminism* (Rowman & Littlefield, 1996).

James Hughes, PhD, is Director, Institutional Research and Planning, Trinity College. He authored *Citizen Cyborg: Why Democratic Societies Must Respond to the Redesigned Human of the Future* (Basic Books, 2004); and "Embracing Change with All Four Arms: A Post-Humanist Defense of Genetic Engineering" (*Eubios Journal of Asian and International Bioethics* 6, 1996).

Randal A. Koene, PhD, is Founder and CEO, Carboncopies.org. He authored "Fundamentals of Whole Brain Emulation: State, Transition and Update Representations" (*International Journal on Machine Consciousness* 4, 2012); and "Embracing Competitive Balance: The Case for Substrate-Independent Minds and Whole Brain Emulation" (*The Singularity Hypothesis: A Scientific and Philosophical Assessment*, Springer, 2012).

Ray Kurzweil, PhD, is Founder, Kurzweil Technologies, Inc., Co-Founder and Chancellor, Singularity University. He authored *How to Create a Mind: The Secret of Human Thought Revealed* (Viking Adult, 2012); *The Singularity if Near: When Humans Transcend Biology* (Penguin Books, 2006); and *The Age of Spiritual Machines: When Computers Exceed Human Intelligence* (Penguin Books, 2000).

Ralph C. Merkle, PhD, is Senior Research Fellow, Institute for Molecular Manufacturing, Faculty, Singularity University. He authored "Nanotechnology: What Will It Mean?" (*Spectrum*, 2001); "It's a Small, Small, Small, Small World" (*MIT Technology* Review, 1997); and co-authored with Robert A. Freitas *Kinematic Self-Replicating Machines* (Landes Bioscience, 2004).

Andy Miah, PhD, is Chair of Ethics and Emerging Technologies, University of the West of Scotland. He authored *Genetically Modified Athletes: Biomedical Ethics, Gene Doping and Sport* (Routledge, 2004); and co-authored with Beatriz Garcia *The Olympics: The Basics* (Routledge, 2012); and co-authored with Emma Rich *The Medicalization of Cyberspace* (Routledge, 2008).

Mark S. Miller is Chief Architect, Hewlett-Packard Labs. He authored with K. Eric Drexler "The Agoric Papers" (*The Ecology of Computation*, Elsevier Science, 1988); and *Robust Composition: Towards A Unified Approach to Access Control and Concurrency Control* (PhD dissertation, 2006).

Marvin Minsky, PhD, is co-founder MIT AI Laboratory. He authored *The Society of Mind* (Simon & Schuster, 1988); and *The Emotion Machine: Commonsense Thinking, Artificial Intelligence, and the Future of the Human Mind* (Simon & Schuster, 2007).

Hans Moravec, PhD, is Research Professor at Robotics Institute, Carnegie Mellon University. He authored *Robot: Mere Machine to Transcendent Mind* (Oxford University Press, 2000); and *Mind Children: The Future of Robot and Human Intelligence* (Harvard University Press, 1990).

Max More, PhD, is President of Alcor Life Extension Foundation and Co-Editor of *The Transhumanist Reader*. He authored "The Overhuman in the Transhuman" (*Journal of Evolution and Technology* 21, 2010); "True Transhumanism" (*Global Spiral* 2009); and "The Extropian Principles" (*Extropy: The Journal of Transhumanist Thought* 8).

Michael Nielsen is one of the pioneers of quantum computing. He is an essayist, speaker, and advocate of open science. His most recent book is *Reinventing Discovery: The New Era of Networked Science* (2012).

Ravi Pandya is Systems Software Architect, Microsoft. He co-authored with Sergey Bykov, Alan Geller, Gabriel Kliot, et al. "Orleans: Could Computer for Everyone" (ACM Symposium on Cloud Computing, 2011); and with Sergey Bykov, Alan Geller, Gabriel Kliot, et al. "Orleans: A Framework for Cloud Computing" (Microsoft Research, 2010).

Giulio Prisco, is a physicist, and former Senior Manager, European Space Agency. He authored "Transcendent Engineering" (*The Journal of Personal Cyberconsciousness* 6, 2011); "Let a Thousand Turtles Fly" (*Quest for Joyful Immortality*, 2012); and "Transhumanist Avatars Storm Second Life" (*H+Magazine*, 2011).

Michael R. Rose, PhD, is Professor and Director of NERE, Ecology & Evolutionary Biology, School of Biological Sciences, University of California Irvine. He authored *Evolutionary Biology of Aging* (Oxford University Press, 1994); and *The Long Tomorrow: How Advances in Evolutionary Biology Can Help Us Postpone Aging* (Oxford University Press, 2005).

Martine Rothblatt, PhD, JD, is Chief Executive Officer, United Therapeutics and Inventor, Sirius Satellite Radio. She authored *Apartheid of Sex: A Manifesto on the Freedom of Gender* (Crown, 1995); and *Your Life or Mind: How Geoethics Can Resolve the Conflict between Public and Private Interests in Xenotransplantation* (Ashgate Publishing, 2004).

Anders Sandberg, PhD, is a James Martin Research Fellow, Future of Humanity Institute, Oxford University. He co-authored with Nick Bostrom "Converging Cognitive Enhancements" (*Annals of the New York Academy of Science*, 2006); and "Whole Brain Emulation: A Roadmap" (*Technological Report*, 2008).

Wrye Sententia, PhD, is Postdoctoral Lecturer, University of California Davis. She authored "Neuroethical Considerations: Cognitive Liberty & Converging Technologies for Improving Human Cognition" (*Annals of the New York Academy of Sciences* 1013, 2004); and "Written Comments to the President's Council on Bioethics on the Topic of Mind Enhancing Technologies and Drugs" (*Journal of Cognitive Liberties* 4, 2003).

Michael H. Shapiro, PhD, is Professor of Law, University of Southern California. He authored *Cases, Materials, and Problems on Bioethics and Law* (Thomson West, 2003); edited and authored *Biological and Behavioral Technologies and the Law* (Praeger, 1982); and "The Identity of Identity: Moral and Legal Aspects of Technological Self-Transformation" (*Social Philosophy and Policy* 22, 2005).

Marc Stiegler is a Researcher, Intelligent Infrastructure Lab, Hewlett-Packard. He authored *The Gentle Seduction* (Baen Books, 1990); and *David's Sling* (Baen Books, 1987); and co-authored with Joseph H. Delaney *Valentina: Soul in Sapphire* (Baen Books, 1984).

Gregory Stock, PhD, is Chief Executive Officer, Signum Biosciences, former Director of Medicine, Technology and Society, University of California Los Angeles. He authored *Redesigning Humans: Choosing Our Genes, Changing Our Future* (Mariner Books, 2003; and *Metaman: The Merging of Humans and Machines into a Global Superorganism* (Simon & Schuster, 1993).

J. Storrs Hall, PhD, is Founding Chief Scientist, Nanorex, Inc. He authored *Beyond AI: Creating the Conscience of the Machine* (Prometheus Books, 2007); and *What's Next for Nanotechnology* (Prometheus Books, 2005).

E. Dean Tribble is Principal Architect, Microsoft. He authored nine patents, including: with Mark S. Miller, Norman Hardy, and Christopher T. Hibbert "Diverse goods arbitration system and method for allocation resources in a distributed computer system" (Sun Microsystems, 1997); and with Norman Hardy, Linda L. Vetter "System and method for generating unique secure values for digitally signing documents" (2000).

Vernor Vinge, PhD, is former Professor of Mathematics, University of California San Diego. He authored *A Fire Upon the Deep* (Tor, 1993, 2011); "The Coming Technological Singularity: How to Survive in the Post-Human Era" (*Whole Earth Review*, 1993); and *True Names … and Other Dangers* (Baen Book, 1987).

Natasha Vita-More, PhD, is Professor of Design University of Advancing Technology, co-founder, Institute for Transhumanism, chairman of Humanity+, and co-editor of *The Transhumanist Reader*. She authored "Epoch of Plasticity" (*Metaverse Creativity* 1, 2010); and "Aesthetics of the Radically Enhanced Human" (*Technoetic Arts: A Journal of Speculative Research* 8, 2003).

Brian Wowk, PhD, is Senior Scientist, 21st Century Medicine, Inc. He authored "Thermodynamic aspects of vitrification" (*Cryobiology* 60, 2010), "Cryopreservation of complex systems (*Cryobiology*, 2007) and "Cryonics Revived: Verification Unjustly Vilified" (*Skeptic*, 2005).

The Philosophy of Transhumanism

Max More

I. The Philosophy

To write of "the" philosophy of transhumanism is a little daring. The growth of transhumanism as a movement and philosophy means that differing perspectives on it have formed. Despite all the varieties and interpretations we can still identify some central themes, values, and interests that give transhumanism its distinct identity. This coherence is reflected in the large degree of agreement between definitions of the philosophy from multiple sources.

According to my early definition (More 1990), the term refers to:

> Philosophies of life (such as extropian perspectives) that seek the continuation and acceleration of the evolution of intelligent life beyond its currently human form and human limitations by means of science and technology, guided by life-promoting principles and values.

According to the Transhumanist FAQ (Various 2003), transhumanism is:

> The intellectual and cultural movement that affirms the possibility and desirability of fundamentally improving the human condition through applied reason, especially by developing and making widely available technologies to eliminate aging and to greatly enhance human intellectual, physical, and psychological capacities.

A corollary definition (also from the FAQ) focuses on the activity rather than the content of transhumanism:

> The study of the ramifications, promises, and potential dangers of technologies that will enable us to overcome fundamental human limitations, and the related study of the ethical matters involved in developing and using such technologies.

The Transhumanist Reader: Classical and Contemporary Essays on the Science, Technology, and Philosophy of the Human Future, First Edition. Edited by Max More and Natasha Vita-More.
© 2013 John Wiley & Sons, Inc. Published 2013 by John Wiley & Sons, Inc.

Thus transhumanism is a life philosophy, an intellectual and cultural movement, and an area of study. In referring to it as a life philosophy, the 1990 definition places transhumanism in the company of complex worldviews such as secular humanism and Confucianism that have practical implications for our lives without basing themselves on any supernatural or physically transcendent belief. Transhumanism could be described by the term "eupraxsophy," coined by secular humanist Paul Kurtz, as a type of nonreligious philosophy of life that rejects faith, worship, and the supernatural, instead emphasizing a meaningful and ethical approach to living informed by reason, science, progress, and the value of existence in our current life.

What is the core content of this philosophy? A simple yet helpful way to grasp its nature is to think of transhumanism as "trans-humanism" plus "transhuman-ism." "Trans-humanism" emphasizes the philosophy's roots in Enlightenment humanism. From here comes the emphasis on progress (its possibility and desirability, not its inevitability), on taking personal charge of creating better futures rather than hoping or praying for them to be brought about by supernatural forces, on reason, technology, scientific method, and human creativity rather than faith.

While firmly committed to improving the human condition and generally optimistic about our prospects for doing so, transhumanism does not entail any belief in the inevitability of progress nor in a future free of dangers and downsides. The same powerful technologies that can transform human nature for the better could also be used in ways that, intentionally or unintentionally, cause direct damage or more subtly undermine our lives. The transhumanist concern with rationality and its concomitant acknowledgment of uncertainty implies recognizing and proactively warding off risks and minimizing costs.

"Trans-human" emphasizes the way transhumanism goes well beyond humanism in both means and ends. Humanism tends to rely exclusively on educational and cultural refinement to improve human nature whereas transhumanists want to apply technology to overcome limits imposed by our biological and genetic heritage. Transhumanists regard human nature not as an end in itself, not as perfect, and not as having any claim on our allegiance. Rather, it is just one point along an evolutionary pathway and we can learn to reshape our own nature in ways we deem desirable and valuable. By thoughtfully, carefully, and yet boldly applying technology to ourselves, we can become something no longer accurately described as human – we can become posthuman.

Becoming posthuman means exceeding the limitations that define the less desirable aspects of the "human condition." Posthuman beings would no longer suffer from disease, aging, and inevitable death (but they are likely to face other challenges). They would have vastly greater physical capability and freedom of form – often referred to as "morphological freedom" (More 1993; Sandberg 2001). Posthumans would also have much greater cognitive capabilities, and more refined emotions (more joy, less anger, or whatever changes each individual prefers). Transhumanists typically look to expand the range of possible future environments for posthuman life, including space colonization and the creation of rich virtual worlds. When transhumanists refer to "technology" as the primary means of effecting changes to the human condition, this should be understood broadly to include the design of organizations, economies, polities, and the use of psychological methods and tools.

As a philosophy, transhumanism does not intrinsically commend specific technologies. Even so, certain technologies and areas of current and projected future technological development clearly are especially relevant to transhumanist goals. These include information technology, computer science and engineering, cognitive science and the neurosciences, neural-computer interface research, materials science, artificial intelligence, the array of sciences and technologies involved in regenerative medicine and life extension, genetic engineering, and nanotechnology. A genuine understanding of the goals and potentials of transhumanism requires taking an interdisciplinary view, integrating the physical and social sciences.

The first fully developed transhumanist philosophy was defined by the Principles of Extropy, the first version of which was published in 1990. The concept of "extropy" was used to encapsulate the core values and goals of transhumanism. Intended not as a technical term opposed to entropy but instead as a metaphor, extropy was defined as "the extent of a living or organizational system's intelligence, functional order, vitality, and capacity and drive for improvement."

The Principles were formulated to "use current scientific understanding along with critical and creative thinking to define a small set of principles or values that could help make sense of the confusing but potentially liberating and existentially enriching capabilities opening up to humanity" (More 2003). The goal was not to specify particular beliefs, technologies, or policies. The Principles of Extropy consist of a handful of principles (or values or perspectives) that codify proactive, life-affirming, and life-promoting ideals supportive of transhumanism.

Although the Principles of Extropy define a specific form of transhumanism, that document is both the first comprehensive and explicit statement of transhumanism and embodies several crucial elements shared by all extant forms of transhumanism. The 2003 (and still current) version included the principles of perpetual progress, self-transformation, practical optimism, intelligent technology, open society, self-direction, and rational thinking.

Perpetual progress is a strong statement of the transhumanist commitment to seek "more intelligence, wisdom, and effectiveness, an open-ended lifespan, and the removal of political, cultural, biological, and psychological limits to continuing development. Perpetually overcoming constraints on our progress and possibilities as individuals, as organizations, and as a species. Growing in healthy directions without bound." The individual element of this is expressed in the principle of self-transformation, which means "affirming continual ethical, intellectual, and physical self-improvement, through critical and creative thinking, perpetual learning, personal responsibility, proactivity, and experimentation. Using technology – in the widest sense to seek physiological and neurological augmentation along with emotional and psychological refinement." Both of these principles clearly express the implementation of transhumanism as being a continual process and *not* about seeking a state of perfection.

All transhumanists to date would likely also have no disagreement with the principles of intelligent technology, self-direction, or rational thinking. Intelligent Technology "means designing and managing technologies not as ends in themselves but as effective means for improving life. Applying science and technology creatively and courageously to transcend 'natural' but harmful, confining qualities derived from our biological heritage, culture, and environment." Self-direction means "valuing independent thinking, individual freedom, personal responsibility, self-direction, self-respect, and a parallel respect for others." And rational thinking means "favoring reason over blind faith and questioning over dogma. It means understanding, experimenting, learning, challenging, and innovating rather than clinging to beliefs."

An emphasis on "transhuman-ism" at the expense of "trans-humanism" might lead some transhumanists to reject the principle of open society, although so far it remains highly compatible with the vast majority of transhumanist views. That principle recommends "supporting social orders that foster freedom of communication, freedom of action, experimentation, innovation, questioning, and learning. Opposing authoritarian social control and unnecessary hierarchy and favoring the rule of law and decentralization of power and responsibility. Preferring bargaining over battling, exchange over extortion, and communication over compulsion. Openness to improvement rather than a static utopia. Extropia ("ever-receding stretch goals for society") over utopia ("no place")."

All the slightly varied statements of transhumanism gravitate around some core values, goals, and commitments. Even so, as with any complex philosophy that is no longer completely new, it is always possible to find one or two representatives who will disagree with some aspects of the view as originally stated. One or two transhumanist writers have, for instance, questioned or challenged at least some interpretations of the perpetual progress and practical optimism principles (Verdoux 2009). A distinct yet highly concordant statement of transhumanism can be found in the Transhumanist Declaration (Various 2002).

In terms of the traditional areas of philosophy, we can inquire about the main transhumanist views of ethics, metaphysics, and epistemology. I will address ethics in the third section of this essay, since transhumanists disagree over the meta-ethical basis of transhumanist values far more than they differ over basic matters of metaphysics and epistemology.

It would not be accurate to speak of a universally accepted "transhumanist epistemology," if that is taken to mean a detailed theory of the acquisition and validation of knowledge. However, transhumanists over the last almost quarter-century have practically always identified themselves as strong rationalists. A healthy legacy of the humanist roots of transhumanism is its commitment to scientific method, critical thinking, and openness to revision of beliefs. A remarkably large number of transhumanists are preoccupied with understanding and attempting to avoid the cognitive biases and deficient cognitive shortcuts to which the human brain is inherently vulnerable. That preoccupation is especially evident on the Overcoming Bias and Less Wrong community blogs.

Except for a widespread commitment to rationalism and a self-critical drive to overcome endemic human cognitive biases, transhumanists' epistemological views range widely (where these are explicitly stated – not all transhumanists delve into such recondite areas of philosophy). Some form of Piercean pragmatism seems to be quite popular while others may accept some form of externalism, explicitly or implicitly.

Another approach with substantial support (which I presented at the first conference organized by Extropy Institute) is pancritical rationalism (PCR), also known as comprehensively critical rationalism (Bartley 1962; More 1994). This epistemology, based on the work of philosopher of science Karl Popper, differs radically from much Enlightenment epistemology. Many Enlightenment thinkers defended some form of foundationalism, starting with Descartes' quest for utterly certain foundations for knowledge which he located in his supposedly clear and distinct idea of God. Empiricists and idealists (other than Bishop Berkeley) usually left God out of the picture yet still sought certain foundations in the form of unquestionable sense impressions or self-evident concepts or intellectual intuition.

Critical rationalism, by contrast, rejects this "justificationism" – the view that beliefs must be justified by appeal to an authority of some kind – in favor of the view that nothing is justified or beyond question. There are no foundations to knowledge. Acquiring and improving knowledge is based essentially on conjecture and criticism. According to critical rationalism, we can give up justification while retaining a respect for objectivity, argumentation, and the systematic use of reason. Despite the popularity of critical rationalism and its obviously close fit with the transhumanist drive toward continual improvement and challenging of limits, it must be acknowledged that there exists a small contingent of Ayn Rand-inspired transhumanists who remain committed to a foundationalist epistemology. Rand's foundationalist view explicitly claims that knowledge is hierarchical in nature, being based on undeniable axioms (Rand 1979).

Any discussion of transhumanist concerns quickly raises multiple issues in the area of metaphysics. Several of these revolve around the nature and identity of the self. With few exceptions, transhumanists describe themselves as materialists, physicalists, or functionalists. As such, they believe that our thinking, feeling selves are essentially physical processes. While a few transhumanists believe that the self is tied to the current, human physical form, most accept some form of functionalism, meaning that the self has to be instantiated in *some* physical medium but not necessarily one that is biologically human – or biological at all. If one's biological neurons were gradually replaced, for example, with synthetic parts that supported the same level of cognitive function, the same mind and personality might persist despite being "in" a non-biological substrate (Koene 2012; Merkle 2012).

Some critics who read discussions of "uploading" minds to non-biological substrates claim that transhumanists are dualists. Those critics are confusing dualism with functionalism. A functionalist holds that a particular mental state or cognitive system is independent of any specific physical instantiation, but must always be physically instantiated at any time in *some* physical form. Functionalism is a form of physicalism that differs from both identity theory (a mental state is identical to a specific brain state) and behaviorism (mental terms can be reduced to behavioral descriptions). According to functionalism, mental states such as beliefs and desires consist of their causal role. That is, mental states are causal relations to other mental states, sensory inputs, and behavioral outputs. Because mental states are constituted by their functional role, they can be realized on multiple levels and manifested in many systems, including non-biological systems, so long as that system performs the appropriate functions.

Functionalism comes in several versions, and transhumanists vary in their stands. One extension of functionalism is known as revisionary materialism or, at its extreme, eliminative materialism. Eliminativism (Churchland 1992) holds that the common-sense view of the mind ("folk psychology") is false, and that some kinds of mental states do not exist. The idea is that some of our common psychological concepts such as belief, desire, or intention are so poorly defined that they will be found to lack any coherent neurological basis – just as the concept of "caloric" was thrown out completely in favor of a thermodynamic conception of heat. Revisionary materialism (or what could equally well be called revisionary functionalism) takes the intermediate position that mental states may be reducible to physical phenomena, but only after some significant changes and refinements are made to the folk psychological concept. Given transhumanists' interest in using scientific knowledge to reconceptualize and revise human cognitive architecture, transhumanists may be uniquely open to this position in the philosophy of mind.

Transhumanists' commitment to technologically mediated transformation naturally generates great interest in the nature and limits of the self. The high level of interest in philosophy and neuroscience among transhumanists has led to a wide acknowledgment that the simple Cartesian view of the mind or self as a unitary, indivisible, and transparent entity is unsupportable. As we store more of our memories externally and create avatars, it is also becoming increasingly apparent that the boundaries of the self are unclear and may not be limited to the location of a single body. Complementing these questions about the nature and identity of the self at any one time are questions about the identity of the self over time, especially for a self that undergoes major cognitive and somatic changes over an extended lifespan. Discussions of theories of personal identity have long been a mainstay in transhumanist forums and publications (Parfit 1984; More 1995; Hughes 2012).

Another particularly relevant area of metaphysics concerns the idea of the world as simulation. As computers have become ever more powerful, simulations for both scientific and ludic purposes have proliferated and rapidly grown in sophistication. Although humans have always lived their lives entirely in the physical world as revealed by the unmediated senses, we may come to spend much of our time in simulated environments, or in "real" environments with virtual overlays. Simulated worlds raise questions about what we value. For instance, we do value the experience of achieving something or *actually* achieving it, and how clear is the distinction (Nozick 1974)? Taking this line of thinking further, transhumanists from Hans Moravec to Nick Bostrom have asked how likely it is that we are *already* living in a simulation (Moravec 1989; Bostrom 2003).

An obvious metaphysical question to raise here is the compatibility or otherwise of religion and transhumanism. In my 1990 essay that first set forth modern transhumanism as a distinct philosophy under that name, I explained how transhumanism (like humanism) can act as a philosophy of life that fulfills some of the same functions as a religion without any appeal to a higher power, a supernatural entity, to faith, and without the other core features of religions (More 1990). The central place accorded to rationalism suggests a tension between transhumanism and religion. But are they actually incompatible?

Since rationalism is an approach to acquiring knowledge and says nothing about the content of knowledge, it is possible in principle for a transhumanist to hold some religious beliefs. And some do. The content of some religious beliefs is easier to reconcile with transhumanism than the content of others. Christian transhumanists, while not completely unknown, are very rare (and I know of none who are fundamentalists, and such a combination would surely indicate deep confusion). There are more Mormon transhumanists (although some of these are cultural rather than religious Mormons), perhaps because that religion allows for humans to ascend to a higher, more godlike level, rather than sharply dividing God from man. Several transhumanists describe themselves as Buddhists (presumably of the secular, philosophical type), and there seem to be few obstacles to combining transhumanism with liberal Judaism. However, the vast majority of transhumanists do not identify with any religion. A pilot study published in 2005 found that religious attitudes were negatively correlated with acceptance of transhumanist ideas. Those with strong religious views tended to regard transhumanism as competing with their beliefs (Bainbridge 2005).

II.   History

Before outlining the precursors, roots, and formation of transhumanism, a brief note is in order on the origin of the term itself. Many terms have been independently coined multiple times – although not necessarily with precisely the same meaning, and this is true of "transhumanism." In 1312, in his *Divine Comedy*, Dante Alighieri uses the term *transumanare*, meaning to pass beyond the human, but his usage was religious or spiritual in nature. T.S. Eliot's used of "transhumanized" in his 1935 *The Cocktail Party* is about "illumination" rather than technologically mediated transformation.

A closer fit is Julian Huxley's brief chapter "Transhumanism" in his 1957 book, *New Bottles for New Wine*. He used it to mean "man remaining man, but transcending himself, by realizing new possibilities of and for his human nature." He did not, however, develop this evolutionary view into a philosophical position, and his usage came to light years after the term was independently coined as part of the contemporary transhumanist movement.

F.M. Esfandiary had written a chapter using the term "transhuman" in a 1972 book, and went on to develop a set of transhumanist ideas in which transhuman was a transition from human to posthuman, yet he never referred to them as "transhumanism." The term was introduced explicitly to label a deliberately transhumanist philosophy in the 1990 essay, "Transhumanism: Toward a Futurist Philosophy" (More 1990).

The current section is able to provide only a brief outline of the roots and history of transhumanism. Different scholars will emphasize differing aspects of the history, so it's important to consider multiple sources (Jones 1995; Bostrom 2005). We should be careful to distinguish precursors and proto-transhumanists from early transhumanists proper. For instance, we can easily regard the European alchemists of the thirteenth to eighteenth centuries as proto-transhumanists. Their search for the Philosopher's Stone or the Elixir of Life looks like the search for a magical form of technology capable of transmuting elements, curing all disease, and granting immortality.

In 1995, at Extro-1 – perhaps the first explicitly and exclusively transhumanist conference – as part of a survey of the roots of the transhumanist concept of extropy, Reilly Jones brought our attention to the renowned Renaissance philosopher Pico della Mirandola. The Judeo-Christian tradition has standardly pictured a gulf between human and God that is absolute and unbreachable. That led Ludwig Feuerbach to accuse that tradition of debasing humanity by transferring all the creative potential of our species into an external, perfect being who we can only worship. But Pico della Mirandola saw a far more mutable distinction between the human and the divine. In his 1486 piece, *Oration on the Dignity of Man*, he portrays God as the Craftsman explaining to humanity its nature in a way that sounds much closer to transhumanism than to the religious worldview it emerged from:

Neither a fixed abode nor a form that is thine alone nor any function peculiar to thyself have we given thee, Adam, to the end that according to thy longing and according to thy judgment thou mayest have and possess what abode, what form, and what functions thou thyself shalt desire. The nature of all other beings is limited and constrained within the bounds of laws prescribed by Us. Thou, constrained by no limits, in accordance with thine own free will, in whose hand We have placed thee, shalt ordain for thyself the limits of thy nature. We have set thee at the world's center that thou mayest from thence more easily observe whatever is in the world. We have made thee neither of heaven nor of earth, neither mortal nor immortal, so that with freedom of choice and with honor, as though the maker and molder of thyself, thou mayest fashion thyself in whatever shape thou shalt prefer. Thou shalt have the power to degenerate into the lower forms of life, which are brutish. Thou shalt have the power, out of thy soul's judgment, to be reborn into the higher forms, which are divine.

The realization of transhumanist goals – or perhaps even the full articulation of the philosophy – would not be possible before the development and use of scientific method. In that light, we can see Francis Bacon as a precursor. In *The Advancement of Learning* (1605) and *Novum Organum* (1620), Bacon advocated inductive reasoning and helped Western thought turn away from Scholastic and Platonic approaches and toward empirical methods. As science flowered, some Enlightenment thinkers began to think along proto-transhumanist lines, as in this passage by the Marquis de Condorcet (1743–94) from *Sketch for a Historical Picture of the Progress of the Human Mind* (1795):

In fine, may it not be expected that the human race will be meliorated by new discoveries in the sciences and the arts, and, as an unavoidable consequence, in the means of individual and general prosperity; by farther progress in the principles of conduct, and in moral practice; and lastly, by the real improvement of our faculties, moral, intellectual and physical, which may be the result either of the improvement of the instruments which increase the power and direct the exercise of those faculties, or of the improvement of our natural organization itself? (1795: 319)

Condorcet's immensely influential formulation of the idea of progress placed it at the center of Enlightenment though. With no reference to supernatural forces, he contended that growing knowledge in the natural and social sciences would enable us to create a world of growing material abundance, individual freedom, and moral compassion. He went so far as to make the following transhumanistic statement:

> Would it even be absurd to suppose this quality of melioration in the human species as susceptible of an indefinite advancement; to suppose that a period must one day arrive when death will be nothing more than the effect either of extraordinary accidents, or of the flow and gradual decay of the vital powers; and that the duration of the middle space, of the interval between the birth of man and this decay, will itself have no assignable limit? (Condorcet 1795: 368)

Enlightenment thought contained a range of views about the nature of progress, ranging from a sense of its inevitability to the view that humanity had to work hard and persistently to maintain it. To this day, some transhumanists seem attracted to the iron logic of progress, often expressed in graphs showing accelerating technological progress. However, no one goes so far as to believe in genuine inevitability in the sense often attributed to Hegel and Marx. Some formulations of transhumanism explicitly address the issue. The Principles of Extropy include the concept of "practical optimism" or "dynamic optimism" which tempers an optimistic sense of radical possibility with an insistence that we actively create the future we desire.

For several decades, it has been fashionable in some circles (especially the postmodernists and poststructuralists) to sneer at Enlightenment ideas, to declare that they are outdated, human-centric, or naive. Transhumanism continues to champion the core of the Enlightenment ideas and ideals – rationality and scientific method, individual rights, the possibility and desirability of progress, the overcoming of superstition and authoritarianism, and the search for new forms of governance – while revising and refining them in the light of new knowledge. The search for absolute foundations for reason, for instance, has given way to a more sophisticated, uncertain, and self-critical form of critical rationalism. The simple, unified self has been replaced by the far more complex and puzzling self revealed by the neurosciences. The utterly unique status of human beings has been superseded by an understanding that we are part of a spectrum of biological organisms and possible non-biological species of the future.

Before Enlightenment ideas fed into transhumanism, they were filtered through an evolutionary perspective. With the 1859 publication of Darwin's *Origin of Species*, the traditional view of humans as unique and fixed in nature gave way to the idea that humanity as it currently exists is one step along an evolutionary path of development. Combined with the realization that humans are physical beings whose nature can be progressively better understood through science, the evolutionary perspective made it easy to see that human nature itself might be deliberately changed. In a philosophical rather than scientific form, Friedrich Nietzsche picked up this idea and declared that humans are something to be overcome, and asked "What have you done to overcome him?" (Nietzsche 1896). Although Nietzsche seemed not to see a role for technology in this transformation, his bold language inspired some modern transhumanists (More 2010).

One of the more interesting precursors to transhumanism was Nikolai Fedorovich Fedorov (1829–1903), a Russian Orthodox Christian philosopher and participant in the Russian cosmism movement, who advocated using scientific methods to achieve radical life extension, physical immortality, resurrection of the dead, and space and ocean colonization. According to Fedorov, the evolutionary process led to increased intelligence culminating, so far, in human beings. Humans must use reason and morality to shape further evolution. Especially crucial was to overcome mortality and even to restore everyone who had ever died to life. They would be restored not in their former physical forms, but in a self-creating, immortal form. Shortly after Fedorov another, less known, thinker took up the immortalist, transhumanizing cause. Jean Finot (1856–1922) advocated using science to engineer life and fabricate living matter in his book, *The Philosophy of Long Life*.

The first part of the twentieth century saw other proto-transhumanists who may have had an indirect influence on later transhumanism. These include British geneticist and evolutionary biologist J.B.S. Haldane who, in his 1924 book, *Daedalus; or, Science and the Future*, envisioned scientific advances including *in vitro* fertilization ("ectogenesis") and foresaw a world where humans direct their own evolution to their benefit. J.D. Bernal's 1929 book, *The World, the Flesh and the Devil*, developed visionary ideas about space colonization (including the Bernal sphere), and the enhancement of human intelligence and lifespan. The turn of the century and early twentieth century saw other proto-transhumanists, such as Charles Stephens and Alexander Bogdanov (Stambler 2010) as well as the beginnings of modern science fiction, which has helped expand our sense of the possible.

Transhumanism as we know it today finally began to take form in the latter part of the twentieth century. Champions of life extension played a central and persistent part in this development. Not all advocates of extending the maximum human lifespan had well-developed ideas beyond that single goal, but many had at least some sense that the same technological advances that could deliver longer, healthier lives could also enable us to change ourselves in other ways. The "father of cryonics," Robert Ettinger, was one of the latter. After explaining in his first book, *The Prospect of Immortality* (1964), that we could have another chance at life by preserving ourselves at ultra-low temperatures at the point of clinical death, his 1972 *Man into Superman* explored other transformative possibilities, and explicitly used the term "transhuman." Another enduring supporter of life extension and cryonics, Saul Kent, not only wrote practically and speculatively about extending the human lifespan, but also about other possibilities in his 1974 book, *Future Sex*.

One of the most comprehensively (if sometimes idiosyncratic) transhumanist thinkers of this period was F.M. Esfandiary (later known as FM-2030). Esfandiary's approach was more literary than academic, even though he taught at the New School for Social Research in New York in the 1960s. Starting in 1966, while teaching classes in "New Concepts of the Human," he outlined a vision of an evolutionary transhuman future. He also brought together optimistic futurists in a loosely organized group known as UpWingers. In his 1989 book, *Are You a Transhuman?*, he defined a transhuman as a "transitional human," whose use of technology, way of living, and values marked them as a step toward posthumanity. FM-2030's writing and social activity importantly underscored the practical elements of the philosophy. The idiosyncratic and personal nature of FM-2030's transhumanism was displayed in his book, which contained extensive questionnaires, then rated the reader as more or less transhuman. Some of his measures included how much someone traveled, what alterations they had made to their body (even though the existing technology remained primitive), the degree to which they rejected traditional family structures and exclusive relationships, and so on.

The dependence of transhumanist goals on major technical and scientific advances means that technically oriented visionaries have played an influential role. One central and persistent concern has been with the development of greater than human intelligence and the possibility of an "intelligence explosion." In 1970, Marvin Minsky made what turned out to be highly optimistic forecasts of the advent of super-intelligent artificial intelligence (AI), then in a 1994 *Scientific*

American article explained why vastly extended lives will require replacing our biological brains with superior computational devices.

The idea of accelerating technological progress driven by machine super-intelligence dates back several decades. This idea, now frequently referred to as "the singularity," was explicitly pondered in a 1958 conversation between Stanislaw Ulam and John von Neumann during which they discussed "the ever accelerating progress of technology and changes in the mode of human life, which gives the appearance of approaching some essential singularity in the history of the race beyond which human affairs, as we know them, could not continue" (Ulam 1958). In 1965, I.J. Good argued that AI development would lead to an intelligence explosion. These ideas were taken up and elaborated and extended by several other influential writers (Bostrom 1998; Broderick 2001; Kurzweil 1990, 1999; Moravec 1989; Vinge 1993). Although numerous techno-logical pathways have informed transhumanist projections, nanotechnology as envisioned by Eric Drexler has been especially influential (Drexler 1986).

Philosophy, science, and technology are not the only influences on the development of tran-shumanist thinking. The arts have also enriched our appreciation of what is possible and what is important. The role of science fiction in elaborating on possible transhumanist futures is clear, but a topic too large to even touch on here. Other art forms and art theory have played a role since around 1982, when Natasha Vita-More wrote the Transhuman Manifesto (Vita-More 1983), followed by the Transhuman Arts Statement (Vita-More 1992, revised 2002). In 1997, a later version of the manifesto was released first onto the Internet and signed by hundreds of creative thinkers and then placed aboard the Cassini Huygens spacecraft.

The activities of the first fully, explicitly, and exclusively transhumanist organization, Extropy Institute (ExI), shaped the intellectual and cultural movement of transhumanism starting in the late 1980s. *Extropy* magazine (subtitled "Vaccine for Future Shock" and then "The Journal of Transhumanist Thought") was first published in 1988 by Max More and Tom W. Bell (the latter coined the term "extropy"). That publication, in its paper and online versions, presented ideas from numerous leading transhumanists, and included the 1990 essay "Transhumanism: Toward a Futurist Philosophy." A vast amount of discussion focused on transhumanism started taking place when ExI created an early (and still existing) email list in 1991. This was followed by a series of influential conferences starting in 1994, a website in 1996, and an online Vital Progress Summit in 2004, which led to the development of the Proactionary Principle (More 2004). The history of ExI has been detailed further elsewhere (Extropy Institute 2005).

In 1998, the Transhumanist Declaration was crafted by an international group of authors. Other groups sprang up in the 1990s, including Aleph in Sweden, De:Trans in Germany, and Transcedo in the Netherlands. In the same year, another general-purpose transhumanist organi-zation – the World Transhumanist Association – was founded. After Extropy Institute was closed, the WTA – renamed Humanity+ – became and remains the central organization of the move-ment in general, although organizations such as the Institute for Ethics and Emerging Tech-nologies (IEET) and the Future of Humanity Institute play a strong role in the academic arena.

III.   Currents

At this point in its development, it is probably impossible to list necessary and sufficient conditions for transhumanism that would be accepted by all self-described transhumanists. At the start of this essay, some of the core elements were identified, including the view that it is both possible and desirable to overcome biological limitations on human cognition, emotion, and physical and sensory capabilities, and that we should use science, technology, and experimentation guided by critical and creative thinking to do so. Beyond these shared and rather general views, transhumanists vary widely in their assumptions, values, expectations, strategies, and attitudes.

In addressing moral and ethical concerns, transhumanists typically adopt a universal standard based not on membership in the human species but on the qualities of each being. Creatures with similar levels of sapience, sentience, and personhood are accorded similar status no matter whether they are humans, animals, cyborgs, machine intelligences, or aliens. Yet the meta-ethical basis for making moral decisions and according rights can be consequentialist, deontological, or virtue-based. A genuinely pure deontological ethics appears to be uncommon. At least since the advent of the extropian transhumanism, many transhumanists have established their morality on a virtue foundation. In recent years, some prominent transhumanists have assumed a consequentialist foundation, in the form of various kinds of utilitarian – most radically in David Pearce's "hedonistic imperative."

Transhumanism supports a rich diversity of political perspectives. Given shared goals, it is unsurprising that transhumanists all support personal choice in the use of self-directed technological transformations, including anti-aging treatments and cryonics, cognition-enhancers, and mood-modifiers. From the late 1980s and through the 1990s, many and perhaps most transhumanists evinced a broadly libertarian politics. This perspective continues to receive far more support among transhumanists than in the general population, but over the previous decade or so, liberal democrats have become just as well recognized, some adopting the term "technoprogressive." Only the latter are likely to favor some form of world government which, in one scenario, might be controlled by a machine super-intelligence. Interestingly, even some libertarian transhumanists share this scenario, although typically seeing the super-intelligent mind acting as a guide or local governor rather than a planetary authority.

Transhumanists of multiple varieties share the view that we can make radical changes to the human condition. Major scientific and technological progress is both possible and desirable. Beyond that, consensus immediately dissolves, with differences over the expected rate, shape, and risks of progress. Those who expect a technological singularity anticipate a drastic acceleration in the rate of change, either as a one-time jump caused by the advent of super-intelligence, or as a continuous acceleration driven by exponential trends in computing power. Others expect technology to advance at different rates in various sectors and to go through faster and slower periods, depending not only on technologies themselves but on economic and social conditions.

An optimistic flavor necessarily permeates transhumanism. Someone cannot believe that radical transformations of the human condition are both possible *and* desirable while also believing that we are doomed to failure or disaster. In the early days as a self-aware movement, transhumanist discussions tended to emphasize the positive – arguing, against the cultural consensus, that technology-enabled transformations were plausible and that we should pursue them vigorously and look forward to the resulting future. (Although consideration of risk has never been entirely absent. An early book of note here is Jonathan Glover's 1984 *What Sort of People Should There Be?*) As the movement has grown, much more of the population has come to accept the plausibility of many of the technological pathways described (AI, advanced biotechnology, nanotechnology, and so on). That facilitated a shift within transhumanism to more fully consider potential risks and downsides.

While transhumanists all continue to resist "bioconservatives" and other opponents of the transhumanist vision, some emphasize the enormous uncertainties of the future. At the extreme, this has become a focus on the risks that AI or runaway self-replication or other technologies might lead to the extinction of the human race. Bill Joy brought these kinds of dangers to the attention of a wide audience with his 2000 *Wired* article, "Why the Future Doesn't Need Us." The philosophy is enriched by a clear-eyed view of potential risks. At the same time, a heavy and persistent focus on catastrophes can make them appear inevitable and even, in some cases, desirable (the "sweet lemons" phenomenon). So far, unlike Joy, the more risk-focused transhumanists remain supportive of strong yet cautious technological advancement, believing that attempts to block advance will only increase risks.

IV.   Misconceptions

Philosophies can be clarifying not only by explaining what they *are*, but also by clarifying what they are *not*. As with any controversial view, critics often take the easy path by constructing straw men then proceed gleefully to burn them down and dance around the ashes. I have addressed several misconceptions elsewhere (More 2010b) but here will very briefly comment on some of the more common, involving notions of perfection, prediction, the body, and the attitudes toward what is "natural" but unchosen.

The frequency with which critics talk of transhumanists as wanting to "perfect" human beings or to achieve a state of perfection or to bring about a utopian society suggests that they haven't actually read much transhumanist literature. More likely, they read it with cognitive blinders on, distorting what they read to fit their preconceptions. For instance, Don Ihde (in Hansell and Grassie 2011) characterizes transhumanists as looking forward to a future posthuman world that would be a utopia. (He labels this purported goal "The Idol of Paradise.") This criticism, and the others like it, confuse the goal of continual improvement or enhancement with the longing for a state of final perfection. These are actually radically different. The former is essentially a process of perpetual change whereas the latter is a state of stasis.

Transhumanism reflects the Enlightenment commitment to meliorism and rejects all forms of apologism – the view that it is wrong for humans to attempt to alter the conditions of life for the better. Nothing about this implies that the goal is to reach a final, perfect state. The contrary view is made explicit in the transhumanist concept of extropy – a process of perpetual progress, not a static state. Further, one of the Principles of Extropy is Perpetual Progress. This states that transhumanists "seek continual improvement in ourselves, our cultures, and our environments. We seek to improve ourselves physically, intellectually, and psychologically. We value the perpetual pursuit of knowledge and understanding."

In my own formulations of transhumanism, I found the Idol of Paradise and the idea of a Platonically perfect, static utopia, is so antithetical to true transhumanism that I coined the term "extropia" to label a conceptual alternative. Transhumanists seek not utopia, but perpetual progress – a never-ending movement toward the ever-distant goal of extropia. If the transhumanist project is successful, we may no longer suffer some of the miseries that have always plagued human existence. But that is not reason to expect life to be free of risks, dangers, conflicts, and struggle. Outside, perhaps, of David Pearce's goal of eliminating all suffering, you will have to search far and wide to find any suggestion of utopia or perfection in transhumanist writing. This is why such a mischaracterization typically is not supported by quotations from relevant sources.

Another misconception – one which is somewhat more justifiable than the last – is that transhumanism essentially makes predictions about the future. Certainly some transhumanists (whether or not they apply that term to themselves) do make predictions. In recent years the most well-known example is Ray Kurzweil, who has provided numerous detailed predictions based on his analysis of exponential trends in computer-based technologies. Beyond the forecasts made by particular individuals, it's reasonable to say that transhumanism depends on very general expectations about continued technological advance.

No specific predictions, however, are essential to transhumanism. Transhumanism is defined by its commitment to shaping fundamentally better futures as defined by values, goals, and general direction, not specific goals. Even to the extent that a goal is somewhat specific – say, abolishing aging, becoming post-biological, or enhancing cognitive abilities to some arbitrary degree – the means and time frame in which these might be achieved are open to differing views. Transhumanism per se says much about goals but nothing about specific means or schedules.

A third common misconception is that transhumanists loathe their biological bodies. The origin of this mistaken view is hard to fathom. Transhumanists do seek to improve the human body, by making it resistant to aging, damage, and disease, and by enhancing its senses and sharpening the cognition of our biological brains. Perhaps critics have made a flying leap from the idea of being dissatisfied with the body to hating it, despising it, or loathing it. In reality, transhumanism doesn't find the biological human body disgusting or frightening. It does find it to be a marvelous yet flawed piece of engineering. It could hardly be otherwise, given that it was designed by a blind watchmaker, as Richard Dawkins put it. True transhumanism *does* seek to enable each of us to alter and improve (by our own standards) the human body and champions morphological freedom. Rather than denying the body, transhumanists typically want to choose its form and be able to inhabit different bodies, including virtual bodies.

A related misconception is the reflexive assumption that, because we seek to overcome biological aging and the inevitability of death that we are terrified of death. While some transhumanists – like anyone else – may fear a painful, prolonged death, we understand that death is not something to be feared. It is nothing. It is simply the end of experience. What makes death extremely undesirable is not that it is a bad condition to be in, it is that it means the end of our ability to experience, to create, to explore, to improve, to live.

I have attempted to provide as accurate a view of the philosophy of transhumanism as is possible at present. The philosophy will continue to grow and develop, and various individuals will emphasize certain aspects of it. But these elaborations and emphases should not be confused with the core elements.

References

Bacon, Francis (1620) *Novum Organum*, trans. R.L. Ellis and J. Spedding, in J. Robertson, ed., *The Philosophical Works of Francis Bacon*. London: Routledge (1905).

Bainbridge, William S. (2005) "The Transhuman Heresy." *Journal of Evolution and Technology* 14/2 (August), pp. 1–10.

Bartley, William Warren (1962) *The Retreat to Commitment*. New York: Knopf.

Bostrom, Nick (1998) "How Long Before Superintelligence?" *International Journal of Futures Studies* 2.

Bostrom, Nick (2003) "Are You Living in a Computer Simulation?" *Philosophical Quarterly* 53/211, pp. 243–255.

Bostrom, Nick (2005) "A History of Transhumanist Thought." *Journal of Evolution and Technology* 14 (April).

Churchland, Paul M. (1992) *A Neurocomputational Perspective: The Nature of Mind and the Structure of Science*. Cambridge, MA: MIT Press.

Condorcet, Jean Antoine Nicolas de Caritat (1795) *Sketch for a Historical Picture of the Progress of the Human Mind*. Google digitized edition, pp. 319, 368.

Drexler, K. Eric (1986) *Engines of Creation: The Coming Era of Nanotechnology*. London: Fourth Estate.

Ettinger, Robert (1964) *The Prospect of Immortality*. New York: Doubleday.

Ettinger, Robert (1972) *Man into Superman*. New York: St. Martin's Press.

Extropy Institute (2005) "History and Achievements of ExI from 1988 – 2005." http://www.extropy.org/history.htm (accessed January 15, 2012).

FM-2030 (1989) *Are You a Transhuman?* New York: Warner Books.

Glover, Jonathan (1984) *What Sort of People Should There Be?* London: Pelican.

Hansell, Gregory R. and Grassie, William, eds. (2011) *H+/–: Transhumanism and Its Critics*. Bloomington, IN: Xlibris Corporation.

Hughes, James (2012) "Transhumanism and Personal Identity." In M. More and N. Vita-More, eds., *The Transhumanist Reader*. Oxford: Wiley-Blackwell.

Huxley, Julian (1957) *New Bottles for New Wine*. London: Chatto & Windus.

Jones, Reilly (1995) "A History of Extropic Thought: Parallel Conceptual Development of Technicism and Humanism," *EXTRO-2 Proceedings*, Extropy Institute.

Koene, Randal A. (2012) "Uploading to Substrate-Independent Minds." in M. More and N. Vita-More, eds., *The Transhumanist Reader*. Oxford: Wiley-Blackwell.

Kurzweil, Ray (1990) *The Age of Intelligent Machines*. Cambridge, MA: MIT Press.

Kurzweil, Ray (1999) *The Age of Spiritual Machines: When Computers Exceed Human Intelligence*. New York: Viking.

Merkle, Ralph (2012) "Uploading." in M. More and N. Vita-More, eds., *The Transhumanist Reader*. Oxford: Wiley-Blackwell.

Minsky, Marvin (1994) "Will Robots Inherit the Earth?" *Scientific American* (October).

Moravec, Hans (1989) *Mind Children*. Cambridge, MA: Harvard University Press.

More, Max (1990) "Transhumanism: Toward a Futurist Philosophy." *Extropy* 6 (Summer), pp. 6–12. Revised June 1994 and 1996.

More, Max (1993) "Technological Self-Transformation: Expanding Personal Extropy." *Extropy* 10, 4/2 (Winter/Spring), pp. 15–24.

More, Max (1994) "Pancritical Rationalism: An Extropic Metacontext for Memetic Progress." *EXTRO-1 Proceedings*, Extropy Institute.

More, Max (1995) *The Diachronic Self: Identity, Continuity, Transformation*. Ann Arbor, MI: A. Bell & Howell. http://www.maxmore.com/disscont.htm.

More, Max (1997) "Mind Morph: Technologically Refined Emotion and Personality." *EXTRO-3 Proceedings*, Extropy Institute.

More, Max (2003) "Principles of Extropy, Version 3.11.2003." http://www.extropy.org/principles.htm. Original version: "The Extropian Principles." *Extropy* 5/5 (May 1990).

More, Max (2004) "The Proactionary Principle" (May). http://www.maxmore.com/proactionary.htm, http://www.extropy.org/proactionaryprinciple.htm.

More, Max (2009) "Hyperagency and Hope: Critiquing Human Limitationism." Metanexus Institute, July 19. vimeo.com/9860229.

More, Max (2010a) "The Overhuman in the Transhuman." *Journal of Evolution and Technology* 21/1 (January), pp. 1–4.

More, Max (2010b) "True Transhumanism." In Gregory R. Hansell and William Grassie, eds., *H+/–: Transhumanism and Its Critics*. Bloomington, IN: XLibris Corporation.

Nietzsche, Friedrich W. (1896) *Thus Spake Zarathustra*, trans. Alexander Tille. New York: Macmillan.

Nozick, Robert (1974) *Anarchy, State, and Utopia*. New York: Basic Books.

Parfit, Derek (1984) *Reasons and Persons*. Oxford: Clarendon Press.

Pico della Mirandola, Giovanni (1486) *Oration on the Dignity of Man.*

Rand, Ayn (1979) *Introduction to Objectivist Epistemology.* Denver: Mentor.

Sandberg, Anders (2001) "Morphological Freedom – Why We Not Just Want It, but Need It." http://www.nada.kth.se/~asa/Texts/MorphologicalFreedom.htm. Retrieved November 21, 2011.

Stambler, Ilia (2010) "Life Extension: A Conservative Enterprise? Some Fin-de-Siècle and Early Twentieth-Century Precursors of Transhumanism." *Journal of Evolution and Technology* 21/1 (March), pp. 13–26.

Ulam, Stanislaw (1958) "John von Neumann 1903–1957." *Bulletin of the American Mathematical Society* (May), part 2, pp. 1–49.

Various (2002) "The Transhumanist Declaration." http://humanityplus.org/philosophy/transhumanist-declaration/.

Various (2003) "The Transhumanist FAQ: v 2.1." World Transhumanist Association. http://humanityplus.org/philosophy/transhumanist-faq/.

Verdoux, Philippe (2009) "Transhumanism, Progress and the Future." *Journal of Evolution and Technology* 20/2 (December), pp. 49–69.

Vinge, Vernor (1993) "The Coming Technological Singularity." *Whole Earth Review* (Winter).

Vita-More, Natasha (1983) "Transhuman Manifesto." http://www.transhumanist.biz/transhumanmanifesto.htm.

Vita-More, Natasha (1992) "Transhumanist Arts Statement." Revised 2002. http://www.transhumanist.biz/transhumanistartsmanifesto.htm.

Further Reading

Bell, T. W. and Murashige, K.H. (1999) "Who Owns Your Genes?" EXTRO-4: Biotech Futures Conference, Berkeley, CA.

Moravec, Hans (1999) *Robot: Mere Machine to Transcendent Mind.* New York: Oxford University Press.

Sandberg, Anders (1997) "Amplifying Cognition: Extending Human Memory and Intelligence." *EXTRO-3 Proceedings*, Extropy Institute.

Sandel, Michael (2004) "The Case Against Perfection." *The Atlantic* (April).

Stock, Gregory (2002) *Redesigning Humans: Our Inevitable Genetic Future.* New York: Houghton Mifflin.

Part I

Roots and Core Themes

Transhumanism developed as a philosophy that became a cultural movement, and now is regarded as a growing field of study. It is often confused with, compared to, and even equated with posthumanism. Transhumanism arrived during what is often referred to as the postmodernist era, although it has only a modest overlap with postmodernism. Ironically, transhumanism shares some postmodernist values, such as a need for change, reevaluating knowledge, recognition of multiple identities, and opposition to sharp classifications of what humans and humanity ought to be. Nevertheless, transhumanism does not throw out the entirety of the past because of a few mistaken ideas. Humanism and scientific knowledge have proven their quality and value. In this way, transhumanism seeks a transmodernity or hypermodernism rather than arguing explicitly against modernism. One aspect of transhumanism that we hope to explore and elucidate throughout this book is the need for inclusivity, plurality, and continuous questioning of our knowledge, as we are a species and a society that is forever changing. The roots and core themes of transhumanism address some of the underlying themes that have formed its philosophical outlook.

The first section of the book presents a definitive overview of transhumanism. Transhumanism is a class of philosophies that seeks the continued evolution of human life beyond its current human form as a result of science and technology guided by life-promoting principles and values. Transhumanism promotes an interdisciplinary approach to understanding and evaluating the opportunities for enhancing the human condition and the human organism opened up by the advancement of technology.

To begin this section, philosopher Max More sets forth the core values, goals, and principles shared by transhumanists and outlines commonly shared epistemological and metaphysical views, while noting the various distinct schools of transhumanist thought. More provides a briefing on the historical roots of the philosophy from the ancients through to the

The Transhumanist Reader: Classical and Contemporary Essays on the Science, Technology, and Philosophy of the Human Future, First Edition. Edited by Max More and Natasha Vita-More.
© 2013 John Wiley & Sons, Inc. Published 2013 by John Wiley & Sons, Inc.

twentieth-century precursors, explains transhumanism's relationship to humanism and to other concepts including extropy and the technological singularity, and then outlines contemporary variations. He concludes by identifying several misconceptions about transhumanism.

Although the philosophical, scientific, technological, and even political aspects of transhumanism have received much attention over the past decades, the aesthetic aspects have often been treated as secondary, especially to technology. Natasha Vita-More fills that gap. Vita-More explores the artistic, design-based approaches to the classical human form stemming from the Renaissance and on to the cyborg and the transhuman and asks: "What might be concerns of artistic works and design-based practices that approach human enhancement and life extension?"

In his essay "Why I Want to be a Posthuman When I Grow Up," philosopher Nick Bostrom notes that extreme human enhancement could result in "posthuman" modes of being. Being posthuman would mean possessing a general central capacity (healthspan, cognition, or emotion) greatly exceeding the maximum attainable by any current human being. Bostrom argues that some possible posthuman modes of being would be very good, and that it could be very good *for us* to become posthuman.

The Transhumanist Declaration sets forth values and practical goals for transhumanism and the many organizations and scholarly research associated with transhumanism that largely evolved out of the seminal work of Extropy Institute, an educational non-profit organization and, more recently, Humanity+. The Declaration was co-authored by a collection of transhumanists with diverse backgrounds.

Part I concludes with an essay by Anders Sandberg arguing that we have sound reasons to affirm a right to morphological freedom. A right to freedom and the right to one's own body implies that one has a right to modify one's body. Morphological freedom is a negative right – it is the right to be able to do certain things without interference but it does not create any claim on others to support one's exercise of that right. Sandberg argues that we want morphological freedom because of an ancient drive for self-creation through self-definition. We *need* morphological freedom because not accepting it as a basic right would have negative effects. Sandberg concludes by briefly considering some implications for the future of healthcare.

Aesthetics
Bringing the Arts & Design into the Discussion of Transhumanism

Natasha Vita-More

"Transhumans want to elevate and extend life … let us choose to be transhumanist not only in our bodies, but also in our values … toward diversity, multiplicity … toward a more humane transhumanity …"[1]

Imagine a future designed by Frank Gehry that models elements of a "great logistic game" as conceived by Buckminster Fuller, within a monumental Christo installation, kinetically lit by James Turrell, scored by Philip Glass, and sung by Adele.

Introduction

The emergent course of technology is at once explicable and baffling. It has precipitated questions about a shifting human paradigm that remain unanswered by postmodernism. Considering the climate, discussions about speculative and emerging technologies need to include scientific realism *and* cosmic chance – a unity *and* plurality. Transhumanism's[2] proposed elevation of the human condition involves technology *and* the arts. New media's interpretations of the human form, visual landscapes, literary narratives, and musical scores move us from one mental state to another – offering experiences that shift perceptions of ourselves and the world around us. A predominant area where the arts interface with transhumanism is at the transformative human stages – the cyborg, transhuman, and posthuman and in altering elements of time – real time, virtual time, and hyper-reality. Integrating the scope of emergent technology outside the traditional framework of human perception is well suited to the arts and design.

Originally published in Gregory R. Hansell and William Grassie, eds., *H+/−: Transhumanism and Its Critics* (Bloomington, IN: Xlibris, 2011). Copyright © 2011, Metanexus Institute.

The Transhumanist Reader: Classical and Contemporary Essays on the Science, Technology, and Philosophy of the Human Future, First Edition. Edited by Max More and Natasha Vita-More.
© 2013 John Wiley & Sons, Inc. Published 2013 by John Wiley & Sons, Inc.

Current Discussion

The current discussion of transhumanism largely focuses on human enhancement,[3] a domain recognized by its technological advances rather than by its artistic pursuits. Rather than the cyborgization of the body, whose value lies in appending physical attributes, transhumanization proposes an intervention of biology in modifying corporeality, extending the biological lifespan, and preserving the brain by transfer onto non-biological platforms.

The cyborg,[4] transhuman, prosthetic being,[5] posthuman,[6] and upload[7] are a few of the posited outcomes resulting from human–computer interaction and body variation. Perceiving what it might be like to be any one of these agents is imagined in literary and filmic narratives, although often scripted with depraved or overtly optimistic futures. Thus, here is the dilemma: how can we thoughtfully assess and critique the advantages and obstacles of a transhuman if we cannot now build such an existence – in other words, be *in* the experience? Could this untapped area be enough of an enticement to compel artistic and design-based works toward the domain of life expansion?[8]

Looking back to the Lascaux Caves prehistoric imagery and to Greek mythology, and even alchemy, as foreseeing narratives that, while lacking scientific reason, our ancestors added significantly to our species' history of drama, intrigue, romance, fiction, and fantasy. Painters layered pigment upon pigment in depicting the human figure as regal, noetic, and humbled through the Baroque era following the Renaissance and post-Enlightenment Romanticism. Narratives have characterized the human as an object of desire, a phantom of disdain, a ridiculous fool, and a cunning artisan – from Shakespeare's conventional style to Joyce's stream-of-consciousness technique. Music has taken the human metaphorically outside its skin with the tonal scale of harmony and timbre in what Schopenhauer wrote as "the answer to the mystery of life. The most profound of all the arts, it expresses the deepest thoughts of life" (Schopenhauer 1966 [1819]). Looking forward onto social networking as public performance art, to metaverse avatars as sub-identities with tales of their own, and even to bioart, as manipulating and reconstructing matter as a blood-based symbol in our conquering organisms, we have become the creators, users, and players of our own engineering.

Our physical and perceptual experiences are heightened by the urge to push their boundaries. We are handlers of our connections by selecting what media and which combinations to put together in creating our alternative worlds. This self-identification of social media offers a glimpse of how we might select and combine platforms, systems, and substrates of our form, and all its attributes. Eric Drexler's *Engines of Creation* (1986), the primer for nanotechnology, can also be seen as a conceptual manifesto of life expansion and a world of engineered abundance and elaborate creative possibilities. "Nanotechnology will make possible vivid art forms and fantasy worlds far more absorbing than any book, game, or movie (1986: 233). Frank Popper's *Art of the Electronic Age* (1993), constructs a timeline of works framing advances in electronic practices which cover the telematic, interactive, immersive, sensorial, and performative spheres in intimately connecting the machine and man. As Popper writes, "although technological art is clearly the art form most representative of our Electronic Age, its full implications lie in the future. The artists share an exploration into a vast spectrum of aesthetics with the various electronic technologies" (1993: 181).

Form and Perception

The human form continues to be one of the predominant themes in the arts. Its image symbolizes the core of human nature. Michelangelo's *David* and da Vinci's *Mona Lisa* reflect the deep-rooted sentiment of Pico della Mirandola when he said "there is nothing to be seen more wonderful than the image of man" (Fleming 1966: 284).

The late Archaic, early Classical period's *Kritios Boy* was sculpted with a perceived ideality of physical proportion and muscular strength. Varied representations of the human form continued into the Golden Age's melding of chiaroscuro and what Rembrandt called "beweech-gelickhijt" (Slive 1952: 261–264). Proportion and physical strength evolved into Impressionism's ease of interpretation and spontaneity through visual experience and effects of light. In contrast, the human form was pulled apart and broken down in Cubism's reassembled pieces. Dada reached past the form and while fleeing from conventional aesthetics produced a new sensibility – one that eschewed the machine as essential to art. Its tentacles were, as Hans Richter described, "anti-art" (1965) in ignoring traditionalized aesthetics and encouraging an assessment of industrialized culture, mechanized and somewhat surreal. Pop Art's larger-than-life portraits from Mao to Monroe turned icons into overly exaggerated commodities. Removing the icon from popularity and rendering the banal, Fluxus blurred the interpretational form with performative art where the performance became the form. New Media's digitally extended platforms furthered performance as interconnected and net-based, as in "Ping Body" (Stelarc 1995) and the emerging technologies aroused transbiosymbiotic conceptions, as in "Primo Posthuman" (Vita-More 1997).

The aggregate of practices that share creative uses of electronics and computers also seeks to augment the sensorial experience and reality – including the artist, the viewer, and the works themselves. Sensory expansion affects the viewer's reality through uses of light and space in impacting perceptions, as in Turrell's architectural illusion of *Skyscape* (2008). Altered reality in the medium of video offers a different sensorial exchange, by evoking emotional narratives through the sheer magnitude of the figures, their movements and gestures, as in Viola's *The Greeting* (1995). Presence and realness of connectivity between computer and corporeal interaction bring the virtual and real into a shared, augmented space as in Ascott's *Aspects of Gaia: Digital Pathways Across the Whole Earth* (Ascott 1989).

Human enhancement may impact traditional notions of classical style as contextualized by history in experiencing, examining, and understanding works of art. Merleau-Ponty's phenomenological theory suggests that human perception stylizes what it perceives, "because it cannot help but to constitute and express a point of view" (Merleau-Ponty 1968). An individual's frame of reference may be typical or vastly atypical depending on his sensory and cognitive augmented attributes and capabilities, suggesting a richer sensorial and cognitive reaction to style. Virtually enhanced head displays, such as *EyeTap* (Mann 1998), enable augmented visual attributes by replacing the field of vision of one eye with camera and computer which manipulate the real-time images with preferential stylized images. In a cognitively enhanced environment, reality turns the viewer into a participator by providing the tools to build her own personalized reality, first-hand (Broderick 1997; Chislenko 2000).

The cyborg "will not only make a significant step forward in man's scientific progress, but may well provide a new and larger dimension for man's spirit as well" (Clynes and Kline 1960: 33).

While cybernetic posthuman combines the alchemic past and a future noosphere by implying immateriality of consciousness, the transhumanist view of the human form is not differentiated by association with a metal cyborg or disembodied human. Rather, it is a synergistic being, comprising a fluid continuity of self over time and suggesting distributed identity over disembodiment – to enhance rather than to erase.

Unlike the classical human form, this prototype takes the ideal of "man" and incorporates the transhumanist value of elevating the human condition (in particular, the limited lifespan). Unlike the cyborg, the prototype's unfolding nature is based on expanding choices. Unlike the disembodied entity, the prototype suggests a distributed entity. Rather than an erasure of the human form, the prototype suggests a trans-biological form and the continuation of personal existence as "a living organism is an open system in which matter and energy are exchanged within the environment," (Prigogine and Stengers 1984) and for the human system, consciousness is intrinsic and instrumental. (However, for the purposes of transhumanism, "the environment" is understood as "an environment" to clarify that there may be a number of environments where living organisms could exchange matter and energy.)

Further, the idea of matter is not limited to biological matter, but different types of substrates, which could contain a living presence or process of life in non-biological systems and on non-biological platforms. Here, the transformative human disposition emphasizes regenerative existence as a primary aim and the construction of its mass, or body, whether semi-biological or synthetic, as a secondary aim.

Adaptation

Design and process

Humans need change as a result of evolutionary cravings for stimuli. But how will our senses be satisfied in the future? A group of designers at ID Fuel agree that "it could be argued that the reason humans have come so far so fast where technology is concerned is that we've never been satisfied with our own physical abilities. Our arms weren't fast enough to catch fish, so we whittled fishhooks. Our feet got cut when we worked tending crops, so we covered them with shoes. Our eyes went blind in the glaring snow, so we carved slitted goggles from wood to protect them. And, as our command of tools continues to improve, so do the items we develop to augment ourselves" (ID Fuel).

State of the art

Consider a field of human biosculpture, where the human body, mind, and identity are modified by the user. If design is a social process then the art of human enhancement can be viewed as a process of adaptation. For artists and designers in the biological arts, the idea of molding or sculpting the human form has enormous potential. For media artists in interactive, immersive environments, the idea of virtuality as a constructed identity has continuing value regardless of its user/creator. Tom Ray, creator of the "Tierra" artificial life simulation, suggests that "the idea of creating life is exciting but extending life of humans for the purposes of continued and regenerative existence may not be realized as a mode of aesthetic creation in traditional works of art" (Ray 2007).

Regenerative art

Even if we accept the 2,480-year-old *Kritios Boy* as a traditional aesthetic creation, over time it broke down and was restructured – its body in 1965 and its head in 1988. Like the metamorphic rock, humans are made of atoms which systems deconstruct over time. We too need to be restructured when our parts break down.

Identity art

"what matters to me in ordinary survival is not identity over time, but something else. Further, since the only thing of significance in common between fission and ordinary survival is the psychological connectedness/continuity ..." (Parfit 1971: 3–27). Parfit suggests that persons are themselves separate and distinct from their bodies, but that persons' existence is, in fact, nothing other than the existence of a brain and body, the foundation of Parfit's constitutive reductionism. An analogy between identity and an artistic, yet alchemic, assemblage of matter can applied to this understanding, as suggested by Carsten Korfmacher:

> Cellini's *Venus* is made of bronze. Although the lump of bronze and the statue itself surely exist, these objects have different persistence conditions: if melted down, *Venus* ceases to exist while the lump of bronze does not. Therefore, they are not identical; rather, so the suggestion, the lump of bronze constitutes the statue. The same is true of persons, who are constituted by, but not identical with, a physiology, a psychology, and the occurrence of an interrelated series of causal and cognitive relations. (Korfmacher 2006)

Relationship

According to Popper the full implications of technology's use lie in the future. Popper suggests that those who create share a "preoccupation with exploiting a vast spectrum of aesthetic categories" with advanced technologies and an "awareness of the extent of social and cultural change produced by the latest technological developments ... to bring about a significant relationship between basic human experiences ... and the radical and global intrusion into them of the new technologies, in all walks of life, with all the beneficial effects, potential hazards and immense possibilities they offer" (Popper 1993: 181).

There are many questions and concerns about whether or not enhancing the human is advantageous, and there is deep interest in the ratio of positive to negative outcomes of human enhancement. Nevertheless, most of the relevant literature reports a consensus of opinion that biotechnology, nanotechnology, and information technology – separately or together – will inevitably affect human biology and increase human lifespan. Neither over-enthusiasm nor overwhelming negativity offers a solution because the either-or scenario pigeonholes views and offers little resolve other than to choose between them. This is not good enough. We might develop a field of new media approaches to human enhancement and bring about more inclusive discussion, research, and study.

In *H+/H-: Transhumanism and Its Critics* (2011), Katherine Hayles, in her essay "H-: Wrestling with Transhumanism" that "there is little discussion of how access to advanced technologies would be regulated or of the social and economic inequalities entwined with the questions of access." However, socio-political issues are one of the most often discussed transhumanist topics, as evidenced by the numerous transhumanist venues expressly developed for this purpose. Hayles continues with "or at least that transhumanist individuals will be among the privileged elite that can afford the advantages advanced technologies will offer." While I have admiration and respect for Hayles' scholarship on many topics, I do not agree with her on this point.[9] By way of explanation, Extropy Institute formed Macy-like conferences, bringing leading thinkers together to discuss bioethics and economics from 1992 through 2008. At its 2004 Vital Progress Summit, the press release stated "[n]o organization, no policy, no person should have the absolute power and authority to hinder scientific and medical advances that can and do help millions of people throughout the world" (Vita-More 2004, 2009).

A Field

Over the past five or more decades, artists have created new ways to interpret the cyborg, avatar, transhuman, and posthuman. Designers, such as Vivian Rosenthal, have also developed alternative environments to exist within, such as the virtual atmosphere of gaming, interactivity, virtuality, and others – such as Tom Ray – are conceptualizing new environments not yet realized. Artists, such as Roy Ascott, have also developed corresponding theoretical views such as telematics and technoetics, and other artists have thorough philosophical worldviews such as transhumanism. These efforts reflect an anticipated awareness of the sciences and technologies of biological and artificial modification, and issues of consciousness and identity.

Computer-generated works, including robotics, AI, and virtuality, as well as biological arts in altering cell structures, signify the developing artistic field of human enhancement. New media, in offering further technologies as potential media for artistic options, will expand in creating new practices for designing biosynthetic bodies, sensorial extension, cognitive enrichment, gender diversity, identity transfer, and radical life extension.

The modification of biological life systems, from single cells to organisms, increases the transdisciplinarity of the arts and sciences. As noted, some practices have reached far into the uncomfortable zone of bioengineering and genetics, where science and medicine reside, in aptly creating bio-experiments and offering opinions on the meaning of life. On another side of the creative spectrum, exploratory creations with nanotechnological robots have become a molecular vehicle for establishing artistic practice and theory. The transhumanist art arises when we combine biodesign and nanodesign, along with information technology and cognitive/neuro science for life expansion, converging nanotechnology, biotechnology, information technology, and artificial general intelligence to provide the transdisciplinary media for investigating the continuation of life by enhancing, extending, and regenerating life in biological, synthetic, and cybernetic forms.

A Study

Lowry Burgess of Carnegie Mellon's "Studio for Creative Inquiry" offers a pedagogical approach to the future. The program's mission elegantly states, "interdisciplinary projects bring together the arts, sciences, technology, and the humanities, and impact local and global communities" (Burgess 2008). It seems that a wide-open view of the arts and personal responsibility ties in nicely to the field of Future Studies.

Cultivating observational "polis pods" for discourse on the future, including transhumanism, is timely. The impacts of change affect everyone, regardless of what domain the changes originally occur in and where the impacts are first felt.

Considering the evolving human form as a research objective is imperative because of the intersection of human enhancement and the future, as well as academic discourse pertaining to theories concerning this intersection. For the past twenty years I have engaged in the fields of media arts and the social science of futurology concerning human enhancement technologies. Through this immersion, my insights have developed beyond the bio-technological attributes toward ideological viewpoints and the worldview of transhumanism, including the body biopolitic and personal bio-freedom of human enhancements. Of course this is directly affected by issues of when life begins and ends, identity in simulated environments, and the conjectured transhuman and posthuman. I have come to understand that a developed approach to human enhancement reaches beyond electronic media, bioart, and immersive design. I propose that what is needed is a field focusing on radical life extension, especially at the convergence of NBIC (nanotechnology, biotechnology, infotechnology, and cognitive science). These technologies and the supporting science relate to the push beyond limited lifespan, senescence, and apoptosis toward regenerative existence and optional death. To balance out the discussion between disenchanted spectators and transhumanism, we need more creative inquiry. Let's adjust our caps at a slight tilt and engage with more information and experience of constructive creative thinking, for "ideas evolve just as do living things" (Salk 1972: 77–78).

Concluding Thoughts

We could start off asking the question: What might be concerns of artistic works and design-based practices that approach human enhancement and life extension? Addressing this question would imply that possible questions from artistic practices are different than the questions tackled by science. It also implies that there are borders/boundaries that need to be mediated. Another question might be: If human–computer interaction is now a developed field of study, and bioart has become a promising field within the arts curriculum, is there potential that human enhancement and life extension might follow suit? Possibly.

Relatedly, one might ask: Is there a rapport between aesthetics and enhancement which makes enhancement superficial and artificial, rather than being aligned with the notion of the beauty of nature and natural? The ethical concerns of enhancement have populated literature on human futures, and research into this area may help to allay such concerns in developing principles, policies, and/or ethical, artistic, and design-based groups for engaging enhancement issues – forming ideologies that affect and are affected by the arts.

Bringing arts and design into the discussion of transhumanism reflects the idea of the human as transformative. Over time, the approach has been to augment, extend, modify, and enhance human communication, mobility, and experienciality. As Popper observed, artists share a preoccupation with exploiting a vast spectrum of aesthetic categories in works of art with numerous advanced technologies and:

> [an] awareness of the extent of social and cultural change produced by the latest technological developments ... to bring about a significant relationship between basic human experiences ... and the radical and global intrusion into them of the new technologies, in all walks of life, with all the beneficial effects, potential hazards and immense possibilities they offer. (Popper 1993: 181)

Notes

An earlier version of this essay was included in *The Global Spiral* (June 2008); http://www.metanexus.net/essay/h-bringing-artssciences-and-design-discussion-transhumanism. The essay was later included in Gregory R. Hansell and William Grassie, eds., *H+/–: Transhumanism and Its Critics* (Bloomington, IN: Xlibris Corporation, 2011).

1   "Transhuman Manifesto" (1983) preceded the Transhumanist Arts Statement (1992, revised 2002).

2   Where the word "transhumanism" came from, no one is quite sure, as variations of it can be located at different times. However, the very first known reference to transhumanism was written by Durante degli Alighieri (Dante Alighieri) in his magnum opus *Paradiso* of the *Divina Commedia* (1312). It is here that Dante used the term as *transumanare* (to transhumanize, to pass beyond the human). In 1935, T.S. Eliot used the term "transhumanized" in *The Cocktail Party* (republished 1964: 147). Here Eliot wrote about the isolation of the human condition. "You and I don't know the process by which the human is Transhumanized: what do we know of the kind of suffering they must undergo on the way of illumination?" In 1957, Julian Huxley wrote the chapter "Transhumanism" in his book *New Bottles for New Wine* (1957: 13–17). F.M. Esfandiary wrote a chapter on "Transhuman" as the final chapter in *Woman, Year 2000* (1972: 291–298). The philosophy and worldview known as modern transhumanism was written by Max More in 1990, "Transhumanism: Toward a Futurist Philosophy."

   To clear up the misunderstanding that "transhumanism" was originated by Julian Huxley: Huxley might have borrowed ideas and/or been inspired by the works of Teilhard de Chardin (1881–1955) because, in 1929, Teilhard de Chardin took part in the discovery of both Piltdown Man and Peking Man (Wikipedia), and Huxley stated: "human species will be on the threshold of a new kind of existence, as different from ours as ours is from that of Peking man" (1957: 13–17). Huxley may also have been influenced by T.S. Eliot and/or Dante because their works preceded his own. Such observation is not intended to reduce the scholarship of Huxley in relation to transhumanism, but to clear up misconceptions that that Huxley coined the philosophy of transhumanism (Vita-More 1994).

3   In this essay, human enhancement means improving physical performance, increasing cognitive abilities, and radically extending human lifespan. Human enhancement technologies include biotechnology, nanotechnology, information technology, and cognitive and neuro sciences. The most referred to methods for enhancement include regenerative medicine, nanomedicine, and brain preservation.

4   Primarily as suggested by Manfred Clynes and Nathan Kline in "Cyborgs and Space" (1960) and tangentially as suggested by Donna Haraway in *Simians, Cyborgs, and Women: The Reinvention of Nature* (Haraway 1990).

5   As suggested in *The Prosthetic Impulse: From a Posthuman Present to a Biocultural Future* (Smith and Morra 2007).

6   Primarily as understood by transhumanists as a stage of human transformation, succeeding transhuman, and tangentially as suggested in *How We Became Posthuman: Virtual Bodies in Cybernetics, Literature, and Informatics* (Hayles 1999).

7   As understood by Randal Koene as "whole brain emulation" and more recently "substrate-independent minds." http://www.kurzweilai.net/pattern-survival-versus-gene-survival.

8   Life expansion means increasing the length of time a person is alive and diversifying the matter in which a person exists (Vita-More 1997 [revised 2011]).

9   "Transcentury UPdate," a cable public TV show aired in Los Angeles and Telluride, Colorado, from 1986 through 1993, and broadcast numerous segments on the political and ethical issues of technology and segments on building scenarios for the global distribution of technology (green energy etc.), the latter largely based on Buckminster Fuller's distribution plan (Fuller 1982).

References

Ascott, Roy (1989) *Aspects of Gaia: Digital Pathways Across the Whole Earth*. Paper presented at annual Ars Electronica, Linz, Austria.

Broderick, Damien (1997) *The White Abacus*. New York: Avon Books.

Burgess, Lowry (2008) Studio for Creative Inquiry, Carnegie Mellon University. http://www.cmu.edu/studio/fellowships/index.html.

Chislenko, Alexander "Sasha" (1996) "Intelligent Information Filters and Enhanced Reality." http://penta.ufrgs.br/edu/telelab/10/enhanced.htm.

Clynes Manfred E. and Kline, Nathan S. (1960) "Cyborgs and Space." In *Astronautics*. New York: American Rocket Society.

Drexler, Eric (1986) *Engines of Creation*. New York: Doubleday.

Eliot, T.S. (1935) *The Cocktail Party*. London: Faber & Faber; republished 1964.

Esfandiary F.M. (aka FM-2030) (1972) "Transhumans – 2000." In *Woman, Year 2000*. New York: Arbor House, pp. 291–298.

Extropy Institute (2004) "Vital Progress Summit 2004." Extropy Institute Conference Library. http://www.extropy.org/summitabout.htm.

Fleming, William (1966) *Arts and Ideas*. Fort Worth, TX: Harcourt Brace.

Fuller, Buckminster R. (1982) *Critical Path*. New York: St. Martin's Griffin.

ID Fuel, "Humansys: Further Human Enhancement," http://www.idfuel.com/index.php?blog=2&p=451&more=1&c=1&tb=1&pb=1.

Haraway, Donna (1990) *Simians-Cyborgs-Women-Reinvention-Nature*, 1st edn. New York: Routledge.

Hayles, N. Katherine (1999) *How We Became Posthuman: Virtual Bodies in Cybernetics, Literature, and Informatics*. Chicago: University of Chicago Press.

Hayles, N. Katherine (2008) "H-: Wrestling with Transhumanism." In *The Global Spiral* (June). http://www.metanexus.net/Magazine/tabid/68/id/10543/Default.aspx

Hayles, N. Katherine (2011) "Wrestling with Transhumanism." In Gregory R. Hansell and William Grassie, eds., *H+/-: Transhumanism and Its Critics*. Bloomington, IN: Xlibris Corporation.

Huxley, J. (1957) *New Bottles for New Wine*. London: Chatto & Windus.

Korfmacher, Carsten. (2006) "Personal Identity." In *The Internet Encyclopedia of Philosophy*. Linacre College, University of Oxford. http://www.iep.utm.edu/p/person-i.htm.

KurzweilAI. "RadicalbodyDesignbyNatashaVita-More."KurzweilAI.net.http://www.kurzweilai.net/radical-body-design-primo-posthuman.

Merleau-Ponty, Maurice (1968) *The Visible and the Invisible*, trans. Alphonso Lingis. Evanston: Northwestern University Press.

Mann, Steve (1998, 2008) The EyeTap Lab. http://www.eyetap.org/.

More, M. (1990) "Transhumanism: Toward a Futurist Philosophy." *Extropy* 6 (Summer). Revised June 1994 and 1996.

Parfit, Derek A. (1971) "Personal Identity." *The Philosophical Review* 80/1 (January), pp. 3–27. http://mind.ucsd.edu/syllabi/06-07/Phil285/readings/parfit-personal-identity.pdf.

Popper, Frank (1993) *Art of the Electronic Age*. London: Thames & Hudson.

Prigogine, Ilya and Stengers, Isabelle (1984) *Order Out of Chaos: Man's New Dialogue with Nature*. New York: Bantam New Age Books.

Ray, Tom (2007) Email interview with author.

Richter, Hans (1965) *Dada: Art and Anti-Art*. London: Oxford University Press.

Salk, Jonas (1972) *Man Unfolding*. New York: Harper & Row.

Schopenhauer, Arthur (1966 [1819]) *The World as Will and Representation*, part IV, trans. E.F.J. Payne. Mineola, NY: Dover Publications.

Slive, Seymour (1952) "Art Historians and Art Critics – II Huygens on Rembrandt." *The Burlington Magazine* 594, pp. 261–264.

Smith, Marguard and Morra, Joanne (2007) *The Prosthetic Impulse: From a Posthuman Present to a Biocultural Future*. Cambridge, MA: MIT Press.

Stelarc (1997) "Parasite: Event for Invaded and Involuntary Body." Ars Electronica Festival. http://www.stelarc.va.com.au/.

Stelarc (1995) "Ping Body". Performed at Telepolis Fractal Flesh event, Paris. See http://www.medienkunstnetz.de/works/ping-body/ (accessed August 3, 2011).

Turrell, James (2008) *Skyscape*. Pomona University, Claremont, CA. http://www.arcspace.com/exhibitions/turrell/turrell.html.

Viola, Bill (1995) *The Greeting*. http://www.medienkunstnetz.de/works/the-greeting/.

Vita-More, Natasha (1983) "Transhuman Manifesto." http://www.transhumanist.biz/transhumanmanifesto.htm.

Vita-More, Natasha (1994) "Transhuman History." http://www.transhuman.org/transhistory.htm.

Vita-More, Natasha (1997) "Primo Posthuman." http://www.natasha.cc/primo.htm. Revised 2011.

Vita-More, N. (2002) "Transhumanist Arts Statement." http://www.transhumanist.biz/transhumanistartsmanifesto.htm.

Vita-More, Natasha (2004) "Vital Progress (VP)." Summit press release. http://www.extropy.org/summit.htm (accessed August 7, 2011).

Vita-More, Natasha (2009) "Transhuman Statement (Manifesto)." In Alex Danchev, ed., *100 Artists' Manifestos: From the Futurists to the Stuckists*. New York: Penguin Modern Classics.

Further Reading

Carnegie Mellon School of Design. http://www.idsa.org/index.htm.

MIT Media Lab. MIT University. http://h20.media.mit.edu/about.html.

MIT University (2007) "H2.0 – New Minds, New Bodies, New Identities: Ushering a New Era for Human Capability," MIT University Conference. http://h20.media.mit.edu/about.html (accessed June 2, 2008).

More, Max (1995) "The Diachronic Self: Identity, Continuity, Transformation." PhD diss., University of Southern California.

Roco, Mihail C. and Bainbridge, William, eds. (2003) *Converging Technologies for Improving Human Performance: Nanotechnology, Biotechnology, Information Technology and Cognitive Science*. New York: Springer.

Wiener, Norbert (1954) *The Human Use of Human Beings*. Boston: Da Capo Press.

Why I Want to be a Posthuman When I Grow Up

Nick Bostrom

I am apt to think, if we knew what it was to be an angel for one hour, we should return to this world, though it were to sit on the brightest throne in it, with vastly more loathing and reluctance than we would now descend into a loathsome dungeon or sepulchre.

Bishop Berkeley (1685–1753)[1]

I. Setting the Stage

The term "posthuman" has been used in very different senses by different authors.[2] I am sympathetic to the view that the word often causes more confusion than clarity, and that we might be better off replacing it with some alternative vocabulary. However, as the purpose of this essay is not to propose terminological reform but to argue for certain substantial normative theses (which one would naturally search for in the literature under the label "posthuman"), I will instead attempt to achieve intelligibility by clarifying the meaning that I shall assign to the word. Such terminological clarification is surely a minimum precondition for having a meaningful discussion about whether it might be good for us to become posthuman.

I shall define *a posthuman* as a being that has at least one posthuman capacity. By *a posthuman capacity*, I mean a general central capacity greatly exceeding the maximum attainable by any

Originally published in Bert Gordijn and Ruth Chadwick, eds., *Medical Enhancement and Posthumanity* (Springer, 2008), pp. 107–137. With kind permission of Springer Science + Business Media B.V.

current human being without recourse to new technological means. I will use *general central capacity* to refer to the following:

- *healthspan* – the capacity to remain fully healthy, active, and productive, both mentally and physically
- *cognition* – general intellectual capacities, such as memory, deductive and analogical reasoning, and attention, as well as special faculties such as the capacity to understand and appreciate music, humor, eroticism, narration, spirituality, mathematics, etc.
- *emotion* – the capacity to enjoy life and to respond with appropriate affect to life situations and other people.

In limiting my list of general central capacities to these three, I do not mean to imply that no other capacity is of fundamental importance to human or posthuman beings. Nor do I claim that the three capacities in the list are sharply distinct or independent. Aspects of emotion and cognition, for instance, clearly overlap. But this short list may give at least a rough idea of what I mean when I speak of posthumans, adequate for present purposes.

In this essay, I will be advancing two main theses. The first is that some possible posthuman modes of being would be very good. I emphasize that the claim is not that *all* possible posthuman modes of being would be good. Just as some possible human modes of being are wretched and horrible, so too are some of the posthuman possibilities. Yet it would be of interest if we can show that there are some posthuman possibilities that would be very good. We might then, for example, specifically aim to realize those possibilities.

The second thesis is that it could be very good *for us* to become posthuman. It is possible to think that it could be good to be posthuman without it being good *for us* to become posthuman. This second thesis thus goes beyond the first. When I say "good for us," I do not mean to insist that for every single current human individual there is some posthuman mode of being such that it would be good for that individual to become posthuman in that way. I confine myself to making a weaker claim that allows for exceptions. The claim is that for *most* current human beings, there are possible posthuman modes of being such that it could be good for these humans to become posthuman in one of those ways.

It might be worth locating the theses and arguments to be presented here within a broader discourse about the desirability of posthumanity. Opponents of posthumanity argue that we should not seek enhancements of a type that could make us, or our descendants, posthuman. We can distinguish at least five different "levels" on which objections against posthumanity could be launched: see Box 3.1. This essay focuses on levels 3 and 4. I am thus setting aside issues of feasibility, costs, risks, side-effects, and social consequences. While those issues are obviously important when considering what we have most reason to do all things considered, they will not be addressed here.

Some further terminological specifications are in order. By *a mode of being* I mean a set of capacities and other general parameters of life. A posthuman mode of being is one that includes at least one posthuman capacity.

I shall speak of the value of particular modes of being. One might hold that primary value-bearers are some entities other than modes of being; e.g. mental states, subjective experiences, activities, preference-satisfactions, achievements, or particular lives. Such views are consistent with this essay. The position I seek to defend is consistent with a wide variety of formal and substantive theories of value. I shall speak of the value of modes of being for the sake of simplicity and convenience, but in doing so I do not mean to express a commitment to any particular controversial theory of value.

Box 3.1   Levels of objection to posthumanity

Level 0. "It can't be done"
Objections based on empirical claims to the effect that it is, and will remain, impossible or infeasible to create posthumans.

Level 1. "It is too difficult/costly"
Objections based on empirical claims that attempts to transform humans into posthumans, or to create new posthuman beings, would be too risky, or too expensive, or too psychologically distracting. Concerns about medical side-effects fall into this category, as do concerns that resources devoted to the requisite research and treatment would be taken away from more important areas.

Level 2. "It would be too bad for society"
Objections based on empirical claims about social consequences that would follow from the successful creation of posthuman beings, for example concerns about social inequality, discrimination, or conflicts between humans and posthumans.

Level 3. "Posthuman lives would be worse than human lives"
Objections based on normative claims about the value of posthuman lives compared to human lives.

Level 4. "We couldn't benefit"
Objections based on agent-relative reasons against human beings transforming themselves into posthuman beings or against humans bringing new posthuman beings into existence. Although posthuman lives might be as good as or better than human lives, it would be bad *for us* to become posthuman or to create posthumans.

We might interpret "the values" of modes of beings as proxies for values that would be realized by particular lives instantiating the mode of being in question. If we proceed in this way, we create some indeterminacy. It is possible for a mode of being (and even more so for a *class* of modes of being) to be instantiated in a range of different possible lives, and for some of these lives to be good and others to be bad. In such a case, how could one assign a value to the mode of being itself?

Another way of expressing this concern is by saying that the value of instantiating a particular mode of being is context-dependent. In one context, the value might be high; in another, it might be negative. Nevertheless, it is useful to be able to speak of values of items other than those we accord basic intrinsic value. We might for example say that it is valuable to be in good health and to have some money. Yet neither having good health nor having some money is guaranteed to make a positive difference to the value of your life. There are contexts in which the opposite is true. For instance, it could be the case that because you had some money you got robbed and murdered, or that because you were always in rude health you lacked a particular (short, mild) disease experience that would have transformed your mediocre novel into an immortal masterpiece. Even so, we can say that health and money are good things without thereby implying that they are intrinsically valuable or that they add value in all possible contexts. When we say that they are valuable we might merely mean that these things would *normally* make a positive contribution to the value of your life; they would add value in a very wide range of plausible contexts. This mundane meaning is what I have in mind when I speak of modes of being having a value: i.e., in a very wide range of plausible contexts, lives instantiating that mode of being would tend to contain that value.[3]

A life might be good or bad because of its causal consequences for other people, or for the contribution it makes to the overall value of a society or a world. But here I shall focus on the value that a life has for the person whose life it is: how good (or bad) it is for the subject to have this life. The term "wellbeing" is often used in this sense.[4]

When I speak of the value of a life here, I do not refer to the moral status of the person whose life it is. It is a separate question what the moral status would be of human and posthuman beings. We can assume for present purposes that human and posthuman persons would have the same moral status. The value of a life refers, rather, to how well a life goes for its subject. Different human lives go differently well, and in this sense their lives have different values. The life of a person who dies from a painful illness at age 15 after having lived in extreme poverty and social isolation is typically worse and has less value than that of a person who has an 80-year-long life full of joy, creativity, worthwhile achievements, friendships, and love. Whatever terminology we use to describe the difference, it is plain that the latter kind of life is more worth having. One way to express this platitude is by saying that the latter life is more valuable than the former.[5] This is consistent with assigning equal moral status to the two different persons whose lives are being compared.

Some pairs of possible lives are so different that it is difficult – arguably impossible – to compare their value. We can leave aside the question of whether, for every pair of possible lives, it is true either than one is better than the other, or that they are equally good; that is, whether all pairs of possible lives have commensurable value. We shall only assume that at least for some pairs of possible lives, one is definitely better than the other.

To supply our minds with a slightly more concrete image of what becoming posthuman might be like, let us consider a vignette of how such a process could unfold.

II.   Becoming Posthuman

Let us suppose that you were to develop into a being that has posthuman healthspan and posthuman cognitive and emotional capacities. At the early steps of this process, you enjoy your enhanced capacities. You cherish your improved health: you feel stronger, more energetic, and more balanced. Your skin looks younger and is more elastic. A minor ailment in your knee is cured. You also discover a greater clarity of mind. You can concentrate on difficult material more easily and it begins making sense to you. You start seeing connections that eluded you before. You are astounded to realize how many beliefs you had been holding without ever really thinking about them or considering whether the evidence supports them. You can follow lines of thinking and intricate argumentation farther without losing your foothold. Your mind is able to recall facts, names, and concepts just when you need them. You are able to sprinkle your conversation with witty remarks and poignant anecdotes. Your friends remark on how much more fun you are to be around. Your experiences seem more vivid. When you listen to music you perceive layers of structure and a kind of musical logic to which you were previously oblivious; this gives you great joy. You continue to find the gossip magazines you used to read amusing, albeit in a different way than before; but you discover that you can get more out of reading Proust and *Nature*. You begin to treasure almost every moment of life; you go about your business with zest; and you feel a deeper warmth and affection for those you love, but you can still be upset and even angry on occasions where upset or anger is truly justified and constructive.

As you yourself are changing you may also begin to change the way you spend your time. Instead of spending four hours each day watching television, you may now prefer to play the saxophone in a jazz band and to have fun working on your first novel. Instead of spending the weekends hanging out in the pub with your old buddies talking about football, you acquire new friends with whom you can discuss things that now seem to you to be of greater significance than sport. Together with some of these new friends, you set up a local chapter of an international non-profit to help draw attention to the plight of political prisoners.

By any reasonable criteria, your life improves as you take these initial steps towards becoming posthuman. But thus far your capacities have improved only within the natural human range. You can still partake in human culture and find company to engage you in meaningful conversation. Consider now a more advanced stage in the transformation process...

You have just celebrated your 170th birthday and you feel stronger than ever. Each day is a joy. You have invented entirely new art forms, which exploit the new kinds of cognitive capacities and sensibilities you have developed. You still listen to music – music that is to Mozart what Mozart is to bad Muzak. You are communicating with your contemporaries using a language that has grown out of English over the past century and that has a vocabulary and expressive power that enables you to share and discuss thoughts and feelings that unaugmented humans could not even think or experience. You play a certain new kind of game which combines VR-mediated artistic expression, dance, humor, interpersonal dynamics, and various novel faculties and the emergent phenomena they make possible, and which is more fun than anything you ever did during the first hundred years of your existence. When you are playing this game with your friends, you feel how every fiber of your body and mind is stretched to its limit in the most creative and imaginative way, and you are creating new realms of abstract and concrete beauty that humans could never (concretely) dream of. You are always ready to feel with those who suffer misfortunes, and to work hard to help them get back on their feet. You are also involved in a large voluntary organization that works to reduce suffering of animals in their natural environment in ways that permit ecologies to continue to function in traditional ways; this involves political efforts combined with advanced science and information-processing services. Things are getting better, but already each day is fantastic.

As we seek to peer farther into posthumanity, our ability to concretely imagine what it might be like trails off. If, aside from extended healthspans, the essence of posthumanity is to be able to have thoughts and experiences that we cannot readily think or experience with our current capacities, then it is not surprising that our ability to imagine what posthuman life might be like is very limited. Yet we can at least perceive the outlines of some of the nearer shores of posthumanity, as we did in the imaginary scenario above. Hopefully such thought experiments are already enough to give plausibility to the claim that becoming posthuman could be good for us.

In the next three sections we will look in a little more detail at each of the three general central capacities that I listed in the introduction section. I hope to show that the claim that it could be very good to be posthuman is not as radical as it might appear to some. In fact, we will find that individuals and society already in some ways seem to be implicitly placing a very high value on posthuman capacities – or at least, there are strong and widely accepted tendencies pointing that way. I therefore do not regard my claim as in any strong sense revisionary. On the contrary, I believe that the denial of my claim would be strongly revisionary in that it would force us to reject many commonly accepted ethical beliefs and approved behaviors. I see my position as a conservative extension of traditional ethics and values to accommodate the possibility of human enhancement through technological means.

III.   Healthspan

It seems to me fairly obvious why one might have reason to desire to become a posthuman in the sense of having a greatly enhanced capacity to stay alive and stay healthy.[6] I suspect that the majority of humankind already has such a desire implicitly.

People seek to extend their healthspan, i.e. to remain healthy, active, and productive. This is one reason why we install air bags in cars. It may also explain why we go to the doctor when we are sick, why higher salaries need to be paid to get workers to do physically dangerous work, and why governments and charities give money to medical research.[7] Instances of individuals sacrificing their lives for the sake of some other goal, whether suicide bombers, martyrs, or drug addicts, attract our attention precisely because their behavior is unusual. Heroic rescue workers who endanger their lives on a dangerous mission are admired because we assume that they are putting at risk something that most people would be very reluctant to risk, their own survival.

For some three decades, economists have attempted to estimate individuals' preferences over mortality and morbidity risk in labor and product markets. While the tradeoff estimates vary considerably between studies, one recent meta-analysis puts the median value of the value of a statistical life for prime-aged workers to about $7 million in the United States (Viscusi and Aldy 2003). A study by the EU's Environment Directorates-General recommends the use of a value in the interval €0.9 to €3.5 million (Johansson 2002). Recent studies by health economists indicate that improvements in the health status of the U.S. population over the twentieth century have made as large a contribution to raising the standards of living as all other forms of consumption growth combined (Murphy and Topel 2003; Nordhaus 2003). While the exact numbers are debatable, there is little doubt that most people place a very high value on their continued existence in a healthy state.

Admittedly, a desire to extend one's healthspan is not necessarily a desire to become posthuman. To become posthuman by virtue of healthspan extension, one would need to achieve the capacity for a healthspan that greatly exceeds the maximum attainable by any current human being without recourse to new technological means. Since at least some human beings already manage to remain quite healthy, active, and productive until the age of 70, one would need to desire that one's healthspan were extended greatly beyond this age in order that it would count as having a desire to become posthuman.[8]

Many people will, if asked about how long they would wish their lives to be, name a figure between 85 and 90 years (Cohen and Langer 2005). In many cases, no doubt, this is because they assume that a life significantly longer than that would be marred by deteriorating health – a factor from which we must abstract when considering the desirability of healthspan extension. People's stated willingness to pay to extend their life by a certain amount does in fact depend strongly on the health status and quality of that extra life (Johnson et al. 1998). Since life beyond 85 is very often beset by deteriorating health, it is possible that this figure substantially underestimates how long most people would wish to live if they could be guaranteed perfect health.

It is also possible that a stated preference for a certain lifespan is hypocritical. Estimates based on revealed preferences in actual market choices, such as fatality risk premiums in labor markets or willingness to pay for healthcare and other forms of fatality risk reduction might be more reliable. It would be interesting to know what fraction of those who claim to have no desire for healthspan extension would change their tune if they were ever actually handed a pill that would reliably achieve this effect. My conjecture would be that when presented with a real-world choice, most would choose the path of prolonged life, health, and youthful vigor over the default route of aging, disease, and death.

One survey asked: "Based on your own expectations of what old age is like, if it were up to you, how long would you personally like to live – to what age?" Only 27 percent of respondents said they would like to live to 100 or older (Cohen and Langer 2005). A later question in the same survey asked: "Imagine you could live to 100 or older, but you'd have to be very careful about your diet, exercise regularly, not smoke, avoid alcohol, and avoid stress. Would it be worth it, or not?" To this, 64 percent answered in the affirmative! Why should *more* people want to live beyond 100 when restrictions on activity are imposed? Is it because it frames the question more as if it were a real practical choice rather than as an idle mind game? Perhaps when the question is framed as a mind game, respondents tend to answer in ways which they believe expresses culturally approved attitudes, or which they think signal socially desirable personal traits (such as having "come to terms" with one's own mortality), while this tendency is diminished when the framing suggests a practical choice with real consequences. We do not know for sure, but this kind of anomaly suggests that we should not take people's stated "preferences" about how long they would wish to live too seriously, and that revealed preferences might be a more reliable index of their guiding values.

It is also worth noting that only a small fraction of us commit suicide, suggesting that our desire to live is almost always stronger than our desire to die.[9] Our desire to live, *conditional on our being able to enjoy full health*, is even stronger. This presumption in favor of life is in fact so strong that if somebody wishes to die soon, even though they are seemingly fully healthy, with a long remaining healthy life expectancy, and if their external circumstances in life are not cata-strophically wretched, we would often tend suspect that they might be suffering from depression or other mental pathology. Suicidal ideation is listed as a diagnostic symptom of depression by the American Psychiatric Association.[10]

Even if a stated preference against healthspan extension were sincere, we would need to question how well considered and informed it is. It is of relevance that those who know most about the situation and are most directly affected by the choice, namely the elderly, usually prefer life to death. They usually do so when their health is poor, and overwhelmingly choose life when their health is at least fair. Now one can argue that a mentally intact 90-year-old is in a better position to judge how their life would be affected by living for another year than she was when she was 20, or 40. If most healthy and mentally intact 90-year-olds prefer to live for another year (at least if they could be guaranteed that this extra year would be one of full health and vigor), this would be evidence against the claim that it would be better for these people that their lives end at 90.[11] Similarly, of course, for people of even older age.

One can compare this situation with the different case of somebody becoming paraplegic. Many able-bodied people believe that their lives would not be worth living if they became paraplegic. They claim that they would prefer to die rather than continuing life in a paraplegic state. Most people who have actually become paraplegic, however, find that their lives are worth living.[12] People who are paraplegic are typically better judges of whether paraplegic lives are worth continuing than are people who have never experienced what it is like to be paraplegic. Similarly, people who are 90 years old are in a better position to judge whether their lives are worth continuing than are younger people (including themselves at any earlier point in their lives).[13]

One study assessed the will to live among 414 hospitalized patients aged 80 to 98 years, presumably representing the frailer end of the distribution of the "old old." 40.8 percent of respondents were unwilling to exchange any time in their current state of health for a shorter life in excellent health, and 27.8% were willing to give up at most 1 month of 12 in return for excellent health.[14] (Patients who were still alive one year later were even less inclined to give up life for better health, but with continued large individual variations in preferences.) The study also found that patients were willing to trade significantly less time for a healthy life than their surrogates assumed they would.

Research shows that life-satisfaction remains relatively stable into old age. One survey of 60,000 adults from 40 nations discovered a slight upward trend in life-satisfaction from the twenties to the eighties in age (Diener and Suh 1998). Life satisfaction showed this upward trend even though there was some loss of positive affect. Perhaps life-satisfaction would be even higher if positive affect were improved (a possibility we shall discuss in a later section). Another study, using a cross-sectional sample (age range 70–103 years), found that controlling for functional health constraints reversed the direction of the relationship between age and positive affect and produced a negative association between age and negative affect (Kunzmann et al. 2000). These findings suggest that some dimensions of subjective wellbeing, such as life-satisfaction, do not decline with age but might actually increase somewhat, and that the decline in another dimension of subjective wellbeing (positive affect) is not due to aging per se but to health constraints.

Most people reveal through their behavior that they desire continued life and health,[15] and most of those who are in the best position to judge the value of continued healthy life, at any age, judge that it is worth having. This constitutes prima facie support for the claim that extended life is worth having even when it is not fully healthy. The fact that this holds true at all currently realized ages suggests that it is not a strongly revisionary view to hold that it could be good for many people to become posthuman through healthspan extension. Such a view might already be implicitly endorsed by many.

IV. Cognition

People also seem to be keen on improving cognition. Who wouldn't want to remember names and faces better, to be able more quickly to grasp difficult abstract ideas, and to be able to "see connections" better? Who would seriously object to being able to appreciate music at a deeper level? The value of optimal cognitive functioning is so obvious that to elaborate the point may be unnecessary.[16]

This verdict is reflected in the vast resources that society allocates to education, which often explicitly aims not only to impart specific items of knowledge but also to improve general reasoning abilities, study skills, critical thinking, and problem-solving capacity.[17] Many people are also keen to develop various particular talents that they may happen to have, for example musical or mathematical, or to develop other specific faculties such as aesthetic appreciation, narration, humor, eroticism, spirituality, etc. We also reveal our desire for improving our cognitive functioning when we take a cup of coffee to increase our alertness or when we regret our failure to obtain a full night's sleep because of the detrimental effects on our intellectual performance.

Again, the fact that there is a common desire for cognitive improvement does not imply that there is a common desire for becoming posthuman. To want to become posthuman through cognitive improvement, one would have to want a great deal of cognitive improvement. It is logically possible that each person would only want to become slightly more intelligent (or musical, or humorous) than he or she currently is and would not want any very large gain. I will offer two considerations regarding this possibility.

First, it seems to me (based on anecdotal evidence and personal observations) that people who are already endowed with above-average cognitive capacities are at least as eager, and, from what I can tell, actually *more* eager, to obtain further improvements in these capacities than are people who are less talented in these regards. For instance, someone who is musically gifted is likely to spend more time and effort trying to further develop her musical capacities than is somebody who lacks a musical ear; and likewise for other kinds of cognitive gifts.

This phenomenon may in part reflect the external rewards that often accrue to those who excel in some particular domain. An extremely gifted musician might reap greater rewards in terms of money and esteem from a slight further improvement in her musicality than would somebody who is not musically gifted to begin with. That is, the difference in external rewards is sometimes greater for somebody who goes from very high capacity to outstandingly high capacity than it is for somebody who goes from average capacity to moderately high capacity. However, I would speculate that such differences in external rewards are only part of the explanation and that people who have high cognitive capacities are usually also more likely (or at least no less likely) to desire further increases in those capacities than are people of lower cognitive capacities even when only the intrinsic benefits of capacities are considered. Thus, if we imagine a group of people placed in solitary confinement for the remainder of their lives, but with access to books, musical instruments, paints and canvasses, and other prerequisites for the exercise of capacities, I would hypothesize that those with the highest pre-existing capacity in a given domain would be more likely (or at least not less likely) to work hard to further develop their capacities in that domain, for the sake of the intrinsic benefits that the possession and exercise of those capacities bestow, than would those with lower pre-existing capacities in the same domain.[18] While $100 brings vastly less utility to a millionaire than to a pauper, the marginal utility of improved cognitive capacities does not seem to exhibit a similar decline.

These considerations suggest that there are continuing returns in the "intrinsic" (in the sense of non-instrumental, non-positional) utility of gains in cognitive capacities, at least within the range of capacity that we find instantiated within the current human population.[19] It would be implausible to suppose that the current range of human capacity, in all domains, is such that while increments of capacity within this range are intrinsically rewarding, yet any further increases outside the current human range would lack intrinsic value. Again, we have a prima facie reason for concluding that enhancement of cognitive capacity to the highest current human level, and probably beyond that, perhaps up to and including the posthuman level, would be intrinsically desirable for the enhanced individuals. We get this conclusion if we assume that those who have a certain high capacity are generally better judges of the value of having that capacity or of a further increment of that capacity than are those who do not possess the capacity in question to the same degree.

V.   Emotion

It is straightforward to determine what would count as an enhancement of healthspan. We have a clear enough idea of what it means to be healthy, active, and productive, and the difference between this state and that of being sick, incapacitated, or dead. An enhancement of healthspan is simply an intervention that prolongs the duration of the former state. It is more difficult to define precisely what would count as a cognitive enhancement because the measure of cognitive functioning is more multifaceted, various cognitive capacities can interact in complex ways, and it is a more normatively complex problem to determine what combinations of particular cognitive competences are of value in different kinds of environments. For instance, it is not obvious what degree of tendency to forget certain kinds of facts and experiences is desirable. The answer might depend on a host of contextual factors. Nevertheless, we do have some general idea of how we might value various increments or decrements in many aspects of our cognitive functioning – a sufficiently clear idea, I suggest, to make it intelligible without much explanation what one might mean by phrases like "enhancing musical ability," "enhancing abstract reasoning ability," etc.

It is considerably more difficult to characterize what would count as emotional enhancement. Some instances are relatively straightforward. Most would readily agree that helping a person who suffers from persistent suicidal depression as the result of a simple neurochemical imbalance so that she once again becomes capable of enjoyment and of taking an interest in life would be to help her improve her emotional capacities. Yet beyond cases involving therapeutic interventions to cure evident psychopathology it is less clear what would count as an enhancement. One's assessment of such cases often depends sensitively on the exact nature of one's normative beliefs about different kinds of possible emotional constitutions and personalities.

It is correspondingly difficult to say what would constitute a "posthuman" level of emotional capacity. Nevertheless, people often do strive to improve their emotional capacities and functionings. We may seek to reduce feelings of hate, contempt, or aggression when we consciously recognize that these feelings are prejudiced or unconstructive. We may take up meditation or physical exercise to achieve greater calm and composure. We may train ourselves to respond more sensitively and empathetically to those we deem deserving of our trust and affection. We may try to overcome fears and phobias that we recognize as irrational, or we may wrestle with appetites that threaten to distract us from what we value more. Many of us expend life-long effort to educate and ennoble our sentiments, to build our character, and to try to become better people. Through these strivings, we seek to achieve goals involving modifying and improving our emotional capacities.

An appropriate conception of emotional capacity would be one that incorporates or reflects these kinds of goal, while allowing perhaps for there being a wide range of different ways of instantiating "high emotional capacity," that is to say, many different possible "characters" or combinations of propensities for feeling and reacting that could each count as excellent in its own way. If this is admitted, then we could make sense of emotional enhancement in a wide range of contexts, as being that which makes our emotional characters more excellent. A posthuman emotional capacity would be one which is much more excellent than that which any current human could achieve unaided by new technology.

One might perhaps question whether there are possible emotional capacities that would be *much* more excellent than those attainable now. Conceivably, there might be a maximum of possible excellence of emotional capacity, and those people who currently have the best emotional capacities might approach so closely to this ideal that there is not enough potential left for improvement to leave room for a posthuman realm of emotional capacity. I doubt this, because aside from the potential for fine-tuning and balancing the various emotional sensibilities we already have, I think there might also be entirely new psychological states and emotions that our species has not evolved the neurological machinery to experience, and some of these sensibilities might be ones we would recognize as extremely valuable if we became acquainted with them.

It is difficult intuitively to understand what such novel emotions and mental states might be like. This is unsurprising, since by assumption we currently lack the required neurological bases. It might help to consider a parallel case from within the normal range of human experience. The experience of romantic love is something that many of us place a high value on. Yet it is notoriously difficult for a child or a prepubescent teenager to comprehend the meaning of romantic love or why adults should make so much fuss about this experience. Perhaps we are all currently in the situation of children relative to the emotions, passions, and mental states that posthuman beings could experience. We may have no idea of what we are missing out on until we attain posthuman emotional capacities.

One dimension of emotional capacity that we can imagine enhanced is subjective wellbeing and its various flavors: joy, comfort, sensual pleasures, fun, positive interest, and excitement. Hedonists claim that pleasure is the only intrinsic good, but one need not be a hedonist to appreciate pleasure as one important component of the good. The difference between a bleak, cold, horrid, painful world and one that is teeming with fun and exciting opportunities, full of delightful quirks and lovely sensations, is often simply a difference in the hedonic tone of the observer. Much depends on that one parameter.

It is an interesting question how much subjective wellbeing could be enhanced without sacrificing other capacities that we may value. For human beings as we are currently constituted, there is perhaps an upper limit to the degree of subjective wellbeing that we can experience without succumbing to mania or some other mental unbalance that would prevent us from fully engaging with the world if the state were indefinitely prolonged. But it might be possible for differently constituted minds to have experiences more blissful than those that humans are capable of without thereby impairing their ability to respond adequately to their surroundings. Maybe for such beings, gradients of pleasure could play a role analogous to that which the scale ranging between pleasure and pain has for us.[20] When thinking the possibility of *posthumanly happy* beings, and their psychological properties, one must abstract from contingent features of the human psyche. An experience that would consume us might perhaps be merely "spicy" to a posthuman mind.

It is not necessary here to take a firm stand on whether posthuman levels of pleasure are possible, or even on whether posthuman emotional capacities more generally are possible. But we can be confident that, at least, there is vast scope for improvements for most of individuals in these dimensions because even within the range instantiated by currently exiting humans, there are levels of emotional capacities and degrees of subjective wellbeing that, for most of us, are practically unattainable to the point of exceeding our dreams. The fact that such improvements are eagerly sought by many suggests that if posthuman levels were possible, they too would be viewed as highly attractive.[21]

VI.   Structure of the Argument, and Further Supporting Reasons

It might be useful to pause briefly to reflect on the structure of the argument presented so far. I began by listing three general central capacities (healthspan, cognition, and emotion), and I defined a posthuman being as one who has at least one of these capacities in a degree unattainable by any current human being unaided by new technology.

I offered some plausibility arguments suggesting that it could be highly desirable to have posthuman levels of these capacities. I did this partly by clarifying what having the capacities would encompass and by explaining how some possible objections would not apply because they rely on a misunderstanding of what is proposed. Furthermore, I tried to show that for each of the three capacities we find that many individuals actually desire to develop the capacities to higher levels and often undertake great effort and expense to achieve these aims. This desire is also reflected in social spending priorities, which devote significant resources to e.g. healthspan-extending medicine and cognition-improving education. Significantly, at least in the cases of healthspan extension and cognitive improvement, the persons best placed to judge the value and desirability of incremental improvements at the high end of the contemporary human capacity distribution seem to be especially likely to affirm the desirability of such additional improvements of capacity. For many cognitive faculties, it appears that the marginal utility of improvements *increases* with capacity levels. This suggests that improvements beyond the current human range would also be viewed as desirable when evaluated by beings in a better position to judge than we currently are.

That people desire X does not imply that X is desirable. Nor does the fact that people find X desirable, even when this judgment is shared among those who are in the best position to judge the desirability of X, prove that X is desirable or valuable. Even if one were to assume some version of a dispositional theory of value, it does not follow from these premises that X is valuable. A dispositional theory of value might assert something like the following (see e.g. Lewis 1989):

> X is valuable for A if and only if A would value X if A were perfectly rational, perfectly well-informed, and perfectly acquainted with X.

The people currently best placed to judge the desirability for an individual of enhancement of her general central capacities are neither perfectly rational, nor perfectly well-informed, nor perfectly acquainted with the full meaning of such enhancements. If these people were more rational or obtained more information or became better acquainted with the enhancements in question, they would perhaps no longer value the enhancements. Even if everybody judged becoming posthuman as desirable, it is a logical possibility that becoming posthuman is not valuable, even given a theory of value that defines value in terms of valuing-dispositions.

The argument presented in the preceding sections is not meant to be deductive. Its ambition is more modest: to remind us of the plausibility of the view that (1) enhancements along the three dimensions discussed are possible in principle and of significant potential intrinsic value, and (2) enhancements along these dimensions large enough to produce posthuman beings could have very great intrinsic value. This argument is defeasible. One way in which it could be defeated would be by pointing to further information, rational reasoning, or forms of acquaintance not accounted for by current opinion, and which would change current opinion if they were incorporated. Critics could for example try to point to some reasoning mistake that very old people commit when they judge that it would be good for them to live another year in perfect health. However, I think the considerations I have pointed to provide prima facie evidence for my conclusions.

There are other routes by which one could reach the position that I have advocated, which supports the above arguments. For instance, one might introspect one's own mind to determine whether being able to continue to live in good health longer, being able better to understand the world and other people, or being able more fully to enjoy life and to react with appropriate affect to life events would seem like worthwhile goals for oneself if they were obtainable (see e.g. Bostrom 2005). Alternatively, one might examine whether having these capacities to an enhanced or even posthuman degree could enable one to realize states and life paths that would have great value according to one's favorite theory of value. (To me, both these tests deliver affirmative verdicts on (1) and (2).)

Yet another route to making the foregoing conclusions plausible is by considering our current ignorance and the vastness of the as-yet unexplored terrain. Let S_H be the "space" of possible modes of being that could be instantiated by someone with current human capacities. Let S_P be the space of possible modes of being that could be instantiated by someone with posthuman capacities. In an intuitive sense, S_P is enormously much larger than S_H. There is a larger range of possible life courses that could be lived out during a posthuman lifespan than during a human lifespan. There are more thoughts that could be thought with posthuman cognitive capacities than with human capacities (and more musical structures that could be created and appreciated with posthuman musical capacities etc.). There are more mental states and emotions that could be experienced with posthuman emotional faculties than with human ones. So why, apart from a lack of imagination, should anybody suppose that the S_H already contains all the most valuable and worthwhile modes of being?

An analogy: For as long as anybody remembers, a tribe has lived in a certain deep and narrow valley. They rarely think of what lies outside their village, and on the few occasions when they do, they think of it only as a mythical realm. One day a sage who has been living apart from the rest, on the mountainside, comes down to the village. He explains that he has climbed to the top of the mountain ridge and from there he could see the terrain stretching far away, all the way to the horizon. He saw plains, lakes, forests, winding rivers, mountains, and the sea. Would it not be reasonable, he says, in lieu of further exploration, to suppose that this vast space is likely to be home to natural resources of enormous value? – Similarly, the sheer size and diversity of S_P is in itself a prima facie reason for thinking that it is likely to contain some very great values (Bostrom 2004).

VII.   Personal Identity

Supposing the previous sections have succeeded in making it plausible that being a posthuman could be good, we can now turn to a further question: whether becoming posthuman could be good *for us*. It may be good to be Joseph Haydn. Let us suppose that Joseph Haydn had a better life than Joe Bloggs so that in some sense it is better to be Haydn and living the life that Haydn lived than to be Bloggs and living Bloggs' life. We may further suppose that this is so from Bloggs' evaluative standpoint. Bloggs might recognize that on all the objective criteria which he thinks make for a better mode of being and a better life, Haydn's mode of being and life are better than his own. Yet it does not follow that it would be good for Bloggs to "become" Haydn (or to become some kind of future equivalent of Haydn) or to live Haydn's life (or a Haydn-like life). There are several possible reasons for this which we need to examine.

First, it might not be possible for Bloggs to become Haydn without ceasing to be Bloggs. While we can imagine a thought experiment in which Bloggs' body and mind are gradually transformed into those of Haydn (or of a Haydn-equivalent), it is not at all clear that personal identity could be preserved through such a transformation. If Bloggs' personal identity is essentially constituted by some core set of psychological features such as his memories and dispositions, then, since Haydn does not have these features, the person Bloggs could not become a Haydn-equivalent. Supposing that Bloggs has a life that is worth living, any transformation that causes the person Bloggs to cease to exist might be bad for Bloggs, including one that transforms him into Haydn.

Could a current human become posthuman while remaining the same person, or is the case like the one of Bloggs becoming Haydn, the person Bloggs necessarily ceasing to exist in the process? The case of becoming posthuman is different in an important respect. Bloggs would have to lose all the psychological characteristics that made him person Bloggs in order to become Haydn. In particular, he would have to lose all his memories, his goals, his unique skills, and his entire personality would be obliterated and replaced by that of Haydn. By contrast, a human being could retain her memories, her goals, her unique skills, and many important aspects of her personality even as she becomes posthuman. This could make it possible for personal identity to be preserved during the transformation into posthuman.[22]

It is obvious that personal identity could be preserved, at least in the short run, if posthuman status is achieved through radical healthspan enhancement. Suppose that I learnt that tonight after I go to bed, a scientist will perform some kind of molecular therapy on my cells while I'm sleeping to permanently disable the aging processes in my body. I might worry that I would not wake up tomorrow because the surgery might go wrong. I would *not* worry that I might not wake up tomorrow because the surgery succeeded. Healthspan enhancement would help *preserve* my personal identity. (If the psychological shock of discovering that my life-expectancy had been extended to a thousand years were so tremendous that it would completely remold my psyche, it is possible that the new me would not be the same person as the old me. But this is not a necessary consequence.[23])

Walter Glannon has argued that a lifespan of 200 years or more would be undesirable because personal identity could not be persevered over such a long life (Glannon 2002). Glannon's argument presupposes that personal identity (understood here as a determinant of our prudential concerns) depends on psychological connectedness. On this view, we now have prudential interests in a future time segment of our organism only if that future time segment is psychologically connected to the organism's present time segment through links of backward-looking memories and forward-looking projects and intentions. If a future time segment of my brain will not remember anything about what things are like for me now, and if I now have no projects or intentions that extend that far into the future, then that future time segment is not part of my person. Glannon asserts that these psychological connections that hold us together as persons could not extend over 200 years or so.

There are several problems with Glannon's argument, even if we accept his metaphysics of personal identity. There is no reason to think it impossible to have intentions and projects that range over more than 200 years. This would seem possible even with our current human capacities. For example, I can easily conceive of exciting intellectual and practical projects that may take me many hundreds of years to complete. It is also dubious to assume that a healthy future self several hundred years older than I am now might be unable remember things from current life stage. Old people often remember their early adulthood quite well, and it is not clear that these memories always decline significantly over time. And of course, the concern about distant future stages being unable to remember their earlier stages disappears completely if we suppose that enhancements of memory capacity become available.[24] Furthermore, if Glannon was right, it would follow that it is "undesirable" for a small child to grow up, since adults do not remember what it was like to be a small child and since small children do not have projects or intentions that extend over time spans as long as decades. This implication would be counterintuitive. It is more plausible that it can be desirable for an agent to survive and continue to develop, rather than to die, even if psychological connections eventually become attenuated. In the same way, it could be desirable for us to acquire the capacity to have a posthuman healthy lifespan, even if we could not remain the same person over time scales of several centuries.

The case that personal identity could be preserved is perhaps less clear-cut with regard to radical cognitive or emotional enhancement. Could a person become radically smarter, more musical, or come to possess much greater emotional capacities without ceasing to exist? Here the answer might depend more sensitively on precisely which changes we are envisaging, how those changes would be implemented, and on how the enhanced capacities would be used. The case for thinking that both personal identity and narrative identity would be preserved is arguably strongest if we posit that (a) the changes are in the form of addition of new capacities or enhancement of old ones, without sacrifice of preexisting capacities; (b) the changes are implemented gradually over an extended period of time; (c) each step of the transformation process is freely and competently chosen by the subject; (d) the new capacities do not prevent the preexisting capacities from being periodically exercised; (e) the subject retains her old memories and many of her basic desires and dispositions; (f) the subject retains many of her old personal relationships and social connections; and (g) the transformation fits into the life narrative and self-conception of the subject. Posthuman cognitive and emotional capacities could in principle be acquired in such a way that these conditions are satisfied.

Even if not all the conditions (a)–(g) were fully satisfied in some particular transformation process, the normatively relevant elements of a person's (numerical or narrative) identity could still be *sufficiently* preserved to avoid raising any fundamental identity-based objection to the prudentiality of undergoing such a transformation. We should not use a stricter standard for technological self-transformation than for other kinds of human transformation, such as migration, career change, or religious conversion.

Consider again a familiar case of *radical* human transformation: maturation. You currently possess vastly greater cognitive capacities than you did as an infant. You have also lost some capacities, e.g. the ability to learn to speak a new language without an accent. Your emotional capacities have also changed and developed considerably since your babyhood. For each concept of identity which we might think has relevant normative significance – personal (numerical) identity, narrative identity, identity of personal character, or identity of core characteristics – we should ask whether identity in that sense has been preserved in this transformation.

The answer may depend on exactly how we understand these ideas of identity. For each of them, on a sufficiently generous conception of the identity criteria, identity was completely or in large part preserved through your maturation. But then we would expect that identity in that sense would also be preserved in many other transformations, including the ones that are *no more profound* than those of a child growing into an adult; and this would include transformations that would make you posthuman. Alternatively, we might adopt conceptions that impose more stringent criteria for the preservation of identity. On these conceptions, it might be impossible to become posthuman without wholly or in large part disrupting one form of identity or another. However, on such restrictive conceptions, identity would also be disrupted in the transformation of child into adult. Yet we do not think it is bad for a child to grow up. Disruptions of identity in those stringent senses form part of a normal life experience and they do not constitute a disaster, or a misfortune of any kind, for the individual concerned.

Why then should it bad for a person to continue to develop so that she one day matures into a being with posthuman capacities? Surely it is the other way around. If this had been our usual path of development, we would have easily recognized the failure to develop into a posthuman as a misfortune, just as we now see it as a misfortune for a child to fail to develop normal adult capacities.

Many people who hold religious beliefs are already accustomed to the prospect of an extremely radical transformation into a kind of posthuman being, which is expected to take place after the termination of their current physical incarnation. Most of those who hold such a view also hold that the transformation *could* be very good for the person who is transformed.

VIII. Commitments

Apart from the concern about personal identity, there is a second kind of reason why it might be bad for a Bloggs to become a Haydn. Bloggs might be involved in various projects or relationships, and may have undertaken commitments that he could not or would not fulfill if he became Haydn. It would be bad for Bloggs to fail in these undertakings if they are important to him. For example, suppose that Mr. Bloggs is deeply committed to Mrs. Bloggs. His commitment to Mrs. Bloggs is so strong that he would never want to do anything that contravenes any of Mrs. Bloggs' most central preferences, and one of her central preferences is that Mr. Bloggs not become posthuman. In this case, even though becoming posthuman might in some respects be good for Mr. Bloggs (it would enable him to understand more, or to stay healthy longer, etc.) it might nevertheless be bad for him all things considered as it would be incompatible with fulfilling one of the commitments that are most important to him.[25]

This reason for thinking that it might be bad for a person to become posthuman relies on the assumption that it can be very bad for a person to forfeit on commitments that would be impossible to fulfill as a posthuman.[26] Even if we grant this assumption, it does not follow that becoming a posthuman would necessarily be bad for us. We do not generally have commitments that would be impossible to fulfill as posthumans. It may be impossible for Mr. Bloggs to become posthuman without violating his most important commitment (unless, of course, Mrs. Bloggs should change her mind), but his is a special case.

Some humans do not have any commitments of importance comparable to that of Mr. Bloggs to his wife. For such people the present concern does not apply. But even for many humans who do have such strong commitments, becoming posthuman could still be good for them. Their commitments could still be fulfilled if they became posthuman. This is perhaps clearest in regard to our commitments to projects and tasks: most of these we could complete – indeed we could complete them better and more reliably – if we obtained posthuman capacities. But even with regard to our specific commitments to people, it would often be possible to fulfill these even if we had much longer healthspans or greatly enhanced cognitive or emotional capacities.

IX. Ways of Life

In addition to concerns about personal identity and specific commitments to people or projects, there is a third kind of reason one might have for doubting that it could be good for us to become posthuman. This third kind of reason has to do with our interpersonal relations more broadly, and with the way that the good for a person can be tied to the general circumstances and conditions in which she lives. One might think that the very concept of a good life for a human being is inextricably wound up in the idea of flourishing within a "way of life" – a matrix of beliefs, relationships, social roles, obligations, habits, projects, and psychological attributes outside of which the idea of a "better" or "worse" life or mode of being does not make sense.

The reasoning may go something like this: It would not be good for a clover to grow into a rhododendron, nor for a fly to start looking and behaving like a raven. Neither would it, on this view, be good for a human to acquire posthuman capacities and start living a posthuman life. The criterion for how well a clover is doing is the extent to which it is succeeding in realizing its own particular nature and achieving the natural "telos" inherent in the clover kind; and the equivalent might be said of the fly. For humans, the case may be more complicated as there is a greater degree of relevant individual variation among humans than among other species. Different humans are pursuing different "ways of life," so that what counts as flourishing for one human being might differ substantially from what counts as such for another. Nevertheless, as we are all currently pursuing human ways of life, and since what is good for us is defined by reference to our way of life, it is not the case for any human that it would be good for her to become posthuman. It might be good for posthumans to be posthumans, but it would not be good for humans to become posthuman.

This third concern seems to be a conglomerate of the two concerns we have already discussed. Why could it not be good for a human to become posthuman? One possible reason is if her personal identity could not be preserved through such a transformation. The comparison with the clover appears to hint at this concern. If a clover turned into a rhododendron, then the clover would presumably cease to exist in the process. If a fly started looking and behaving like a raven, would it still be a fly? So part of what is going on here seems to be that the assertion that the relevant form of identity could not be preserved in the transformations in question. But we have already addressed this concern insofar as it pertains to humans becoming posthuman.

There might be more at stake with this third concern than identity. The problem with a clover becoming a rhododendron is not just that the clover might cease to exist in the process, but that it seems a mistake to think that being a rhododendron is in any sense better than being a clover. There might be external criteria of evaluation (such as economic or aesthetic value to the human owner) according to which a rhododendron is better or more valuable than a clover. But aside from such extrinsic considerations, the two plants seem to be on a par: a thriving clover thrives just as much as a thriving rhododendron, so if the good for a plant is to thrive then neither kind is inherently better off or has a greater potential for realizing a good life than the other. Our challenger could claim that the same holds vis-à-vis a human and a posthuman.

I think the analogy is misleading. People are not plants, and the concept of a valuable mode of being for a person is fundamentally different from that of the state of flourishing for a plant. In a metaphorical sense we can ascribe interests to plants and other non-sentient objects: this clover "could use" some water; that clock "needs" winding up; the squeaky wheel "would benefit" from a few drops of oil. Defining interests relative to a functionalist basis might be the only way we can make sense of these attributions. The function of the clock is to indicate the time, and without being wound up the clock would fail to execute this function; thus it "needs" to be wound up. Yet sentient beings may have interests not only in a metaphorical sense, based on their function, but in a quite literal sense as well, based on what would be normatively good for them. A human being, for example, might have interests that are defined (partially) in terms of what she is actually interested in, or would be interested in given certain conditions.[27] So from the fact that we could not make sense of the claim that it would be good for a clover to become a rhododendron, it does not follow that we would similarly be unable to make sense of the claim that it would be good for a human to become a posthuman. Even if the successful execution of "the function" of a human were not facilitated by becoming posthuman, there would be other grounds on which one could sensibly attribute to a human an interest in becoming posthuman.

It is at any rate highly problematic that something as complex and autonomous as a human being has any kind of well-defined "function." The problem remains even if we relativize the function to particular ways of life or particular individuals. We might say that the function of the farmer is to farm, and that of the singer is to sing, etc. But any particular farmer is a host of other things as well: e.g. a singer, a mother, a sister, a homeowner, a driver, a television watcher, and so forth *ad infinitum*. Once she might have been a hairdresser; in the future she might become a shopkeeper, a golfer, a person with a disability, a transsexual, or a posthuman. It is difficult to see how any strong normative conclusions could be drawn from the fact that she currently occupies a certain set of roles and serves a certain set of functions. At most we could conclude that when and insofar as she acts as a farmer, she ought to tend to her crops or livestock; but from the fact that she is a farmer, nothing follows about whether she ought to be or remain a farmer. Likewise, the most we could conclude from the fact that she is currently a human person is that she ought to do things that are good for humans – brush her teeth, sleep, eat, etc. – but only so long as she remains human. If she became a posthuman who did not need to sleep, she would no longer have any reason so sleep. And the fact that she currently has a reason to sleep is not a reason for her not to become a sleepless posthuman.

At this point, an objector could attempt an alternative line of argumentation. Maybe there are some crucial interests that we have that are not conditional on us occupying particular social roles or having particular personal characteristics or serving particular functions. These interests would be unlike our interest in sleep, which does not provide us with a reason not to change in such a way that we no longer need to sleep. Rather these unconditional ("categorical") interests would be such as to give us reason not to change in ways that would make us no longer have those interests.

I have already admitted that individuals can have such interests, and in some cases this might make it the case for some possible individuals that it would not be good for them to become posthuman. I discussed this above as the "second concern." This is not a problem for my position since it is compatible with it being true for other individuals (and perhaps for the overwhelming majority or even all actual human persons) that it could be good for them to become posthuman. But our hypothetical objector might argue that there are certain categorical interests we all have *qua* humans. These interests would somehow derive from human nature and from the natural ends and ideals of flourishing inherent in this essential nature. Might not the existence of such universally shared categorical human interests invalidate the thesis that it could be good for us to become posthuman?

X. Human Nature

Let us consider two different candidate ideas of what a human "telos" might be.

If we seek a telos for human individuals within a naturalistic outlook, one salient candidate would be the maximization of that individual's inclusive fitness. Arguably, the most natural way to apply a functional characterization of a human individual from an evolutionary perspective is as an inclusive fitness maximizer (tuned for life in our ancestral environment). From this perspective, our legs, our lungs, our sense of humor, our parental instincts, our sex drive and romantic propensities subserve the ultimate function of promoting the inclusive fitness of an individual. Now if we define the telos of a human individual in this way, as a vehicle for the effective promulgation of her genes, then many of the seemingly most attractive posthuman possibilities would be inconsistent with our successfully realizing this alleged telos, in particular those possibilities that involve radical alteration of the human genome. (Replacing our genes with other genes does not seem to be an effective way to promulgate the genes we have.)

As a conception of the human good, however, the telos of maximizing inclusive fitness is singularly lacking in plausibility. I do not know of any moral philosopher who advocates such a view. It is too obvious that what is good for a person can, and usually does, diverge from what would maximize that person's inclusive fitness.[28] Those who attempt to derive a theory of the human good from the telos inherent in a conception of human functioning will need to start from some conception of human functioning other than the evolutionary one.

One starting point that has had more appeal is the doctrine that a human being is essentially a rational animal and that the human telos is the development and exercise of our rational faculties. Views of this sort have a distinguished pedigree that can be traced back at least to Aristotle. Whatever the merits of this view, however, it is plainly not a promising objection to the claims I advance in this essay, since it would be perfectly possible for a posthuman to realize a telos of rationality as well as a human being could. In fact, if what is good for us is to develop and exercise our rational nature, this implies that it would be good for us to become posthumans with appropriately enhanced cognitive capacities (and preferably with extended healthspan too, so that we may have more time to develop and enjoy these rational faculties).

One sometimes hears it said that it is human nature to attempt to overcome every limit and to explore, invent, experiment, and use tools to improve the human condition.[29] I don't know that this is true. The opposite tendency seems to be at least as strong. Many a great invention was widely resisted at the time of its introduction, and inventors have often been viciously persecuted. If one wished to be provocative, one might even say that humanity has advanced technologically *in spite of anti-technological tendencies in human nature*, and that technological advancement historically has been due more to the intrinsic utility of technological inventions and the competitive advantages they sometimes bestow on their users than to any native preference among the majority of mankind for pushing boundaries and welcoming innovation.[30] Be that as it may; for even if it were "part of human nature" to push ever onward, forward, and upward, I do not see how anything follows from this regarding the desirability of becoming posthuman. There is too much that is thoroughly unrespectable in human nature (along with much that is admirable), for the mere fact that X is a part of human nature to constitute any reason, even a prima facie reason, for supposing that X is good.

XI.   Brief Sketches of Some Objections and Replies

Objection. One might think that it would be bad for a person to be the only posthuman being since a solitary posthuman would not have any equals to interact with.
Reply. It is not necessary that there be only one posthuman.

I have acknowledged that capacities may not have basic intrinsic value and that the contribution to wellbeing that having a capacity makes depends on the context. I suggested that it nevertheless makes sense to talk of the value of a capacity in a sense similar to that in which we commonly talk of the value of e.g. money or health. We can take such value ascriptions as assertions that the object or property *normally* makes a positive contribution to whatever has basic value. When evaluating posthuman attributes, the question arises what we should take to be the range of circumstances against which we assess whether something "normally" makes a positive contribution. As we do not have a concrete example in front of us of a posthuman civilization, there is a certain indeterminacy in any assertion about which things or attributes would "normally" make a positive contribution in a posthuman context. At this point, it may therefore be appropriate to specify some aspects of the posthuman context that I assume in my value-assertions. Let me here postulate that the intended context is one that includes a society of posthuman beings.

What dialectical constraints are there on what I am allowed to stipulate about the posthuman context? The main cost to making such stipulations is that if I end up defining a gerrymandered "posthuman context," which is also extremely unlikely ever to materialize, then the significance of any claims about what would normally be valuable in that context would tend to wane. It is simply not very interesting to know what would "normally" be valuable in some utterly bizarre context defined by a large number of arbitrary stipulations. I do not think that by postulating a society of posthumans I am significantly hollowing out my conclusions. I do, in fact, assume throughout this essay more generally that the postulated posthuman reference society is one that is adapted to its posthuman inhabitants in manners similar to the way current human society is adapted to its human inhabitants.[31] I also assume that this reference society would offer many affordances and opportunities to its posthuman inhabitants broadly analogous to those which contemporary society offers humans. I do not intend by this postulation to express any prediction that this is the kind of posthuman society that is most likely to form, nor do I mean to imply that being a posthuman could not be valuable even outside of the context of such a kind of society. The postulation is merely a way of delimiting the claims I am trying to defend in this essay.

Objection. The accumulated cultural treasures of humanity might lose their appeal to somebody whose capacities greatly exceeded those of the humans who produced them. More generally, challenges that seemed interesting to the person while she was still human might become trivial and therefore uninteresting to her when she acquires posthuman capacities. This could deprive posthumans of the good of meaningful achievements.

Reply. It is not clear why the ability to appreciate what is more complex or subtle should make it impossible to appreciate simpler things. Somebody who has learnt to appreciate Schoenberg may still delight in simple folk songs, even bird songs. A fan of Cézanne may still enjoy watching a sunrise.

Even if it were impossible for posthuman beings to appreciate some simple things, they could compensate by creating new cultural riches. I am assuming that the reference society would offer opportunities for doing this – see above.

If some challenges become too easy for posthumans, they could take on more difficult challenges. One might argue that an additional reason for developing posthuman cognitive capacities is that it would increase the range of interesting intellectual challenges open to us. At least within the human range of cognitive capacity, it seems that the greater one's capacity, the more numerous and meaningful the intellectual projects that one can embark on. When one's mind grows, not only does one get better at solving intellectual problems – entirely new possibilities of meaning and creative endeavor come into view.

Objection. A sense of vulnerability, dependence, and limitedness can sometimes add to the value of a life or help a human being grow as a person, especially along moral or spiritual dimensions.

Reply. A posthuman could be vulnerable, dependent, and limited.

A posthuman could also be able to grow as a person in moral and spiritual dimensions without those extrinsic spurs that are sometimes necessary to affect such growth in humans. The ability to spontaneously develop in these dimensions could be seen as an aspect of emotional capacity.

Objection. The very desire to overcome one's limits by the use of technological means rather than through one's own efforts and hard work could be seen as expressive of a failure to open oneself to the unbidden, gifted nature of life, or as a failure to accept oneself as one is, or as self-hate.[32]

Reply. This essay makes no claims about the expressive significance of a desire to become post-human, or about whether having such a desire marks one as a worse person, whether necessarily or statistically. The concern here rather is about whether being posthuman could be good, and whether it could be good for us to become posthuman.

Objection. A capacity obtained through a technological shortcut would not have the same value as one obtained through self-discipline and sacrifice.

Reply. I have argued that the possession of posthuman capacities could be extremely valuable even where the capacities are effortlessly obtained. It is consistent with what I have said that achieving a capacity through a great expenditure of blood, sweat, and tears would further increase its value. I have not addressed what would be the *best* way of becoming posthuman. We may note, however, that is unlikely that we *could* in practice become posthuman other than via recourse to advanced technology.

Objection. The value of achieving a goal like winning a gold medal in the Olympics is reduced and perhaps annulled if the goal is achieved through inappropriate means (e.g. cheating). The value of possessing a capacity likewise depends on how the capacity was acquired. Even though having posthuman capacities might be extremely valuable if the capacities had been obtained by appropriate means, there are no humanly possible means that are appropriate. Any means by which humans could obtain posthuman capacities would negate the value of having such capacities.

Reply. The analogy with winning an Olympic medal is misleading. It is in the nature of sports competitions that the value of achievement is intimately connected with the process by which it was achieved. We may say that what is at stake in the analogy is not really the value of a medal, nor even the value of winning a medal, but rather (something like) winning the medal by certain specified means in a fair competition, in a non-fluke-like way, etc. Many other goods are not like this. When we visit the doctor in the hope of getting well, we do not usually think that the value of getting well is strongly dependent on the process by which health is achieved; health and the enjoyment of health are valuable in their own right, independently of how these states come about. Of course, we are concerned with the value of the means to getting well – the means themselves can have negative value (involving perhaps pain and inconvenience), and in evaluat-ing the value of the consequences of an action, we take the value of the means into account as well as the value of the goal that they achieve. But usually, the fact that some means have negative value does not reduce the value of obtaining the goal state.

One possible exception to this is if the means are in a certain sense *immoral*. We might think that a goal becomes "tainted," and its value reduced, if it was achieved through deeply immoral means. For example, some might hold that the medical findings obtained by Nazi doctors in concentration camps have reduced or no value because of the way the findings were produced. Yet this radical kind of "taint" is a rather special case.[33] Having to use bad means might be good reason not to pursue a goal, but *typically* this is not because the use of bad means would reduce the value of the attainment of the goal, but rather it is either because the means themselves have more negative value than the goal has positive value, or (on a non-consequentialist view) because it is morally impermissible to use certain means independently of the total value of the consequences.[34]

The values that I have alleged could be derived from posthuman capacities are not like the value of an Olympic gold medal, but rather like the value of health. I am aware of no logical, metaphysical, or "in principle" reason why humans could not obtain posthuman capacities in ways that would avoid recourse to immoral means of the sort that would "taint" the outcome (much less that would taint the outcome to such a degree as to annul its extremely high surplus value). It is a further question to what extent it is *practically feasible* to work towards realizing posthuman capacities in ways that avoid such taint. This question lies outside the scope of the present essay. My conclusion may therefore be understood to implicitly contain the proviso that the posthuman capacities of which I speak have been obtained in ways that are non-Faustian.

Objection. Posthuman talent sets the stage for posthuman failure. Having great potential might make for a great life if the potential is realized and put to some worthwhile use, but it could equally make for a tragic life if the potential is wasted. It is better to live well with modest capacities than to life poorly with outstanding capacities.

Reply. We do not lament that a human is born talented on grounds that it is possible that she will waste her talent. It is not clear why posthuman capacity would be any more likely to be wasted than human capacity. I have stipulated that the posthuman reference society would offer affordances and opportunities to its posthuman inhabitants broadly analogous to those that contemporary society offers humans. If posthumans are more prone to waste their potential, it must therefore be for internal, psychological reasons. But posthumans need not be any worse than humans in regard to their readiness to make the most of their lives.[35]

XII.   Conclusion

I have argued, first, that some posthuman modes of being would be extremely worthwhile; and, second, that it could be good for most human beings to become posthuman.

I have discussed three general central capacities – healthspan, cognition, and emotion – separately for most of this essay. However, some of my arguments are strengthened if one considers the possibility of combining these enhancements. A longer healthspan is more valuable when one has the cognitive capacity to find virtually inexhaustible sources of meaning in creative endeavors and intellectual growth. Both healthspan and cognition are more valuable when one has the emotional capacity to relish being alive and to take pleasure in mental activity.

It follows trivially from the definition of "posthuman" given in this essay that we are not posthuman at the time of writing. It does not follow, at least not in any obvious way, that a posthuman could not also remain a human being. Whether or not this is so depends on what meaning we assign to the word "human." One might well take an expansive view of what it means to be human, in which case "posthuman" is to be understood as denoting a certain possible type of human mode of being – if I am right, an exceedingly worthwhile type.

Notes

I am grateful to Ross Beaton, Bert Gordijn, Guy Kahane, Toby Ord, David Pearce, David Rodin, Anders Sandberg, Julian Savulescu, Harrosh Shlomit, and Elena Patigo Solana for helpful comments. Earlier versions of this essay were presented at the James Martin Advanced Research Seminar (Oxford, January 30, 2006), and at the Institute for Science, Innovation & Society (Nijmegen, February 21, 2006). The essay is published in Bert Gordijn and Ruth Chadwick, eds., *Medical Enhancement and Posthumanity* (Springer, 2008), pp. 107–137. First circulated: 2006.

1 Berkeley et al. 1897: 172.
2 The definition used here follows in the spirit of Bostrom 2003. A completely different concept of "posthuman" is used in e.g. Hayles 1999.
3 Compare this take on "mundane values" with the notion of mid-level principles in applied ethics. The principle of respecting patient autonomy is important in medical ethics. One might accept this if one holds that respect for patient autonomy is an implication of some fundamental ethical principle. But equally, one might accept patient autonomy as an important mid-level principle even if one merely holds that this is a way of expressing a useful rule of thumb, a sound policy rule, or a derived ethical rule that is true in a world like ours because of various empirical facts even though it is not necessarily true in all possible worlds. For the role of mid-level principles in applied ethics, see e.g. Beauchamp and Childress 2001.
4 I am thus not concerned here with global evaluations into which individuals' wellbeing might enter as a factor, e.g. evaluations involving values of diversity, equality, or comparative fairness.
5 I do not assume that the value of a life, or wellbeing, supervenes on the mental experiences of a person, nor that it supervenes on a thin time-slice of a person's life. It could represent a wider and more global evaluation of how well a person's life is going.
6 Having such a capacity is compatible with also having the capacity to die at any desired age. One might thus desire a capacity for greatly extended healthspan even if one doubts that one would wish to live for more than, say, 80 years. A posthuman healthspan capacity would give one the option of much longer and healthier life, but one could at any point decide no longer to exercise the capacity.
7 Although on the last item, see Hanson 2000 for an alternative view.
8 At least one human, Jeanne Calment, lived to 122. But although she remained in relatively fair health until close to her death, she clearly suffered substantial decline in her physical (and presumably mental) vigor compared to when she was in her twenties. She did not retain the capacity to be *fully* healthy, active, and productive for 122 years.
9 For some, the reluctance to commit suicide might reflect a desire not to kill oneself rather than a desire not to die, or alternatively a fear of death rather than an authentic preference not to die.
10 DSM-IV American Psychiatric Association 2000.
11 This is a kind of Millian best-judge argument. However, if fear of death were irrational, one could argue that people who are closer to death are on average worse judges of the value for them of an extra year of life, because their judgments would tend to be more affected by irrational fear.
12 This basic result is reflected in many chronic disease conditions (Ubel et al. 2003). The discrepancy of attitudes seems to be due to non-patient's failure to realize the extent to which patients psychologically adapt to their condition (Damschroder et al. 2005).

13 The analogy with paraplegia is imperfect in at least one respect: when the issue is healthspan extension, we are considering whether it would be worth living an extended life in perfect health and vigor. If anything, this discrepancy strengthens the conclusion, since it is more worth continuing living in perfect health than in poor health, not less worth it.

14 Tsevat et al. 1998. See also McShine et al. 2000. For a methodological critique, see Arnesen and Norheim 2003.

15 This is fully consistent with the fact that many people knowingly engage in risky behaviors such as smoking. This might simply mean that they are unable to quit smoking, or that they desire the pleasure of smoking more than they desire a longer healthier life. It does not imply that they do not desire longer healthier life.

16 One might even argue that a desire for cognitive improvement is a constitutive element of human rationality, but I will not explore that hypothesis here.

17 U.S. *public* expenditure on education in 2003 was 5.7 percent of its GDP (World Bank 2003).

18 Complication: if high capacity were solely a result from having spent a lot of effort in developing that capacity, then the people with high capacity in some domain might be precisely those that started out having an unusually strong desire for having a strong capacity in that domain. It would then not be surprising that those with high capacity would have the strongest desire for further increases in capacity. Their stronger desire for higher capacity might then not be the result of more information and better acquaintance with what is at stake, but might instead simply reflect a prior inclination.

19 It would be more difficult to determine whether the marginal intrinsic utility of gains in capacity are constant, or diminishing, or increasing at higher levels of capacity, and if so by what amount.

20 Pearce 2004.

21 The quest for subjective wellbeing, in particular, seems to be a powerful motivator for billions of people even though arguably none of the various means that have been attempted in this quest has yet proved very efficacious in securing the goal Brickman and Campbell 1971.

22 See also DeGrazia 2005. DeGrazia argues that identity-related challenges to human enhancement largely fail, both ones based on considerations of personal identity and ones based on narrative identity (authenticity), although he mainly discusses more moderate enhancements than those I focus on in this essay.

23 It is not a psychologically plausible consequence even within the limitations of current human psychology. Compare the case to that of a man on death row who has a remaining life expectancy of 1 day. An unexpected pardon suddenly extends this to 40 years – an extension by a factor of 14,610! He might be delighted, stunned, or confused, but he does not cease to exist as a person. If he did, it would presumably be *bad* for him to be pardoned.

Even if one believed (erroneously in my view) that mortality or aging were somehow essential features of the persons we are, these features are consistent with vastly extended healthspan.

24 It is clear that in order for an *extremely* long life to not become either static or self-repeating, it would be necessary that mental growth continues.

25 We may include under this rubric any "commitments to himself" that Mr. Bloggs might have. For example, if he has a firm and well-considered desire not to become posthuman, or if he has solemnly sworn to himself never to develop any posthuman capacities, then it could perhaps on grounds of these earlier desires or commitments be bad for Mr. Bloggs to become posthuman.

26 One may also hold that a person in Mr. Bloggs' situation has additional reasons for not becoming posthuman that don't rely on it being worse for him to become posthuman. For instance, he might have moral reasons not to become posthuman even if it would be good for him to become one. Here I am concerned with the question whether it would necessarily be bad *for* Bloggs to become posthuman, so any moral reasons he might have for declining the transition would only be relevant insofar as they would make the outcome worse *for Mr. Bloggs*.

27 Compare dispositional theories of value, discussed above.

28   For example, for a contemporary man the life plan that would maximize inclusive fitness might be to simply donate as much sperm to fertility clinics as possible.

29   The quest for posthuman capacities is as old as recorded history. In the earliest preserved epic, the Sumerian *Epic of Gilgamesh* (approx. 1700 B.C.), a king sets out on a quest for immortality. In later times, explorers sought the Fountain of Youth, alchemists labored to concoct the Elixir of Life, and various schools of esoteric Taoism in China strove for physical immortality by way of control over or harmony with the forces of nature. This is in addition to the many and diverse religious traditions in which the hope for a supernatural posthuman existence is of paramount importance.

30   As J.B.S. Haldane wrote: "The chemical or physical inventor is always a Prometheus. There is no great invention, from fire to flying, which has not been hailed as an insult to some god. But if every physical and chemical invention is a blasphemy, every biological invention is a perversion. There is hardly one which, on first being brought to the notice of an observer from any nation which has not previously heard of their existence, would not appear to him as indecent and unnatural" (Haldane 1924).

31   But I do not assume that the reference society would only contain posthuman beings.

32   Compare Sandel 2004, although it is not clear that Sandel has an expressivist concern in mind.

33   Even in the Nazi doctor example, it is plausibly the *achievement* of the doctors (and of Germany etc.) that is tainted, and the *achievement's* value that is reduced. The value of the *results* is arguably unaffected, although it might always be appropriate to feel uncomfortable when employing them, appropriate to painfully remember their source, regret the way we got them, and so forth.

34   It might help to reflect that we do not deny the value of our current human capacities on grounds of their evolutionary origin, even though this origin is (a) largely not a product of human achievement, and (b) fairly drenched in violence, deceit, and undeserved suffering. People who are alive today also owe their existence to several thousands of years of warfare, plunder, and rape; yet this does not entail that our capacities or our mode of existence are worthless.

Another possibility is that the result has positive value X, the way you get it has negative value Y, but the "organic whole" comprising both the result and the way it was obtained has an independent value of its own, Z, which also might be negative. On a Moorean view, the value of this situation "on the whole" would be $X + Y + Z$, and this might be negative even if X is larger than $(-Y)$ (Moore 1903). Alternatively, Z might be incommensurable with $X + (-Y)$. In either case, we have a different situation than the one described above in the text, since here X could invariant under different possible ways in which the result was obtained. However, I do not know of any reason to think that this evaluative situation, even if axiologically possible, would necessarily obtain in the sort of case we are discussing. (I'm indebted to Guy Kahane for this point.)

35   If they have enhanced emotional capacity, they may be *more* motivated and more capable than most humans of realizing their potential in beautiful ways.

References

American Psychiatric Association (2000) *Diagnostic Criteria from DSM-IV-TR*. Washington, D.C.: American Psychiatric Association.

Arnesen, Trude M. and Norheim, Ole Frithjof (2003) "Quantifying Quality of Life for Economic Analysis: Time Out for Time Trade Off." *Medical Humanities* 29/2, pp. 81–86.

Beauchamp, Tom L. and Childress, James F. (2001) *Principles of Biomedical Ethics*. New York: Oxford University Press.

Berkeley, George, Sampson, George, et al. (1897) *The Works of George Berkeley, D.D., Bishop of Cloyne*. London: G. Bell and Sons.

Bostrom, Nick (2004) "Transhumanist Values." In F. Adams, ed., *Ethical Issues for the 21st Century*. Charlottesville: Philosophical Documentation Center Press.

Bostrom, Nick (2005) "The Fable of the Dragon-Tyrant." *Journal of Medical Ethics* 31/5, pp. 273–277.

Brickman, Philip and Campbell, Don T. (1971) "Hedonic Relativism and Planning the Good Society." In M.H. Apley, ed., *Adaptation-Level Theory: A Symposium*. New York: Academic Press, pp. 287–301.

Cohen, Jon and Langer, Gary (2005) "Most Wish for a Longer Life – Despite Broad Aging Concerns." ABC News/USA Today Poll. http://abcnews.go.com/images/Politics/995a1Longevity.pdf.

Damschroder, Laura J., Zikmund-Fisher, Brian J., et al. (2005) "The Impact of Considering Adaptation in Health State Valuation." *Social Science & Medicine* 61/2, pp. 267–277.

DeGrazia, David (2005) "Enhancement Technologies and Human Identity." *Journal of Medicine and Philosophy* 30, pp. 261–283.

Diener, Edward and Suh, Eunkook M. (1998) "Subjective Well-Being and Age: An International Analysis." *Annual Review of Gerontology and Geriatrics* 17, pp. 304–324.

Glannon, Walter (2002) "Identity, Prudential Concern, and Extended Lives." *Bioethics* 16/3, pp. 266–283.

Haldane, John Burdon S. (1924) *Daedalus; or, Science and the future*. London: K. Paul, Trench, Trubner & Co.

Hanson, Robin (2000) "Showing That You Care: The Evolution of Health Altruism." http://hanson.gmu.edu/showcare.pdf.

Hayles, N. Katherine (1999) *How We Became Posthuman: Virtual Bodies in Cybernetics, Literature, and Informatics*. Chicago: University of Chicago Press.

Johansson, Per-Olov (2002) "On the Definition and Age-Dependency of the Value of a Statistical Life." *Journal of Risk and Uncertainty* 25/3, pp. 251–263.

Johnson, F. Reed, Desvousges, William H., et al. (1998) "Eliciting Stated Health Preferences: An Application to Willingness to Pay for Longevity." *Medical Decision Making* 18/2, S57–S67.

Kunzmann, Ute, Little, Todd D., et al. (2000) "Is Age-Related Stability of Subjective Well-Being a Paradox? Cross-Sectional and Longitudinal Evidence from the Berlin Aging Study." *Psychology and Aging* 15/3, pp. 511–526.

Lewis, David (1989) "Dispositional Theories of Value." *Proceedings of the Aristotelian Society, supp.* 63, pp. 113–137.

McShine, Randall, Lesser, Gerson T., et al. (2000) "Older Americans Hold on to Life Dearly." *British Medical Journal* 320/7243, pp. 1206–1207.

Moore, George E. (1903) *Principia Ethica*. Cambridge: Cambridge University Press.

Murphy, Kevin and Topel, Robert (2003) "The Economic Value of Medical Research." In Kevin Murphy and Robert Topel, eds., *Measuring the Gains from Medical Research: An Economic Approach*. Chicago: University of Chicago Press.

Nordhaus, William (2003) "The Health of Nations: The Contribution of Improved Health to Living Standards." In K.M. Murphy and R.H. Topel. eds., *Measuring the Gains from Medical Research: An Economic Approach*. Chicago: University of Chicago Press, p. 263.

Pearce, David (2004) "The Hedonistic Imperative." http://www.hedweb.com/hedab.htm.

Sandel, Michael (2004) "The Case Against Perfection." *The Atlantic Monthly* 293/3, pp. 50–62.

Tsevat, Joel, Dawson, Neal V., et al. (1998) "Health Values of Hospitalized Patients 80 Years or Older." *Jama-Journal of the American Medical Association* 279/5, pp. 371–375.

Ubel, Peter A., Loewenstein, George, et al. (2003) "Whose Quality of Life? A Commentary Exploring Discrepancies between Health State Evaluations of Patients and the General Public." *Quality of Life Research* 12/6, pp. 599–607.

Viscusi, Kip and Aldy, Joseph E. (2003) "The Value of a Statistical Life: A Critical Review of Market Estimates throughout the World." *Journal of Risk and Uncertainty* 27/1, pp. 5–76.

World Bank (2003) "EdStats – the World Bank's Comprehensive Database of Education Statistics." http://www.worldbank.org/education/edstats/index.html.

4

Transhumanist Declaration (2012)

1. Humanity stands to be profoundly affected by science and technology in the future. We envision the possibility of broadening human potential by overcoming aging, cognitive shortcomings, involuntary suffering, and our confinement to planet Earth.

2. We believe that humanity's potential is still mostly unrealized. There are possible scenarios that lead to wonderful and exceedingly worthwhile enhanced human conditions.

3. We recognize that humanity faces serious risks, especially from the misuse of new technologies. There are possible realistic scenarios that lead to the loss of most, or even all, of what we hold valuable. Some of these scenarios are drastic, others are subtle. Although all progress is change, not all change is progress.

4. Research effort needs to be invested into understanding these prospects. We need to carefully deliberate how best to reduce risks and expedite beneficial applications. We also need forums where people can constructively discuss what could be done and a social order where responsible decisions can be implemented.

5. Reduction of risks of human extinction, and development of means for the preservation of life and health, the alleviation of grave suffering and the improvement of human foresight and wisdom, be pursued as urgent priorities and generously funded.

6. Policy making ought to be guided by responsible and inclusive moral vision, taking seriously both opportunities and risks, respecting autonomy and individual rights, and showing solidarity with and concern for the interests and dignity of all people around the globe. We must also consider our moral responsibilities towards generations that will exist in the future.

7. We advocate the well-being of all sentience, including humans, non-human animals, and any future artificial intellects, modified life forms, or other intelligences to which technological and scientific advance may give rise.

The Transhumanist Reader: Classical and Contemporary Essays on the Science, Technology, and Philosophy of the Human Future, First Edition. Edited by Max More and Natasha Vita-More.
© 2013 John Wiley & Sons, Inc. Published 2013 by John Wiley & Sons, Inc.

8. We favor morphological freedom – the right to modify and enhance one's body, cognition, and emotions. This freedom includes the right to use or not to use techniques and technologies to extend life, preserve the self through cryonics, uploading, and other means, and to choose further modifications and enhancements.

The "Transhumanist Declaration" has been modified over the years by several organizations and individuals, although there is little record of the specific modifications and their respective authors. Nevertheless, the original "Transhumanist Declaration" was crafted in 1998 by, in alphabetical order: Alexander Sasha Chislenko, Anders Sandberg, Arjen Kamphuis, Bernie Staring, Bill Fantegrossi, Darren Reynolds, David Pearce, Den Otter, Doug Bailey, Eugene Leitl, Gustavo Alves, Holger Wagner, Kathryn Aegis, Keith Elis, Lee Daniel Crocker, Max More, Mikhail Sverdlov, Natasha Vita-More, Nick Bostrom, Ralf Fletcher, Shane Spaulding, T.O. Morrow, Thom Quinn.

5

Morphological Freedom – Why We Not Just Want It, but Need It

Anders Sandberg

Over the years, I have lectured about various enhancements and modifications of the human body; now I am going to deal more with the whys than the hows. I am hoping to demonstrate why the freedom to modify one's body is essential not just to transhumanism, but also to any future democratic society.

Morphological Freedom as a Right

This essay will largely be based on a rights ethics framework, although I am fairly certain most of the arguments easily carry over to other ethical frameworks.

What is morphological freedom? I would view it as an extension of one's right to one's body, not just self-ownership but also the right to modify oneself according to one's desires. Different human rights can be derived from each other (many of the arguments in this section are from Nordin 1992 and Machan 1987).

The right to life, the right to not have other people prevent oneself from surviving, is a central right, without which all other rights have no meaning. But to realize the right to life we need other rights.

Another central right for any humanistic view of human rights is the right to seek happiness. Without it human flourishing is unprotected, and there is not much point in having a freedom to live if it will not be at least a potentially happy life. In a way the right to life follows from it, since death or the threat of it is one of the main threats to the pursuit of happiness.

From the right to seek happiness and the right to life the right of freedom can be derived. If we seek to survive, we must be able to act freely in our own interest. Similarly, since we are different and have different conceptions of happiness (which is after all a deeply personal thing that

The Transhumanist Reader: Classical and Contemporary Essays on the Science, Technology, and Philosophy of the Human Future, First Edition. Edited by Max More and Natasha Vita-More.
© 2013 John Wiley & Sons, Inc. Published 2013 by John Wiley & Sons, Inc.

cannot be separated from the person pursuing happiness) we need freedom to practice these. Also, since values differ and uncertainties in knowledge and intelligence make people come to opposing conclusions about the best way of acting even when their goals are exactly the same, there is a need for freedom to enable different approaches to be tested, compared, and pursued.

The right to freedom and life imply a right to one's body. If we have a right to live and be free, but our bodies are not free, then the other rights become irrelevant. If my body is coerced or threatened, I have no choice to obey whatever demands the coercer makes on me if I wish to continue to survive. Even worse, changes to my body can be used to affect my pursuit of happiness.

Similarly, a right to ownership can be derived in the same way. We are technological beings who cannot survive without the tools and resources we employ, and if we are denied them we cannot thrive.

From the right to freedom and the right to one's own body follows that one has a right to modify one's body. If my pursuit of happiness requires a bodily change – be it dying my hair or changing my sex – then my right to freedom requires a right to morphological freedom. My physical welfare may require me to affect my body using antibiotics or surgery. On a deeper level, our thinking is not separate from our bodies. Our freedom of thought implies a freedom of brain activity. If changes of brain structure (as they become available) are prevented, they prevent us from achieving mental states we might otherwise have been able to achieve. There is no dividing line between the body and out mentality, both are part of ourselves. Morphological freedom is the right to modify oneself.

Morphological freedom can of course be viewed as a subset of the right to one's body. But it goes beyond the idea of merely passively maintaining the body as it is and exploiting its inherent potential. Instead it affirms that we can extend or change our potential through various means. It is strongly linked to ideas of self-ownership and self-direction (More 1998).

Morphological freedom is, like the others, a negative right. It is a right to be able to do certain things, but it does not in itself imply others are morally obliged to support exercise of it. It would after all be unreasonable to demand others to support changes in my body that they would not see as beneficial or even ethical according to their personal moral. If I want to have green skin, it is my own problem – nobody has the moral right to prevent me, but they do not have to support my ambition. Of course, other ethical principles such as compassion would imply a moral obligation to help, but I will here mainly concentrate on the skeletal rights framework.

As a negative right, morphological freedom implies that nobody may force us to change in a way we do not desire or prevent our change. This maximizes personal autonomy.

This talk will only deal with the basic case of informed consenting adults as regards to morphological change. There exist a number of special cases where volition becomes problematic, such as mentally ill people, pre-persons, or deliberate changes in the motivational systems of the brain. That these cases are troublesome cannot be held as an argument against morphological freedom or any other freedom, since any ethical system will have its limits and messy borderlands. What is important is how well the general principle can be applied, and if it can be adapted with as little contrivance as possible to the special cases. In the case of this kind of rights ethics many liberal thinkers have analyzed the rights of deranged persons, embryos, or the dead (cf. Nordin 1992).

In current debate and legal systems the right to one's body and morphological freedom has been divided into a large number of subject fields, weakening the underlying right. Debates rage about medical privacy, women's right to their bodies, doping, reproductive rights, euthanasia, and the appropriateness of various medical procedures while largely ignoring that they are all based on a common issue: our right to modify (or allow others to modify) our bodies in various ways. It is important to assert the underlying unity before looking at the various special cases and considerations that have to go into the different issues. Otherwise there is a risk that the right to one's body and morphological freedom will vanish from the ethical debate, to be replaced by a patchwork of largely independent ethical judgments with no overall coherence. In the face of rapid technological and social change we need robust basic ethical principles to build on.

What Possibilities Do We See Today and Tomorrow?

Being technological animals we have a long tradition of both integrating artificial components into ourselves or our personal space, as well as deliberately modifying ourselves to fit personal or cultural aims (Weber 2000). Clothing, ornamentation, cosmetics, tattoos, piercing, and plastic surgery have all long traditions. They have mainly been intended to affect our appearance and social impression, rather than actual bodily functions.

Today we have the technological means to modify functions in addition to appearance, making morphological changes far more profound. Various chemical methods of adjusting or enhancing physical or mental efficacy exist and many more are under development (Sandberg 1997). Sex changes have gone from something extremely rare and outrageous to something still rare, but merely unusual (it was amusing to notice that when asked few in the 2001 audience even remembered the transsexual Israeli artist Dana International, who in 1998 won the Eurovision song contest).

We are already seeing suggestions for human genetic modifications (either somatic or germline) for not just treating disease but to enhance quality of life through increased DNA repair, decreases in age-related muscular decline, cancer, and AIDS prevention as well as possibly cognitive enhancements (Stock and Campbell 1999; Migliaccio et al. 1999; Tang et al. 1999; Barton-Davis et al. 1998). While implants are currently only used for treating illness, it seems reasonable to assume that implants for preventing illness or enhancing health or other functions are possible, for example ways of maintaining or controlling homeostatic functions and interfacing with external information sources.

In the past medicine was mainly curative and palliative. Today there is an emphasis of preventative medicine. But the edges are being blurred between the areas. A more heath-conscious public is integrating preventative medicine in the form of exercise, nutrition, and functional food into their lifestyle. Methods intended for one field, such as hormone replacement therapy, can be applied to enhance quality of life outside the field. Techniques are rapidly becoming cheaper and available to more people. We are rapidly approaching a time where there is not just curative, palliative, and preventative medicine, but also augmentative medicine.

Technology and morphological freedom go hand in hand. Technology enables new forms of self-expression, creating a demand for the freedom to exercise them. The demand drives further technological exploration. It is not just a question of a technological imperative, but a very real striving of people towards self-actualization.

Morphological Freedom and Society

It should be noted that morphological freedom is not atomic. Although it has been stated, as is common with a rights ethics, from the perspective of individuals, morphological freedom is part of human interactions. That individuals have rights does not absolve them from their obligations to each other or their need of each other. But these obligations and needs cannot ethically overrule the basic rights. No matter what the social circumstances are, it is never acceptable to overrule someone's right to life or morphological freedom. For morphological freedom – or any other form of freedom - to work as a right in society we need a large dose of tolerance.

Morphological freedom does not threaten diversity, as has been suggested repeatedly by critics of genetic modification or other forms of physical modification, but in my opinion would have quite the opposite effect.

Today we see in Western societies an increasing acceptance and cherishing of individual self-expression and diversity (Brin 1998; Weber 2000). Although peer pressure, prejudices, and societal biases still remain strong forces, they are being actively battled by equally strong ideas of the right to "be oneself," the desirability of diversity and an interest in the unusual, unique, and exotic. These ideas are being expressed through organizations and institutions that are affecting our culture in pervasive ways (Brin 1998).

If new tools for expressing individuality and uniqueness become available, there are always some people willing to embrace them regardless of risks and societal condemnation, just as there are always others who refrain from them for different reasons, including wanting to retain their individuality. While a large majority may choose practical or popular tools, be they telephones or plastic surgery, that only enhances the self-definition of those who refrain from them, which is attractive to a noticeable fraction of people. There is little risk in a diversity-valuing society that everybody is going to jump on a bandwagon, because we also value the critics, conservatives, and opponents highly (Brin 1998).

It is sometimes argued that morphological freedom, for example genetic therapy, would increase class differences, possibly leading to a strongly stratified world of haves and have-nots. This argument is based on the assumption that any morphology-changing procedures are going to be costly and remain so. However, this is not borne out in economic experience where the costs of technology in general decrease exponentially compared to the average wages. In addition the rate of technological diffusion is getting faster, both within Western societies and between rich and poor societies. Especially regarding technologies that may affect future generations such as germline therapy or life extension it is important to remember that the time constant of technology diffusion appears to be much shorter than the human generation time. Issues of value differences may be far stronger determinants of inequalities, in addition to regulations artificially keeping prices up. The best way of making actual morphological freedom an option is not to restrict it, but rather to encourage the use and development of it among a wide variety of people.

Why Do We Want It?

Why do we want morphological freedom? As has already been suggested, humans have an old drive for self-creation through self-definition. It is not done just through creating narratives of who we are and what we do (Hardcastle 2001) but by selecting aspects of our selves we cultivate, changing our external circumstances and physical bodies (Weber 2000). We express ourselves through what we transform ourselves into.

This is a strong drive, motivating and energizing us in many fields. From an evolutionary perspective it improves the fitness of an intelligent being if that being actively seeks to explore and achieve its potential rather than passively wait until a need or circumstances arise. The highly pleasurable flow state we experience when we are doing (to us) purposeful and challeng-ing tasks (Csíkszentmihályi 1990) might be an evolved incentive towards self-improvement. Since self-definition is often challenging and by its nature intensely personal, it is not surprising that it is deeply motivating to most people.

A common criticism against ideas of morphological freedom is that there exists a natural human nature that is disrupted by morphological freedom. But even if one accepts the idea of a particular human nature this nature seems to include self-definition and a will to change as important aspects; a humanity without these traits would be unlike any human culture ever encountered. It is rather denying these traits to oneself or others that would go against human nature. Also, there is no contradiction in having a nature that implies a seeking of its own over-throw; it would rather be a transitory nature that would change as humans change.

Another kind of reason for morphological freedom is practical benefits. Although people have a broad range of views and personal projects, a sizeable fraction experience various forms of self-transformation as beneficial for their personal lives. It may range from improvements in health or life quality to specific desires such as enhanced skills.

We change as humans not because we are unhappy about who we are, but rather because we desire to become better. Self-transformation is not a search for some imaginary state of perfec-tion, as is sometimes suggested, but rather an open-ended process. As we grow as people our ideals and values also grow and change.

Why Do We Need Morphological Freedom?

Just as there are positive arguments for morphological freedom, implying why it would be beneficial to regard as a basic human right, there are also negative arguments showing why not accepting morphological freedom as a basic right would have negative effects.

A strong negative argument, possibly the most compelling argument for the acceptance of morphological freedom as a basic right that may not be infringed, is to protect from coercive biomedicine.

Many have expressed fears that technologies such as genetic modifications would be used in a coercive manner, enforcing cultural norms of normality or desirability. Preventing the devel-opment of technology cannot hinder this efficiently, since the technology is being developed for a large number of legitimate reasons on a broad front in many different cultures and jurisdic-tions. But misuse can be prevented by setting up strong ethical safeguards in our culture and institutions.

Seeing morphological freedom as a basic right is one such safeguard. If it is widely accepted that we have the right to control how our bodies are changed both in the positive sense (using available tools for self-transformation) and in the negative sense of being free to not change, then it becomes harder to argue for a compulsory change.

The desirability to many of the possibilities allowed by morphological freedom also helps support the right to not change, as people see that they are two sides of the same coin. This can be compared to purely negative expressions, such as the statement in the UNESCO Declaration on the Human Genome and Human Rights that children have the right to be born with an unmodified genome. In this example there is already an inherent conflict between the positive demand for giving children the best possible health that is mentioned elsewhere in the document and the negative right. The positive demand is sometimes expressed through *in utero* surgery for certain congenital defects, a process that changes the body and the potential person far more than any present form of genetic modification could hope to achieve (see Mauron and Thévoz 1991 and Stock and Campbell 1999 for further debate and criticism of the genetic heritage concept).

If protection from coercion and ill-advised procedures is the only goal of laws and norms, then they will only gain support proportional to how strongly people feel their rights are being threatened. As various potentially transforming technologies become available, common, and eventually familiar, it is very likely that the familiarity would erode the fear and suspicion that today underlie many bans on applying new biomedical procedures leaving very little support for these regulations, even when they provide a protection against real possibilities of abuse. However, if the regulations are instead based on both the positive and negative aspects of morphological freedom, then they gain continually renewed relevance as they are being supported both by the desire to prevent abuses and the desire to reap the benefits from the technologies.

Without morphological freedom, there is a serious risk of powerful groups forcing change upon us. Historically the worst misuses of biomedicine have always been committed by governments and large organizations rather than individuals. The reason is simply that centralized power broadcast error: if the power makes an erroneous or malign decision, the decision will affect the lives of many individuals who have little recourse against the power and the consequences will encompass the whole of society. Individuals may make mistakes equally often, but the consequences remain on the individual level rather than affecting society as a whole. It hence makes sense to leave decisions on a deeply personal ethical level to individuals rather than making them society-wide policies. Global ethical policies will by necessity both run counter to the ethical opinion of many individuals, coercing citizens to act against their beliefs and hence violating their freedom, and also contain the temptation to adjust the policies to benefit the policymakers rather than the citizens.

As an example, we can imagine that in a near future treatments exist to restore function to many currently handicapped people. In countries with national healthcare systems it becomes very tempting for cost-conscious government officials to reduce costs by curing people – being handicapped is a very expensive "lifestyle" from the perspective of the official.

There clearly exist many people who deeply wish to be cured from various disabilities. But there are also many people who over time have become used to them and instead integrated them into their self-image. The investment of personal growth and determination necessary to accept, circumvent, or overcome a disability is enormous. Suggesting a cure to them implies a change to themselves on a far deeper level than just "fixing" a broken tool, and quite often is experienced as an attack on their human dignity.

The government official would from his perspective do society good by enforcing a cure. But he would deeply violate the self-image and autonomy of a large number of people in doing so. In a society where individual freedom is not viewed as essential, such a violation would be acceptable.

A simple ban on coercive medical procedures would not be enough, even if it is better than nothing. The reason is that it does not imply any right to have an alternative body or protect differently bodied people. The official could encourage "normal" bodies through various means, including officially pronouncing disabled people who did not change as irresponsible and wasting public resources. Without any protection of the right to have a different body, both in the legal sense to prevent discrimination and in the ethical sense as a part of public ethics guiding acceptance and tolerance, the disabled would be in a very disagreeable situation.

It should be noted that the disability movement has been a strong supporter of the right to determine one's body just for this reason. This seems to be a natural point of agreement between transhumanists and the disability movement which might prove fruitful in future debate. The postmodern critique of the normal body also supports the right to be differently bodied, although in this case rather by dethroning normality than by supporting any ethical project.

It might be argued that what is needed here is merely the protection of those whose bodily state is the result of accidents and illness, rather than the full morphological freedom I have discussed. But as the lines blur between curative and augmentative treatments, self-expression moves further into the realm of self-transformation and treatments that might be seen as desirable by some people but not others (such as cochlear hearing implants or genetic therapy) become more available, it becomes increasingly hard to define what constitutes a natural body and what is a body modified in a volitional way. Attempting to set up regulations based on any such distinction will lead to a situation where the dividing line is constantly challenged due to new technological advances, experienced as arbitrary and not protecting people in need of protection. Taking the step to full morphological freedom creates a far simpler ethical guideline, which both protects those who do not wish to change, those who are differently bodied, and those wanting to change their bodies.

Morphological Freedom and Future Healthcare

The health official example points at a relevant issue regarding healthcare in the future. As new and often initially expensive biomedicine becomes available it is not obvious what to make available in national healthcare. The blurring of the lines between curative and augmentative medicine compounds the issue.

As an example, at the time of writing the earlier subsidies of Viagra and Xenical treatments in Sweden have been withdrawn as they are regarded as "lifestyle medication" rather than normal medication. However, it is possible to be granted exception for this, but the Cabinet will handle the case! This not only makes the details of the case public according to Swedish law, but also puts politicians rather than medical professionals in the position to judge the medical needs of a person. This odd situation will unfortunately likely become more and more common as traditional healthcare must deal with ever more advanced options for morphological change. Even without a public or legal acceptance of morphological freedom the mere existence of such options will force healthcare systems to consider them.

Morphological freedom implies that healthcare systems must be able to deal with not just wishes for health but different kinds of health. Since the purpose of healthcare is to be life-enhancing but the amount of resources is always finite, the allocation issue is a dilemma. It might be possible to define a baseline health everyone is entitled to, with further treatments left to the private sector. Voucher systems might entitle to a certain amount of healthcare, and so on. These issues are complex and controversial, but not unsolvable. Although to my knowledge there does not exist any healthcare system – private or nationalized – that is unanimously agreed to work well, societies can and do reach more or less workable compromises. Morphological freedom just adds another factor to this issue.

Morphological freedom implies the need to redefine concepts of health and illness.

A possible model for how to do this might be the volitional normative model of disease of Robert Freitas, which implicitly includes morphological freedom. In the volitional normative view health is the optimal functioning of a biological system. Normal and optimal function is defined from the patient's own genetic instructions rather than by comparing with the rest of the population or some Platonic ideal of function, making health something individual. The physical condition of the patient is viewed as a volitional state, and the desires of the patient are crucial elements in the definition of the health. Disease is a failure of optimal functioning or desired functionality (Freitas 1999).

This fits in well with the new view of patients not as clients but rather as customers. Patients participate in the health process as active partners rather than passive subjects of the physician. Emphasizing this new view and shoring it up with a strong system of individual rights will likely help people gain access to individually life-enhancing tools and to avoid or at least counteract the paternalism that is currently common in healthcare.

Conclusions

I have sketched a core framework of rights leading up the morphological freedom, showing how it derives from and is necessary for other important rights. Given current social and technological trends issues relating to morphological freedom will become increasingly relevant over the next decades. In order to gain the most from new technology and guide it in beneficial directions we need a strong commitment to morphological freedom.

Morphological freedom implies a subject that is also the object of its own change. Humans are ends in themselves, but that does not rule out the use of oneself as a tool to achieve oneself. In fact, one of the best ways of preventing humans from being used as means rather than ends is to give them the freedom to change and grow. The inherent subjecthood of humans is expressed among other ways through self-transformation.

Some bioethicists such as Leon Kass (Kass 2001) has argued that the new biomedical possibilities threaten to eliminate humanity, replacing current humans with designed, sanitized clones from Huxley's *Brave New World*. I completely disagree. From my perspective morphological freedom is not going to eliminate humanity, but to express what is truly human even further.

Note

This essay is based on a talk given at the TransVision 2001 conference, Berlin, June 22–24, 2001.

References

Barton-Davis, Elisabeth R., Shoturma, Daria I., Musaro, Antonio, Rosenthal, Nadia, and Sweeney, H. Lee (1998) "Viral Mediated Expression of Insulin-Like Growth Factor I Blocks the Aging-Related Loss of Skeletal Muscle Function." *Proceedings of the National Academy of Sciences USA* 95 (December), pp. 15603–15607.

Brin, David (1998) *The Transparent Society*. Reading: Perseus.

Csíkszentmihályi, Mihaly (1990) *Flow: The Psychology of Optimal Experience*. New York: Harper & Row.

Freitas, Robert A. Jr. (1999) *Nanomedicine*, vol. 1. Austin: Landes Bioscience.

Hardcastle, Valerie Gray (2001) "The Development of the Self." *Journal of Cognitive Systems Research* 1, pp. 77–86.

Kass, Leon R. (2001) "Preventing a Brave New World." *The New Republic*, May 21.

Machan, Tibor R. (1987) *Freedom Philosophy*. Stockholm: Timbro.

Mauron, A. and Thévoz, J. (1991) "Germ-Line Engineering: A Few European Voices." *The Journal of Medicine and Philosophy* 16, pp. 649–666.

Migliaccio, Enrica, Giorgio, Marco, Mele, Simonetta, Pelicci, Giuliana, Reboldi, Paolo, Pandolfi, Pier Paolo, Lanfrancone, Luisa, and Pelicci, Pier Giuseppe (1999) "The p66shc Adaptor Protein Controls Oxidative Stress Response and Life Span in Mammals." *Nature* 402, pp. 309–313.

More, Max (1998) "Self-Ownership: A Core Extropian Virtue." *Extropy Online* (January), http://www.maxmore.com/selfown.htm.

Nordin, Etik Ingemar (1992) *Teknik & Samhälle: Ett Rättighetsetiskt Alternativ*. Stockholm: Timbro.

Sandberg, Anders (1997) "Amplifying Cognition: Extending Memory and Intelligence." *Extropy Online*. Based on a talk given at the Extro 3 conference, San José, August 9–10.

Stock, Gregory and Campbell, John, eds. (1999) *Engineering the Human Germline*. New York: Oxford University Press.

Tang, Ya-Ping, Shimizu, Eiji, Dube, Gilles R., Rampon, Claire, Kerchner, Geoffrey A., Min Zhuo, Guoasang Liu, and Joe Z. Tsien (1999) "Genetic Enhancement of Learning and Memory in Mice." *Nature* 401, pp. 63–69.

Weber, Robert J. (2000) *The Created Self: Reinventing Body, Persona and Spirit*. New York: W.W. Norton.

Part II

Human Enhancement
The Somatic Sphere

Enhancement can be corrective – as in the case of eyeglasses, contact lenses, robotic limbs, and dental implants. The history of corrective enhancement reaches back to the invention of crescent lenses dating back to the fifth century BC, the prosthetic foot of an Egyptian mummy, and even to the prehistoric ingenuity of dental drillings, carbon-dated to 9,000 years ago. Enhancement can also augment capabilities beyond the limits of purely biological, non-technologically altered humanity. The second section of the book turns from philosophy and aesthetics toward the more practical side of human enhancement by addressing the nature of the human body, alternative biologies, and technological transformations of the human, including hybrids and virtual bodies.

Robert Freitas explores a technology highly relevant to this field which he calls "nanomedicine" – a well-developed approach that includes precise assemblies of nanorobot structures for repairing human physiology. He emphasizes the disastrous outcomes for life and wellbeing due to the current limited level of medical technology development and commercialization. An immediate large-scale investment in medical nanorobots could save up to 52 million lives a year. Freitas explains the essence of nanotechnology and how it could lead to a 1,000-fold improvement over our current human biological abilities. Nanomedicine would not only save and extend lives but enable us to transform our biology in radical and desirable ways. Whether or not Freitas's specific vision is realized exactly, the direction of technology suggests that level of fine control over biological processes is almost inevitable.

Natasha Vita-More's design theory introduces the idea of life expansion as "increasing the length of time a person is alive and diversifying the matter in which a person exists," but it is the act of being alive that is the core theme throughout the essay. Vita-More asks: "what core elements of life are to be expanded and what type of matter might we live within?" She draws upon several views on what is life, including that of cybernetics. Stemming from Aristotle's psyche and

The Transhumanist Reader: Classical and Contemporary Essays on the Science, Technology, and Philosophy of the Human Future, First Edition. Edited by Max More and Natasha Vita-More.
© 2013 John Wiley & Sons, Inc. Published 2013 by John Wiley & Sons, Inc.

Lynn Margulis' symbiogenesis, Vita-More echoes Dylan Thomas' rage against the "dying of the light" by suggesting a transmutation of matter.

In the field of wearable technology, artist Laura Beloff proposes human agency as a virtual "Hybronaut," which forms a continuous existence while being connected to real-time and virtual space. Beloff writes: "An individual can be seen as a mesh of links crisscrossing with the body and between the body and technological devices, and further, to other bodies and surrounding environment." Beloff suggests that the relationship between user and wearable becomes a hybronautic application of technology, uniquely engaging society, and foresees the human as a system that forgoes thinking of humans as framed by clearly defined bodies.

William Bainbridge points out that enhancement of human abilities can be accomplished in several ways, and need not require modification of the person's biological body. We can already make use of avatars in virtual worlds and, in future, we are likely to have the option of teleoperation of personal robots. Enhancement means increasing the effectiveness of a person in taking action, but avatars show that it can also mean "an altered form of consciousness that expands opportunities for experiences, and escape from the conventional system of moral constraints." Part of the human condition (except in rare pathological cases) has been the equation: one body = one person. Now we can already see that one individual may have many different avatars, which is a step along the way to possibly becoming a multiplex or protean personality. Bainbridge also considers how users can build posthumous avatars in virtual worlds and develop unique relationships with their human users.

Concluding this section, medical doctor and artist Rachel Armstrong explores cutting-edge "metabolic materials" such as the protocell as one way to extend biological systems to create novel architectural structures and alternative biologies. Armstrong suggests that new living technologies, such as protocells, offer novel ways to imagine the relationships between humans and the environment. According to Armstrong, living technology may help us create architecture that could form regenerative systems for humans and the ecosphere.

6

Welcome to the Future of Medicine

Robert A. Freitas Jr.

Introduction

I never met my maternal grandfather, Irving Lincoln Smith. I understand he was a good man, a kind and loving father, a hard worker. He died in 1935, at the age of 39, when my mother was only 12.

Irving died of encephalitis, or "sleeping sickness." It is a horrible disease with many possible causes which has up to a 50 percent untreated mortality rate in some population subgroups. Encephalitis is an inflammation of the brain. Prolonged fevers over 106 Fahrenheit are not uncommon. There is a pounding headache, unending nausea, stiff muscles, then drowsiness, coma, and sometimes death.

Irving's passing was a great hardship on the family, which now consisted solely of my mother and grandmother. The Great Depression, you may recall, hit bottom in 1935, the year Irving died. My scrappy grandmother, who had never worked, managed to find a job and held on to the house. She and my mother burned player piano rolls in the fireplace that winter, to keep warm. The piano had been delivered just days before Irving fell ill. As a matter of fact, I still have that once-prized piano, and the last two surviving rolls, in my own house today.

What Irving's wife and daughter did not know, what none of Irving's doctors knew, what almost no one in the entire world knew, was that almost a decade earlier, in 1928, an obscure Scottish microbiologist named Alexander Fleming had first reported the antibacterial activity of a common blue-green mold. By 1929, Fleming had isolated the antibiotic substance and named it: "penicillin." Tests showed that penicillin was not toxic to humans.

Reprinted from Renata G. Bushko, ed., *Studies in Health Technology and Informatics* 149 (2009). © 2009, with permission from IOS Press.

But that was 1929. Irving died in 1935, six years later. Almost nothing was done to promote the use or production of penicillin until 1938.

That's when two British biochemists, Florey and Chain, began an intensive study to define the range of bacteria affected by penicillin. They discovered, among other things, that penicillin was an effective treatment for some bacterial forms of encephalitis.

By 1941–1944, in cooperation with American industry and the War Department, up to a ton of penicillin was being manufactured and distributed to Allied troops fighting in World War II. Penicillin, a true wonder in its day, saved millions of wounded soldiers from dying of gangrene and other common battlefield bacterial infections that just a few years earlier would have been fatal. But all this good news came a decade too late for Irving.

My grandfather may have died, not because the cure he needed had yet to be discovered, and not because the FDA had taken too long to approve a new drug, but simply because the development and commercialization of a new technology took too long. As a result, I never knew my grandfather, and my life has been forever impoverished as a result.

Each of us similarly has friends and loved ones we care deeply about – children, spouses, parents, and friends. Two of them die every second, somewhere on Earth, totaling 52 million worldwide annually. But almost all of these deaths are, in principle, medically preventable – not by the methods of present-day medicine, but by a new form of medicine, called nanomedicine, that now lurks on the technological horizon.

What is Nanomedicine?

What is nanomedicine? The concept is fairly easy to understand. The only important difference between the carbon atoms in a plain lump of coal and the carbon atoms in a stunning crystal of diamond is their molecular arrangement, relative to each other. Future technology currently envisioned will allow us to rearrange all atoms exactly the way we want them, consistent with natural laws, thus permitting the manufacture of artificial objects of surpassing beauty and strength that are far more valuable than diamonds. This is the essence of nanotechnology: the control of the composition and structure of matter at the atomic level. The prefix "nano-" refers to the scale of these constructions. A nanometer is one-billionth of a meter, the width of about 5 carbon atoms nestled side by side. Nanomedicine is the application of nanotechnology to the field of medicine.

Nanorobotics

In decades to come, nanotechnologists will build nanoscale molecular parts like gears, bearings, and ratchets. Each nanopart may comprise a few thousand precisely placed atoms. These mechanical nanoparts will then be assembled into larger working machines such as nanopumps, nanocomputers, and even complete nanorobots. With medical nanorobots in hand, doctors will be able to quickly cure most diseases that hobble and kill people today, rapidly repair most physical injuries our bodies can suffer, and vastly extend the human healthspan. This application of nanotechnology to the improvement of human health is the most visionary branch of nanomedicine, called medical nanorobotics.

Microscale robots are already being investigated for *in vivo* medical use. In 2002, researchers at Tohoku University tested magnetically driven spinning screws intended to propel drug payloads through veins and into infected tissues, or even to burrow into tumors and destroy them with heat. In 2005 a team at the Swiss Federal Institute of Technology in Zurich fabricated a similarly powered microrobot small enough to be injected into the body through a syringe. The team hopes their device might be used to deliver drugs or to perform minimally invasive eye surgery. Moving still smaller in scale, experimentalists have used a rapidly vibrating micropipette to slice individual dendrites from single neurons without damaging cell viability. Other researchers have wielded tightly focused femtosecond lasers as nano-scissors to perform nanosurgery on individual chromosomes inside a live cell nucleus, and have dissected the cell wall of a single bacterium, layer by layer, using an atomic force microscope.

Medical nanorobots would be even smaller and would be constructed entirely of atomically precise mechanical components. The first and most famous scientist to voice the possibility of nanorobots traveling through the body, searching out and clearing up diseases, was the late Nobel physicist Richard P. Feynman. In his remarkably prescient 1959 talk "There's Plenty of Room at the Bottom," Feynman proposed employing machine tools to make smaller machine tools, these to be used in turn to make still smaller machine tools, and so on all the way down to the atomic level, noting that this is "a development which I think cannot be avoided."

With these small machine tools in hand, small mechanical devices, including nanorobots, could be constructed. This technology, said Feynman, "suggests a very interesting possibility for relatively small machines. Although it is a very wild idea, it would be interesting in surgery if you could swallow the surgeon. You put the mechanical surgeon inside the blood vessel and it goes into the heart and looks around. (Of course the information has to be fed out.) It finds out which valve is the faulty one and takes a little knife and slices it out. … [Imagine] that we can manufacture an object that maneuvers at that level! … Other small machines might be permanently incorporated in the body to assist some inadequately functioning organ" (Feynman 1960).

What is a medical nanorobot? Like a regular robot, a nanorobot may be made of many thousands of mechanical parts such as bearings and gears composed of strong diamond-like material. A nanorobot will have motors to make things move, and perhaps manipulator arms or mechanical legs for mobility. It will have a power supply for energy, sensors to guide its actions, and an onboard computer to control its behavior. But unlike a regular robot, a nanorobot will be very small. A nanorobot that would travel through the bloodstream must be tiny enough to squeeze through even the narrowest capillaries in the human body. Such machines must be smaller than the red cells in our blood. A convenient measure of size is the micron, or one-millionth of a meter. A red cell is about 7 microns wide. A bloodborne medical nanorobot will typically be no larger than 2–3 microns in its largest dimension. The mechanical parts that make up a nanorobot will be much smaller still, typically 1–10 nanometers in size.

Nanorobotics Revolution by the 2020s

We cannot build such tiny robots today. But perhaps by the 2020s, we will. These future devices may be made of rigid diamondoid nanometer-scale parts and subsystems including onboard sensors, motors, manipulators, and molecular computers. They will be fabricated in a nanofactory via positional assembly: picking and placing nanoscale parts one by one, then moving them along controlled trajectories much like the robot arms that manufacture cars on automobile assembly lines. These steps will be repeated over and over with all the different parts until the final product, such as a medical nanorobot, is fully assembled.

The ability to build nanorobots cheaply and in therapeutically useful numbers will revolutionize the practice of medicine. Performance improvements up to 1,000-fold over natural biological systems of similar function appear possible. For example, the respirocyte is an artificial mechanical red blood cell just 1 micron in diameter having 1/100th the volume of a natural red cell. Red cells carry oxygen to our tissues and remove carbon dioxide. Respirocytes do too, but would be made of much stronger diamond-like materials, not floppy lipids and proteins as we find in living cells. This allows respiratory gases to be safely stored within the respirocyte at tremendous pressures – up to 1,000 atmospheres – and to be loaded or unloaded, molecule by molecule, using mechanical pumps on the device's surface. This simple nanorobot is regulated by onboard computers, powered by glucose fuel cells, and controlled by a physician who communicates with the device via ultrasound signals beamed into the body from outside. A therapeutic 5 cc. injection of respirocytes, just 1/1000th of total blood volume, duplicates the oxygen-carrying ability of the entire human blood mass. Such a dose could instantly revive emergency victims of carbon monoxide poisoning at the scene of a fire.

Artificial mechanical white blood cell devices called microbivores are nanorobots that would seek and digest harmful bloodborne pathogens including bacteria, viruses, or fungi. The pathogens are completely digested into harmless sugars, amino acids, and the like, which are the only effluents from this 3-micron nanorobot. No matter that a bacterium has acquired multiple drug resistance to antibiotics or to any other traditional treatment – the microbivore will eat it anyway. Microbivores would completely clear even the most severe bloodborne infections in hours or less, then be removed from the body. This is 1,000 times faster than the weeks or months often needed for traditional antibiotic-based cures.

Related medical nanorobots with enhanced tissue mobility could similarly consume tumor cells with unmatched speed and surgical precision, eliminating cancer. Other devices could be programmed to remove circulatory obstructions in just minutes, quickly rescuing even the most compromised stroke victim from near-certain brain damage.

The most advanced types of nanomedical devices could perform surgery on your individual cells. In one procedure, a nanorobot called a chromallocyte, controlled by a physician, would extract existing chromosomes from a diseased tissue cell in a living patient, then insert fresh new ones in their place. This process is called chromosome replacement therapy. The replacement chromosomes would be manufactured earlier, outside of the patient's body, by a desktop nanofactory that includes a molecular assembly line, using the patient's individual genome as the blueprint. If the patient chooses, inherited defective genes could be replaced with nondefective base-pair sequences, permanently curing any genetic disease and permitting cancerous cells to be reprogrammed to a healthy state. Each chromallocyte is loaded with a single copy of the digitally corrected chromosome set. After injection, each device travels to its target tissue cell, enters the nucleus, replaces old worn-out genes with new chromosome copies, then exits the cell and is removed from the body.

The implications for extension of healthy lifespan are profound. Perhaps most importantly, chromosome replacement therapy could be used to correct the accumulating genetic damage and mutations that lead to aging in every one of your cells. With annual checkups and cleanouts, and some occasional major cellular repairs, your biological age could be restored once a year to a more or less constant physiological age that you select. Nanomedicine thus may permit us first to arrest, and later to reverse, the biological effects of aging and most of the current medical causes of natural death, severing forever the link between calendar time and biological health.

This sounds almost miraculous, but getting there is primarily an engineering and R&D challenge. Building nanorobots requires the ability to fabricate strong, rigid, nanoscale diamond or diamond-like machine parts that are atomically precise, and then to assemble them into working machinery. Reminiscent of Alexander Fleming's early experiments with blue-green mold in 1928, an obscure Japanese research group led by Oscar Custance at Osaka University in Japan reported, in 2003, the first atomically precise bonding and unbonding of a single silicon atom, on a single spot on a silicon surface, using purely mechanical forces. This was the first laboratory demonstration of a mechanically forced chemical reaction – called mechanosynthesis – in history. And mechanosynthesis is the key manufacturing technology that must be developed in order to build medical nanorobots, atom by atom.

Several years ago, Ralph Merkle and I founded the Nanofactory Collaboration to coordinate a combined experimental and theoretical R&D program to design and construct the first working diamondoid nanofactory, which could then build medical nanorobots. This long-term effort must start by developing the initial technology of positionally controlled mechanosynthesis of diamondoid structures using engineered tooltips and simple molecular feedstock. Our collaboration has led to continuing efforts involving direct collaborations among more than two dozen researchers at a dozen organizations in 5 countries – the U.S., U.K., Russia, Australia, and Belgium. A dozen peer-reviewed papers are published or in progress as of 2008.

Most recently, after working closely for three years with Philip Moriarty, one of the leading scanning probe microscopists in the U.K., in 2008 our international colleague received a five-year $3 million grant to undertake direct experiments to build and validate several of our proposed mechanosynthesis tooltips in his laboratory. We're also preparing a separate research program proposal of our own to solicit additional funding from various U.S. public or private sources to support further mechanosynthesis-related experimental and theory work on a greatly accelerated schedule. We expect these efforts will ultimately lead to the design and manufacture of medical nanorobots for life extension, perhaps during the 2020s.

Conclusions

This new medical technology needs to be moved forward as quickly as possible. Every year we delay, 52 million of our fellow travelers on the river of life fall overboard and are lost forever to the rest of us. Every decade that we delay, half a billion people perish who could have been saved. The stupendous loss of knowledge and human capital is unquestionably the greatest catastrophe that humankind has ever faced. This catastrophe continues tormenting us year after year. We have a moral obligation to minimize the number of people who die unnecessarily between now and the day that nanorobotic medicine is first introduced for therapeutic purposes.

Let's not repeat the mistakes of the past. Let's not take too long to develop this important new medical technology. I'm sure – though I never had the pleasure of meeting him – that my grandfather Irving Smith would have heartily agreed.

References

Web references

Personal website of Robert A. Freitas Jr.: http://www.rfreitas.com
Nanomedicine website: http://www.nanomedicine.com
Nanofactory Collaboration website: http://www.MolecularAssembler.com/Nanofactory
Nanomedicine Art Gallery: http://www.foresight.org/Nanomedicine/Gallery/index.html

Literature references (popular)

Feynman, Richard P. (1960) "There's Plenty of Room at the Bottom." *Engineering and Science*, California Institute of Technology (February), pp. 22–26.

Freitas, Robert A. Jr., (2000) "Say Ah!" *The Sciences* 40 (July/August), pp. 26–31. http://www.foresight.org/Nanomedicine/SayAh/index.html.

Freitas, Robert A. Jr., (2002) "Death is an Outrage!" Invited Lecture delivered at the Fifth Alcor Conference on Extreme Life Extension, November, 16, Newport Beach, CA. http://www.rfreitas.com/Nano/DeathIsAnOutrage.htm.

Freitas, Robert A. Jr., (2003) "Nanomedicine," KurzweilAI.net, November 17. http://www.kurzweilai.net/meme/frame.html?main=/articles/art0602.html.

Literature references (technical)

First book on nanomedicine ever published: Robert A. Freitas Jr. (1999) *Nanomedicine*, vol. 1: *Basic Capabilities*. Georgetown, TX: Landes Bioscience. http://www.nanomedicine.com/NMI.htm. See also: Robert A. Freitas Jr. (2003) *Nanomedicine*, vol. 2A: *Biocompatibility*. Georgetown, TX: Landes Bioscience. http://www.nanomedicine.com/NMIIA.htm.

First medical nanorobot design paper ever published: Robert A. Freitas Jr. (1998) "Exploratory Design in Medical Nanotechnology: A Mechanical Artificial Red Cell." *Artificial Cells, Blood Substitutes, and Immobil. Biotech.* 26, pp. 411–430. http://www.foresight.org/Nanomedicine/Respirocytes.html.

Published design paper on the microbivores: Robert A. Freitas Jr. (2005) "Microbivores: Artificial Mechanical Phagocytes using Digest and Discharge Protocol." *Journal of Evolution and Technology* 14 (April), pp. 55–106. http://www.jetpress.org/volume14/freitas.pdf.

First technical description of a cell repair nanorobot ever published: Robert A. Freitas Jr. (2007) "The Ideal Gene Delivery Vector: Chromallocytes, Cell Repair Nanorobots for Chromosome Replacement Therapy." *Journal of Evolution and Technology* 16 (June), pp. 1–97. http://jetpress.org/v16/freitas.pdf.

7

Life Expansion Media

Natasha Vita-More

Life expansion means increasing the length of time a person is alive and diversifying the matter in which a person exists. For human life, the length of time is bounded by a single century and its matter is tied to biology. We might ask: What core elements of life are to be expanded and what type of matter might we live within? Taking the core elements of life, time, and matter into consideration, life expansion then becomes an issue of how to regenerate biological cells, extend personal identity, and preserve the brain, whether through cryonics,[1] connectomics,[2] or computations.[3] Taking its media into consideration, it then becomes an issue of the semi-biological and non-biological substrates[4] we might exist within (whether virtual, synthetic, and/or computational), the potential of a connective mind,[5] what we might look like and what form we might take, and how to sustain our human species as a whole.

Living

Aristotle (350 BC) described essence, form, and matter as components of living things. In *De Anima*, his inquiry of *psyche* [ψυχη] proposed that "[t]he [psyche] is the cause or source of the living ... it is (a) the movement, it is (b) the end, it is (c) the essence of the whole living body" (Ross 1931). Intrinsic to all living matter is this psyche – "the first principle of living things" (*De anima*, 402a) (Goetz and Taliaferro 2011: 19).

According to Eugene Thacker in *After Life* (Thacker 2010), a particular "problem for philosophy" is based on two concepts that are relevant to life expansion: (1) the "time and temporality" of life and (2) the "form and finality" of life (Thacker 2010: xii). Thacker looks at life outside the scientific-biological-medical perspective and the mechanical-technological sphere. Nevertheless, his study on "after life" is significant. While it may not pertain to the issues of brain preservation and/or future

The Transhumanist Reader: Classical and Contemporary Essays on the Science, Technology, and Philosophy of the Human Future, First Edition. Edited by Max More and Natasha Vita-More.
© 2013 John Wiley & Sons, Inc. Published 2013 by John Wiley & Sons, Inc.

types of matter for existence, it does relate to questioning what might be "life" after biological life – the point where "living" becomes something other than biological. As such, "life after life" (2010: xiv) links to the issue of being "alive" after biological cells reach their divisional limits, as in the Hayflick Limit Theory of Aging. Interpreting it this way, the posthuman as a computational upload could be "life after life." However, on this point I do not assume Thacker might agree with me.

Notably, Thacker introduces an ontology of life by identifying two aspects that parallel life expansion. First, that life manifests in instances and, second, that those who are living denote the manifestations of particular instances (Thacker 2010: 17). This observation is derived from Aristotle's use of life as the concept of "life-in-itself" and the "now" that you live as "the living", including "any and all the instances of life" (2010: 17). For life expansion, the idea is to stay alive. Life in and of itself is necessary, to be sure, but it is you – your personhood – the "now" of being alive, and the continuation of the instances of "living", that denotes life. Thus, any and all instances of life could be experienced in a posthuman virtual, synthetic, and/or computational matter.

Matter

In *What is Life?*, Lynn Margulis brings us directly into body matter as an evolutionary conglomeration of bacterial strains where life is "the transmutation of energy and matter" in an autopoietic process (Margulis and Sagan 2000: 215).[6]

The theory of "symbiogenesis"[7] suggests that we are comprised of a conglomerate of life forms – that as animals, humans are nucleated cells (Margulis and Sagan 2000) descended not just from a Darwinian theory of common ancestry (Darwin 1859), but from ancient bacteria, which are themselves comprised of different strains of bacteria (Margulis and Sagan 2000). The idea of a symbiogenesis is an underlying theme of life expansion,[8] in relation to a "biotechnogenesis"[9] of emerging and speculative technologies, which form the media of life expansion.

The biotechnogenesis media of life expansion for the human and transhuman include biotechnology (genetic engineering, and methods of regenerative medicine, i.e., stem cell cloning and regenerative cells growing organs), nanotechnology (nanomedicine, nanorobotics, and molecular manufacturing) and human–computer interaction, including artificial intelligence (artificial general intelligence), and processes for whole brain emulation. The quintessence of being alive – that element of you, the *psyche* according to Aristotle, form the biotechnogenesis of matter as they repeatedly collapse and expand into each other. In doing so, they form something other than a linear time-based process (as proposed in the horizontality of Darwin), and begin to reflect what Margulis suggests in symbiogenesis, and what this essay suggests is a process of life expansion. Molecules, at their finest point known to date, are comprised of atoms. How atoms form in making molecules and how molecules form in making matter is relevant to life expansion, especially the media of molecular nanotechnology. "Molecular manufacturing will eventually transform our relationship to molecules and matter as thoroughly as the computer changed our relationship to bits and information. It will enable precise, inexpensive control of the structure of matter" (Neil Jacobstein, personal communication).

Degeneration/Regeneration

If the goal of life expansion is increasing the length of time a person is alive and diversifying the matter or substrates in which a person exists, then the process of decomposition is at the center of the process of regeneration. They go hand in hand, as one cannot exist without the other.

Whether or not death itself is good or bad is irrelevant. What is relevant is that prior to being alive there is no physically recorded recollection of existence and, likewise, after death existence is supposed, but nevertheless unknown. Life expansion, in terms of biology, is mostly concerned with existence now, not prior to birth or after death's biological finality. And it is this "now" of being alive that forms the motivation for defeating death, as passionately summed up in the Dylan Thomas poem "Do not go gentle into that good night" and its refrain " … rage, rage against the dying of the light" (Thomas 1951).

Thomas' rage, however vocally expressed or silently confirmed by transhumanists, reflects, in part, the biopolitics of human enhancement. The culture of new-agers, life extensionists, feminists, cyberpunks, posthumanists, transhumanists, grrrls, avatars, transsexuals, bio-hackers, geeks, and others, has displayed a vocal and/or silent rage over body and gender diversity. The transhumanist rage against the dying of the light is largely fostered by an urgency to change dictums of "normal" and "normalcy" that prescribe not just what a man and woman are, and their respective gender and genitalia, but also what life and death are. Gender choice, body image, ownership of body, and certain rights of bodily modification are impassioned by an insistence for certain human rights. Extending life, prolonging personhood, and morphological freedom are certain transhuman rights.

But let me clarify that the issue is not just about body enhancement and life expansion. It concerns the larger environment in which enhancement takes place and the idea that humans might and can append their bodies and expand their lives. If our ancestors augmented the body for millions of years, since the *Homo habilis* and the Oldowan people and their tools, then the phenotype of appending the body is an innate and/or a learned expression. This interrelationship between the organism, the appendage, and the environment is an evidenced observation that needs to be understood, whether accepted or not, by all sides engaged in the socio-economics and biopolitics of body enhancement issues.

Transmutation

In *De Divisione Naturae*, Johannes Scotus Eriugena[10] envisioned the universe as an "emanation" of life itself. If life is the universe, and if the whole of nature is alive, is death not just a transmutation of matter, thereby affirming that nothing is dead or inanimate? If the universe is infinite and eternal, if all of nature is based on interactions between atoms in perpetual movement, then it seems all elements within nature are in motion, including life and death. These issues are highly consequential to life expansion because the biotechnogenesis of life expansion media will, inevitably, address the dialectics of life and death. As human–computer interface, virtuality, bioarts, synthetic life, and other means begin to link to extending life over time and onto/into nonbiological platforms, the issue of transmutation of matter will need to be further developed, debated, and articulated, especially in theoretical and practice-based models. One such model is "Platform Diverse Body" (a system autonomous self) (Figure 7.1). This conceptual design referred to as a new human genre is based on a scientific study of potential of emerging and speculative technologies.[11]

Dialectics of Desirability and Viability

The dialectic between the desire for life expansion and the viability of enhancement technology is often approached in relation to the research climate, costs of technological developments, the ethical issues, and legal ramifications – in other words, the environment in which the

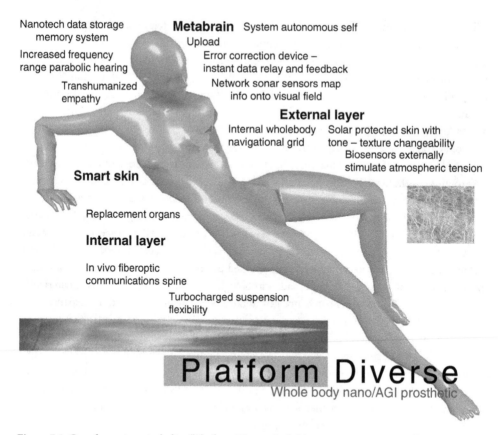

Nanotech data storage
memory system

Increased frequency
range parabolic hearing

Transhumanized
empathy

Metabrain System autonomous self
Upload
Error correction device –
instant data relay and feedback
Network sonar sensors map
info onto visual field

External layer
Internal wholebody   Solar protected skin with
navigational grid   tone – texture changeability
                           Biosensors externally
                           stimulate atmospheric tension

Smart skin

Replacement organs

Internal layer

In vivo fiberoptic
communications spine

Turbocharged suspension
flexibility

Platform Diverse
Whole body nano/AGI prosthetic

Figure 7.1 Complex systems including "Platform Diverse Body" (a system autonomous self) by Natasha Vita-More, 1977; "Primo Posthuman," revised 2011.

technology is lodged. It is necessary for objectivity that the dialectics include both the desire for technological advancements[12] and a realistic overview of enhancement technologies,[13] as sought by the proponents of enhancement technologies and those who might be adverse to the proposition.

How is the desire to expand life technologically viable? At one end of the spectrum is caution, where rational concerns reside, but there is also unreasonable resistance, religious dogmatism, and science fiction's exploitative exaggerations. At the other end of the spectrum is creativity where innovation and a growing degree of enthusiasm persist, but there are also broad claims and absurd propositions. Where is the balance? Without a doubt, "we need to guide ourselves … in all our assembled forms and multiple selves right between the two towers of promise and danger, of desire and technology" (Stone 2001: 183).

"In the arts, the desire to find new things to say and new ways of saying them is the source of all life and interest" (Wiener 1949: 134). But, as Wiener duly notes, this is often derailed in the "arid correctness and limitation to scope" (1954: 134–135). Life expansion is indeed based on a particular desire – that of extending life and expanding personal identity beyond the current biological lifespan. Notably, Wiener recognized a desire to "find new things to say and new ways of saying them" as the "source of life and interest" (1954: 134), with which this study wholeheartedly agrees, and with the observation of Stone that "we need to guide ourselves" in what can be looked at as the desirability and viability of technology than might alter our biological bodies.

Cybernetics

The province of life expansion can be seen as having emerged from cybernetics, and most directly from n-order cybernetics. It is here where concepts of the human and machine integrate[14] and the computer interacts with human biology. Homeostasis[15] most directly reflects the cybernetic idea of control and feedback. Our attempt to obtain control over physiological abilities, psychological attributes, and the extension of life is homeostasis. The "[o]rganism is opposed to chaos, to disintegration, to death, as message is to noise" (Wiener 1954: 95). It is apropos that Wiener's theory of messages ultimately relates to the entropy of life and the transhumanist, extropic aim to extend it.

Like the explorer's stick, "[t]he chisel in a sculptor's hand can be regarded ... as a part of the complex biophysical mechanism that is shaping the marble ..." (Ashby 1954: 39–40). Humans and machines have furthered their relationship through the interdependent and varied branches of science and technology. This union forms a province for human-directed enhancement, sustainability, and evolution. The single most essential resource of being human is giving and maintaining life. Without giving and maintaining life, the species could not exist. The course of existence of a human involves its organic, biological orientation and behavioral expression. It is personal continuity[16] in relation to the length of time a person is alive and diversifying the matter in which a person exists that forms the primary basis of life expansion. The medium – how it might come about – is secondary, but certainly consequential.

Human-machine Interfaces and the Prosthetic Body

Human-machine interfaces directly link to cybernetics but were not born out of cybernetics. Instead, they were a concept envisioned by Julien Offray de La Mettrie, who penned *L'Homme machine* (*Machine Man*) (La Mettrie 1996 [1747]). La Mettrie wrote *Machine Man* for two reasons: (1) to offer an alternative to the view of Cartesian thought, and (2) to "expound a materialistic philosophy" (La Mettrie 1996 [1747]: xix). By contrasting the moral religious ideals of the eighteenth century, including the attention given to Descartes and dualism, La Mettrie was criticized by many of his peers as someone who wrote for the elite with little consideration for the needs of society (La Mettrie 1996 [1747]: x). Of interest to this essay is that La Mettrie emphasized the most significant characteristic of the human as that of his [or her] "organization" (Wellman 1992: 201), a quantifiable distinction between human and other animals.[17] Perhaps this "organization" links La Mettrie's view of a machine human with human-machine interface. If organization is what distances the human from other animals, then it can also be also be understood that organization is what separates a human from a machine. The close proximity of humans and other animals, according to La Mettrie is not only viable, its proposition places man *near* to rather than *above* other animals (Wellman 1992: 201). Likewise, the close proximity of the human and the machine elicits an understanding that both have organization, but the machine, especially the computer, can be seen as more apt at organizational quantitative infor-mation-gathering than the human. However, as Wellman notes:

> the analogy of the robot or even the computer, frequently associated with La Mettrie's *L'Homme machine*, is quite foreign to the spirit of the text itself. In sum, the evolution of the concept of man-machine may be a better way to assess La Mettrie's subsequent influence than to discuss his text itself. (Wellman 1992: 172)

Rather than focusing on which one is more apt in its organizational performance, the human coalescence with the machine is increasing. If the relationship furthers adjunct appendages, then the human-machine interface is at the core of human homeostasis.[18]

> I'm titanium, carbon, silicon, a bunch of nuts and bolts … [m]y limbs that I wear have 12 computers, five sensors and muscle-like actuator systems that able me to move throughout my day. (Herr 2011)

> [w]hat really matters might be just the fluidity of the human-machine integration and the resulting transformation of human capacities, projects and lifestyles. (Clark 2004: 24)

Significantly, "the process for fitting, tailoring, and factoring in leads to the creation of extended computational and mental organizations: reasoning and thinking systems distributed across the brain, body, and world" (Clark 2004: 32–33). By this, one can combine the La Mettrie machine man as being the necessary and consequential organization of the human, which is furthered by the extended organization of computation-biology (or vice versa: biology-computation as in human-machine) as a means to distribute thinking processes as a type of appendage of the brain, and perhaps a quintessential "you."

Could there be a prosthetic you? (See Figure 7.2.) Perhaps the avatar is a prosthetic agent, just as an upload might be thought of as a prosthetic agency. The point being that the prosthetic is no longer merely a "replacement of a missing part of the body with an artificial one" (Willis 1995: 218). Its structure – its robotic electronics, AI-generated programming, lightweight silicone, titanium, alu-minum, plastics, and carbon-fiber composites, and aesthetic streamline design – and its future varied formations of bodies and other platforms for existence – have already altered the realm of "normal."

Life Expansion

The universe is in constant flux, changing its physical and spatial composition of matter and energy but never truly dying. For humans, biology has a time frame and even though we are elements of the universe and its many transformations, and molecules never really die, our memory of the past, experience in the present, and projection of the future, suggest that we are an agent with sentience that is fully aware of its pending morality.

Nikolai Fedorovich Fedorov (1827–1903), in his plight for the end of dying for humankind in the late nineteenth century, claimed that the dead are atoms vibrating in their graves. He asserted that the common task of humanity was not only to unite to prevent death, as an everlasting enemy, but to resurrect the dead. Fedorov's proposed universal project was to "regulate the forces of nature, to defeat death and bring ancestors back to life" (Koutaissoff 1990: 11). The pas-sion of Fedorov may have sprung from his Christian faith, or may have been an instinctive or fictional vision of the future – a Promethean utopia. Fedorov asked "What is man created for?"

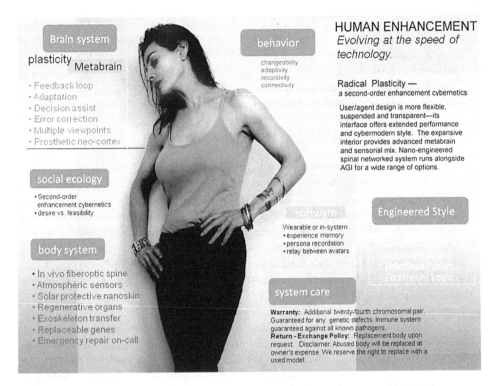

Figure 7.2 "System Autonomous Self" (for upload and whole body prosthetic avatar) by Natasha Vita-More (2010).

in the posthumous book of his writings *What Was Man Created For? The Philosophy of the Common Task*, a salvo that continues today deep in the minds of agents with sentience who are faced with the realization that they may be able to do something about it, and in doing so confront the difficult problems that are yet to be solved.

Chemistry and physics, according to Jean Finot (1856–1922), along with reducing a living organism to its most basic elements or molecules, are the basis of life, and in order to prolong life science needs to engineer life. Finot surmised that the "fabrication of living matter" (Finot 2009 [1923]: 277) would be the creative endeavor of man's sculpting of sentient beings.

"Why has evolution crafted a sentient species? Why did our consciousness, our realization of our very existence, evolve? What purpose does it serve?" Niles Eldredge asks in the forward to *What is Life?* (Margulis and Sagan 2000: xi). Human life is just one species in tens of millions that current inhabit Earth. Life is "matter which, like crystal – a strange 'aeriodic crystal' – repeats its structure as it grows" (2000: 1). Yet Margulis and Sagan pause to consider Schrödinger's view of the world – that structures differ and that repetitious, periodic patterns exemplify not a dull repetition but an "elaborate, coherent, meaningful design" (Schrödinger and Penrose 1992: 5).

Life is a "controlled, artistic chaos, a set of chemical reactions so staggeringly complex that more than eighty million years ago it produced the mammalian brain that now, in human form, composes love letters and uses silicon computers to calculate the temperature of matter at the origins of the universe" (Margulis and Sagan 2000: 31).

Notes

1   In reference to cryonics whereby a patient is suspended in liquid nitrogen.

2   Kenneth J. Hayworth's research with connectomics (the science of mapping the brain) is one way in which life expansion media could emerge.

3   In relation to uploads, otherwise known as whole brain emulation or substrate-independent minds.

4   In relation to non-biological computational platforms.

5   In relation to Teilhard de Chardin's "noosphere" or what is suggested to be computational life of a posthuman.

6   Margulis states that "[c]hanging to stay the same is the essence of autopoiesis. It applies to the biosphere as well as the cell. Applied to species, it leads to evolution" (Margulis and Sagan 2000: 31). To contextualize this statement, Margulis mentions de Kooning's reflections on abstract expressionism and that "If you write down a sentence and you don't like it, but that's what you wanted to say, you say it again in another way. … You have to change to stay the same" (Willem de Kooning, cited in Marshall and Mapplethorpe 1986). The continuous analysis and reanalysis of what is life and living in philosophy and science has evolved over time, change and change again.

7   Symbiogenesis is a term coined by the Russian biologist Merezhkovsky and developed by others such as Kozo-Poliansky (see Khakhina 1979).

8   Margulis references Ivan Wallin's seminal work in developing the theory of "symbionticism" also referred to as "the formation of microsymbiotic complexes" as a process by which new species form (he meant new species form by the permanent acquisition of symbiotic bacteria) (Margulis and Sagan 2000: 133). Wallin's theory is concretized in his book *Symbionticism and the Origin of the Species* (Wallin 1927).

9   Although I suggest the term "biotechnogenesis" for the process by which biology and technology synthesize in producing an origin by which new transmutations might emerge, Keith Ansell-Pearson refers to the phrase "bio-technogenesis" in relation to the "collapsing of bios and technos into each other" as "politically naïve" and what he calls a "spurious claim that with the coming of computers and the arrival of robot intelligence the planet is now entering a 'silicon age.'" Notably, Ansell-Pearson has a good point because if this statement were a standalone, it in itself would be luddite, but Ansell-Pearson shows a clear understanding of the influence of Margulis and, as he writes: "the fact that metallurgy has an ancient pre-human history, with human metalworking following the bacterial use of magnetite for internal compasses by almost three thousand million years (Margulis and Sagan 1995: 194)" (Ansell-Pearson 1997: 182) Of note in this thesis is the angst noted by not just Ansell-Pearson, but through his book *Deleuze and Philosophy: The Difference Engineer*, that when it comes to life and extending life, morphing life, and the symbiotechno-genesis, a certain disdain is present.

10   As a note of reference, *De Divisione Naturae* is interpreted as "The division of nature" and Johannes Scotus Eriugena, a ninth-century theologian, is often referred to as John Erigena. Erigena read *De Anima*, and was influenced enough to contemplate issues on "being" and "non-being." Although this essay is not influenced by any one religion regarding the philosophical issues of life and death, it does interpret early writings concerning life and being as philosophical, and even ideological, rather than theological. The proposition of Erigena concerning being and non-being is significant in this study because the four classes of nature, as described by Erigena, concern that which creates and that which is created, and its converse. Because this thesis suggests human enhancement and the explicit pursuit of life expansion stems from cybernetics, and especially second-order cybernetics, and the cyborg has a relationship with the transhuman, what is being and nonbeing and what creates and is created is significant from a philosophical perspective.

11   This project resulted through the collaborative advice of Drs. Robert Freitas, Michael Rose, Greg Fahy, Marvin Minsky, Roy Walford, Max More, Robin Hanson, Vernor Vinge, Hans Moravec, and Gregory Benford.

12   In this essay, the desire for technological enhancement relates to proponents of human enhancement, which include those who seek to resolve physical damage due to injury and disease (therapeutic

enhancement) and those who seek to append human physiological and cognitive abilities (what this study refers to as alternative enhancement), including extending the human lifespan and expanding agency onto semi- and non-biological platforms and/or substrates.

13   Human enhancement technologies include genetic engineering, nanomedicine, and artificial intelligence, what this study refers to as the "biotechnogenesis."

14   In the last chapter of *The Human Use of Human Beings*, Wiener discusses "semi-medical purposes for the prosthesis and replacement of human functions which have been lost or weakened" in certain people (Wiener 1949: 163).

   This integration is recognized through the notion of "feedback", electronic "turtles," and "learning machines."

15   Homeostasis originated from the term *milieu intérieur* or interior milieu, from the French (the environment within), coined by Claude Bernard to refer to the extra-cellular fluid environment, and its physiological capacity to ensure protective stability for the tissues and organs of multicellular living organisms. "The fixity of the milieu supposes a perfection of the organism such that the external variations are at each instant compensated for and equilibrated. … All of the vital mechanisms, however varied, they may be, have always one goal, to maintain the uniformity of the conditions of life in the internal environment. … The stability of the internal environment is the condition for the free and independent life" (Bernard 1974). One issue that this essay disputes is the notion of "perfection," which is often misconstrued to imply that pursuing human enhancement is synonymous with a modernist attempt to seek perfection. For the transhumanist, a post-postmodernist view is more fitting in pursuing betterment, which stems from a combined perspective of scientific realism and radical constructivism and as such pertains to the issues of efficacy of human enhancement and obtainable betterment, rather than perfection.

16   Personal continuity here refers to personhood as a diachronic process, of continuing and changing over time (Parfit 1982; More 1995).

17   Of note is La Mettrie's disparaging of Descartes, who he proposed was a "closet atheist and materialist" (Wellman 1992: 229). It is unknown whether there is reliable evidence to support this conjecture.

18   Homeostasis is the "tendency of a system, especially the physiological system of higher animals, to maintain internal stability, owing to the coordinated response of its parts to any situation or stimulus that would tend to disturb its normal condition or function." In relation to the human and homeostasis as comparable to mechanical automata, Wiener notes: "These mechanisms [internal biological processes] constitute what is known as homeostasis, and are negative feedback mechanisms of a type that we find exemplified in mechanical automata" (Wiener 1949: 96).

References

Alberts B., Johnson A., Lewis J., et al. (2002) *Molecular Biology of the Cell*, 4th edn. New York: Garland Science, pp. 134–135. http://www.ncbi.nlm.nih.gov/books/NBK26873/ (accessed October 2, 2011).

Ansell-Pearson, Keith (1997) *Deleuze and Philosophy: The Difference Engineer*. New York: Routledge.

Aristotle (1930). *De anima* (ca. 350 B.C.), trans. J.A. Smith. In *The Works of Aristotle*, ed. W.D. Ross, vol. 3. Oxford: Clarendon Press.

Ashby, William Ross (1954) *Design for a Brain*. New York: John Wiley & Sons, Inc.

Ashby, William Ross (1956) "Cybernetics and Requisite Variety." In *An Introduction to Cybernetics*. http://www.panarchy.org/ashby/variety.1956.html.

Bernard, C. (1974) *Lectures on the Phenomena Common to Animals and Plants*, trans. H.E. Hoff, R. Guillemin, and L. Guillemin. Springfield, IL: Charles C. Thomas.

Clark (2003) *Natural-Born Cyborgs: Minds, Technologies, and the Future of Human Intelligence*. Oxford: Oxford University Press.

Darwin, Charles (1859) *On the Origin of Species by Means of Natural Selection*. http://darwin-online.org.uk/EditorialIntroductions/Freeman_OntheOriginofSpecies.html.

Fedorov, N.F. (1990 [1881]) *What Was Man Created For?* New York: Hyperion Books. http://www.regels. org/N-Fedorov-1.htm.

Finot, Jean (2009 [1923]) *The Philosophy of Long Life,* trans. Harry Roberts. Whitefish, MT: Kissinger Publishing, LLC. Originally published London: John Lane, The Bodley Head (1909).

Goetz, Stewart and Taliaferro, Charles (2011) *A Brief History of the Soul.* Malden, MA: Wiley-Blackwell.

Herr (2011) http://www.npr.org/2011/08/10/137552538/the-double-amputee-who-designs-better-limbs (accessed August 30, 2011).

Jacobstein, Neil. See http://thenanoage.com/molecular-manufacturing.htm. (accessed August 10, 2011).

Khakhina, Liya N. (1979) *Concepts of Symbiogenesis.* USSR: Akademie NAUK.

Koutaissoff, Elisabeth (1990), "Introduction." In *What Was Man Created For?* New York: Hyperion Books.

La Mettrie, Julien Offray de (1996 [1747]) *Man a Machine and Man a Plant,* ed. and trans. Ann Thomson. New York: Cambridge University Press.

Margulis, L. and Sagan, D. (2000) *What is Life?* Berkeley: University of California Press.

Marshall, Richard and Mapplethorpe, Robert (1986) *Fifty New York Artists.* San Francisco: Chronicle Books.

More, Max (1995) *The Diachronic Self: Identity, Continuity, Transformation.* http://www.maxmore. com/disscont.htm.

National Public Radio® (2011) Terry Gross Host. Interview with Herr, Hugh. "The Double Amputee Who Designs Better Limbs." (Audio recording August 10). NPR Arts & Life, Books. http://www.npr.org/ 2011/08/10/137552538/the-double-amputee-who-designs-better-limbs?ft=1&f=1032&sc=tw&utm_ source=twitterfeed&utm_medium= twitter (accessed October 13, 2011).

Parfit, Derek. (1982) *Reasons and Persons.* New York: Oxford University Press.

Ross, M.A. (1931) *The Works of Aristotle Translated into English under the Editorship of W.D. Ross.* "De Anima," trans. J.A. Smith. Oxford: Clarendon Press. http://etext.virginia.edu/etcbin/toccer-new2?id=AriSoul. xml&images=images/modeng&data=/texts/english/modeng/parsed&tag=public&part=2&division=div2 (accessed September 27, 2011).

Schrödinger, Erwin and Penrose, Roger (1992) *What is Life? With "Mind and Matter" and "Autobiographical Sketches".* Cambridge: Cambridge University Press.

Stone, Allucquère Rosanne (2001) *The War of Desire and Technology at the Close of the Mechanical Age.* Cambridge, MA: MIT Press.

Thacker, Eugene (2010) *After Life.* Chicago: University of Chicago Press.

Thomas, Dylan (1951) "Do not go gentle into that good night." http://www.bbc.co.uk/wales/arts/sites/ dylan-thomas/pages/do-not-go-gentle.shtml.

Thomas, Dylan (1971) *Collected Poems of Dylan Thomas 1934–1952.* New York: W.W. Norton.

Wallin, Ivan (1927) *Symbionticism and the Origin of Species.* London: Baillière, Tindall & Cox.

Wellman, Kathleen. (1992) *La Mettrie: Medicine, Philosophy, and Enlightenment.* Durham, NC: Duke University Press.

Wiener, Norbert. (1954) *The Human Use of Human Beings: Cybernetics.* New York: Da Capo Press.

Willis, David (1995) *Prosthesis.* Stanford, CA: Stanford University Press.

Further Reading

Carabine, Deirdre (2000) *John Scottus Eriugena.* Oxford: Oxford University Press.

Cecconi, F., Alvarez-Bolado, G., Meyer, B., Roth, K., and Gruss, P. (1998) "Apaf1 (CED-4 Homolog) Regulates Programmed Cell Death in Mammalian Development." *Cell* 94 (September 18), pp. 727–737. Published 5-10092. Göttingen: Max Planck Institute for Biophysical Chemistry.

Conway, Flo and Siegelman, Jim (2005) *Dark Hero of the Information Age: In Search of Norbert Wiener, the Father of Cybernetics.* New York: Basic Books.

8

The Hybronaut Affair
A Ménage of Art, Technology, and Science

Laura Beloff

Techno-Organic Environment

Alfons Schilling began his long-term investigations on perception during the early 1960s by designing motion paintings,[1] and continued the research with design of optical instruments called Vision Machines.[2] Schilling's experiments were constructed as head-worn objects, or instruments, in various shapes and sizes, which transformed the viewer's perception through first-hand experience. Schilling's aim was to see something that no one had never seen before; he believed that new perceptions and realities could be revealed by a modified and extended perception (Schilling 1975; Reder 1987). The heavy construction of Schilling's optical vision machines hindered the mobility of the user; nevertheless, they created an impressive visual effect produced by the optical manipulation of the user's perception. His art enwrapped the user's whole body in perception of their surroundings. "Similar to experimental enquiries in scientific laboratories Schilling's vision machines create artificial perceptual disturbances in the viewer's visual-motoric realm" (Schuler 2009). However, even if Schilling was aware of the scientific research on perception of the time, he did not rely on the rigor of formally conducted scientific research or its legitimated devices. Instead, he constructed his own instruments for the phenomenological exploration of perception within the realm of the arts.

The experimental Seeing Machines by Alfons Schilling can be seen as an example of the *alterity relation*,[3] in which technology is seen as a focal other and with which humans might and do interact. Everyday life events of this relation are, for example, taking money out of an ATM machine and the ensuing relationship between the human and the "other" money-giving counterpart, or in virtual reality where humans relate to a simulated world not as a machine world, but as a anthropomorphized other world (Ihde 1990; Jørgenssen 2003; Verbeek 2008). To make a distinction here, in Schilling's case the aim is to experience or see the unusual – or something

The Transhumanist Reader: Classical and Contemporary Essays on the Science, Technology, and Philosophy of the Human Future, First Edition. Edited by Max More and Natasha Vita-More.
© 2013 John Wiley & Sons, Inc. Published 2013 by John Wiley & Sons, Inc.

different – in this relationship with technology. Schilling held the concept that parallel worlds could be revealed through this kind of optical instrument.

A recent development in wearable technology is so-called thought-control computing, in which technology is controlled by the brain waves of the user. This kind of technology can and has been used in gaming or other conscious activities, but it can also be used in an involuntary manner. For example, activity in the brain is translated to automated controls, such as the dimming or brightening of lights in an environment depending on user's alertness. In this approach technology is designed to stay in the background of the physical activities of the user. This is close to what Ihde defines as *background relation*, in which technologies are running in the background but in the foreground of our minds they create a context for our perception, e.g. various automated tasks, such as the humming sound of air conditioning (Ihde 1990; Verbeek 2008). Examples of this relation include wearable devices that stay active in the background by being "aware" of their local situation, and which may generate data even without the user's actions. Therefore, through continuous background activity, a device creates a contextual technological environment for the user.

The 2010 Winter Olympics presented an experiment of thought-control computing by Interaxon company, where a user could control the lighting of three public locations: Niagara Falls, Toronto's CN Tower, and Ottawa's parliament buildings. The wearable headset used in this installation measured the user's brain electrical output – the alpha waves associated with relaxation and the beta waves that are associated with concentration. Depending upon how users relaxed or focused their thoughts, the networked computer-controlled lighting on the defined site was changed accordingly. This experiment constructed a very intimate link between a technological environment and a user. In his definition of *background relation* Ihde considered automated technologies, such as air conditioning or automated heating, that are typically controlled externally from the user. Whereas in the case where the user's brain activity is detected and accordingly the lighting (of a room) is adjusted, technology is not only running in the background of the user's immediate physical environment but also running in the background of the user's mental activity. In some ways this scenario can be compared to involuntary bodily functions such as the heart beating or breathing with the noted difference that control is directed outside of the user's physical, mobile body. When the immediate, networked environment becomes firmly linked to a user and his biological body, the idea of borders, what is a part of a user and where his/her body ends and environment begins, start blurring.

This blurring of borders of body and technology is hybridized by the *cyborg relation*,[4] in which "the human and the technological actually merge rather than "merely" being embodied" (Verbeek 2008). Verbeek includes pacemakers, artificial valves, microchips, and antidepressants in his list of examples, which all are within a body and working in the background without our manual and conscious control of them. There is no longer a relation between human and non-human parts, but a new merged human/technology entity appears, which is then in relation to the world (Verbeek, 2008). Even if the above-mentioned brain activity detection device is currently wearable and hence easily detachable from a user's physiological body, it belongs to the same list of examples of body–technology merger. However, the difference is the creation of a connection between internal body functions and external environmental activities, instead of impacting changes internally within a user's body. Verbeek writes: "Technologies used, like telescopes and hearing aids, help to constitute us as different human beings, whereas technologies incorporated constitute a new hybrid being" (Verbeek 2008). In *cyborg relation* human and technology have become a single experiencing entity.

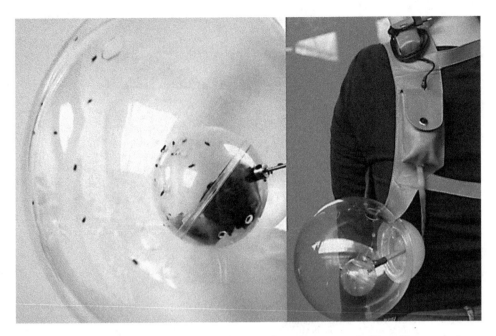

Figure 8.1   "Fruit Fly Farm" (2006) by Beloff. The Fruit Fly Farm is a networked wearable space station designed for fruit flies and humans.

The thought-controlled computing development of wearable technology, as well as Verbeek's formulation of *cyborg relation*, points to a developing scenario where biological humans wear body-embedded and artificially grown, and possibly biosynthetically inherited, abilities to control the techno-organic environment, and in which humans are continuously connected to various human and non-human networks.

The *Umwelt* Bubble

The biologist Jakob von Uexküll's term *Umwelt* refers to a concept about the subjective world of an organism. The world can be imagined as a soap bubble, which surrounds each individual and contains signifying markers relevant only to the world of that specific creature. This soap bubble, or *Umwelt*, is actively created by the individual organism in a process of forming a perception of reality, which is guided by the organism's design, its physiology, and its needs.

According to Uexküll, the physiology and design of an organism impacts its *Umwelt*. For example, it has been proven that fighting fish do not recognize their own reflection if it is shown 18 times per second, but they do recognize their reflection if it is shown at a minimum speed of 30 times per second. This experiment shows that in the world of fighting fish, "who feed on fast-moving prey, all motor processes – as in the case of slow-motion photography – appear at reduced speed" (Uexküll 1934). The *Umwelt* of a fighting fish is based on its need to be able to capture food for its survival. Uexküll's point of view was that biology should study organisms not as objects, but as active subjects, and focus on their ability to integrate into complex environments.

According to the dictionary entry on extracellular matrix in the Biology Online resource, biologists have recently become aware of the fact that an organism's environment or substrate (e.g. extracellular matrix) can influence the behavior of cells quite markedly, possibly even more

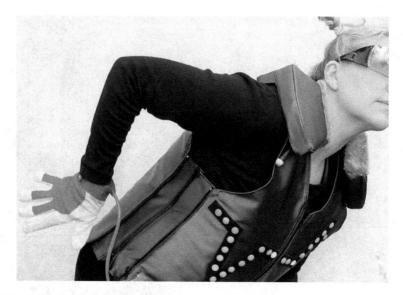

Figure 8.2   "Heart-Donor" (2007) by Beloff and Berger with Mitrunen. A vest addressing one's presence and social network in a hybrid environment.

significantly than DNA in the development of complex organisms. The removal of cells from their usual environment to another environment can have far-reaching effects. This notion, as well as Uexküll's concept of the *Umwelt*, both lay weight on the importance of the environment as a crucial factor for the development of an organism. Uexküll proposes that an organism actively creates its own environment – the *Umwelt* – and includes in it only what is necessary for its survival. In other words survival, or staying alive, in relation to an organism's environment, is the defining factor for an organism's biological and physiological design.

However, when considering humans, the idea of an organism's design for survival only holds together when biological survival is at stake. In contemporary Western societies staying alive or the basic biological survival of a human is mainly solved through man-made social infrastructures that offer the prerequisites for living. Therefore, it is no longer necessary to consider the development of a human and his physiology from a traditional perspective of survival. Biological survival concerning the human is being replaced by self-defined design of a human body, of which wearable technology is one example. The current wearable technology projects and devices can be considered as exercises that help us to adjust for future changes and possibilities concerning the human.

Network and the Hybronaut

Wearable technology is an area of experimentation with networks, spatiality, and the design of the human body, and often steered by a diversity of relations between humans and their environment. In spite of the fact that wearable technology is *wearable* and is (currently) located outside the body it nevertheless suggests a view of the body as a techno-organic entity, which is constructed from various connected parts and a multiplicity of relations. The growing number of projects from wearable computing industry and academic research in design and the arts present a trajectory of changes in cultural attitudes concerning the human, the body, identity, and its created and recreated connections to the world. In comparison to science and engineering perspectives, which often tackle single detailed problems concerning the improvement or enhancement of a human (body), many artistic experiments in the field of wearable technology often take a more holistic approach. They concentrate on experiential factors and the emergence of undefined possibilities of a human within a ménage of art, technology, and science. These artistic projects may appear to lack purposefulness or clearly defined goals; features that are often intentionally left open in them. They are more about the creation of experiments; open lab work with a possibility of revealing new insights into the issues at hand.

It has become obvious that technologically constructed networks are here to stay in one form or another. Network has become our primary connection to a temporally and spatially fragmented world and constitutes part of our personal *Umwelt*. Network and abiding connectedness is our new umbilical cord, which is pulling the information society's digital infrastructure into our physical bodies (Townsend 2001).

I have developed a concept that attempts to emphasize, cross, and further blur the borders of technology and the human. My artistic research work experiments with a networked human, whose body and environment are characteristically techno-organic. This concept developed as the techno-organic figure, what I call "the Hybronaut." The Hybronaut proposes an "action" state of a human, whose existence and identity are deeply intertwined with its networked hybrid environment. It is understood as an entity which is constructed of physical, social, technological, and other relations formed in a hybrid environment, and which suggests a perception of a human as a system that breaks away from thinking of a human as a clearly framed whole with defined borders.

The Hybronaut's living environment – hybrid environment – is a mesh of links and connections that constitute a network of relations, actions, humans, and diverse materials in a heterogeneous assembly and in which the Hybronaut is seen simultaneously as the middle from which relations expand and simultaneously, simply, as one of the nodes in a large network of connections. In other words, the Hybronaut is a figure whose existence is profoundly based on a hybrid environment and various kinds of relations formed in this environment. In this situation technology is no longer considered solely as a communication channel for taking care of tasks or delivering messages, but has become one dimension of an environment, as well as an essential element of a networked human. The Hybronaut is not an enhanced isolated body, but an entity that is in close connection with its environment.

The actual experiments are constituted in the form of wearable equipment that is offered for public testing. These wearable artworks offer a possibility of entering into the Hybronaut's perspective and experience his/her *Umwelt*. The experiments investigate what happens when network-ability is embedded in a human. How will I feel and how will I see the world around me? And what does it mean for my existence as a human?

The Hybronaut is part of a practical and critical investigation into the merger of the organic and the technological and their relation to the human and his perception of the world. In a sense the Hybronaut and the created situations can be seen as conceptual prototypes and rehearsals for possible future circumstances.

The Appendix-tail

The project Appendix (2011) by the author is a wearable, networked tail for the human body (for the Hybronaut). Conventionally, the appendix, an organ that is within the human body, has been regarded as a potentially troublesome, redundant organ without any beneficial aspects. However, currently some scientists believe that the appendix is a place for good bacteria to localize as a reserve in case of a sudden disorder caused by malevolent bacteria. This function is nevertheless still under debate, due to the fact that humans who have their appendix removed appear to carry on with life without problems.

In the core of the author's constructed Appendix-tail are the relations between body and technology and between the human and his/her surrounding environment; all elements which are increasingly based on technological, or artificially created, features and connections.

In a sense comparable to way in which the function of the inner appendix is not fully understood by science, the precisely defined functional goal of the Appendix-tail is purposely left open. Rather than aiming at being an enhanced function or ability of human, the work creates a situation, which attaches the user (the Hybronaut) to a relational network within a hybrid environment. The work presents an aesthetic experiment in which it is not known beforehand what the benefit of it is, or what kind of experience it will create. Even if the structure of the work is based on technology, it purposely lacks an instrumental use of technology as a means for achieving a predefined goal.

Parallel to its physical existence, the Appendix-tail extends the Hybronaut with an invisible "tail" of relations, which are impacting his evolving worldview and defining his identities. The Appendix-tail makes visible humans' dependency and connectedness to things, nature, people, and various systems. It presupposes that many of the connections to various human, non-human, artificial, and organic entities will be increasingly (re)constructed and modified by technology in the future.

Conclusion

In the field of wearable technology, the very basic concept of network enables an understanding of a body and a wearable device as a networked structure that contains body parts, biological functions, machine parts, and technological functions. An individual can be seen as a mesh of links criss-crossing within the body and between the body and technological devices, and further, to other bodies and the surrounding environment.

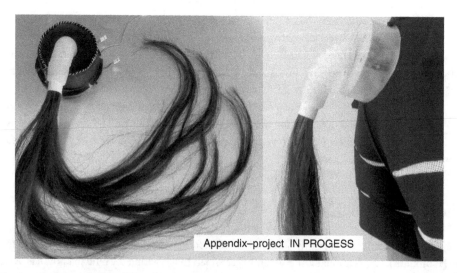

Figure 8.3 "Appendix" (2011) by Beloff. A networked tail designed for a human.

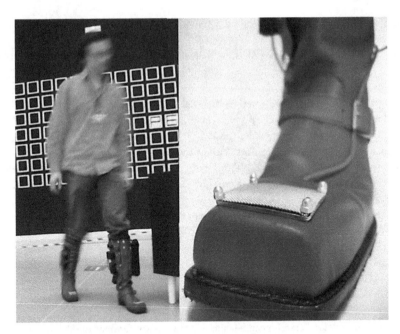

Figure 8.4 "Seven Mile Boots" (2003–2004) by Beloff–Berger–Pichlmair. Boots that enable one to walk through the Internet. With kind permission of Laura Beloff.

The author's developed concept of the Hybronaut is an instantiation of this kind of human. It is an art and research experiment, which creates situations with the help of designed equipment that can potentially reveal something new or unexpected within the experiences they offer the user. "As the tools and ideas of our art continue to evolve, so too shall we" (Vita-More 1983, 2003).

Notes

1 Schilling is considered to be one of the representatives of Action Painting. Action Painting dates to the 1940s through early 1960s and is associated with abstract expressionism, which formed a major shift in aesthetics, which cited the physicality of painting or the introduction as "art as a process" as consequential.

2 Schilling developed several large-scale, body-worn vision machines that focused on the optical-physical act of seeing and can be considered as precursors of virtual cyberspace. http://www.alfons-schilling. com/home.html (accessed October 15, 2011).

3 Alterity relation is a term coined by Don Ihde as relations and communications between human and technology that are described by the personification of the machine as an "other."

4 Cyborg relation is a term coined Peter-Paul Verbeek developed to reflect the merging of the human and technology.

References

Beloff, Laura (2009) "The Hybronaut, An Early Protonaut of the Future." In G. Beiguelman, L. Bambozzi, M. Bastos, and R. Minelli, eds., *Appropriations of the (Un)common: Public and Private Space in Times of Mobility*. Sao Paulo: Institute Sergio Motta, pp. 74–82.

Ihde, Don (1990) *Technology and the Lifeworld: From Garden to Earth.* Bloomington and Indianapolis: Indiana University Press.

Jørgenssen, Jari Friis (2003) "A Garden Meeting: Ihde and Pickering." In Don Ihde and Evan Selinger, eds., *Chasing Technoscience; Matrix for Materiality.* Bloomington and Indianapolis: Indiana University Press, p. 249.

Reder, Christian (1987) "Über Sehen sprechen: Im Dialog mit Alfons Schilling." In Peter Noever and Oswald Oberhuber, eds., *Alfons Schilling Sehmaschinen.* Vienna: Hochschule für angewandte Kunst und Österreichischen Museum für angewandte Kunst.

Schilling, Alfons (1975) *Binocularis.* New York, Vienna, and Cologne: Galerie Ariadne.

Schuler, Romana (2009) "Experimentelle Wahrnehmung in Psychologie und Kunst Von Umkehrbrillen und Sehmaschinen." In Elisabeth von Samsonov, ed., *Unzipping Philosophy.* Vienna: Passagen, pp. 46–75.

Townsend, Anthony (2001) "Mobile Communications in the 21st-Century City." In Barry Brown, ed., *The Wireless World: Social and Interactional Aspects of the Mobile Age.* Berlin: Springer.

Uexküll, Jacob von (1934) "A Stroll Through the Worlds of Animals and Men: A Picture Book of Invisible Worlds." In Claire H. Schiller, ed., *Instinctive Behavior: The Development of a Modern Concept,* New York: International Universities Press, pp. 5–76.

Verbeek, Peter-Paul (2008) "Cyborg Intentionality: Rethinking the Phenomenology of Human-Technology Relations." *Phenomenology and the Cognitive Sciences* 7, pp. 387–395.

Vita-More, Natasha (1983) "Transhuman Manifesto." http://www.transhumanist.biz/transhumanmanifesto.htm.

Vita-More, Natasha (1992, revised 2002) "Transhumanist Arts Statement." http://www.transhumanist.biz/transhumanistartsmanifesto.htm (accessed October 15, 2011).

Vita-More, Natasha (2011) "Transhuman Statement." In Alex Danchev, ed., *100 Artists' Manifestos: From the Futurists to the Stuckists.* New York: Penguin Modern Classics.

Websites

http://www.realitydisfunction.org – The author's personal website
http://www.alfons-schilling.com/home.html – Alfons Schilling's personal website
http://www.interaxon.ca – Thought-controlled computing
http://www.biology-online.org – Life science reference – Biology Online
http://www.transhumanist.biz – Transhumanist arts and culture

9

Transavatars

William Sims Bainbridge

Enhancement of human abilities can be accomplished in several ways, and need not require modification of the person's biological body. Avatars in virtual worlds are a contemporary example, and in future teleoperation of personal robots or entirely fresh alternatives may become popular. Avatars point out to us that enhancement is not merely a matter of increasing the effectiveness of a person in taking action, but also can mean an altered form of consciousness that expands opportunities for experiences, and escape from the conventional system of moral constraints. Especially noteworthy is the fact that one individual may have many different avatars, thereby becoming a *multiplex* or *protean personality*. Decades ago, psychiatrists described this as multiple personality neurosis or some form of split personality (Thigpen and Cleckley 1957; Lifton 1971), but in future we may decide that the most effective mode of being is pluralism. Buckminster Fuller (1970) used to say, "I seem to be a verb." Perhaps today we should say, "I am a plural verb in future tense."

Avatars and Simulation

Under the right conditions an avatar in a virtual world can substantially enhance the abilities of the user – the person who owns and operates it. Since ancient times, philosophers have debated the meaning of reality. Transhumanist philosophers have suggested varied viewpoints of simulation, consciousness, and existence, and notably argued whether humans could or do reside within a simulation (Moravec 1998; Bostrom 2003). Social scientists tend to be satisfied by the so-called Thomas theorem: "If men define situations as real, they are real in their consequences" (Thomas and Thomas 1929: 572). The inverse of this theorem is at least as true: Whatever has consequences is real.

The Transhumanist Reader: Classical and Contemporary Essays on the Science, Technology, and Philosophy of the Human Future, First Edition. Edited by Max More and Natasha Vita-More.
© 2013 John Wiley & Sons, Inc. Published 2013 by John Wiley & Sons, Inc.

Virtual world has become the generic term for a computer-generated environment in which humans, through its user-avatar, can act and interact, and where their actions have consequences. Some of these are marketed as massively multiplayer online games (MMOs), notably *World of Warcraft*, a gameworld with more than ten million subscribers (Bainbridge 2010a, 2010c). A few are presented as artificial environments where the user may own territory, create objects and architecture, and perform useful work. The prime current example is *Second Life*, where I have held serious panels of experts to evaluate scientific research proposals, on an "island" belonging to the National Science Foundation (Bainbridge 2007; Bohannon 2011).

In *World of Warcraft*, my avatar can ride a horse much better than I can in the "real world," and I twice swam under water there for an hour without coming up for air or needing diving equipment. In *Second Life*, my avatar has sat next to people who were thousands of miles away, and whenever I wish I can fly across my island rather than walking. These examples may be trivial, but considering my thousands of hours exploring virtual worlds, I see five main ways they can be real for transhumanists:

1. *Subjectivity.* The experience of virtually transcending my ordinary limitations "feels real" in some positive sense, for example giving pleasure, so it is valuable to me quite apart from any wider significance it might or might not have.
2. *Consequentiality.* Through my avatar, my actions in the virtual world have unusual consequences outside it, whether by influencing other people, in terms of economic resources that can be transferred across the reality boundary, or in terms of ideas and information that can be applied in other contexts.
3. *Prototype.* Whatever significance gameworlds may have today, they are early steps toward much more significant future developments, for example technology in which my avatar is a powerful robot in the material world, rather than a mere image on a computer screen.
4. *Education.* Through operating an avatar in one of the more sophisticated current gameworlds, I gain valuable skills that enhance my abilities in the material world, for example in learning how to use geographic information systems, realtime teamwork groupware systems, graphic computer programming languages, and inventory information systems.
5. *Transference.* Aspects of my identity are offloaded onto multiple avatars, including semi-autonomous agents possessing a measure of artificial intelligence, which can function as me simultaneously, when I am not currently logged into a computer, and even after my death.

The fifth of these is clearly the most radical, yet the first syllable of *transference* suggests some connection to transhumanism, and to transcendence, thus evoking the word *transavatar*. Before considering the more controversial implications, it is necessary to survey some of the variations in how people currently employ avatars, using two of the well-established gameworlds, *Star Wars Galaxies* and *EverQuest II*. These were both hosted by Sony Online Entertainment, a company with an admirable reputation for cooperating with academic scientists, for example in giving a major research team access to primary *EverQuest II* data (Williams et al. 2011). The following section is more modest, based on my own ethnographic observation in the two gameworlds, and on manual tabulation of two kinds of quantitative data gained without any special cooperation from Sony.

Avatar Censuses

Among well-established MMOs, perhaps the most intellectually accessible one with special relevance to transhumanism is *Star Wars Galaxies* (SWG), which launched on June 26, 2003, and was closed down after eight successful years on December 15, 2011 (Ducheneaut and Moore 2004; Bainbridge 2011). The setting was a dozen planets, at the point in history just hours after the destruction of the Death Star in the original 1977 *Star Wars* movie. While SWG offered many conventional game quests, plus battles between players representing the Galactic Empire or the Rebel Alliance, it is remarkable for having devoted much of its energy to living in virtual worlds, where players would not only have their own homes and businesses, but build their own cities. Especially relevant for transhumanists was the fact that Jedi are depicted in the *Star Wars* mythos as having a commitment to ethics and justice, opposing negation of human potential, and possessing innate biological attributes, enhanced by intensive training. When SWG launched in 2003, only after extreme achievement could a player earn the right to have a Jedi avatar, and they were forced to begin as ordinary citizens of the galaxy, but a major redesign in 2005 allowed even lazy players to operate Jedi avatars (McCubbin 2005; McCubbin et al. 2005).

A perspective on the options available to players in creating and developing an avatar can be gained from a census of 532 avatars in the FarStar galaxy during the early part of July 2011. At that time, there were 13 SWG Internet servers, or *galaxies* as they were called, and FarStar was the more popular of the two for European users. To get the data, I created an avatar in FarStar, then at 10 separate points in time when there were many people online, I used the in-game system for assembling teams to catalog their avatars.

When creating an SWG avatar, selection of race and gender is permanent. The player also selects the class or profession (such as Jedi or bounty hunter), but this can be changed later, albeit at some cost, and after playing several hours most avatars become allied with either the Empire or the Rebels. Researchers in the field debate whether any significant fraction of MMO players experiment with gender switching (Huh and Williams 2010), and I can speak from my own experience that having run something close to 75 avatars I naturally give the new ones characteristics very different from my own, without worrying about what that says about me. I had four main SWG avatars, each of which reached the maximum experience level of 90; three were female and one of those was a huge, hairy Wookiee, fit to be the bride of Chewbacca, the Wookiee in the movies. Just 149 of the 532 FarStar avatars (28 percent) were female.

Including Humans and Wookiees, there were 10 races, all humanoid in form but having evolved separately on their own planets. Fully 282 (53.2 percent) of the avatars were Human and only 17 (3.2 percent) were Wookiees. Second most popular, with 93 (17.5 percent), were Zabraks, fierce, horned, carnivorous humanoids who look like devils and were represented by Darth Maul, the formidable villain of *The Phantom Menace*, first of the prequel movies (Reaves 2001). Third most popular with 59 (11.1 percent) were the Twi-leks, clever aliens whose brains have tails, represented by Jabba's administrative assistant Bib Fortuna and by a seductive dancing girl named Oola in *Return of the Jedi*, both of which could be found near Jabba in SWG. Thus, the two most popular alternatives to Humans represented intensification of two very different human qualities: obsessive ferocity and artful calculation.

For present purposes, it is especially interesting to look at the professions chosen by players for their avatars, because they reflect players' wishes to have abilities and accomplish goals rather different from those available in everyday life. Table 9.1 shows some statistics about the nine

Table 9.1   The ten classes of avatar in *Star Wars Galaxies*.

Profession	Cases	Female	Human	Zabrak	Twi-lek
Combat-oriented:					
Bounty Hunter	56	20%	54%	23%	5%
Commando	69	13%	67%	12%	4%
Jedi	140	21%	51%	28%	10%
Medic	37	39%	46%	14%	11%
Officer	39	13%	67%	5%	10%
Smuggler	16	19%	50%	19%	6%
Spy	20	20%	45%	35%	0%
Non-combat:					
Entertainer	70	63%	39%	14%	27%
Trader	85	34%	56%	7%	12%

primary professions, and we immediately see that the most popular profession is Jedi, with 26.3 percent of the avatars.

The gender differences across the nine professions help us understand their meanings, because female avatars have no practical disadvantage in any of them, so what we see is gender preferences and stereotypes. Entertainers dance and play musical instruments in cantinas, at least one of which is located in every town on every planet, and other avatars gain strength for their coming battles by watching their performances. We see that 63 percent of entertainers are female, as are 39 percent of medics. Medics can also give strength to warriors, but more often do so on the battlefield. Both are support jobs, and across many MMOs female avatars tend to be more numerous in such nurturant roles. Traders mine resources from the environment and then construct things they can sell to others, including droids (robots), vehicles, munitions, furniture, and architecture. Although Medics are listed among the combat professions, and they can employ biological weapons in combat, none of the three with the highest female percentages require violent behavior. The two professions with the lowest percentages female, commando and officer at 13 percent female, are most similar to combat ranks in the army.

The two professions with the highest percentage Human among its avatars, commando and officer both at 67 percent, are the two least imaginative. Zabraks like Darth Maul are violent but control their violence under great skill, and would make good bounty hunters or spies. Humans are always a plurality, but weakest among entertainers, where Twi-leks are at their peak, suggesting that this is a creative, non-violent profession that places a priority on exoticism.

A very different MMO in which to explore personal enhancement is *EverQuest II*. On October 7, 2011, the EverQuest II community website leaderboards listed 15 guilds which had at least 1,000 avatar members each, for a total of 22,237 avatars. The leaderboard also tabulated how many players had avatars in each guild. There are two different ways to calculate an average, summing across guilds before producing a ratio or calculating a ratio for each guild and then averaging them, but the results were quite similar. The average player in a large guild had 2.03 or 2.12 avatars in it.

To get a fuller picture of how avatars varied, I manually downloaded descriptions of 3,676 belonging to the largest EQII guild, Blackhawks on the Antonia Bayle server. The EQII database connects the avatars belonging to each player, so we can determine that these 3,676 avatars represent 1,782 people, for an average of 2.06 guild-member avatars per player. Often, players have additional avatars, some on other servers, some belonging to other guilds, and some lacking guild membership. Because the immediate focus here will be on how multiple avatars increase the range of roles a person can play in cooperation with other people, the analysis will concern the division of labor among the Blackhawks members.

EverQuest II has a very complex system of avatar classes and subclasses, each customizing the avatar with different abilities, but primarily there are four categories. The game's instruction manual describes them thus (with the numbers of cases in parentheses):

> *Fighters* enjoy the thick of the fray, often absorbing the brunt of attacks while taking the battle to the enemy directly. Fighters can wear a variety of armor, and employ a host of weapons and combat arts to defeat enemies. (1,145 cases = 31.1%)
>
> Wise and steadfast, *Priests* use spells and blessings to strengthen their comrades. They are able to heal wounds, bolster defenses, and even return life to fallen friends, while still being able to hold their own on the field of battle. (802 cases = 21.8%)
>
> Intelligent and dexterous, *Mages* wield spells as their primary offense and defense. Mages are not suited for melee combat. Instead, they use their magic to bolster the power of their comrades and devastate enemies from the rear ranks. (1,005 cases = 27.3%)
>
> Stealth and speed are the hallmarks of *Scouts*, and they employ them to sneak up on their enemies to take them out quickly. Though agile, sharp-witted, and skilled in a variety of combat types, Scouts are not well-suited to the harsh, blow-by-blow of a frontal assault. (724 cases = 19.7%)

Note that these four describe not only sets of abilities, but personality types. Each is an ideal type of person, who may be very different from the real-life persona of the player. The first three fit the three standard roles in MMOs: (1) *tanks* who are heavily armored and engage the enemy in melee combat, (2) *healers* who stand back and provide assistance to the tank when he is wounded, and (3) *DPS* (damage per second) bowmen, marksmen, or mages who stand back and do damage to the enemy from a distance while letting the tank monopolize the enemy's attention. The scout role is less standard, but comparable to rogues in *World of Warcraft*, possibly better for solo play.

Table 9.2 examines the 786 different players who had at least two avatars in Blackhawks, focusing on the two highest-level avatars, breaking ties by use of random numbers. Of these 786, 335 had 2 avatars, 182 had 3, 105 had 4, 72 had 5, and 92 had more than 5 avatars in the guild. In the special language of game players, the avatar in which the player invests most time is a *main*, and another avatar is an *alt* (alternate). The table is organized in terms of the class of a player's main, and the main tends to be about 20 experience levels more advanced than the alt.

For three of the classes – fighter, mage, and scout – players are less likely to pick the same class for the alt as they did for the main, but this is not true for priests. Players whose mains are mages and scouts are slightly more likely to pick a fighter for the alt than players whose mains are priests. Mages and priests both wield supernatural powers, which some players may love, thus explaining why mage mains are often accompanied by priest alts. Given that each class has six sub-sub specialties, even when the main and alt are the same class, they may be significantly different. For example, among mages, both conjurors and necromancers operate magical assistants, but the conjuror can call for help upon the four elements (earth, air, fire, water), while the necromancer reanimates corpses. Thus, the table only hints at the diversity of avatars.

There are three "race" factions in *EverQuest II* – Good, Evil, and Neutral – and players with priest mains are more likely to select Good. In *World of Warcraft*, we know that priests are much

Table 9.2 Two highest guild avatars for 786 *EverQuest II* players.

| | Class of Main Avatar | | | |
	Fighter	Mage	Priest	Scout
Main Avatar cases	261	232	164	129
Main Avatar percent of 786	33.2%	29.5%	20.9%	16.4%
Mean Experience Level of Main	52.2	57.9	58.5	60.0
Mean Experience Level of Alt	32.2	37.4	36.9	41.8
Alt is a Fighter	21.8%	34.5%	29.8%	45.0%
Alt is a Mage	33.7%	19.0%	28.7%	28.7%
Alt is a Priest	20.3%	31.0%	22.0%	14.7%
Alt is a Scout	24.1%	15.1%	19.5%	11.6%
Main is in Good Faction	16.5%	20.3%	43.9%	28.7%
Main is in Evil Faction	32.6%	36.2%	27.4%	18.6%
Alt is in Same Faction as Main	42.1%	44.0%	44.5%	42.6%
Main Has Craft Specialization	75.1%	70.3%	80.5%	69.0%
Alt Has Craft Specialization	67.8%	74.4%	58.5%	50.4%

Created by the author.

more likely than avatars of other classes to be female, and whatever the biological gender of the player, the healing role of a priest implies a different player personality on average. Quite apart from the other decisions, any avatar can learn one of many mutually exclusive craft specializations, such as carpenter or alchemist, but self-sufficient players tend to select crafts that support their avatar's call. For example, fighters are more likely to have the armorer skill so they can make their own armor for tanking. However, members of guilds often select crafts that are needed by their friends' avatars rather than by their own avatars. This table demonstrates the key point that players do seek diversity, but decisions in creating multiple avatars are shaped by multiple factors. For my general research on MMOs, I suggest there are at least the following six considerations.

1. *Division of labor.* Two avatars of different *classes* have a greater range of abilities than either one of them, so players often have more than one in order to perform different practical functions at different times. Among other uses, this gives a player the opportunity to join temporary teams that need different specialties. For example, a player may have two avatars, one a tank and the other a healer, logging into one or the other depending upon the momentary needs of a team that is in the process of assembling. Even without other players, division of labor can be an important motivation for having two avatars.

2. *Diversity of experience.* Avatars of different *races* often enter the virtual world in different geographic regions, experiencing a different set of initial conditions and completing different missions. Different *classes* experience even the same quest and territory in a different way. Game designers encourage this diversity of experiences, because they want players to persist in subscribing to the gameworld, effectively combining many games into one to accomplish this commercial goal. Very popular games like *World of Warcraft* run many *instances* of the game simultaneously, on different servers, which may be fundamentally different in their rules, as well as being inhabited by different players who give each a distinct

quality. As of September 28, 2011, *World of Warcraft* had 241 of these realms for primarily North American users, and 23 of them officially encourage role-playing as if one really were one's avatar. Of the 218 ordinary WoW realms, fully 103 had rule sets that encouraged player-versus-player combat by allowing one character to attack another without permission in most geographic areas, and the same was true for six of the role-playing realms. Notably, FarStar and Starsider in SWG are inhabited primarily by players who live on different continents.

3. *Multiple affiliations.* Most gameworlds incorporate sophisticated groupware systems not only to allow temporary teams to cooperate, but also to support long-term guilds or similar groups, many of which survive for years. With few exceptions, notably *A Tale in the Desert*, it is impossible for an avatar to belong to more than one guild, so a player who has friends in two guilds will need at least two avatars. Like many other gameworlds, *World of Warcraft* divides avatars into competing factions, usually two, but three factions in the case of *Dark Age of Camelot*. To study WoW adequately, I needed to have avatars in both factions, the Horde and the Alliance. The cultures and virtual territories of the two factions are quite different, but being in both also allows one to experience their conflict from both perspectives.

4. *Achievement of perfection.* It is said that practice makes perfect, but online gameworlds have a second way through which players may develop superior avatars, namely using resources obtained elsewhere to give a low-level avatar the highest-quality gear, which usually consists of armor, weapons, and consumable resources like magic potions. In most gameworlds, high-level avatars experience much higher incomes in terms of virtual resources, and are permitted to transfer this wealth to lower-level avatars called *twinks*. This is a controversial point, because twinks can defeat ordinary low-level characters in player-versus-player combat, allowing players effectively to buy victories. The controversy has increased recently, as many games moved to a "free-to-play, pay-to-win" system in which players could invest dollars to outfit their characters, thereby importing into the gameworld the wealth differentials that exist in the surrounding world.

5. *Trial and error.* Most gameworlds set narrow limits on how much an avatar can be changed after it has been created. For Algorithma to become a Jedi, she would need to drop from level 90 to level 5, and invest a couple of hundred hours building up her lightsaber skills. No amount of prayer will turn a *World of Warcraft* warrior into a priest. Thus, after creating an avatar and running it for a few hours, a player may decide it has the wrong qualities, and start a new one from scratch with a better understanding of what decisions to make. However, in many gameworlds there is no particular reason to erase the earlier character. Some large fraction of the low-level avatars in such gameworlds are really failed experiments, but they do continue to exist.

6. *Multiboxing.* A few rare players are so avid and so skilled that they use two computers and two subscription accounts to run two avatars simultaneously. I have done this *multiboxing* myself in both *World of Warcraft* and *Second Life*, partly to study closely the technical details of how avatars interact with each other, but also to be able to collect more data during important events. For example, when I organized the first major scientific conference in a gameworld, in WoW in May 2008, two of the 120 avatars in the three mains sessions were operated by me on two computers, side by side, each connected to the Internet by a different path (Bohannon 2008; Bainbridge 2010b). This reduced the possibility that a technical glitch would prevent me from running the meeting, or from recording the text chat which

became the basis for two chapters of the book that resulted from the conference. In *World of Warcraft*, I once observed four avatars operated simultaneously by a multiboxer who had four computers.

Secondary and Posthumous Avatars

The fact that many players have multiple avatars, and that a small minority run two or more simultaneously via multiboxing, suggests that giving avatars a degree of autonomy could allow anybody to operate several at once, thereby becoming more than just a single person. In fact, most successful MMOs provide the opportunity to run one secondary avatar in addition to the primary avatar. For example, in SWG Algorithma Teq constructed a *super battle droid* for Socio Path, and he used it in attacking small installations of the Rebel Alliance, given that he was loyal to Darth Vader and the Empire. The droid could be used as a decoy, taught to roam a specified area to draw the fire of enemies, or simply increasing Scio's firepower. After killing two or three Rebels, the final task was to destroy a Rebel flag, which took a long time, so Socio would assign this tedious task to the droid while he went about other business.

Several much more recent gameworlds allow a player to operate multiple secondaries at once, typically as substitutes for friends when a mission requires a team to complete but other players are not available. Three prominent examples are *Guilds Wars*, *Star Trek Online*, and *Dungeons and Dragons Online*. My primary avatar is Sagittarius; the lioness is a rather stupid secondary avatar, who merely accompanies him and bites enemies if they get too near, and five others are sophisticated *hirelings*, which I could rent for actual money, each with its own set of abilities. I could control each of the hirelings directly, or give them very general instructions and allow them to function semi-autonomously. *Star Trek Online* has an even more complex system, because the secondaries are members of the starship crew commanded by the primary avatar, so each can be given a personal name, provided with whatever equipment is desired, and even trained to cultivate unique abilities.

Dungeons and Dragons Online also illustrates the profound issue of how avatar technology can deal with death. The tomb of Dave Arneson, who with Gary Gygax invented the original *Dungeons and Dragons* table-top game. Both are deceased today, but many players of WoW, EQII, and DDO have named avatars after Gygax. Elsewhere in this virtual world is the tomb of Gygax, and a nearby mission is narrated by the recorded voice of Gygax, literally a voice from the grave. Reflecting on my own life and family, I have created virtual representations of 17 deceased members of my family in a research project on ancestor veneration avatars (AVAs). One creates an avatar somehow related to the deceased relative, and then has that relative's real personality in mind while operating the avatar, as I did for over 700 hours with Maxrohn, the posthumous avatar representing my deceased uncle Max Rohn.

Conclusion

As noted in the introduction, enhancement of human abilities need not require modification of the person's biological body. Avatars in virtual worlds are a contemporary example, and in future teleoperation of personal robots or entirely fresh alternatives may become popular. Avatars point out to us that enhancement is not merely a matter of increasing the effectiveness of a person in taking action, but also can mean an altered form of consciousness that expands opportunities for experiences, and escape from the conventional system of moral constraints. Especially noteworthy is the fact that one individual may have many different avatars, thereby becoming a *multiplex* or *protean personality*. And, lastly, that users have and will most likely consider building posthumous avatars of Virtual Worlds and develop unique relationships with their human users.

Note

The views expressed in this essay do not necessarily represent the views of the National Science Foundation or the United States; exploration of the gameworlds was conducted outside the hours of federal employment.

References

Bainbridge, William Sims (2007) "The Scientific Research Potential of Virtual Worlds." *Science* 317 (July 27), pp. 472–476.
Bainbridge, William Sims (2010a) *Online Multiplayer Games*. Morgan and Claypool.
Bainbridge, William Sims, ed. (2010b) *Online Worlds*. London: Springer.
Bainbridge, William Sims (2010c) *The Warcraft Civilization*. Cambridge, MA: MIT Press.
Bainbridge, William Sims (2011) "Star Wars Galaxies." In *The Virtual Future*. London: Springer, pp. 131–148.
Bohannon, John (2008) "Scientists Invade Azeroth." *Science* 320, pp. 1592.
Bohannon, John (2011) "Meeting for Peer Review at a Resort that's Virtually Free." *Science* 331, p. 27.
Bostrom, Nick (2003) "Are We Living in the Matrix? The Simulation Argument." In Glenn Yeffeth, ed., *Taking the Red Pill: Science, Philosophy and Religion in The Matrix*. Dallas: BenBella, pp. 233–241.
Ducheneaut, Nicolas and Moore, Robert J. (.2004) "The Social Side of Gaming: A Study of Interaction Patterns in a Massively Multiplayer Online Game." In *Proceedings of Computer Supported Cooperative Work '04*. New York: ACM, pp. 360–369.
Fuller, R. Buckminster (1970) *I Seem To Be a Verb*. New York: Bantam.
Huh, Searle and Williams, Dmitri (2010) "Dude Looks Like a Lady: Gender Swapping in an Online Game." In W.S. Bainbridge, ed., *Online Worlds*. London: Springer, pp. 161–174.
Lifton, Robert Jay (1971) "Protean Man." *Archives of General Psychiatry* 24/4, pp. 298–304.
McCubbin, Chris (2005) *Star Wars Galaxies: The Complete Guide*. Roseville, CA: Prima Games.
McCubbin, Chris, Ladyman, David, and Frase, Tuesday, eds. (2005) *Star Wars Galaxies: The Total Experience*. Roseville, CA: Prima Games.
Merrick, Kathryn E. and Maher, Mary Lou (2009) *Motivated Reinforcement Learning: Curious Characters for Multiuser Games*. New York: Springer.
Moravec, Hans (1998) "Simulation, Consciousness, Existence." http://www.frc.ri.cmu.edu/~hpm/project.archive/general.articles/1998/SimConEx.98.html (accessed October 28, 2011).
Reaves, Michael (2001) *Darth Maul: Shadow Hunter*. New York: Del Rey.
Thigpen, Corbett H. and Cleckley, Hervey M. (1957) *The Three Faces of Eve*. New York: McGraw-Hill.
Thomas, William I. and Thomas, Dorothy (1929) *The Child in America*. New York: Alfred Knopf.
Williams, Dmitri, Kennedy, Tracy L.M., and Moore, Robert J. (2011) "Behind the Avatar: The Patterns, Practices, and Functions of Role Playing in MMOs." *Games and Culture* 6/2, pp. 171–200.

10

Alternative Biologies

Rachel Armstrong

Those who have taken upon them to lay down the law of nature as a thing already searched out and understood, whether they have spoken in simple assurance or professional affectation, have therein done philosophy and the sciences great injury for as they have been successful in inducing belief, so they have been effective in quenching and stopping inquiry; and have done more harm by spoiling and putting an end to other men's efforts than good by their own.

(Francis Bacon, 1620)

Biology is the spontaneous set of carbon-based self-replicating structures that persist on earth, and conventionally biology has been regarded as an unregulated product of "nature." Over the last 50 years biotechnology has provided insights into the workings of natural cells that have revolutionized our understanding of what biological systems are capable of. Manipulating these biological processes produces technologies that can directly or indirectly influence human enhancement. Increasingly, researchers are thinking of biological systems as a technology and applying them to address global challenges in the advancement of human development in areas such as stem cell research, cloning, genetic modification, *in vitro* fertilization, the science of aging, and tissue grafting.

Human enhancement can be achieved by direct interventions where the body hosts the technology, such as in the case of neural implants. However, indirect methods in human enhancement are possible, although seldom considered in transhumanist discussions. They draw from the intrinsic relationship that exists between organisms and their environment, which was first described by Charles Darwin and later expressed as an iterative interaction by biologist Richard Lewontin. In modifying the environment, human advancement results from the increasing quality of life that comes from improved living conditions.

The Transhumanist Reader: Classical and Contemporary Essays on the Science, Technology, and Philosophy of the Human Future, First Edition. Edited by Max More and Natasha Vita-More.
© 2013 John Wiley & Sons, Inc. Published 2013 by John Wiley & Sons, Inc.

Biology as Technology

Using biology in a technological context is not a new perspective. The products of nature were harnessed to the service of the environment during the agrarian revolution, most notably through the spatial and temporal organization of plants. This provided an abundance of food to increasing numbers of human settlers and enabled positive development in a resource-rich natural environment. The deliberate enhancement of animals and plants during this period was achieved by various breeding programs where desirable characteristics such as the size of cattle were selected favorably so that these traits would be passed to offspring. It was also noticed that the actual design of farms and gardens would impact on the characteristics of livestock: for example, fish grew larger in a lake than in a pond.

The Rise of Machines

The agrarian revolution was succeeded by the industrial revolution, which effectively created a worldview of machines that were powered by natural resources, which were converted into a ready source of energy by the combustion engine. The increased control that these technologies wielded over nature enabled humans to shape and orchestrate their environment to a degree and on a scale that literally changed the face of the earth. Industrialists became exceedingly wealthy and industrialized nations saw a rise in the standard of living. Indeed, this worldview is so successful it pervades every aspect of our existence and machines shape our world to such a degree that they influence the way that we solve problems. The machine thinking, or Cartesian perspective, underpinning the problem solving capabilities of modern technology even extends to the way that we think about biological systems. Currently biology has been regarded as a kind of "natural capital" that fuels industrial processes and is set to work as if plants and organisms are just micro-machines and parts made of "soft stuff," instead of silicon chips and metal.

Complexity

An important shift in the way that reality is framed is taking place. Over the last decade, Western societies have experienced a vast change in the way they work and are organized because of complex global, cultural, and technological developments. Whilst the machine metaphor was adequate for describing the world in the last millennium it is not sufficient to navigate twenty-first-century phenomena, which impact upon everyday experience through a panoramic range of media such as, telecommunications, social networking, world travel, and the evolution of world markets. At the start of the twenty-first century, society draws from a world that is less determined by objects and increasingly shaped by connectivity. The clear either/or distinctions that formerly informed experience are being replaced by a much more fluid understanding of the world. In a twenty-first-century society identity is not fixed but shaped by networks where people and "things" can coherently exist in many states. In other words the dualistic either/or distinction that characterizes the machine worldview is being replaced by a complex system of networks that are able to explain perpetual transience, omnipresence, and parallel identities through inclusive relationships that can best be represented as and/and/and. So whilst in the previous century it was common to have a particular job, a particular identity, and live in a discrete geographic location, in the twenty-first century people are multiskilled, have many identities and exist "glocally" (simultaneously locally and globally). This constantly changing environment is managed through the continual navigation and reshaping of networks in which these fluid realities exist and embraces other transgressions between borders such as the crossing over of disciplines, geographies, languages, and cultures. Despite the world being in flux, greatly expanded, and somewhat chaotic there are patterns that help describe and navigate this constantly evolving existence paradigm.

The Science of Complexity

Science has also noted the change in the way that the world is being experienced and described. Complexity Science, or Systems Science, is concerned with the study of networks and systems. Systems thinking offers a different strategic way of problem-solving to the Cartesian, object-based perspective that mechanical technologies have to offer. Complexity considers the physical world to exist as the result of an interconnected set of complex and simple systems rather than as a series of objects that are hierarchically connected. Network connections are shared by different organizing systems through information flow where linkages are made and broken around sites of localizing activity. Complex systems do not acquire complexity but fundamentally possess it and may be composed of only a few ingredients that when combined are irreducible. The unexpected universality of the principles governing these complex systems suggests that the same laws govern complex networks in both artificial and natural systems. These common organizational principles allow the characterization of poorly understood complex systems, such as those that govern biological and cellular functions, from principles that are already well characterized in large and well-mapped non-biological systems such as the Internet.

Synthetic Biology – Complex Embodied Technology

Living systems are complex and operate according to the world of systems thinking as opposed to Cartesian reality. They possess fundamental properties that mechanical technologies cannot offer, being flexible, robust, adaptable, and able to respond to continual changes in their environment. They are also able to deal with unpredictability, the converse of this being that living technologies may also behave in unpredictable ways. Synthetic biology embodies the principles of complex systems using real-world technologies that can connect with ecology as flexible chemical networks. It is a new kind of technology that can be thought of as "living technology" (Armstrong 2009). Living systems are not made of components, nor can they be reduced to "parts," so different approaches are needed to design and construct living technologies. Although biology cannot be componentized, significant "hubs" of activity, such as DNA can be modified and rebooted in a network setting. This makes the engineering of complex systems a technical challenge producing unreliable results. The advantage of developing complex systems is that they participate in a problem-solving process to meet ongoing challenges rather than searching for a preconceived outcome.

Synthetic biology can be created using direct top-down interventions where existing systems are modified through instrumentation or using bottom-up approaches that engage with chemical self-assembly.

Top-Down Synthetic Biology

Synthetic biology is often equated with the genetic modification of biological systems as a top-down design practice. Genes are found in a membrane-bound region in the center of cells called the nucleus. This houses the large information-containing molecule DNA, which plays a key role in governing cellular design processes through regulating protein expression. If changed in the chemical sequences encoded in the DNA are engineered, often using new fragments of information carried by viruses, then the way that a gene is read, or expressed, can be changed, which can give a cell new capability. Today genetic engineering approaches are able to take very particular sequences of DNA that encode for various characteristics. These can then be modified and designed to create very specific changes and expressed in a new way, which often takes place in a host organism – normally a bacterium as they are more genetically robust than "higher," multicellular organisms. Genetic engineering reduces the element of "chance" in biological systems, which underpins the process of evolution and enables designers to effectively choose new biological functions, giving rise to notions of "designer biology" and even "artificial evolution." Genetic engineering has been placed firmly on the cultural map by biotechnologist J. Craig Venter, who not only beat the United States government to the sequencing of the human genome but also created the first entirely synthetic genome earlier this year that was dubbed "Synthia" by the popular media. His outspoken confidence, technical abilities, commercial skills, and ability to deliver amazing results have ensured his high profile and controversial status. Venter has developed a whole lexicon of possibilities for precision engineering the genetic information of organisms, which he calls "genomics," the science of combinatorial gene sequencing where gene sequences can be mixed and matched to suit the intended application. Venter's remarkable achievements have heralded a new era in the potential of synthetic biology to rewrite the code of nature and ultimately create new genetic species.

In practice, genetic engineering is not as precise as the theory suggests, as it is technically challenging and typically expensive, since it requires special laboratories with sterile conditions. Moreover from a public health and safety perspective genetically modified organisms are also heavily regulated owing to concerns about their unknown impact on natural systems, should they contaminate a local environment.

Bottom-Up Synthetic Biology

The astonishing feats of molecular biology in the second half of the twentieth century have downstaged scientific advances in a broader field of investigation that examines many different kinds of molecular self-assembly. Whilst most attention has been focused on the role of DNA in the cell, it does not actually self-form, or regulates itself but requires the action of many other chemical systems to achieve its effects, whose interactions are not fully characterized. However, other non-genetic molecules *are* capable of chemical self-organization in both biological and non-biological contexts and are being explored in a range of scientific fields of research, including chemistry, biochemistry, and the origins of life sciences. These scientific disciplines examine the phenomenology of non-genetic self-organization and investigate how an inert substance can acquire life-like properties, which is an ancient quest that is steeped in history, alchemy, magic, and religion. From a scientific perspective, self-organization is the outcome of a complex phenomenon called emergence, where new features arise from the collective interaction of more simple systems that takes place *en masse*, at the molecular level. Over the last couple of centuries some interesting observations and developments have been made, suggesting that molecular systems that do not contain specific information encoding molecules, such as DNA, are able to exhibit life-like properties. This field of research originates in the mid-nineteenth century when scientists were trying to disprove the notion of "vitalism." This was a viewpoint championed by the eminent scientist Louis Pasteur, who argued that the living essence in organism was a "special" quality that was preformed and could not be created by physical means. A number of scholars disagreed proposing that life was "merely" chemistry and not "special'" at all. Life-like qualities of chemical systems were demonstrated in non-biological systems as early as the latter half of the nineteenth century when nonliving systems exhibited some properties that appeared rather "biological" in their manifestation but were not based on cells, or even cell extracts. In 1867, Moritz Traube described the first inorganic plant-like cell (Traube 1867), using a copper hexacyanoferrate semi-permeable membrane that was formed by placing a crystal of copper sulfate into a weak solution of potassium hexacyanoferrate. The membrane enabled the selective passage of water molecules from the weak to the strong salt solution, resulting in an increase in osmotic pressure. Under tension, the thin membrane split and was repaired by the further mixing of the salts, which allowed further expansion of the cell, so more water could pass. This process continued, producing a gelatinous, seaweed-like knot of matter, until one of the ingredients necessary for the repair of the inorganic membrane was depleted.

In 1907, Stephane Leduc also produced inorganic "cells" that were similar to those described by Traube (Leduc 1907). He placed a crystal of calcium chloride in a strong potassium salt solution to create a membrane of calcium phosphate, which is a mineral found in bone, which had a cell-like appearance. Just like the Traube Cell, Leduc's system also seemed to be governed by the movement of water molecules. Leduc also coined the term "synthetic biology" in 1911 and proposed that this field of study would provide insights into the origins of life and cell organization. Over the twentieth century, research by scientists such as Alexander Oparin and Sidney Fox delved deeper into the search for chemical processes that could have led to the formation of cellular life. However, the discovery of DNA and the new field of biotechnology in the second half of the twentieth century looked to genetics as the key to understanding life. Genetics became the main focus for biological research, though there is much common ground emerging between these scientific fields as researchers are applying their knowledge of the genetic code to create artificial life.

Protocells

In 2007 two researchers, chemist Martin Hanczyc and artificial life scientist Takashi Ikegami, who were collaborating across disciplines agreed to test a hypothesis about the earliest forms of life (Hanczyc et al. 2007). They hypothesized that life's precursors would need to move around their environment to take advantage of a resource-rich situation on early Earth. Hanczyc made a model system to test this hypothesis using an oil droplet that he bestowed with an internal chemical reaction, or "metabolism," that propelled it through water. All living systems have a "metabolism," which is a specific set of chemical reactions that allow living systems to remain in constant conversation with the natural world. These reactions involve the chemical conversion of one group of substances into another, either through the production or the absorption of energy, and this enables living systems to make the most of their local resources in an adaptable, sustainable way. Designing a chemical system that could move around was a significant scientific break-through, but Hanczyc's "proto-cell" did more than this: it also behaved in a life-like way, being able to sense its environment (Toyota et al. 2009) and show complex "behaviors," and is the first experimental system that has so clearly possessed life-like qualities without needing instructions from DNA. This protocell represented an entirely new kind of technology that operates in a way that is completely different to machines that can distribute matter in time and space.

Protocells are self-assembling agents that are based on the chemistry of oil and water. They assemble themselves from a spontaneous field of self-organizing energy and can exist as oil droplets in a water medium or water-based droplets in an oil medium as a range of different kinds of "species" being composed from different recipes. Where oil/water interfaces occur there is a spontaneous self-assembly of molecules owing to the chemical basis for energy exchange at the droplet interface. The consequences of mass interactions are observed in the system as emergent phenomena that typically exhibit life-like behavior such as movement. Even when the initial conditions are the same the various protocell species show a range of possible types in any given environment because of the emergence in the system, and these can be characterized.

Protocells are not thought to be alive since they do not possess DNA, so although they possess a metabolism and a container they do not pass any specific information to their "offspring." Protocells do not replicate through any recognizable deliberate strategy but occasionally fuse and divide by "random" means without the need for DNA. This adds more intrigue to their indeterminate identity between living and non-living states. Ultimately protocells cannot self-replicate autonomously and depend on the participation of humans for their effective propagation. The spontaneously occurring processes of increasing population density observed in the laboratory are slow and simply too inefficient to be used as an effective method of replication.

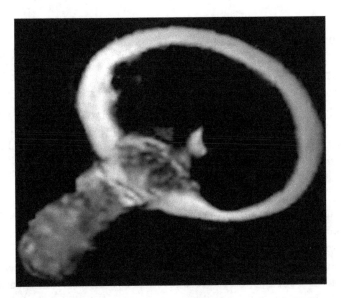

Figure 10.1 "Protocells" by Rachel Armstrong. A protocell possessing a fundamental metabolism that produces soft, insoluble crystals moves around its environment, senses changes in its surroundings, and is gradually producing a skin of crystals that will exert a physical change on the system, which responds through changing shape and method of locomotion. This kind of developmental change takes place over several seconds. Photograph by Rachel Armstrong.

Living technologies are very new and we're still trying to figure out how they work and how to best apply them, but they are very different to machines. When we look at them we probably won't even recognize them as technology, as they are not built like the machines that we are familiar with, which are cold, and hard and dry to the touch, whereas living technology is soft and warm and soggy.

> Protocells *do not have parts and they are not objects. They may act more improbably and organically than any technology that we know, but they represent a chance to replace the outdated practice of designing buildings as environmental barriers using a more constructive and harmonious approach.* (*ICON Magazine*, Oceans Issue, 096, June 2011)

Artificial Biology

Currently self-assembling chemical systems can be used to create DNA-less, complex materials that can be thought of as artificial biologies since they do not possess the same kinds of chemistries as natural biology does, nor are they modified versions of existing cells. They are made from dynamic, programmable chemical agents such as the "protocell" (oil in water-based droplet system), or "chell" (Traube cell-like vesicles with inorganic membranes). These agents are not alive but embody some of the complex properties of living systems, therefore offering a robust complex medium for manipulation and possible successful linkage to the NBIC (nanotechnology, biotechnology, information technology, and cognitive technologies) converging technologies to improve human performance through direct or indirect methods.

From Proposition to Reality

Currently artificial biologies exist only as research models in the laboratory, and commercial applications have not yet been produced. The technological potential of these technologies, such as protocells to perform useful work, relates to their programmable self-assembly, and their ability to carry chemicals in a droplet "container" and release the contents in an environmentally specific manner. Ongoing research (Schmidt et al. 2010) explores the potential for protocell systems and eventually fully artificial cells, to participate in sustainable manufacturing and environmental practices in a number of ways.

Protocells can be used as a delivery system for "environmental pharmaceuticals," such as the development of smart "paints" or surface coatings, that can fix carbon dioxide into inorganic carbonate. This application serves a dual function as an accretion technology that can build up the thermal insulation qualities of existing buildings to improve their energy efficiency. Protocells could also be used as a self-limiting system to treat chemical imbalances in the environment since they have limited capacity for survival, such as cleaning up environmental waste toxins like cyanide and converting them into harmless thiocyanide that can be absorbed into the natural ecological system. Protocell technologies may also support synthetic biology in achieving some of its environmental goals, such as assisting extremophile bacteria to perform under extreme conditions by providing a slow-release system of inorganic nutrients.

Paint companies are currently considering research into protocells as "smart" environmentally friendly agents for use in exterior emulsion-based paints, and the first commercially available applications of protocell-based technologies are likely to be around five to ten years away when carbon-fixing building coatings become available. In these systems the protocells will not be fully artificial cells but will function over a period of months to produce an accretion of carbonate on the surface that the paint is applied to. These paints may be coupled to a color-change indicator that reveals when the process has consumed the active ingredient. Since protocells cannot replicate the surface will need to be replenished by painting it again. Further applications of the "paint" would need to be applied in order to keep the growing surface "active." Smart self-maintaining surface coatings that are self-regenerating are probably another 20 years away.

Future Venice

Speculative applications for artificial biology that may help human enhancement via indirect methods are being envisaged through architectural design projects (Armstrong and Spiller 2011). Research is ongoing to develop them as alternative approaches to challenges in sustainability that have not been satisfactorily solved by machine-based methods. A suitable site would offer ready access to water, require a material solution, benefit from environmental responsiveness, and warrant an intervention that could clearly be distinguished from an industrial intervention.

Venice is situated in northeastern Italy where the Po delta meets the Venice lagoon off the Adriatic Sea. It was built on the soft delta soils in the harshest environment on earth, the shore-line, where the fabric of the buildings is repeatedly battered by the elements, flooded by the periodic *aqua alta*, and desiccated by the sun. This ferociously unstable environment poses an insurmountable set of conditions for materials that are effectively inert. On a geological timescale it is worth remembering that the tempestuous forces of nature eventually subsume mountains. Venice has weathered its environment for three centuries and its unique buildings are already being actively eroded. Walking along the waterways reveals buildings that have literally been digested into dust fragments, which has led to all kinds of acts of architectural desperation, where fist-sized holes in the wall are plugged up with concrete, rubble, rubbish, and even chewing gum.

The traditional architectural approach to meeting the challenges of hostile environments is to create the most effective possible barrier between nature and human activity using durable and inert materials, but although this has worked sufficiently effectively for human development, on an evolutionary timescale this is not how the most resilient structures persist.

Along the edges of the waterways is an indigenous system that is able to respond to the con-stant challenges of a hostile environment. Biological residents such as algae, shellfish, and bacte-ria have claimed a construction process within this harsh terrain as their own, accreting, secreting, remolding, and sculpting the materials of their surroundings to create microenviron-ments that are suited to their needs. Although the individual lifespans of organisms are short, from the perspective of persistence, living systems have been around for four and a half billion years. Uniquely, life is able to respond to continual changes in the environment in a flexible and robust manner that gives rise to evolutionary change over large timescales.

Whilst these biological systems are undirected they behave like an unruly garden, finding opportunities to extend into new territories and vigorously pursuing easily accessible sources of nutrients. Consequently, from a human perspective the presence of biological systems in the

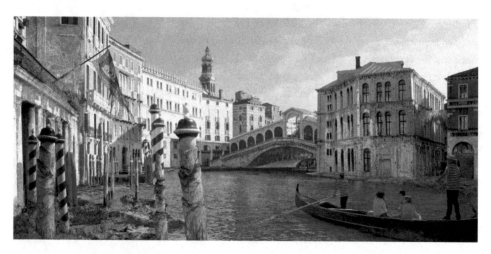

Figure 10.2   "Future Venice" by Dadier Madoc-Jones and Robert Graves (2009). Drawing of a speculative vision of Venice where the city has been sustainably reclaimed through the application of protocell technology to creating an artificial limestone reef underneath the foundations, which are resting on woodpiles. This scheme aims to spread the point load of the city over the soft delta soils on which the city has been founded, across a much broader base provided by an artificial limestone reef. Light-sensitive protocell technology is designed to accrete a mineral layer around the woodpiles by finding its way to the darkened foundations where it fixes carbon dioxide from the water into an insoluble form using local minerals. Drawing by GMJ.

waterways poses a threat to the longevity and integrity of the architecture. Yet if the element of chance could be removed from the actions of these resilient, adaptive, and evolving populations and the processes guided to engage in synthetic activities that could enhance and reinforce the fabric of Venice then the city could effectively acquire a means of patrolling the damage caused at the shoreline and respond to it through biological mechanisms.

Protocell technology working in combination with top-down forms of synthetic biology could offer a new kind of approach to shape these natural processes to improve environmental conditions (Hanczyc and Ikegami 2009) and positively impact on human health. So a project to sustainably reclaim the city of Venice was proposed by using protocell technology and synthetic biology to grow an artificial limestone reef underneath it and stop the city sinking into the soft mud on which its foundations are built, in a way that respects its non-human inhabitants.

For the scheme light-sensitive protocells would be needed so that they would move away from the light in the canals and move towards the darkened foundations of the city that rest on wood-piles, which support the weight of the city over a relatively small weight-bearing area. Protocells have already been engineered in the laboratory to vigorously respond to a light stimulus so it is possible that the energized technology would be able to move against currents and chemical gradients. Once the protocells had reached the woodpiles, a second metabolism would be activated to use dissolved carbon dioxide and create insoluble crystalline skins from minerals in the water. These would be accreted on the woodpiles and gradually petrify them. Over time and with monitoring, an artificial limestone reef would be created jointly by the indigenous marine life such as barnacles and clams. These natural organisms would make use of the bioavailable minerals produced by the protocells and contribute to the synthesis of the reef. The greatly expanded area over which the weight of the city was spread would help prevent the city from sinking. The longevity of the historic city would be extended by literally equipping it with the ability to engage in a struggle for survival against the elements by giving it a technology that conferred life-like properties on it. Additionally the protocell technology would provide other important benefits such as carbon dioxide fixation, adsorption of pollutants, and providing new niches for the local marine ecology which are symbiotic with and beneficial to established environmental systems.

The issues involved with the reclamation of Venice are complex and this particular protocell-based approach addresses just one aspect of a large range of factors that threaten the continued survival of the city. The development of different species of protocells with program-mable metabolisms suggests that an entirely new approach to the production of architecture, and healthy environments that impact positively on humanity, is possible.

Artificial Biology and Human Enhancement

Currently artificial biology exists in laboratories as prototypes and model systems. However, these new living technologies such as protocells help us imagine how it may be possible to change the relationship that exists at the heart of human development, the negative impact that our industrial-ized approaches have on the environment. With living technologies it may be possible for us to create architectures with a positive impact on natural systems, which in turn look out for us in a very architectural way, such as by removing carbon dioxide, or other pollutants, from the environment. These new technologies may indeed be our future guardians against some of the unpredictable consequences of climate change, and may also help us adapt to and survive an unpredictable future and ultimately create a much cleaner, healthier environment that will benefit the wellbeing of many.

References

Armstrong, Rachel (2009) "Systems Architecture: A New Model for Sustainability and the Built Environment Using Nanotechnology, Biotechnology, Information Technology, and Cognitive Science with Living Technology." *Artificial Life (MIT Press)* 16, pp. 1–15.

Armstrong, Rachel and Spiller, Neill (2011) "Synthetic Biology: Living Quarters." *Nature* 467 (October 21, 2010), pp. 916–918.

Hanczyc Martin and Ikegami, Takashi (2009) "Protocells as Smart Agents for Architectural Design." *Technoetic Arts Journal* 7/2.

Hanczyc, Martin and Ikegami, Takashi, et al. (2007) "Fatty Acid Chemistry at the Oil-Water Interface: Self-Propelled Oil Droplets." *Journal of the American Chemical Society* 129/30, pp. 9386–9391.

Leduc, Stéphane (1907) *Les Bases physiques de la vie*. Paris.

Schmidt, Marcus, Mahmutoglu, Ismail, Porcar, Manuel, Armstrong, Rachel, et al. (2010) *Synthetic Biology Applications in Environmental Biotechnology: Assessing Potential Economic, Environmental and Ethical Ramifications*. TARPOL Project Report.

Traube, Moritz (1867) *Archiv für Anatomie Physiologie und wissenschaftliche Medicin*, pp. 87–128, 129–165.

Toyota, Taro, Maru, Naoto, Hanczyc, Martin, Ikegami, Takashi, and Sugawara Tadashi (2009) "Self-Propelled Oil Droplets Consuming "Fuel' Surfactant." *Journal of the American Chemical Society* 131/14, pp. 5012–5013.

Further Reading

Armstrong, Rachel (2011) "Unconventional Computing in the Built Environment." *International Journal of Nanotechnology and Molecular Computation* 3/1, pp. 1–12.

Part III

Human Enhancement
The Cognitive Sphere

Enhancing the human brain's cognitive capacities is another crucial goal of transhumanism. In a new essay Andy Clark, author of *Natural-Born Cyborgs: Minds, Technologies, and the Future of Human Intelligence*, considers how the merging of humans and machines will enable us to redesign ourselves for the better. The options may include not only better bodies and improved senses but also reorganized mental architectures. This will be made possible not only by scientific and technological advancement but also by our native biological plasticity. Clark argues that fear of enhancement results from a fundamentally misconceived vision of our own humanity. A more accurate vision recognizes that human minds and bodies are open to deep and transformative restructuring, in which new physical and cognitive equipment can become literally incorporated into the thinking and acting systems that we identify as minds and persons. Clark calls this aspect of ourselves "profoundly embodied agency." Understanding profound embodiment helps us to address questions and fears concerning converging technologies for improving human performance.

AI researcher Ben Goertzel's new essay explores the implications of artificial general intelligence (AGI). Whereas much AI research has developed computerized cognition for narrow tasks, AGI researchers aim for the original goal of a general machine intelligence of human-level intellect or better. Goertzel sees the next huge leap in humanity's progress as involving the radical extension of technology into the domain of thought. He argues that "our top priority should be the creation of beneficent artificial minds with greater than human general intelligence, which can then work together with us to solve the other hard problems and explore various positive avenues." Given the enormous potential benefits of advanced AGI technology, why is so little work being done on it (as distinct from narrow AI)? After answering that question, Goertzel concludes by laying out the risks and rewards of advanced AGI.

The Transhumanist Reader: Classical and Contemporary Essays on the Science, Technology, and Philosophy of the Human Future, First Edition. Edited by Max More and Natasha Vita-More.
© 2013 John Wiley & Sons, Inc. Published 2013 by John Wiley & Sons, Inc.

Writing just a couple of years after the introduction of the World Wide Web in 1990, former MIT researcher Sasha Chislenko projected technological trends to see how we might use intelligent information filters and enhanced reality (now called "augmented reality") to expand our perceptual and cognitive abilities and to personalize our view of reality. He makes some observations and predictions of the transformations in people's perception of the world and themselves in the course of this technological change. Since Chislenko wrote this essay, we have begun to see the idea being introduced in reality, with early versions of the technology being built into smartphones and heads-up displays on some car windshields. How long will it be before we experience the more intimate and comprehensive versions considered by Chislenko? His essay helps us think through the possibilities and implications.

Transhumanism takes very seriously the goal of extending our lives not just for a few years or even decades, but indefinitely. Even if aging is conquered, our biological bodies are too fragile to ensure our survival against accident and mayhem over very long periods of time. Truly long-term survival will probably require the transfer of our minds and personalities from biological brains and bodies to a different substrate. The last two essays in this section explore the feasibility of doing this.

Randal Koene explores "Uploading to Substrate-Independent Minds" and explains that the goal of substrate-independence is to continue personality, individual characteristics, a manner of experiencing and a personal way of processing those experiences. Of six technology paths through which we may gain substrate-independence for our minds, the most conservative and well-supported by research is Whole Brain Emulation (WBE). Koene notes that, back in 2000, WBE was considered science fiction, since it was beyond what was then considered feasible science and engineering. That is no longer true, as leading scientists and principal investigators tackle projects supporting WBE such as high-resolution connectomics.

In a much-cited 1993 essay, AI and nanotechnology researcher Ralph Merkle delves into the concept of "uploading" – the term most commonly used before "substrate-independent minds." Much discussed in transhumanism, the uploading idea is that we might eventually be able to transfer our minds and personalities from the fleshy neuronal processor of the biological brain to a more durable and extendable synthetic thinking substrate. Merkle analyzes how much computing power would be required to model your brain on a computer, based on his estimate of human memory capacity.

11

Re-Inventing Ourselves
The Plasticity of Embodiment, Sensing, and Mind

Andy Clark

I.   Introduction: Where the Rubber Meets the Road

In a short article in the May 2004 edition of *Wired* magazine (revealingly subtitled "Fear and Loathing on the Human-Machine Frontier") the futurist and science fiction writer Bruce Sterling sounds an increasingly familiar alarm. After warning us of the imminent dangers of "brain augmentation" he adds:

> Another troubling frontier is physical, as opposed to mental, augmentation. Japan has a rapidly growing elderly population and a serious shortage of caretakers. So Japanese roboticists … envision walking wheelchairs and mobile arms that manipulate and fetch.
> But there's ethical hell at the interfaces, The peripherals may be dizzyingly clever gizmos but the CPU is a human being: old, weak, vulnerable, pitifully limited, possibly senile. (Sterling 2004: 116)

This kind of fear is rooted, I shall argue, in a fundamentally misconceived vision of our own humanity. A vision that depicts us as "locked-in agents" – as beings whose minds and physical abilities are fixed quantities, apt (at best) for mere support and scaffolding by their best technologies. In contrast to this view, I have argued (Clark 1997, 2003) that human minds and bodies are essentially open to episodes of deep and transformative restructuring, in which new equipment (both physical and "mental") can become quite literally incorporated into the thinking and acting systems that we identify as minds and persons. In what follows, I pursue this theme with special attention to the very notion of the human-machine interface itself.

It helps to start with the commonplace. Sensing and moving are the spots where the rubber of embodied agency meets the road of the wider world, the world outside the agent's physical

From *The Journal of Medicine and Philosophy* 32/3 (2007), pp. 263–282. Copyright © 2007 Andy Clark.

The Transhumanist Reader: Classical and Contemporary Essays on the Science, Technology, and Philosophy of the Human Future, First Edition. Edited by Max More and Natasha Vita-More.
© 2013 John Wiley & Sons, Inc. Published 2013 by John Wiley & Sons, Inc.

boundaries. The typical human agent, circa 2004, feels herself to be a bounded physical entity in contact with the world via a variety of standard sensory channels, including touch, vision, smell, and hearing. It is a commonplace observation, however, that the use of simple tools can lead to alterations in that local sense of embodiment. Picking up and using a stick, we feel as if we are touching the world at the end of the stick, not (usually) as if we are touching the stick with our hand. The stick, it has sometimes been suggested, is in some way incorporated and the overall effect seems more like bringing a temporary whole new agent-world circuit into being, rather than simply exploiting the stick as a helpful prop or tool.

In these cases there suddenly seem to be two interfaces at play: the place where the stick meets the hand, and the place where the extended system "biological-agent + stick" meets the rest of the world. When we read about new forms of human-machine interface, we are again confronted by a similar duality, and an accompanying tension. What makes such interfaces *appropriate* as mechanisms for human enhancement is, it seems, precisely their potential role in creating whole new agent-world circuits. But insofar as they succeed at this task, the new agent-tool interface itself fades from view, and the proper picture is one of an extended or enhanced agent confronting the (wider) world.

In sections II and III, I shall lightly explore this notion of the interface, and then look at some examples in which new systemic wholes are created by various forms of technological intervention. Section IV asks under what conditions it becomes proper to speak of enhanced agents rather than un-enhanced agents with new props and scaffoldings. Here, I try to show that there is more at issue than a way of speaking, and that there are scientifically and philosophically important differences between the two cases. Next (section V) I extend the discussion from bodily augmentation to mental augmentation, indicating what would need to be done to make the vexed idea of *enhanced human mentality* concrete. The discussion continues (section VI) by developing a notion of the "profoundly embodied agent" as a means of marking the philosophical and scientific importance of our potential for repeated and literal episodes of self-reconfiguration. The essay ends by relating this image of profound embodiment to some questions (and fears) concerning converging technologies for improving human performance.

II.   What's in an Interface?

Haugeland (1998) is, in part, an extended philosophical meditation on the very idea of an interface. The goal is to uncover the underlying principles "for dividing systems into distinct subsystems along nonarbitrary lines" (1988: 211). According to Haugeland, the notions of "component," "system," and "interface" are all interdefined and interdefining. Components are those parts of a larger whole that interact through interfaces. Systems are "relatively independent and self-contained" composites of such interfaced components. And an interface itself is a point of interactive "contact" between components such that the relevant interactions are "well-defined, reliable and relatively simple" (1988: 213).

Haugeland is right, I think, to point to the nature of interactions as the key to the location of an interface. We discern an interface where we discern a kind of regimented, often deliberately designed, point of contact between two or more independently tuneable or replaceable parts. It does not seem correct, however, to insist that flow across the interface be simple. The idea here seems to be that we find genuine interfaces only where we find energetic or informational bottlenecks, as if an interface must be a narrow channel yielding what Haugeland describes as "low bandwidth" coupling. This is important for Haugeland's argumentative purpose, as he means to show (by appeal to broadly speaking Gibsonian characterizations of sensing (see Gibson 1979) that human sensing typically yields very task-variable, high-bandwidth forms of agent-environment coupling, and thus to argue that no genuine interface or interfaces separate agent and world. Instead, there is said to be "intimate intermingling of mind, body and world" (Haugeland 1998: 224).

The Gibsonian angle is useful, as it points to two distinct ways in which we might conceive of our own biological sensory systems. According to the standard (non-Gibsonian) conception, a sensory interface is a point of information transduction. It is a point at which rich energetic input (e.g., visual input) must begin to be somehow transformed into discrete internal action guiding representations. This is the notion of the sensory interface as a kind of fixed veil between an agent and a represented world.

But there is another way to look at (at least some uses of) sensing, which can be introduced by a simple example. Consider running to catch a fly ball in baseball. Giving perception its standard role, we might assume that the job of the visual system is to transduce information about the current position of the ball so as to allow a reasoning system to project its future trajectory. It seems, however, that nature has a more elegant and efficient solution: you simply run so that the ball's trajectory looks straight against the visual background (McBeath et al. 1995). This solution exploits a powerful invariant in the optic flow, discussed in Lee and Reddish (1981). But most importantly for our purposes, it highlights (see Maturana 1980) a very different role for the perceptual coupling itself, Instead of using sensing to get enough information inside, past the visual bottleneck, so as to allow the reasoning system to "throw away the world" and solve the problem wholly internally, it uses the sensor as an open conduit allowing environmental magnitudes to exert a constant influence on behavior. Sensing is here depicted as the opening of a channel, with successful whole-system behavior emerging when activity in this channel is kept within a certain range. What is created is thus a kind of new, task-specific agent-world circuit.[1]

As Randall Beer recently put it,

> The focus shifts from accurately representing an environment to continuously engaging that environment with a body so as to stabilize patterns of coordinated behavior that are adaptive for the agent. (Beer 2000: 97)

This shift in perspective on what sensing is (often) all about will be important later when we consider new sensory channels and their potential impact on the bounds of human agents.

But while agreeing with Haugeland that sensing is often best understood in these terms, his own conclusion that no genuine interfaces then link agent and world seems premature. Haugeland depicts these kinds of "open-channel" solutions as involving "tightly coupled high-bandwidth interaction" (Haugeland 1998: 223) and hence as inimical to the very idea of an agent-world interface.[2] But it seems intuitive that there can be genuine interfaces that support extremely high-bandwidth forms of coupling.

Think, for example, of multiple computers linked into a network by means of super-fast, very high-bandwidth "grid technologies."[3] There is really no doubt but that we here confront a web of distinct intercommunicating component machines. Yet that web, in action, can sometimes function as a single unified resource. Nonetheless, we still think of it as a web of distinct-but-interfaced devices. And we do so not because the point of each machine's contact with the grid is narrow (it isn't), but because there exist, for each machine on the grid, very well-defined points of potential detachment and re-engagement. We discern interfaces at the points at which one machine can be easily disengaged and another engaged instead, allowing the first to join another grid, or to operate in a stand-alone fashion. An interface, I conclude, is indeed a point of contact between two items across which the types of performance-relevant interaction are reliable and well defined. But there is no requirement that such interfaces be narrow-bandwidth bottlenecks.

III.   New Systemic Wholes

Biological systems, from lampreys to primates, display remarkable powers of bodily and sensory adaptability.[4] The Australian performance artist Stelarc routinely deploys a "third hand," a mechanical actuator controlled by Stelarc's brain via commands to muscle sites on his legs and abdomen.[5] Activity at these sites is monitored by electrodes that transmit signals (via a computer) to the artificial hand. Stelarc reports that, after some years of practice and performance, he now feels as if he simply wills the third hand to move. It has become what some philosophers call "transparent equipment," something through which Stelarc (the agent) can act on the world without first willing an action on anything else. In this respect, it now functions much as his biological hands and arms, serving his goals without (generally) being itself an object of conscious thought or effortful control.

Recent experimental work reveals more about the kinds of mechanisms that may be at work in such cases. A much-publicized example is the work by Miguel Nicolelis and colleagues on a BMI (brain-machine interface) that allows a macaque monkey to use thought control to move a robot arm. In the most recent version of this work, Carmena et al. (2003) implanted 320 electrodes in the frontal and parietal lobes of a monkey. The electrodes allowed a monitoring computer to record neural activity across multiple cortical ensembles while the monkey learnt to use a joystick to move a cursor across a computer screen for rewards. As in previous work, the computer was able to extract the neural activity patterns corresponding to different movements (including direction and grip).

Next, the joystick is disconnected. But the monkey is still able to use its neural activity to directly control the cursor for rewards, and learns to do so. Finally (and this is the new element in the work) these commands are diverted to a robot arm whose actual motions are then translated into on-screen cursor movements (including an on-screen equivalent of forceful gripping). This closes the loop. Instead of the monkey merely moving an unseen robot arm by thought control alone, the movements now yield visual feedback in the form of on-screen cursor motion.

When the robot arm was inserted into the control loop, the monkey displayed a striking degradation of behavior. It took two full days of practice for fluent thought-control over the onscreen cursor to be re-established. The reason was that the monkey's brain now had to learn to factor in the mechanical and temporal "friction" created by the new physical equipment: it had to factor in the mechanical and dynamical properties of the robot arm and the time delays (which were substantial, in the 60–90 millisecond range) caused by interposing the motion of the arm between neural command and on-screen feedback. By the time full fluency was achieved, it is reasonable to conjecture that these properties of the (still unseen) distant arm were incorporated into the monkey's own body-schema. In support of this, the experimenters were able to track real long-term physiological changes in the response profiles of fronto-parietal neurons following use of the BMI, leading them to comment that:

the dynamics of the robot arm (reflected by the cursor movements) become incorporated into multiple cortical representations ... we propose that the gradual increase in behavioral performance emerged as a consequence of a plastic reorganization whose main outcome was the assimilation of the dynamics of an artificial actuator into the physiological properties of fronto-parietal neurons. (Carmena et al. 2003: 205)

Creatures capable of this kind of deep incorporation of new bodily (and, as we'll see, sensory and cognitive) structure are examples of what shall call (see section IV) "profoundly embodied agents." Such agents are able constantly to negotiate and renegotiate the agent-world boundary itself.

Although our own capacity for such renegotiation is (I believe) vastly under-appreciated, it really should come as no great surprise, given the facts of biological bodily growth and change. The human infant must learn by "self-exploration" which neural commands bring about which bodily effects, and must then practice until skilled enough to issue those commands without conscious effort. This process has been dubbed (Meltzoff and Moore 1997) "body babbling" and continues until the infant body becomes "transparent equipment." Since bodily growth and change continue, it is simply good design not to permanently lock in knowledge of any particular configuration, but instead to deploy plastic neural resources and an ongoing regime of monitoring and recalibration (for some excellent discussion, see Ramachandran and Blakeslee 1998).

As a second class of examples of recalibration and renegotiation, consider the plasticity revealed by work in sensory substitution. Pioneered in the 1960s and 1970s by Paul Bach-y-Rita and colleagues, the earliest such systems were grids of blunt "nails" fitted to the backs of blind subjects, and taking input from a head-mounted camera. In response to the camera input, specific regions of the grid became active, gently stimulating the skin under the grid. At first, subjects report only a vague tingling sensation. But after wearing the grid while engaged in various kinds of goal-driven activity (walking, eating, etc.) the reports change dramatically. Subjects stop feeling the tickling on the back and start to report rough, quasi-visual experiences of looming objects, etc.

After a while, a ball thrown at the head causes instinctive and appropriate ducking. The causal chain is "deviant": it runs via the systematic input to the back. But the nature of the information carried, and the way it supports the control of action, is suggestive of the visual modality. Performance using such devices can be quite impressive. In a recent review article, Bach-y-Rita and Kercel note that TVSS (Tactile Visual Substitution Systems) have

been sufficient to perform complex perception and "eye"-hand coordination tasks. These have included face recognition, accurate judgment of speed and direction of a rolling ball with over 95% accuracy in batting the ball as it rolls over a table edge, and complex inspection-assembly tasks. (Bach-y-Rita and Kercel 2003: 543)

The key to effective sensory substitution is goal-driven motor engagement. It seems to be crucial that the head-mounted camera be under the subject's motor control. This meant that the brain could, in effect experiment via the motor system, giving commands that systematically varied the input, so as to begin to form hypotheses about what information the tactile signals might be carrying. Such training yields quite a flexible new agent-world circuit. Once trained in the use of the head-mounted camera the motor system operating the camera could be changed, e.g. to a hand-held camera, with no loss of acuity. The touch pad, too, could be moved to new bodily sites, and there was no tactile/visual confusion: an itch scratched under the grid caused no "visual" effects (for these results, again see Bach-y-Rita and Kercel 2003).

Such technologies, though still experimental, are now increasingly advanced. The back-mounted grid is often replaced by a tongue-mounted coin-sized array, and extensions in other sensory modalities. Bach-y-Rita and Kercel (2003) give the nice example of a touch-sensor-rich glove that allows leprosy patients to begin to feel again using their hands. The patient is fitted with the glove that transmits signals to a forehead-mounted tactile disc-array and rapidly reports feeling sensations of touch at the fingertips. This is presumably because the motor-control over the sensors runs via commands to the hand, so the sensation is subsequently projected to that site.

The line between these kinds of rehabilitative strategy and wholly new forms of bodily and sensory enhancement is already thin to the point of non-existence. There is advanced work on night-vision versions of sensory substitution, and (at the more dramatic end of this spectrum) it is possible to bypass the existing sensory peripheries, feeding signals direct to cortex (see Bach-y-Rita and Kercel 2003, and discussion in Clark 2003). Even without penetrating the existing surface of skin and skull, sensory enhancement and bodily extension are a pervasive possibility.

One rather unusual example, reported in Schrope (2001), is a U.S. Navy innovation known as a tactile flight suit. The suit (a kind of vest worn by the pilot) allows even inexperienced helicopter pilots to perform difficult tasks such as holding the helicopter in a stationary hover in the air. It works by generating bodily sensations (via safe puffs of air) inside the suit. If the craft is tilting to the right or left or forward or backward, the pilot feels a puff-induced vibrating sensation on that side of the body. The pilot's own responses (moving in the opposite direction so as to correct the vibrations) can even be monitored by the suit to control the helicopter. The suit is so good at transmitting and delivering information in a natural and easy way that military pilots can use it to fly blindfolded.

While the pilot is wearing the suit, the helicopter behaves very much like an extended body for him or her: it rapidly links the pilot to the aircraft in the same kind of closed-loop interaction that linked Stelarc and the third hand, or the monkey and the robot arm, or the blind person and the TVSS system. What matters, in each case, is the provision of closed-loop signaling so that motor commands affect sensory input! What varies is the amount of training (and hence the extent of deeper neural changes) required to fully exploit the new agent-world circuits thus created.

It is important, in all these cases, that the new agent-world circuits be trained and calibrated in the context of a whole agent engaged in world-directed (goal-driven) activity. Here, too, we encounter a Gibsonian theme, in the form of

> a conception of the senses in terms of Gibson's (1966) perceptual systems (i.e. as a whole and complex system that is functionally constituted as one piece from beginning to end ...) but [going] beyond in allowing for a conception of the senses as contingent modalities that are tributary of the overall perceptual system's performance. (Gonzalez and Bach-y-Rita, manuscript)

One sign of successful calibration is, as we noted earlier, that once fluency is achieved the specific details of the (old or new) circuitry by which the world is engaged feel "transparent" in use. The conscious agent is then aware of the oncoming ball, not of seeing the ball, or (by the same token) of using a tactile substitution channel to detect the ball. In just this way the tactile-vest-wearing pilot becomes aware of the plane's tilt and slant, not of the puffs of air. Perception, as Varela et al. (1991) and O'Regan and Noe (2001) have persuasively argued, just is this open-ended process of actively engaging a world.

To sum up, humans and other primates are integrated but constantly negotiable bodily platforms of sensing, moving, and (as we'll see later) reasoning. Such platforms extend an open invitation to technologies of human enhancement. They are biologically designed so as to fluidly incorporate new bodily and sensory kits, creating brand new systemic wholes.

IV.   Incorporation Versus Use

A very natural doubt to raise, at about this point, would be the following:

> Critic: "You are making quite a song and a dance out of this, what with talk of brand new systemic wholes and so on. But we all know we can use tools, and that we can sometimes learn to use them fluently and transparently. Why talk of new systemic wholes, of extended bodies and reconfigured users, rather than just the same old user in command of a new tool?"

This is the right question to push, and we have already seen a hint of the answer in the comments of Carmena et al. concerning the altered response profile of certain fronto-parietal neurons. To bring the key idea into focus, it helps next to consider a closely related body of research on tool-use by primates. To set the scene requires a brief neuro-scientific excursion.

Recent years have seen the discovery, in primate brains, of a variety of so-called "hi-modal neurons." These are:

> Pre-motor, parietal and putaminal neurons that respond both to somatosensory information from a given body region (i.e., the somatosensory receptive field; sRF) and to visual information from the space (visual receptive field; vRF) adjacent to it. (Maravita and Iriki 2004: 79)

For example, some neurons respond to somatosensory stimuli (light touches) at the hand and to visually presented stimuli near the hand, so as to yield an action-relevant coding of visual space. In a series of experiments, recordings were taken from bi-modal neurons in the intraparietal cortex of Japanese macaques while they (the macaques) learnt to reach for food using a rake. The experimenters found that after just five minutes of rake-use, the responses of some hi-modal neurons whose original vRFs picked out stimuli near the hand had expanded to include the entire length of the tool, "as if the rake was part of the arm and forearm" (Maravita and Iriki 2004: 79).

Similarly, other bi-modal neurons, that previously responded to visual stimuli within the space reachable by the arm, now had vRFs that covered the space accessible by the arm-rake combination, After surveying a number of other related findings (including some fascinating work in which similar effects are observed after experience of reaching with a virtual arm in an on-screen display) Maravita and Iriki conclude that "[s]uch vRF expansions may constitute the neural substrate of use-dependent assimilation of the tool into the body-schema, suggested by classical neurology" (Maravita and Iriki 2004: 80).

It is also noteworthy, especially in the light of our previous discussion, that "any expansion of the vRF only followed active, intentional use of the tool not its mere grasping by the hand" (Maravita and Iriki 2004: 81). In human subjects suffering from unilateral neglect (in which stimuli from within a certain region of egocentrically coded space are selectively ignored) it has been shown that the use of a stick as a tool for reaching actually extends the area of visual neglect to encompass the space now reachable using the tool (see Berti and Frassinetti 2000). Berti and Frassinetti conclude that "[t]he brain makes a distinction between 'far space' (the space beyond reaching distance) and 'near space' (the space within reaching distance)" and that implies "holding a stick causes a remapping of far space to near space. In effect the brain, at least for some purposes, treats the stick as though it were a part of the body" (Berti and Frassinetti 2000: 415).

The plastic neural changes reported by Carmena et al. (section III above), and now further underlined by Maravita and Iriki, and by Berti and Frassinetti, are, I want to suggest, the key to a real (philosophically important and scientifically solid) distinction between true incorporation into the body-schema and mere use. The body-schema, in this sense, is not the same thing as the body-image, though the two can sometimes he related.

As I shall use the terms, the body-image is a conscious construct, able to inform thought and reasoning about the body. The body-schema is a suite of neural settings that implicitly (and non-consciously) define a body in terms of its capabilities for action, for example, by defining the extent of "near space" for action programs.[6] I would speculate, however, that the striking conscious experiential datum of equipment (not just rakes but even cars and violins) falling transparent in use is plausibly one result, in conscious agents, of just these kinds of deeper changes: changes (that may be temporary, context-dependent, or long-term) in the body-schema itself.

We can certainly imagine tool-users (perhaps even fluent tool-users?) whose brains were *not* engineered so as to adapt the body-schema in these ways. Such beings would *always* use tools the way we typically begin: by representing the tool and its features and powers (its length, for example) and calculating effective uses accordingly. We can even imagine (I think) beings who were so fast and good at these calculations as to deploy the tools with the same skill and efficacy as an expert human agent.

The contrast that would remain, even in the latter kind of case, would be between the skilled agent's first representing the shape, dimensions, and powers of the tool and then inferring (consciously or otherwise) that you can now reach such and such, and do such and such, and agents whose brains were so constituted that experience with the tool results in (for example) a suite of altered VRFs such that objects within tool-augmented reaching range are now *automatically* treated as falling within "near space."

These are surely distinct strategies. The latter strategy might be especially recommended for beings whose bodies (like our own) are naturally subject to growth and change. Beings deploying this strategy do not relate to their own bodies the way classical cognitive science depicts the intelligent agent as relating to its world, namely, via a process of objectivist representation and inference. The deep distinction is thus between various forms of knowledge-based use (which involves a lot of explicit representation of features, properties, and inferences based on those features), and genuine episodes of assimilation and integration, which can now be defined as cases in which plastic neural resources are recalibrated (in the context of goal-directed whole agent activity) to reflect new bodily and sensory opportunities. In this way, our own embodied activity brings forth new systemic wholes.

V.   Extended Cognition

Could anything like this notion of "incorporation" (rather than mere use) and new systemic wholes get a grip in the more ethereal domain of mind and cognition? Could human minds be genuinely extended and augmented by cultural and technological tweaks, or is it always (as many evolutionary psychologists, such as Pinker [1997] would have us believe) just the same old mind with a shiny new tool?

Here, the story is murkier by far. My own view, defended at much greater length elsewhere (see Clark and Chalmers 1998; Clark 2003) is that external and non-biological information-processing resources are also apt for temporary or long-term recruitment and incorporation rather than simply knowledge-based use, and that to whatever extent that this holds, we are not just bodily and sensorially but also *cognitively* permeable agents. But whereas we can point, in the case of basic tool-use, to visible neural changes that accompany the genuine assimilation of new bodily structure, it is harder to know what to look for in the case of mental and cognitive routines.

It may be helpful[7] first to display the bare logical possibility of such cognitive extension. For even the bare possibility, some might feel, is ruled out by a simple argument to the effect that "cognitive enhancement requires that the cognitive operations of the prop be intelligible to the agent." If this were so, cognitive enhancement would always be in some clear sense superficial. But the argument is clearly flawed, since the cognitive operations of much of my own brain are not thus intelligible to me, the conscious agent. Yet they surely help make me the cognitive agent I am. It also helps to reflect that biological brains must change and evolve by coordinating old activities and processes with new ones made available by new or subtly altered structures. To insist that such change requires the literal intelligibility of the operations of the new by the old (rather than simply some appropriate integration and coordination) is to miss the potential for new wholes that are *themselves* the determiners of what is and is not intelligible. Certain non-biological tools and structures, I am thus suggesting, can become sufficiently well integrated into our problem-solving activity to count as parts of new wholes in just this way. But just what does such integration (genuine cognitive incorporation) require?

One suggestion (Clark and Chalmers 1998) is that cognitive incorporation occurs when the existing system learns a complex problem-solving routine that makes deep implicit commitments to the robust availability of certain operations and/or bodies of information while carrying out some species of online problem-solving. This is the cognitive equivalent, I would now suggest, of the implicit commitments to bodily shape and potentials for action made by tuning the receptive fields of bi-modal neurons. In the cognitive case, what matters is the delicate temporal tuning of multiple participating elements (including, for example, calls to internal or external information stores) that simply factor in the availability of those operations or bodies of information.

The field of "active vision" provides a nice example. Ballard et al. (1997) studied a task in which subjects copied a pattern of colored blocks by moving them from one on-screen area (the model) to another (the target). Using eye-tracking techniques, the experimenters found that subjects looked to the model both before and after picking up a block. The explanation for the apparently unnecessary repetitions of gaze seems to be that when glancing at the model, the subject stores only one piece of information: either the color or the position of the next block to be copied (not both). The conclusion was that the brain uses repeated visual fixation to link a target location to a type of information (color or position) retrieving that information "just-in-time" for use. In this way, according to the authors, "fixation can be seen as binding the value of the variable currently relevant for the task [and] changing gaze is analogous to changing the memory reference in a silicon computer" (Ballard et al. 1997: 723). In this respect, for this task, the brain simply uses the external scene as its memory store.

This subtle reliance on the external scene is dramatically illustrated by recent work on so-called "change blindness" (see, e.g., Simons 2000) in which simple experimental manipulations (the masking of motion transients while large changes are made to a visually presented scene) suggest[8] the surprising sparseness of our on-the-spot (all in one instant, or "snapshot" [see Noe 2004]) conscious awareness. Subjects seldom see these changes, and are often amazed when they realize what has happened without their noticing it. One diagnosis of why we are not normally aware of any such sparseness is that our feeling of "seeing all the detail" in the scenes (and hence the surprisingness of the demonstrations of unseen changes) is really a reflection of something implicit in the overall problem-solving organization in which vision participates. That organization "assumes" the (ecologically normal) ability to retrieve more detailed information when needed, so we feel (correctly, in an important sense) that we are already in command of the detail.[9]

The point, for present purposes, is that the brain need not actively represent the availability of such-and-such information from any given internal or external location. Instead, it simply deploys a problem-solving routine (that may involve programmed saccades to a visual location, or calls to biological memory) whose fine temporal structure assumes the easy availability of such-and-such information from such-and-such a location. It is in this way (I am suggesting) that non-biological informational resources can become – either temporarily or long-term – genuinely incorporated into the problem-solving whole. Just as the experienced brain need not (though it sometimes can) explicitly represent the shape of a tool and then infer the available reach, so too it need not (though it sometimes can) first represent the availability of specific information at some location, and then infer that it can find what it needs by accessing a given resource.

Instead, a problem-solving routine is delicately "grown" so as to maximally exploit the local informational field.[10] Such a field can include biological resources, environmental structure, and cognitive artifacts such as notebooks and laptops. As we move towards an era of wearable computing and ubiquitous information access, the robust, reliable information fields to which our brains delicately adapt their routines will become increasingly dense and powerful, further blurring the distinction between the cognitive agent and her best tools, props, and artifacts.

VI.   Profound Embodiment

The notion of embodiment[11] plays an increasingly prominent role in philosophy and cognitive science. It is not always clear, however, exactly what it is that matters about embodiment, I shall end, then, by making a concrete (but perhaps somewhat heretical) proposal, and then relating it to the questions concerning the nature of the interface and to the topic of converging technologies for improving human performance.

We can distinguish three "grades" of embodiment. I shall call these (rather unimaginatively) "mere embodiment," "modest embodiment," and "profound embodiment." A "merely embodied" creature or robot would be one equipped with a body and sensors, able to engage in closed-loop interactions with its world, but for whom the body was nothing but a means to implement solutions arrived at by pure reason. Imagine also that this being can control the body only by issuing a complex series of micro-managing commands to every tiny muscle, tendon, spring, and actuator. A close real-world approximation to such a being is the early mobile robot, such as Shakey, built over three decades ago at the Stanford Research Institute.

A "modestly embodied" creature or robot would then be one for whom the body was not just another problem-space, requiring constant micro-managed control, but was rather a resource whose own features and dynamics (of sensor placement, of linked tendons and muscle groups, etc.) could be actively exploited allowing for increasingly fluent forms of action selection and control. Much work in contemporary robotics explores this middle ground of modest embodiment, for example, Barbara Webb's (1996) lovely work on the robot cricket in which sensor placement and time delays caused by signal transmission along internal pathways prove integral to its capacity to identify the song of a mate and locomote in that direction. What makes this an example of only modest embodiment is that the specific solution is "locked in" by the details of the hard-wired architecture itself. Such systems are congenitally unable to learn new kinds of body-exploiting solution "on the fly," in response to damage, growth, or change.

It is perhaps hardly surprising that much (though not all – see Lungarella et al. 2003) work in real-world robotics explores this space of "modest embodiment." After all, robots (so far) don't grow, use tools, or self-repair. By contrast, as we have seen, biological systems (and especially us primates) seem to be specifically designed so as to constantly search for opportunities to make the most of body and world, checking for what is available, and then (at various time-scales and with varying degrees of difficulty) integrating new resources very deeply, creating whole new agent-world circuits in the process. A "profoundly embodied" creature or robot is thus (according to this definition) one that is highly engineered so as to be able to learn to make maximal problem-simplifying use of an open-ended variety of internal, bodily, or external sources of order.

We saw, in previous sections, some hints of the kinds of engineering involved. It includes the use of plastic neural resources to create and update a body-schema, the capacity to factor the availability of information (wherever and however stored) into the heart of temporally fine-tuned problem-solving routines, and the capacity (in conscious beings like ourselves) for equipment to become transparent in use. This is not, of course, an all-or-nothing divide. Profound embodiment comes in many degrees and flavors, all the way from almost (but not quite) fully hard-wired solutions to amazingly plastic and reconfigurable ones. But primates, as we have seen, seem to fall quite close to the more radically reconfigurable end of this spectrum.

But why describe this as "profound embodiment" rather than as a return to the outdated (or so many of us believe – see Clark 1997 for review) image of mind as a disembodied organ of control? The answer is that these kinds of minds are not in the least disembodied. Rather, they are *promiscuously* body-and-world exploiting. They are forever testing and exploring the possibilities for incorporating new resources and structures deep into their problem-solving regimes. They are, to use the jargon of Clark (2003), the minds of Natural-Born Cyborgs: of systems continuously renegotiating their own limits, components, data-stores, and interfaces. On this account, the body (any given biological or bio-technological body) is both critically important and constantly negotiable. It is critically important, as it is a key player on the problem-solving stage. It is not simply the point at which processes of transduction pass the real problems (now rendered in rich internal representational formats) to an inner engine of disembodied reason.

Instead, much of our skilled engagement with the world flows, we saw, from the way subtle neural changes enable the embodied agent to rather directly engage the world, without representing every detail of bodily form and action-taking capacity (a neat example was the way tool-use affects receptive field properties that then implicitly distinguish "near" space and "far" space). But by the same token, all this is now highly negotiable, with the body-schema and other supporting resources apparently able to re-form and reconfigure as components, interfaces, and resources change and shift.

All this matters, both scientifically and philosophically. It matters scientifically since it puts plasticity and adaptability where they belong, at center stage of our best models of minds, agents, and persons. And it matters philosophically since it invites us to take our best present and future technologies very seriously, as quite literally helping to constitute who and what we are. With this picture in mind, those opening fears expressed by Bruce Sterling should seem infinitely less compelling. Sterling paints a truly frightening picture of an augmented agent within whom "the CPU is a human being: old, weak, vulnerable, pitifully limited, possibly senile." Such fears, I hope to have suggested, play upon a deeply misguided image of who and what we *already* are. They play upon an image of the human agent as doubly locked in: as a fixed mind constituted solely by a given biological brain, and as a fixed bodily presence in a wider world.

But human minds are not old-fashioned CPUs trapped in fixed and increasingly feeble corporeal shells. Instead, they are the surprisingly plastic minds of *profoundly* embodied agents: agents whose boundaries and components are forever negotiable, and for whom body, thinking, and sensing are woven flexibly (and repeatedly) from the whole cloth of situated, intentional action.

VII.   Enhancement or Subjugation?

The picture I have painted is meant to be a guardedly optimistic one. It is our basic, biologically grounded nature (or so I have suggested) to be open to a wide variety of forms of technologically mediated enhancement, from sensory substitution to bodily extension to mental extension and cognitive reconfiguration. If this picture is correct, our best tools and technologies literally become us: the human self emerges as a "soft self" (Clark 2003), a constantly negotiable collection of resources easily able to straddle and criss-cross the boundaries between biology and artifact. In this hybrid vision of our own humanity, I see potentials for repair, empowerment, and growth.

But the very same hybrid vision may raise specters of coercion, monstering, and subjugation. For clearly, not all change is for the better, and hybridization (however naturally it may come to us) is neutral rather than an intrinsic good. Uncritical talk of human "enhancement" thus threatens to beg philosophically, culturally, and politically important questions. How do we distinguish genuine enhancement from pernicious encroachment and new horizons from new impositions? Such questions demand sustained, informed debate going far beyond the scope of the present treatment. But there is cause for cautious optimism, and for three interlocking reasons.

First, there is simply nothing new about human enhancement. Ever since the dawn of language and self-conscious thought, the human species has been engaged in a unique "natural experiment" in progressive niche construction (see Sterelny 2003). We engineer our own learning environments so as to create artificial developmental cocoons that impact our acquired capacities of thought and reason. Those enhanced minds then design new cognitive niches that train new generations of minds, and so on, in an empowering spiral of co-evolving complexity. The result is that, as Herbert Simon is reputed to have said, "most human intelligence is artificial intelligence anyway." Technologies of human cognitive enhancement are just one more step along this ancient path.

Second, the conscious mind is perfectly at ease with reliance upon anything that works! The biological brain is itself populated by a vast number of "zombie processes" that underpin the skills and capacities upon which successful behavior depends. There are, for example, a plethora of such unconscious processes involved in activities from grasping an object (see Milner and Goodale 1995) all the way to the flashes of insight that characterize much daily skillful problem-solving. Technology-based enhancements add, to that standard mix, still more processes whose basic operating principles are not available for conscious inspection and control. The patient using a brain-computer interface to control a wheelchair will not typically know just how it all works, or be able to reconfigure the interface or software at will. But in this respect too, the new equipment is simply on a par with much of the old; to fear that this must inevitably lead to dilutions of self-control and diminishment of responsibility is to miss the fact that we are already host to scores of similarly hidden processes. Insofar as this is compatible (in the biological case) with a sufficiently robust notion of self-control and of responsibility, it must at least be possible for the same to be true in the case of well-tuned technologically mediated enhancements.

A third reason for cautious optimism is the power of the hybrid/cyborg image itself as a means of generating public debate. For once we accept that our best tools and technologies literally become us, changing who and what we are, we must surely become increasingly diligent and exigent, demanding technological prostheses better able to serve and promote human flourishing. Empirical science is now beginning (e.g., Layard 2005) systematically to address the sources and wellsprings of human happiness and human flourishing, and the findings of these studies must themselves be taken as important data points for the design and marketing of putative technologies of enhancement. Just as the slogan that "you are what you eat" contributed to the emerging recognition that food, far from simply being fuel, had a finely nuanced impact on our mental and physical health, so the realization that we are soft selves, wide open to new forms of hybrid cognitive and physical being, should serve to remind us to choose our biotechnological unions very carefully, for in so doing we are choosing who and what we are.

VIII.   Conclusions

I have tried to show that we humans are profoundly embodied agents: creatures for whom body, sensing, world, and technology are resources apt for recruitment in ways that yield a permeable and repeatedly reconfigurable agent/world boundary. For the profoundly embodied agent, the world is not something locked away behind the fixed veil of a certain skin-bag, a reasoning engine, and a primary sensory sheath. Rather, it is a resource apt for active recruitment and use, in ways that bring new forms of embodied intelligence into being. Such agents are genuinely of their worlds, and not simply in them. They are not helpless bystanders watching the passing show from behind a fixed veil of sensing, acting, and representing, but the active architects of their own bounds and capacities.[12] Such a perspective invites a cautious optimism concerning converging technologies for improving human performance.

This discussion has emphasized the potential for new forms of human-machine (or brain-machine) interface. But such technologies may also be chemical, computational, genetic, bio-mechanical, or nanotechnological. They may augment and alter mind, sensing, and body. But whatever the form, the key to successful integration and assimilation looks to be the same: the creation of new forms of rich, feedback-driven agent-world circuits, with sensing and acting under active intentional Control.

Recognition of our vast potential for bio-technological mergers and coalitions should, I finally argue, be a source not of fear and loathing but of guarded hope and cautious optimism. It should increase our respect for the deep biological plasticity that makes such mergers possible, reduce our fears of an unnatural "post-human" future, and license greater expectations concerning the answerability of our chosen tools and technologies to our best empirical models of the wellsprings of human happiness and human flourishing.

Notes

This essay is respectfully dedicated to the memory of Francisco Varela. Thanks to all the participants at the "tribute to Francisco Varela" held at the Sorbonne, Paris, in June 2004 for useful comments and criticisms.

1   This is by no means an isolated case. Susan Hurley (1998) argues convincingly that perception typically involves whole cycles of input-output behavior in which sensing and acting dynamically combine to yield ongoing adaptive fit between whole organisms and the world. This perspective also fits well with recent work in so-called interactive vision (see Ballard 1991; Ballard et al. 1997). The theme of active engagement is similarly visible in a variety of recent treatments that stress the importance of motor activity to perception (see e.g. O'Regan and Noe 2001; Churchland et al. 1994; Clark 1999; Noe 2004).

2   In fact, it is rather doubtful that these kinds of Gibsonian invariant detection involve truly high-bandwidth coupling at all. But (given the extreme difficulty of finding a non-controversial measure of objective bandwidth) I am willing to grant this for the sake of argument. My point will be that such high-bandwidth coupling, even if present, does not undermine the idea of interfaces located at just those points.

3   A typical description reads: "Computational Grids enable the sharing, selection, and aggregation of a wide variety of geographically distributed computational resources (such as supercomputers, compute clusters,

storage systems, data sources, instruments, people) and presents them as a single, unified resource for solving large-scale compute and data intensive computing applications" (Quote taken from the GRID computing information center at: http://www.grideomputing.com/, last accessed September 2006).

4   See Bachy-Rita and Kercel 2003; Clark 2003; Mussa-Ivaldi and Miller 2003.

5   See http://www.stelare.va.cornau and full discussion in Clark 2003: ch. 5.

6   Gallagher (1998) expresses the difference like this: "Body schema can be defined as a system of preconscious, subpersonal processes that play a dynamic role in governing posture and movement … There is an important and often overlooked conceptual difference between the subpersonal body schema and what is usually called body image. The latter is most often defined as a conscious idea or mental representation that one has of one's own body."

7   Thanks to an anonymous referee for pressing this issue.

8   But see Simons et al. 2002 for some important provisos.

9   For some more detailed explorations of this idea, see O'Regan and Noe 2001; Clark 2002.

10   For a lovely example of this, see Gray and Fu 2004.

11   See, among many others, Varela et al. 1991; Clark 1997; and O'Regan and Noe 2001.

12   For some important explorations of these themes, see Heidegger 1962 [1927]; Merleau-Ponty 1945 [1962]; Varela et al. 1991; and O'Regan and Noe 2001.

References

Bach-y-Rita, P. and Kercel, S.W. (2003) "Sensory Substitution and the Human-Machine Interface." *Trends in Cognitive Sciences* 7/12, pp. 541–546.

Ballard, Dana. (1991) "Animate Vision." *Artificial Intelligence* 48, pp. 57–86.

Ballard, Dana, Hayhoe, Mary, Pook, Polly, and Rao, Rajesh. (1997) "Deictic Codes for the Embodiment of Cognition." *Behavioral and Brain Sciences* 20, pp. 723–767.

Beer, Randall D. (2000) "Dynamical Approaches to Cognitive Science." *Trends in Cognitive Sciences* 4/3, pp. 1–99.

Berti, Anna and Frassinetti, Francesca (2000) "When Far Becomes Near: Re-Mapping of Space by Tool Use." *Journal of Cognitive Neuroscience* 12, pp. 415–420.

Carmena, Jose, Lebedev, Mikhail, Crist, Roy, et al. (2003) "Learning to Control a Brain-Machine Interface for Reaching and Grasping by Primates." *PloS Biology (Public Library of Sciences: Biology)* 1/2, pp. 193–208.

Churchland, Paul, Ramachandran, V.S., and Sejnowski, Terrence (1994) "A Critique of Pure Vision." In Christof Koch and Joel Davis, eds., *Large-Scale Neuronal Theories of the Brain*. Cambridge, MA: MIT Press, pp. 23–61.

Clark, Andy (1997) *Being There: Putting Brain, Body and World Together Again*. Cambridge, MA: MIT Press.

Clark, Andy (1999) "Visual Awareness and Visuomotor Action." *Journal of Consciousness Studies* 6/11–12, pp. 1–18.

Clark, Andy (2002) "Is Seeing All it Seems? Action, Reason and the Grand Illusion." *Journal of Consciousness Studies* 9/5–6. Reprinted in Alva Noe, ed., *Is the Visual World a Grand Illusion?* Thorverton, UK: Imprint Academic (2002).

Clark, Andy (2003) *Natural-Born Cyborgs: Minds, Technologies and the Future of Human Intelligence*. New York: Oxford University Press.

Clark, Andy and Chalmers, David J. (1998) "The Extended Mind." *Analysis* 58/1, pp. 7–19.

Gallagher, Shaun (1998) "Body Schema and Intentionality." In José Bermudez, ed., *The Body and the Self*. Cambridge, MA: MIT Press, pp. 25–244.

Gibson, James J. (1979) *The Ecological Approach to Visual Perception*. New York: Houghton-Mifflin.

Gonzalez, Juan C. and Bach-y-Rita, Paul "Perceptual Adaptive Recalibration: Tactile Sensory Substitution in Blind Subjects" (manuscript).

Gray, Wayne D. and Fu, Wai-Tat (2004) "Soft Constraints in Interactive Behavior. 2 *Cognitive Science* 28/3, pp. 359–382.

Haugeland, John (1998) "Mind Embodied and Embedded." In John Haugeland, *Having Thought*. Cambridge, MA: MIT Press, pp. 207–237.

Heidegger, Martin (1962 [1927]). *Sein und Zeit*. Trans. J. Macquarrie and E. Robinson, 1962). New York: Harper & Row.

Hurley, Susan L. (1998) *Consciousness in Action*. Cambridge, MA: Harvard University Press.

Layard, Richard (2005) *Happiness: Lessons from a New Science*. London: Allen Lane.

Lee, David N. and Reddish, Paul E. (1981) "Plummeting Gannets: A Paradigm of Ecological Optics." *Nature* 293, pp. 293–294.

Lungarella Max, Metta, Giorgio, Pfeifer, Rolf, and Sandini, Giulio (2003) "Developmental Robotics: A Survey." *Connection Science* 15/4, pp. 151–190.

Maravita, Angelo and Iriki, Atsushi (2004) "Tools for the Body (Schema)." *Trends in Cognitive Sciences* 8/2, pp. 79–86.

Maturana, Humberto (1980) "Biology of Cognition." In Humberto Maturana, and Francisco Varela, *Autopoiesis and Cognition*. Dordrecht: Reidel, pp. 2–62.

McBeath, Michael, Shaffer, Dennis, and Kaiser, Mary (1995) "How Baseball Outfielders Determine Where to Run to Catch Fly Balls." *Science* 268, pp. 569–571.

Meltzoff, Andrew N. and Moore, M. Keith (1997) "Explaining Facial Imitation: A Theoretical Model." *Early Development and Parenting* 6, pp. 179–192.

Merleau-Ponty, Maurice (1945 [1962]) *The Phenomenology of Perception*, trans. Colin Smith. London: Routledge.

Milner, David A. and Goodale, Melvyn A. (1995) *The Visual Brain in Action*. Oxford: Oxford University Press.

Mussa-Ivaldi, Ferdinando and Miller, Lee (2003) "Brain-Machine Interfaces: Computational Demands and Clinical Needs Meet Basic Neuroscience." *Trends in Cognitive Sciences* 26/6, pp. 329–334.

Noe, Alva (2004) *Action in Perception*. Cambridge, MA: MIT Press.

O'Regan, J. Kevin and Noe, Alva (2001) "A Sensorimotor Approach to Vision and Visual Consciousness." *Behavioral and Brain Sciences* 24/5, pp. 883–975.

Pinker, Steven (1997) *How the Mind Works*. New York: Norton.

Ramachandran, Vilayanur S. and Blakeslee, Sandra (1998) *Phantoms in the Brain: Probing the Mysteries of the Human Mind*. New York: Morrow & Co.

Schrope, Mark (2001) "Simply Sensational." *New Scientist* (June 2), pp. 30–33.

Simons, Daniel J., Chabris, Christopher F., Schnur, Tatiana T., and Levin, Daniel T. (2002) "Evidence for Preserved Representations in Change Blindness." *Consciousness and Cognition* 11, pp. 78–97.

Simons, Daniel J. (2000) "Current Approaches to Change Blindness." *Visual Cognition* 7, pp. 1–15.

Sterelny, Kim (2003) *Thought in a Hostile World: The Evolution of Human Cognition*. Oxford: Blackwell.

Sterling, Bruce (2004) "Robots and the Rest of Us: Fear and Loathing on the Human-Machine Frontier." *Wired* (May), p. 116.

Varela, Francisco, Thompson Evan, and Rosch, Eleanor (1991) *The Embodied Mind*. Cambridge, MA: MIT Press.

Webb, Barbara (1996) "A Cricket Robot." *Scientific American* 275, pp. 62–67.

Further Reading

Clark, Andy (2005) *Intrinsic Content, Active Memory, and the Extended Mind Analysis* 65/1 (January), pp. 1–11.

12

Artificial General Intelligence
and the Future of Humanity

Ben Goertzel

What will be the next huge leap in humanity's progress? We cannot know for sure, but I am reasonably confident that it will involve *the radical extension of technology into the domain of thought*.

Ray Kurzweil (2000, 2005) has eloquently summarized the arguments in favor of this position. We have created tools to carry out much of the practical work previously done by human bodies. Next we will create tools to carry out the work currently done by human minds. We will create powerful robots and artificially intelligent software programs – not merely "narrow AI" programs carrying out specific tasks, but AGIs, artificial general intelligences capable of coping with unpredictable situations in intelligent and creative ways. We will do this for the same reason we created hand-axes, hammers, factories, cars, antibiotics, and computers – because we seek to make our lives easier, more entertaining, and more interesting. Nations and corporations will underwrite AGI research and development in order to gain economic advantage over competitors – this happens to a limited extent now, but will become far more dramatic once AGI technology has advanced a little further. And the result will be something unprecedented in human history: At a certain point, we humans will no longer be the most generally intelligent creatures on the planet.

And – supposing this is true – what will be the next step beyond this? Where will the acceleration of technology ultimately lead us? Of course it's impossible for us to say, at this point. By analogy, I like to imagine the first humans to create a language with complex sentences, sitting around the campfire speculating about where the wild new invention of "language" is ultimately going to lead them. They might have some interesting insights, but would they foresee mathematics, Dostoevsky, hip-hop, PhotoShop, supersymmetry, remote-piloted cruise missiles, *World of Warcraft*, or the Internet?

The Transhumanist Reader: Classical and Contemporary Essays on the Science, Technology, and Philosophy of the Human Future, First Edition. Edited by Max More and Natasha Vita-More.
© 2013 John Wiley & Sons, Inc. Published 2013 by John Wiley & Sons, Inc.

However, basic logic lets us draw a few conclusions about the nature of a world including powerful AGIs. One is: If humans can create AGIs more intelligent than themselves, most likely these first-generation AGIs will be able to create AGIs with yet greater intelligence. And so on – these second-generation AGIs will be able to create yet smarter AGIs. This is what mathematician I.J. Good, back in the 1960s, called the "intelligence explosion" (Good 1965). The dramatic potential consequences of this sort of intelligence explosion led science fiction writer Vernor Vinge, in the early 1990s, to speak of a coming "technological Singularity" (Vinge 1993). Ray Kurzweil has done a huge amount to bring the Singularity meme to the world's attention, via his 2005 book *The Singularity Is Near* and his numerous speeches and articles.

Not everyone believes the Singularity is near, of course. On Kurzweil's kurzweilai.net website, you can also find counter-arguments by Kurzweil to many of the complaints made by detractors of the Singularity idea. Transhumanist thinker Max More argues that we're more likely to see a fairly gradual Surge (or series of non-simultaneous Surges) than a Singularity (More 2009).

Philosopher David Chalmers (2010) has laid out a rigorous analytical argument explaining why a Singularity is very likely to happen, following the basic logic of I.J. Good's "intelligence explosion" idea. But Chalmers is a bit more conservative than Kurzweil in the particulars. Kurzweil projects a Singularity sometime around 2045, but Chalmers discusses a Singularity occurring sometime within the next few hundred years, characterized by an explosion from human-level AGI to massively super-intelligent AGI during a period of decades. I respect the care and rigor of Chalmers' analytical approach, but in the end I suspect Kurzweil is probably close to the mark. I even think we could see a Singularity well before Kurzweil's projected 2045, if the right alignment of scientific progress and economic interest comes about.

My own particular focus, in my work as a scientist, is mainly on the AGI aspect. The Singularity (or Surge, or whatever) is going to involve a variety of different technologies, including genetic engineering, nanotech, novel computing hardware and maybe quantum computing, robotics, brain-computer interfacing, and a lot more. No doubt there will be new categories of technology that we can't now envision. However, in the "intelligence explosion" perspective, AGI plays a special role – it's the main technology catalyzing the next wave of radical change, taking us from the state of "humans with advanced tools but old fashioned bodies and brains" to a new condition that includes radically posthuman features.

The Top Priority for Mankind

In early 2009 I was contacted by some folks associated with the World Economic Forum – best known for their annual conference in Davos, Switzerland – to write an article for distribution at the Summer Davos World Economic Forum that summer in Dalian, China. The attendees at Davos are the world's political and business movers and shakers – top politicians and CEOs and philanthropists and so forth. My contribution was to be included in a collection of articles on the theme of "Mankind's Top Priority."

I like to get right to the point, so the title of my article was: "Mankind's Top Priority Should Be the Creation of Beneficent AI with Greater than Human Intelligence." The Summer Davos Forum is also called the "Annual Meeting of the New Champions," so I thought this was particularly appropriate. The "New Champions" phrase was presumably chosen to refer to the leaders of China, India, and other emerging markets. But I wanted to question the assumption that the new champions leading humanity onwards would always continue to be humans.

What I told the Davos participants is that:

Our top priority should be the creation of beneficent artificial minds with greater than human general intelligence, which can then work together with us to solve the other hard problems and explore various positive avenues.

The pursuit of Artificial General Intelligence (AGI) is currently a small niche of the research and development world – most of the AI research done today focuses on the creation of highly specialized "narrow AI" systems solving isolated problems. But my contention is that AGI should receive dramatically more emphasis and should in fact be the human race's top priority going forward. The reasoning behind this contention is simple: whatever the hard problem at hand, a greater than human intelligence with the proper motivational system is going to solve it better than humans can.

This may seem a farfetched notion, but an increasing number of technologists believe that greater than human AI could arrive sooner than most people think, quite plausibly within the next 2–3 decades. Toward this end each year a number of researchers have gathered in an international conference on Artificial General Intelligence. If these optimistic predictions are accurate, clearly this has extremely important implications for the way we think about ourselves and our future.

The potential benefits to be delivered by advanced AGI are difficult to overestimate. Once we are able to create artificial minds vastly more intelligent than our own, there are no clear limits to what we may be able to achieve, working together with our creations. The possibilities quickly start to sound science fictional – but in the era of space travel, the Internet, genetic engineering, nanotech and quantum computing, the boundary between science fiction and reality progressively blurs.

I then proceeded to articulate the massive benefits that advanced AGI technology could offer various areas of endeavor, such as biomedical research, nanotechnology, energy research, cognitive enhancement, and so forth – as well as the possibility of AGIs that program AGIs, intelligence explosion style. Davos is supposed to be about thinking big, and I wanted to encourage the participants to think *really* big. The creation of AGI with general intelligence at the human level or beyond will have a more dramatic, important, and fascinating impact than anything on the program at Davos that year, or any other year so far.

AGI and the Transformation of Individual and Collective Experience

For the Davos audience, I decided to focus on practical business, engineering, and science applications – energy, medicine, and so forth. But I actually think the applications to modifying the inner and social worlds are at least as important and interesting. The advent of AGI, I believe, is ultimately going to lead to the obsolescence – or at least the radical transmogrification – of many of the most familiar features of our inner lives, like the way we conceive of ourselves, the feeling of free will that we have, the sense we have that our consciousness is sharply distinct from the world around us, the sense we have that our mind and awareness is within us rather than entwined in our interactions with other minds and the external environment.

As neurophilosopher Thomas Metzinger (2003) argues brilliantly in his book *Being No One*, the "self" as the human mind constructs and experiences it is actually a "self model" – it's a symbolic and emotional system that is constructed to reflect a judiciously compressed and distorted version of the actual mind of which it's a part. None of us is really our selves. Metzinger demonstrates this beautifully via consideration of people with various brain injuries that affect the way their mind constructs their selves.

The empirical inadequacy of the commonsense notion of "free will" has been pointed out by a host of philosophers over the ages – I've always been particularly partial to Nietzsche's likening of the will to an army commander who takes responsibility for the actions of his troops, after the actions have already been taken, regardless of the fact that he played no direct role in ordering or orchestrating the actions. Philosopher Daniel Wegner has presented very systematic arguments in this direction, in his book *The Illusion of Conscious Will* (Wegner 2002). Taking one step further, in his book *The Neurophilosophy of Free Will*, Henrik Walter (2001) introduces a notion of "natural autonomy" that bears some resemblance to free will and also agrees with scientific data. In essence, natural autonomy amounts to the idea that if we make decisions that depend sensitively on our brain/mind states, that are rationally comprehensible to us, and that are integrally associated with our self-model and sense of agency, then we are "freely willing" in the only scientifically meaningful sense there is – and no further more mystical sense of free will is necessary.

The fallaciousness of the feeling of individuation and separateness we possess – especially in modern Western culture – has been driven home extensively by the "extended mind" and "embodied mind" communities in cognitive science. It's much better grounded to conceive of a human mind as something including various loops of interaction between brain, body, and social and physical environment. But this is not how we normally think of ourselves – it's not how our selves are built, it's not how we model our "willed" actions.

When we are interacting every day with AGIs that, due to their different cognitive architectures, are not defined by these same constructs (self, will, individual awareness), what will happen to the architecture and dynamics of our minds? More dramatically, when we have hybridized our minds with AGI systems – via brain-computer interfacing (Lebedev and Nicolelis 2006) progressively modified and hybridized mind uploads (Sandberg and Bostrom 2008) or other radical technologies that AGIs may help us invent – then what happens? Becoming cyborg-ically fused with an AGI that doesn't confuse its self-model with its actual existence, that doesn't mistake its natural autonomy for free will, and that fully recognizes its embeddedness in its embodied, social and physical surround – will surely be the ultimate head trip. This is at least as interesting as longevity drugs and molecular or even femto-scale assemblers.

AGI and the Global Brain

Also key to note is the relation between AGI and the emerging global brain. Francis Heylighen (2011) and others have posed articulate arguments that, due mainly to the advance of computing and communication technologies, the various human minds on Earth are gradually becoming incorporated into a greater Earth-level mind that may be thought of as a "Global Brain." Just as each neuron in a human brain is, in a sense, free to be a neuron and make its individual choices as to when to fire or not based on its surround, so we are free to be individual humans and to act according to our own natural autonomy – but just as the neuron acts as part of the overall self-coordinated activity of the human brain, so does each human act as part of the overall self-coordinated activity of the global brain.

I believe the Global Brain, in some sense, already exists – and that it will get more and more intelligent and intense as computing and communication technologies develop, even without AGI. But I think that the unleashing of advanced AGI on the Net will cause a massive increase in the power of the Global Brain. A network of advanced AGIs may come to serve as the "central cortex" of the Global Brain, with the rest – including humans and narrow AI programs – serving as additional processing units. The particulars of this are yet to unfold, and may be hard for us, as individual humans, to understand as they do.

What is a Mind that We Might Build One?

But why am I so confident that building a powerful AGI is really a plausible thing to do in the near future?

There are five big reasons why I think advanced AGI is quite plausibly just around the corner:

1. **Computers and computer networks are very powerful** now, and getting more and more so.
2. **Computer science has advanced greatly**, providing all manner of wonderful algorithms, many wrapped up in easily accessible code libraries (like STL, Boost, and GSL, to name three libraries I use in my own work), and many already engineered so as to be capable of running on distributed networks of multiprocessor machines.
3. **Robots and virtual worlds have matured significantly**, making it feasible to interface AI systems with complex environments at relatively low cost.
4. **Cognitive science has advanced tremendously**, so that we now have a pretty strong basic understanding of what the different parts of the human mind are, what sorts of things they do, and how they work together (even though we still don't understand that much about the internal dynamics of the various parts of the mind, nor how they're implemented in the brain).
5. **The Internet provides fantastic tools for collaboration** – both in terms of sharing of ideas among groups of people (email lists, wikis, Web repositories of research papers), and in terms of collaborative software code creation (e.g. version control systems used by open source projects).

Putting these five factors together, one has a situation where a distributed, heterogeneous group of passionate experts can work together, implementing collections of advanced algorithms on powerful computers, within software architectures modeled on human cognitive science. This is, I strongly suspect, how AGI is going to get created.

In all four of these areas, there has been quite amazing progress in the last two decades. There's no comparison between the situation now and the situation back in the 1960s and 1970s, or the late 1950s when the AI field was founded.

Putting together advances in computing hardware, robots and virtual worlds, algorithms and cognitive science, one arrives, I suggest, at a systematic and viable approach to advanced AGI. You start with a diagram explaining how the human mind works – what the main processes are and how they interact. You look at the assemblage of existing algorithms and data structures, and figure out a set of algorithms and data structures that will do everything specified in the cognitive science diagram. Then you implement these algorithms and data structures in a way that can operate scalably on modern networks of multiprocessor machines. Since this is a rather large job, you don't do it yourself, but you rely on a team of people communicating via the Internet, and drawing on expertise from others outside your team, in the form of Internet communications, online research papers, and so forth.

This is what my colleagues and I are doing now with our OpenCog project (Goertzel et al. 2010, 2011). It's what a number of other research teams are doing too. According to my best understanding, it's how powerful AGI is going to get created.

Of course this isn't the only possible path to creating advanced AGI. As Kurzweil and others have noted, it's possible that detailed brain emulation will get there first. I'm focusing on the integrative cognitive and computer science-based approach here, because it's the one I'm following in most of my own work, and it's the one that I personally intuit has the greatest chance of rapid success. But ultimately, if either approach succeeds it will enable the other one. An AGI built via integrative cognitive and computer science will be a huge help in unraveling the mysteries of the brain; and an AGI built via emulating the brain would enable all sorts of experimentation that can't be done on biological brains, thus leading us to various less brainlike AGI architectures incorporating various computer science advances.

As all these allied areas advance, AGI research will get easier and easier. So, if we AGI researchers wanted to make our lives easier, we would just wait for the technology infrastructure to mature, and then start working on AGI some number of years from now.

So what's the big hurry? Of course, many researchers are pushing fast toward AGI just because they want to be the first, or out of the sheer passion of the pursuit. But there is also, in some circles, a concern that if AGI is developed too *late*, the risk of a dangerous outcome for humanity may be far greater.

If we can develop advanced AGI *soon*, the argument goes, then the chance of a young AGI somehow spiraling out of human control – or being rapidly deployed by evil humans for massive destruction – seems fairly low. For a new AGI to be used in destructive ways now, or in the near future, would require use of a lot of complex, slow-moving infrastructure involving the participation of a lot of people. On the other hand, once there is a lot more advanced technology of various sorts around, it could well be possible for a young AGI to wreak a lot of damage.

Why So Little Work on AGI?

One natural question to ask is: if advanced AGI is possible, and maybe even achievable with current hardware technology – and if its rapid achievement has palpable ethical benefits – then how come it isn't the focus of a trillion-dollar industry right now? How come AGI isn't the largest, best-funded department at MIT and Caltech and so forth?

Peter Voss, an AI theorist, entrepreneur, and futurist, has summarized the situation well. His observation, back in 2002, was that, of all the scientists and engineers working in the AI field:

1. 80 percent don't believe in the concept of General Intelligence (but instead, in a large collection of specific skills and knowledge).
2. Of those that do, 80 percent don't believe it's possible – either ever, or for a long, long time.
3. Of those that do, 80 percent work on domain-specific AI projects for reasons of commercial or academic politics (results are a lot quicker).

4. Of those left, 80 percent have the wrong conceptual framework.
5. And nearly all of the people operating under basically correct conceptual premises lack the resources to adequately realize their ideas.

I think Peter's argument is basically on-target. Of course, the 80 percent numbers are crude approximations, and most of the concepts involved are fuzzy in various ways. But an interesting observation is that, whatever the percentages actually are, most of them have decreased considerably since 2002. Today, compared to in 2002, many more AI researchers believe AGI is a feasible goal to work towards, and that it might arise within their lifetimes. The researchers participating in the AGI conference series have mostly bypassed the first two items on Peter's list. And while funding for AGI research is still very difficult compared to some other research areas, the situation has definitely improved in the last 10 years.

From my personal point of view as an AGI researcher, the most troubling of Peter's five points is the fifth one. Most AI researchers who believe AGI is feasible – and would like to be spending their lives working on it – are still working on highly domain-specific AI projects with much of their time, because that's where the funding is. Even scientists need to eat, and AGI research requires computers and programmers and so forth. I'm among the world's biggest AGI advocates, and I myself spend about half my time on AGI research and the other half on narrow-AI projects that bring me revenue to pay my mortgage and put my kids through college.

Narrow AI gets plenty of money, in forms like Google's and Microsoft's expenditure on AI-based Web search and ad placement, and the military's expenditure on AI-based intelligence analysis and unmanned vehicle control. But AGI is relatively minimally funded.

Indeed, at this stage AGI is research with at best a medium-term payoff – it's not going to make anyone's quarterly profits higher next quarter. One can potentially chart paths that transition from Narrow AI to AGI, and this may be a viable way to get to advanced AGI, but it's certainly not the fastest or easiest way – and it's different than what would happen if society were to explicitly fund AGI research in a big way.

The relatively paltry funding of AGI isn't just due to its speculative nature – society is currently willing to fund a variety of speculative science and engineering projects: billion-dollar particle accelerators, space exploration, the sequencing of human and animal genomes, stem cell research, and so forth. If these sorts of projects merit Big Science-level funding, why is AGI research left out? After all, the potential benefits should AGI proceed and get done right are obviously tremendous. There are potential dangers too, to be sure – but there are also clear potential dangers of particle physics research (discovering better bombs is arguably a hazardous pursuit), and that doesn't stop us.

Any social phenomenon has multiple intertwined causes, but the main reason for the AGI field's relatively paltry funding stream is probably negative momentum from the failures of the original generation of AI researchers. The AI gurus of the 1960s were claiming they could create human-level AI within a decade or less. They were wrong – they lacked the needed hardware, their software tools were primitive, and their conceptual understanding of intelligence was too crude. Just because they were wrong then, doesn't mean the current AGI field is similarly wrong – but the "guilt by association" lingers.

An interesting analogy is the early visionaries who foresaw the Web – Vannevar Bush in the 1950s, Ted Nelson in the 1960s, and others. They understood the potential computer technology held to give rise to something like today's Web – and Ted Nelson even tried to get something Web-like built, back before 1970. But the technology just wasn't there to support his vision. In principle it might have been doable given the technology of that era, but it would have been insanely difficult – whereas by the time the Web came about in the 1990s it seemed almost a natural consequence of the technological infrastructure existing at that time. Similarly, in the 1960s, even if someone had come up with a workable design for human-level AGI, it would have been extraordinarily difficult to get it implemented and working using the hardware and software tools available. But now, with cloud computing, multiprocessor machines with terabytes of RAM, powerful algorithm libraries and debuggers, and a far more mature theory of cognitive science, we are in a whole different position. The conceptual and technological ecosystem is poised for AGI, in the same sense that it was poised for the Web in the 1990s. And just as the Web spread faster than almost anybody foresaw – so, once it gets started, will AGI.

The crux of the matter is: it's not 1970 anymore. We have astoundingly more powerful computers, we have the Internet, we have far better brain-imaging tools and a much better understanding of neuroscience, and we have a cross-disciplinary field of cognitive science which tells us a lot about the overall structure of human cognition. We have single-molecule electric motors, we can do origami with DNA, we can build synthetic organisms via stringing together amino acids, and there are commercially available quantum computers. We can search over a trillion Web pages almost instantly from our laptops or mobile phones. We can hook tens of thousands of insanely fast multiprocessor computers together into functional units. Our guided missiles can fly in the dark to precisely specified locations and destroy precisely what they want to, with remarkably few errors (though our decisions about what to destroy are often quite questionable). We can measure brains using nuclear magnetic resonance and see which regions are most active during which sorts of mental activity. We can clone animals, and cause human organ regeneration via stem cell injections. All these things, and many, many more current realities, would have seemed wildly science fictional in 1970 – or even in 1982 when I first dug into the AI research literature. Technology and science have been advancing dramatically, and in many ways directly relevant to advance AI. The AGI field hasn't advanced as fast as some others so far, but my prediction is that – leveraging a host of related advances – the artificial intelligence explosion will be coming along soon.

Why the "AGI Sputnik" Will Change Things Dramatically and Launch a New Phase of the Intelligence Explosion

Shifting to a different historical analogy, I think about the future of AGI as falling into two phases – before and after the "AGI Sputnik" event.

When the Russians launched Sputnik, this sent a message to the world: "Wow! Going into space is not only a possibility; it's a dramatic reality! The time for humanity to explore space is now!" The consequence was the space race, and the rise of modern space technology.

Similarly, at some point, some AGI research team is going to produce a computer program or robot that does something that makes the world wake up and say: "Wow! Genuinely smart AI is not just a possibility; it's a dramatic reality! The time for humanity to create smart machines is now!" At that point, government and industry will put themselves fully behind the creation of advanced AGI – and progress will accelerate tremendously. The potential of AGI to benefit humanity, and every nation and corporation, is evidently humongous – and all that's needed to shift things dramatically from the current funding regime to something overwhelmingly different is one single crystal-clear demonstration that human-level AGI is feasible in the near term.

We don't have that demonstration right now, but I – and a number of other AGI researchers – believe we know how to do it – and I'm betting it will happen within the lifetimes of most people reading this book.

In the late 1960s and early 1970s, in the era of the Apollo moon missions, I and every other little American kid wanted to grow up and be an astronaut. After the AGI Sputnik event, kids will want to grow up and be AGI developers – or AGIs!

I believe the OpenCog AGI approach has what it takes to get us to an AGI Sputnik event – in the form, perhaps, of a video game character or a humanoid robot that holds meaningful conversations about the things in its environment. Imagine talking to a robot that really gives you sense that it knows what it's talking about – that it understands what it's doing, and knows who it is and who you are. That will be a damn strange feeling – and a wonderful one. And everyone who gets that feeling will understand that humanity is about to take the next, huge, step.

But my main point here isn't to sell my own particular approach to AGI, but to talk about AGI in general. Many of my colleagues have their own different perspectives on the optimal technical approach to create AGI. My main goal here is, first, to get across the points that AGI is probably coming fairly soon, and it's going to be a huge change and quite possibly a fantastic one for all of us.

The Risks and Rewards of Advanced AGI

There are a lot of science fiction movies about AIs going insane and killing everyone or taking over the world. And indeed, if you take the prospect of advanced AGI seriously, it's hard to rule these possibilities out – even though now, at the current stage of technology development, it's hard to understand exactly which of the many possible risks are the most realistic ones, and how the risks and rewards will balance.

In fact there are (at least) *two* major threats related to advanced AGI. One is that people might use AGIs for bad ends; and the other is that, even if an AGI is made with the best intentions, it might reprogram itself in a way that causes it to do something nasty. If it's smarter than us, we might be watching it carefully while it does this, and have no idea what's going on.

One key point, though, is that the risks and rewards of AGI must be considered in the broader context of all the other technologies currently under development, and all the social, psychological, and technological change likely to come in the next decades and centuries. It's not as though our choices are "life goes on exactly as is" versus "life as it is plus super-powerful AI." Various technologies are advancing rapidly and society is changing accordingly, and the rate of advancement of AGI is just one aspect in the mix.

I don't think there are any magic bullets to resolve the dilemmas of AGI ethics. There will almost surely be no provably Friendly AI, in spite of the wishes of Eliezer Yudkowsky (2008) and some others. Nor, in my best guess, will there be an Artilect War in which pro-AGI and anti-AGI forces battle to the death with doomsday machines, as Hugo de Garis (2005) foresees. But I don't pretend to be able to see exactly what the outcome will be. The important thing, as I see it, is that the human race as a whole engages as closely and intelligently as possible with AGI as it evolves – so that, as AGI comes about, it's not a matter of "us versus them", but rather a matter of AGIs and humans, that have become inseparable on various levels, moving forward together into new realms of science, technology, interaction, and experience.

References

Chalmers, David (2010) "The Singularity: A Philosophical Analysis." *Journal of Consciousness Studies* 17, pp. 7–65.

de Garis, Hugo (2005) *The Artilect War*. Pittsburgh: ETC Press.

Goertzel, Ben et al. (2010) "An Overview of the OpenCogBot Architecture." *Proceedings of ICAI-10*, Beijing.

Goertzel, Ben, Pitt, Joel, Wigmore, Jared, Geisweiller, Nil, Cai, Zhenhua, Lian, Ruiting, Huang, Deheng, and Yul, Gino (2011) "Cognitive Synergy between Procedural and Declarative Learning in the Control of Animated and Robotic Agents Using the OpenCogPrime AGI Architecture." *Proceedings of AAAI-11*, pp. 1436–1441.

Good, I.J. (1965) "Speculations Concerning the First Ultraintelligent Machine." *Advances in Computers* 6 (Waltham, MA: Academic Press), pp. 31–88.

Heylighen, Francis (2011) "Conceptions of a Global Brain: An Historical Review." In Leonid E. Grinin, Robert L. Carneiro, Andrey V. Korotayev, and Fred Spier, eds., *Evolution: Cosmic, Biological, and Social*. Volgograd, Russia: Uchitel Publishing, pp. 274–289.

Kurzweil, Ray (2000) *The Age of Spiritual Machines*. New York: Viking Press.

Kurzweil, Ray (2005) *The Singularity Is Near*. New York: Viking Press.

Lebedev, A and Nicolelis M. (2006) "Brain-Machine Interfaces: Past, Present and Future," *Trends in Neurosciences* 29/9, pp. 536–546.

Metzinger, Thomas (2003) *Being No One*. Rockville, MD: Springer.

More, Max (2009) "Singularity and Surge Scenarios." http://strategicphilosophy.blogspot.com/2009/06/how-fast-will-future-arrive-how-will.html (accessed October 30, 2011).

Sandberg, Anders and Bostrom, Nick (2008) *Whole Brain Emulation: A Roadmap*. Technical Report #2008-3. Future of Humanity Institute, Oxford University.

Vinge, Vernor (1993) "The Coming Technological Singularity: How to Survive in the Post-Human Era." *Whole Earth Review* (Winter).

Walter, Henrik (2001) *The Neurophilosophy of Free Will*. Cambridge, MA: MIT Press.

Wegner, Daniel (2002) *The Illusion of Conscious Will*. Cambridge, MA: MIT Press.

Yudkowsky, E. (2008) "Artificial Intelligence as a Positive and Negative Factor in Global Risk." In Nick Bostrom and Milan Cirkovic, eds., *Global Catastrophic Risks*. Oxford: Oxford University Press.

Further Reading

Drexler, Eric (1992) *Nanosystems*. Cambridge, MA: MIT Press.

Goertzel, Ben and Pennachin, Cassio (2005) *Artificial General Intelligence*. Rockville, MD: Springer.

Nilsson, Nils (2005) "Human-Level Artificial Intelligence? Be Serious!" *AI Magazine* 26/4, pp. 68–75.

13

Intelligent Information Filters and Enhanced Reality

Alexander "Sasha" Chislenko

Preface

I started to think seriously about the ideas of augmented perception and personalized views of reality after reading a number of Internet messages containing proposals to introduce language standards for online communications. Frequently, people suggest restricting certain forms of expression or polishing the language of the posts to make them less offensive and more generally understandable. While looking forward to the advantages of improved communications, I wanted see them provided by tools that would at the same time make the language mix of the Net more free and diverse.

In this essay, I suggest that active information-filtering technologies may help us approach this goal for both textual and multimedia information. I also pursue this concept further, discussing the introduction of augmented perception and Enhanced Reality (ER), and share some observations and predictions of the transformations in people's perception of the world and themselves in the course of the technological progress.

Text Translation and Its Consequences

Many of us are used to having incoming email filtered, decrypted, formatted, and shown in our favorite colors and fonts. These techniques can be taken further. Customization of spelling (e.g., American to British or archaic to modern) would be a straightforward process. Relatively simple conversions could also let you see any text with your favorite date and time formats, use metric or

Originally published in *Extropy: The Journal of Transhumanist Thought* 16 (1996). Copyright © Max More.

imperial measures, implement obscenity filters, abbreviate or expand acronyms, omit or include technical formulas, personalize synonym selection and punctuation rules, and use alternative numeric systems and alphabets (including phonetic and pictographic). Text could also be digested for a given user, translated to his native language, and even read aloud with his favorite actor's voice.

My friend Gary Bean suggested possible implementation of "cliché translators" that would explicitly convey the meaning of a sentence that is known to the translator, but not necessarily to the reader. For example, the phrase "that's an interesting idea" might be translated as "I have serious reservations about this." In the reverse operation, words and phrases can be replaced with politically correct euphemisms.

After the recent Communication Decency Act, Robert Carr developed a remarkable "HexOn Exon" program that allows the user to convert obscene words in the messages into the names of the senators responsible for this Act, and vice versa. Besides presenting a humorous attempt to bypass the new obscenity censorship, this program demonstrates that allocating both responsibilities and rights for the contents of a message among multiple authoring and filtering agencies may not be easy.

Translation between various dialects and jargons, though difficult, should still take less effort than the translation between different natural languages, since only a part of message semantics has to be processed. Good translation filters would give "linguistic minorities" – speakers of languages ranging from Pig Latin to E-Prime and Loglan – a chance to practice their own languages while communicating with the rest of the world.

Some jargon filters have already been developed, and you can benefit from them by enjoying reading Ible-Bay, the Pig Latin version of the Bible, or using Dialectizer program to convert your English texts to Fudd or Cockney.

Such translation agents would allow rapid linguistic and cultural diversification, to the point where the language you use to communicate with the world could diverge from everybody else's as far as the requirement of general semantic compatibility may allow. It is interesting that today's HTML Guide already calls for the "divorce of content from representation," suggesting that you should focus on what you want to convey rather than on how people will perceive it.

Some of these features will require full-scale future artificial intelligence, such as "sentient translation programs" described by Vernor Vinge in "A Fire Upon The Deep"). In the meantime, they could be successfully emulated by human agents.

Surprisingly, even translations between different measurement systems can be difficult. For example, your automatic translator might have trouble converting such expressions as "a few inches away," "the temperature will be in the 80s," or "a duck with two feet." A proficient translator might be able to convey the original meaning, but the best approach would be to write the message in a general semantic form which would store the information explicitly, indicating in the examples above where the terms refer to measurements, whether you insist on the usage of the original system, and the intended degree of precision. As long as the language is expressive enough, it is suitable for the task – and this requirement is purely semantic; symbol sets, syntax, grammar, and everything else can differ dramatically.

A translation agent would interactively convert natural-language texts to this semantic lingua franca and interpret them back according to a given user profile. It could also reveal additional parts of the document depending on users' interests, competence in the field, and access privileges.

Currently, we can structure our mental images any way we want so long as we can translate them to a common language. This has led to relatively stable standardized languages and a great variability among minds. Likewise, intelligent software translators could let us make our languages as liberated as our minds and push the communication standards beyond our biologi-cal bodies. (It really means just further exosomatic expansion of the human functional body, but the liberation still goes beyond the traditional human interpretation of "skin-encapsulated" per-sonal identity.)

So will there be more variety or more standardization? Most likely both, as flexible translation will help integrate knowledge domains currently isolated by linguistic and terminological barri-ers, and at the same time will protect linguistically adventurous intellectual excursions from the danger of losing contact with the semantic mainland. Intelligent translators could facilitate the development of more comprehensive semantic architectures that would make the global body of knowledge at the same time more diverse and more coherent.

Information may be stored and transmitted in the general semantic form. With time, an increasing number of applications can be expected to use the enriched representation as their native mode of operation. Client translation software will provide an emulation of the tradi-tional world of "natural" human interactions while humans still remain to appreciate it. The semantic richness of the system will gradually shift away from biological brains, just as data storage, transmission, and computation have in recent history. Humans will enjoy growing ben-efits from the system they launched, but at the expense of understanding the increasingly com-plex "details" of its internal structure, and for a while will keep playing an important role in guiding the flow of events. Later, after the functional entities liberate themselves from the realm of flesh that gave birth to them, the involvement of humans in the evolutionary process will be of little interest to anybody except humans themselves.

Enhanced Multimedia

Similar image-transformation techniques can be applied to multimedia messages. Recently, a video system was introduced that allows you to "soften the facial features" of the person on the screen. Advanced real-time video filters could remove wrinkles and pimples from your face or from the faces of your favorite political figures, caricature their opponents, give your mother-in-law a Klingon persona on your videophone, reclothe people in your favorite fashion, and replace visual clutter in the background with something tasteful.

It also seems possible to augment human senses with transparent external information pre-processors. For example, if your audio/video filters notice an object of potential interest that fails to differ from its signal environment enough to catch your attention, the filters can amplify or otherwise differentiate (move, flash, change pitch, etc.) the signal momentarily, to give you enough time to focus on the object, but not enough to realize what triggered your attention. In effect, you would instantly see your name in a text or find Waldo in a puzzle as easily as you would notice a source of loud noise or a bright light.

While such filters do not have to be transparent, they may be a way to provide a comfortable "natural" feeling of augmented perception for the next few generations of humans, until the forthcoming integration of technological and neural processing systems makes such kludgy patches obsolete.

Some non-transparent filters can already be found in military applications. Called "target enhancements," they allow military personnel to see the enemy's tanks and radars nicely outlined and blinking. More advanced filtering techniques could put consistent dynamic edits into the perceived world. Volume controls could sharpen your senses by allowing you to adjust the level of the signal or zoom in on small or distant objects. Calibration tools could expand the effective spectral range of your perception by changing the frequency of the signal to allow you to hear ultrasound or perceive X-rays and radiowaves as visible light.

Conversions between different types of signals may allow you, for example, to "see" noise as fog while enjoying quiet, or convert radar readings from decelerating pedestrians in front of you into images of red brake lights on their backs.

Artificial annotations to perceived images would add text tags with names and descriptions to chosen objects, append warning labels with skull and crossbones on boxes that emit too much radiation, and surround angry people with red auras (serving as a "cold reading" aid for wanna-be psychics). Reality filters may help you filter all signals coming from the world the way your favorite mail reader filters you messages, based on your stated preferences or advice from your peers. With such filters you may choose to see only the objects that are worthy of your attention, and completely remove useless and annoying sounds and images (such as advertisements) from your view. Perception utilities would give you additional information in a familiar way – project clocks, thermometers, weather maps, and your current EKG readings upon [the image of] the wall in front of you, or honk a virtual horn every time a car approaches you from behind. They could also build on existing techniques that present us with recordings of the past and forecasts of the future to help people develop an immersive trans-temporal perception of reality. "World improvement" enhancements could paint things in new colors, put smiles on faces, "babify" figures of your incompetent colleagues, change night into day, erase shadows, and improve landscapes.

Finally, completely artificial additions could project northern lights, meteorites, and supernovas upon your view of the sky, or populate it with flying toasters, virtualize and superimpose on the image of the real world your favorite mythical characters and imaginary companions, and provide other educational and recreational functions. I would call the resulting image of the world Enhanced Reality (ER).

Structure of Enhanced Reality

One may expect that as long as there are things left to do in the physical world, there will be interest in application of ER technology to improve our interaction with real objects, while Virtual Reality (VR) in its traditional sense of pure simulation can provide us with safe training environments and high-bandwidth fiction. Later, as ER becomes considerably augmented with artificial enhancements, and VR incorporates a large amount of archived and live recordings of the physical world, the distinctions between the two technologies may blur.

Some of the interface enhancements can be made common, temporarily or permanently, for large communities of people. This would allow people to interact with each other using, and referring to, the ER extensions as if they were parts of the real world, thus elevating the ER entities from individual perceptions to parts of shared, if not objective, reality. Some of such enhancements can follow the existing metaphors. A person who has a reputation as a liar could appear to have a long nose. Entering a high-crime area, people may see the sky darken and hear distant funeral music. Changes in global political and economic situations with possible effects on some ethnic groups may be translated into claps of thunder and other culture-specific omens.

Other extensions could be highly individualized. It is already possible, for example, to create personalized traffic signs. Driving by the same place, an interstate truck driver may see a "no go" sign projected on his windshield, while the driver of the car behind him will see a sign saying "Bob's house – next right." More advanced technologies may create personalized interactive illusions that would be loosely based on reality and propelled by real events, but would show the world the way a person wants to see it. The transparency of the illusion would not be important, since people are already quite good at hiding bitter or boring truths behind a veil of pleasant illusions. Many people even believe that their entirely artificial creations (such as music or temples) either "reveal" the truth of the world to them or, in some sense, "are" the truth. Morphing unwashed Marines into singing angels or naked beauties would help people reconcile their dreams with their observations.

Personal illusions should be built with some caution however. The joy of seeing the desired color on the traffic light in front of you may not be worth the risk. As a general rule, the more control you want over the environment, the more careful you should be in your choice of filters. However, if the system creating your personal world also takes care of all your real needs, you may feel free to live in any fairy tale you like.

In many cases, ER may provide us with more true-to-life information than our "natural" perception of reality. It could edit out mirages, show us our "real" images in a virtual mirror instead of the mirror images provided by the real mirror, or allow us to see into – and through – solid objects. It could also show us many interesting phenomena that human sensors cannot perceive directly. Giving us knowledge of these things has been a historical role of science. Merging the obtained knowledge with our sensory perception of the world may be the most important task of Enhanced Reality.

Historical Observations

People have been building artificial symbolic "sur-realities" for quite a while now, though their artifacts (from art to music to fashions to traffic signs) have been mostly based on the physical features of the perceived objects. Shifting some of the imaging workload to the perception software may make communications more balanced, flexible, powerful, and inexpensive.

With time, a growing proportion of objects of interest to an intelligent observer will be entirely artificial, with no inherent "natural" appearance. Image modification techniques then may be incorporated into integrated object designs that would simultaneously interface with a multitude of alternative intelligent representation agents.

The implementation of ER extensions would vary depending on the available technology. At the beginning, it could be a computer terminal, later a headset, then a brain implant. The implant can be internal in more than just the physical sense, as it can actually post- and re-process information supplied by biological sensors and other parts of the brain. The important thing here is not the relative functional position of the extension, but the fact of intentional redesign of perception mechanisms – a prelude to the era of comprehensive conscious self-engineering. The ultimate effects of these processes may appear quite confusing to humans, as emergence of things like personalized reality and fluid distributed identity could undermine their fundamental biological and cultural assumptions regarding the world and the self. The resulting "identity" architectures will form the kernel of transhuman civilization.

The advancement of human input processing beyond the skin boundary is not a novel phenomenon. In the audiovisual domain, it started with simple optics and hearing aids centuries ago and is now making rapid progress with all kinds of recording, transmitting, and processing machinery. With such development, "live" contacts with the "raw world" data might ultimately become rare, and could be considered inefficient, unsafe, and even illegal. This may seem an exaggeration, but this is exactly what has already happened during the last few thousand years to our perception of a more traditional resource – food. Using nothing but one's bare hands, teeth, and stomach for obtaining, breaking up, and consuming naturally grown food is quite unpopular in all modern societies for these very reasons. In the visual domain, contacts with objects that have not been intentionally enhanced for one's perception (in other words, looking at real, unmanipulated, unpainted objects without glasses) are still rather frequent for many people, and the process is still gaining momentum, in both usage time and the intensity of the enhancements.

Rapid progress of technological artifacts and still stagnant human body construction create an imperative for continuing gradual migration of all aspects of human functionality beyond the boundaries of the biological body, with human identity becoming increasingly exosomatic (non-biological).

Truth vs. Convenience

Enhanced Reality could bring good news to privacy lovers. If the filters prove sufficiently useful to become an essential part of the [post]human identity architecture, the ability to filter information about your body and other possessions out of the unauthorized observer's view may be implemented as a standard feature of ER client software. In Privacy-Enhanced Reality, you can be effectively invisible.

Of course, unless you are forced to "wear glasses," you can take them off any time and see the things the way they "are" (i.e., processed only by your biological sensors and filters that had been developed by the blind evolutionary process for jungle conditions and obsolete purposes). In my experience, though, people readily abandon the "truth" of implementation details for the convenience of the interface and, as long as the picture looks pleasing, have little interest in peeking into the binary or HTML source code or studying the nature of the physical processes they observe – or listening to those who understand them. Most likely, your favorite window onto the real world is already not the one with the curtains – it's the one with the controls…

Many people seem already quite comfortable with the thought that their environment might have been purposefully created by somebody smarter than themselves, so the construction of ER shouldn't come to them as a great epistemological shock. Canonization of chief ER engineers (probably well deserved) could help these people combine their split concepts of technology and spirituality into the long-sought-after "holistic worldview."

Biofeedback and Self-Perception

Perception enhancements may also be used for augmenting people's view of their favorite object of observation – themselves. Biological evolution has provided us with a number of important self-sensors, such as physical pain, that supply us with information about the state of our bodies, restrict certain actions, and change our emotional states. Nature invented these for pushing our primitive ancestors to taking actions they wouldn't be able to select rationally. Unfortunately, pain is not a very accurate indicator of our bodily problems. Many serious conditions do not produce any pain until it is too late to act. Pain focuses our attention on symptoms of the disease rather than causes, and is non-descriptive, uncontrollable, and often counterproductive.

Technological advances may provide us with the informational, restrictive, and emotional functions of pain without most of the above handicaps. Indicators of important, critical, or abnormal bodily functions could be put on output devices such as a monitor, watch, or even your skin. It is possible to restrain your body slightly when, for example, your blood pressure climbs too high, and to emulate other restrictive effects of pain. It may also be possible to create "artificial symptoms" of some diseases. For example, showing to a patient a graph demonstrating spectral divergence of his alpha- and delta-rhythms that may indicate some neurotransmitter deficiency may not be very useful. It would be much better to give the patient a diagnostic device that is easier to understand and more "natural-looking":

– "Hello, Doctor, my toenail's turned green!"
– "Don't worry, it's a typical arti-symptom of the XYZ condition, I'm sending you the pills."
(Actually, a watch may serve a lot better than toenails as a display.)

Sometimes, a direct feedback generating real pain may be implemented for patients who do not feel it when their activities approach dangerous thresholds. For example, a non-removable, variable-strength earclip that would cause increasing pain in your ear when your blood sugar climbs too high may dissuade you from having that extra piece of cake. A similar clip could make a baby cry out for help every time its EKG readings go bad. A more ethical solution with improved communication could be provided by attaching this clip to the doctor's ear. "I feel your pain …"

Similar techniques could be used to connect inputs from external systems to human biological receptors. Wiring exosomatic sensors to our nervous systems may allow us to better feel our environments, and start perceiving our technological extensions as parts of our bodies (which they already are). On the other hand, poor performance of your company could now give you a real pain in the neck…

Distant Future

Consequent technological advances in ER, biofeedback and other areas will lead to further blurring of demarcation lines between biological and technological systems, bodies and tools, selves and possessions, personalities and environments. These advances will eventually bring to life a world of complex, self-engineered, interconnected entities that may keep showing emulated "natural" environments to the few remaining (emulations of?) "natural" humans, who would never look behind the magic curtain for fear of seeing that crazy functional soup…

Terminological Exercises: ER < - > EP - > … - > IE - > ?! - > .

You must realize that most ER technologies suggested in this essay have little to do with changing reality and everything to do with changing our perception of it. Though ER techniques still change the-world-as-we-see-it, it would be more accurate to call them EP, for Enhanced Perception, and reserve the term ER for conceptualizing traditional technologies. The traditional technologies have always been aimed at improvement of human perception of the environment, from digestion of physical objects by the stomach (cooking) to digestion of info-features by the brain (time/clock). Since there is hardly any functional difference in how and at what stage the clock face and other images are added to our view of the world, and as the technologies will increasingly intermix, an appropriate general term may be Enhanced Interface of Self with the Environment – and, as in the case of biofeedback, the Enhanced Interface of Self with Self.

With future waves of structural change dissolving the borders between self and environment, the term may generalize into Harmonization of Structural Interrelations. Still later, when interfaces become so smooth and sophisticated that human-based intelligence will hardly be able to tell where the system core ends and interface begins, we'd better just call it Improvement of Everything. Immediately after that, we will lose any understanding of what is going on and what constitutes an improvement, and should not try to name things anymore. Not that it would matter much if we did…

Social Implications

We can imagine that progress in human information-processing will face some usual social difficulties. Your angry "Klingon" relatives may find unexpected allies among "proboscically enhanced" (aka long-nosed) people protesting against using their alternative standard of beauty as a negative stereotype. The girl next door may be wary that your "re-clothing" filters leave her in Eve's dress. Parents could be suspicious that their clean-looking kids appear to each other as tattooed skinheads or bloodthirsty demons, or replace their obscenity masks with the popular "Beavis and Butthead" obscenity-enhancement filter. Extreme naturalists will demand that the radiant icons of the Microsoft logo and Coca-Cola bottle gracefully crossing their sky should be replaced by sentimental images of the sun and the moon that once occupied their place. Libertarians would lobby their governments for the "freedom of impression" laws, while drug enforcement agencies may declare that the new perception-altering techniques are just a technological successor of simple chemical drugs, and should be prohibited for not providing an approved perception of reality.

My readers often tell me that if any version of Enhanced, Augmented, or Annotated Reality gets implemented, it might be abused by people trying to manipulate other people's views and force perceptions upon them. I realize that all human history is filled with people's attempts to trick themselves and others into looking at the world through the wrong glasses, and new powerful technologies may become very dangerous tools if placed in the wrong hands, so adding safeguards to such projects seems more than important.

Unfortunately though, a description of any idea sufficiently complex for protecting the world from such disasters wouldn't fit into an essay that my contemporaries would take time to read. So I just do what I can – clean my glasses and observe the events – and share some impressions.

Note

I am grateful to Ron Hale-Evans, Bill Alexander, and Gary Bean for inspiration and discussions that helped me shape this text.

14

Uploading to Substrate-Independent Minds

Randal A. Koene

In this essay we will use mind as the term to designate the totality and manner in which our thoughts take place. We use the term brain to refer to the underlying mechanics, the substrate and the manner in which it supports the operations needed to carry out thoughts. For example, this includes the raising and lowering of potential across the neural membrane in response to chemical flux.

Your Mind, but not Constrained to the Biological Brain

The difference between the mind that relies on these mechanics of the brain and a substrate-independent mind (SIM) is this: We can consider a mind substrate-independent when its selfsame functions that represent thinking processes can be implemented through the operations available in a number of different computational platforms. For example, if we can carry out the function of a mind both in a biological brain and in a brain that is composed of computer software or neuromorphic hardware (a hardware architecture with design principles based on biological neural systems), then that mind is substrate-independent. The mind continues to depend on a substrate to exist and to operate, of course, but there are substrate choices.

The goal of substrate-independence is to continue personality, individual characteristics, a manner of experiencing, and a personal way of processing those experiences (Koene 2011a, 2011b). Your identity, your memories can then be embodied physically in many ways. They can also be backed up and operate robustly on fault-tolerant hardware with redundancy schemes. Achieving substrate-independence will allow us to optimize the operational framework, the

Originally published in *Extropy: The Journal of Transhumanist Thought* 11 (1993). Copyright © Max More.

The Transhumanist Reader: Classical and Contemporary Essays on the Science, Technology, and Philosophy of the Human Future, First Edition. Edited by Max More and Natasha Vita-More.
© 2013 John Wiley & Sons, Inc. Published 2013 by John Wiley & Sons, Inc.

hardware, to challenges posed by novel circumstances and different environments. Think, instead of sending extremophile bacteria to slowly terraform another world into a habitat, we ourselves can be extremophiles.

Substrate-independent minds is a well-described objective. There are on the present roadmap at least six technology paths (Koene 2012) through which we may enable functions of the mind to move from substrate to substrate (i.e. gaining substrate-independence). Of those six, the path known as Whole Brain Emulation (WBE) is the most conservative one and is receiving the most attention in terms of ongoing projects and researchers directly involved (Sandberg and Bostrom 2008). WBE proposes that we:

1. Identify the scope and the resolution at which mechanistic operations within the brain implement the functions of mind that we experience.
2. Build tools that are able to acquire structural and functional information at that scope in an individual brain.
3. Re-implement the whole structure and the functions in another suitable operational substrate, just as they were implemented in the original cerebral substrate.

Whole Brain Emulation

The biological substrate that is responsible for our present thinking supports all the activity of our experience. That activity is comprised of the interactions, the relevant information transactions of the physiological components of the brain. The list of operant components is certain to include neural membranes and synapses. Possible interactions are constrained by the existing functional connections between the components – the functional connectome, which is in turn reflected by physical neuroanatomy in the structural connectome.

We consider a strategy of straightforward duplication of the activity, and look at the numbers of some of the components. The human brain has up to one hundred billion (10^{11}) neurons and between one hundred trillion (10^{14}) and one quadrillion (10^{15}) synapses. But we have reached a point where for purposes of data acquisition these objects are now considered fairly large (e.g. 200 nm to 2,000 nm for synaptic spines and 4,000 nm to 100,000 nm for the neural soma), at least by the standards of the current nanotechnology industry (working with precision at 10s to 100s of nanometers). And in terms of their activity those components are mostly quiet.

I coined the term whole brain emulation around February/March of 2000 during a discussion on the old "mind uploading research group" (MURG) mailing list, in an effort to remove confusion stemming from the use of the term "mind uploading", which better refers to a process of transfer of a mind from a biological brain to another substrate. It has since found a home in mainstream neuroscience, although the less specific term "brain emulation" is also frequently used when a project does not take on the scope of whole brains. The concept of emulation, as opposed to simulation (a term in common use where models in computational neuroscience are involved), refers to the running of an exact copy of the functions of mind on another processing platform. It is intended to be understood as analogous to the process of taking a computer program from one hardware platform (e.g., an Android cell phone) to an emulator of the same processing operations on a different hardware platform (e.g., a Macintosh computer).

Whole brain emulation differs from modeling and simulation in computational neuroscience and neuroinformatics in that the functions and parameters used for the emulation come from an individual brain, so that the emulated circuitry is identical and represents the same result of development and learning. Within that context, all of the connections, connection strengths, and response functions make sense in that they embody the characteristics that elicit the mind of that specific individual. Many of the underlying details resemble the sort of details that are also included in ambitious large-scale computational models such as in the Blue Brain project (Markram 2006) and the rat vibrissal cortex column model by Oberlaender et al. (2011), but there is that important distinction.

Projects such as Blue Brain are composed of neural circuitry that is generated by sampling stochastically from distributions of reasonable parameter values as obtained by making measurements in the brains of many different animals, and in some cases even different species. This means that the resulting models have many of the gross aspects that would be recognized in the brain of any typical member of the species. They can also display recognizable large-scale activity, such as oscillations and propagated activity. Such models can even be trained to tune their circuitry so that they carry out behaviorally interesting tasks. Yet, as with any highly complex and over-parametrized system, there are many different ways to successfully tune the system to achieve a given task. Such success is not a guarantee that the tuned system is a faithful representation of the implementation in any one specific brain.

Imagine inspecting 50 different computer programs, each with a few hundred lines of code. All of the programs were written to accomplish the same basic task. They go about it in slightly different ways and the results have variations that differ somewhat from program to program. You can either sample and learn from each of those programs and create a representative amalgam that may even be able to carry out some semblance of the same task. Or you can pick a program and copy it line by line. That is where we employ the difference in terminology. We call the stochastically generated models simulations and the faithful copies emulations. In this sense, obtaining a human connectome for WBE relates to neuroscience in a manner analogous to the way in which research in cosmology relates to astrophysics. Where astrophysics focuses on the physical or chemical properties of celestial bodies, cosmology focuses on the properties of our universe as a whole, in the one form in which it exists, of many possible forms allowed by physical properties.

By now, you can probably tell that a whole brain emulation takes a very specific tack in its approach to achieving substrate-independent minds. We consider whole brain emulation the most conservative approach. If we understood a lot more about the way the mind works and how brain produces mind then we might have far more creative or effective ways to achieve a transfer (an "upload") from a biological brain to another substrate. The resulting implementation might then be vastly more efficient, taking the greatest advantage of the new processing substrate at its disposal. When we eventually achieve that, we might (again by analogy) call it "compilation" rather than emulation. When one compiles a computer program with a good compiler instead of running it on an emulator or interpreter then the resulting code is usually much more efficient, faster, and more powerful.

At present, we probably do not know enough to carry out a feasible and practical project towards SIM that aims at such an intelligent extraction of functions and parameters in an individual brain that they could be compiled into a very different, efficient implementation that is the same mind. We do understand enough about neurons, synaptic channels, dendritic computation, diffuse messengers, and other modulating factors that we can concurrently undertake projects to catalog details about the range of those fundamental components and to identify and re-implement that neuro-anatomy and neuro-physiology in another computational substrate.

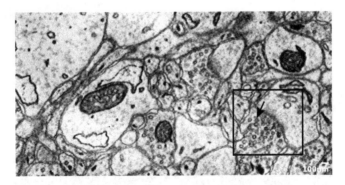

Figure 14.1   A slice of brain tissue collected by the ATLUM and imaged at 5 nm resolution by electron-microscopy.

Whole brain emulation resembles carefully copying each tiny speck on the canvas of a masterpiece instead of attempting to redraw the masterpiece using broad strokes carried out by a different artist.

Figure 14.1 shows one moment in such a process, as carried out using the Automatic Tape-Collecting Lathe Ultramicrotome (ATLUM) that was developed by Ken Hayworth and Jeff Lichtman for exactly this purpose. It is an image taken with an electron microscope from a slice of brain tissue so thin that we can see the individual vesicles (indicated by the white arrow) filled with neurotransmitters within the body of a synaptic terminal (within the red square).

The steps involved in achieving whole brain emulation will involve the development of new tools such as the ATLUM and will undoubtedly teach us many things about the brain. Still, creating a whole brain emulation does not automatically guarantee a full understanding of brain and mind – or require it! What it does give us are the essential requirements of a substrate-independent mind. WBE provides robustness and backup, and it offers total access to every operation being carried out. That access enables exploration. We can then reversibly, gradually, and carefully carry out modifications that augment our capabilities. Augmentation can enable us to keep pace with developments, truly experience that which our tools are capable of, and intimately benefit from those advances.

Main Developments toward SIM

Since the term whole brain emulation was introduced in 2000 several important developments have made substrate-independent minds a feasible project in the foreseeable future. The transistor density and storage available in computing hardware have increased between 50- and 100-fold, at an exponential rate. Now, the rapidly increasing number of processing cores in general-purpose CPUs and GPU arrays are indicative of a drive toward parallel computation. Parallel computation is a more natural fit to neural computation. It is essential for the acquisition and analysis of data from the brain. Of course, compared with a sequential Von Neumann architecture, parallel computing platforms, and in particular neuromorphic platforms, are a much better target for the implementation of a whole brain emulation. An example of neuromorphic processor hardware is the chip developed at IBM as an outcome of research in the DARPA SyNAPSE program led by Dharmendra Modha.

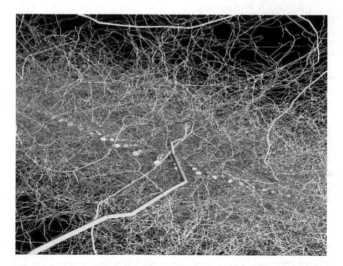

Figure 14.2   Large-scale high-resolution representations of neuronal circuitry in neuroinformatics. The circuitry shown here was generated with NETMORPH (Koene et al. 2009).

The new field of large-scale neuroinformatics emerged during the last decade, taking computational neuroscience toward a focus on greater model detail and model scale. Some of these developments arose from a few highly ambitious projects, such as the Blue Brain project. Organizations such as the International Neuroinformatics Coordinating Facility (INCF) have made a concerted effort to drive neuroinformatics toward shared resources and shared collections of data. Projects in whole brain emulation will require methods of representation and implementation that are well suited to the necessary scale and resolution (e.g., see Figure 14.2). Those requirements closely resemble the ones that neuroinformatics has been addressing.

Systematic investigations have commenced in recent years that test our hypotheses about the scope and resolution that are needed to acquire, transfer, and re-implement the characteristic functions of a mind. Briggman, Helmstaedter, and Denk recently published a study (Briggman et al. 2011) in which they carried out both electrical recording and reconstruction from morphology obtained by electron microscope imaging of the same retinal tissue. They demonstrated that it was possible to determine the correct functional layout from the morphology. Bock et al. carried out similar studies of neurons of the visual cortex (Bock et al. 2011). The technique known as optogenetics was developed by Karl Disseroth and Ed Boyden (Boyden et al. 2005), which enables very specific excitation or inhibition *in vivo* by adding light sensitivity to specific sets of neurons.

These and similar techniques enable testing of hypotheses about the significance of specific groups of neurons with regards to mental function. Projects such as the Blue Brain project, led by Henry Markram, and the cortical column model by Oberlaender et al. (2011) have been mentioned several times in this essay and are prime examples of work in recent years that carries out very specific hypothesis testing about neurophysiology and brain function that is directly meaningful to WBE and SIM. And now David Dalrymple has embarked upon a project to begin the testing of the hypotheses that relate to specific steps in a program to develop WBE. The first hypothesis being tested by Dalrymple is *"Recording of membrane potential is sufficient to enable whole brain emulation of C. Elegans."* Through emulation of the nematode *C. Elegans*, he will determine cases when information at the molecular level is not needed and when it is.

An increasing number of projects are explicitly building the sort of tools that are needed to acquire data from a brain at the large scope and high resolution required. There are by now at least three different versions of the Automated Tape-Collecting Lathe Ultramicrotome that was developed at the Lichtman Lab at Harvard University (Hayworth et al. 2007). Ken Hayworth is presently working on its successor that employs focused ion beam scanning electron microscopy (FIBSEM) to improve accuracy, reliability, and speed of structural data acquisition from whole brains at a resolution of 5 nm (Hayworth 2011). Meanwhile, the Knife-Edge Scanning Microscope (KESM) developed by Bruce McCormick is presently able to acquire neuronal fiber and vasculature data from entire mouse brains at a slightly lower resolution (McCormick and Mayerich 2004).

A number of labs, including the MIT Media Lab of Ed Boyden, are aiming at the development arrays of recording electrodes with tens of thousands of channels. To go beyond this *in vivo*, recent collaborations have emerged to develop ways of recording the connectivity and the activity of millions and billions of neurons concurrently from the inside. There is a range of very different approaches to the design of such internal recording agents. In some cases, the design takes advantage of biological resources that already operate at the requisite scale and density, such as the application of viral vectors for the delivery of specific DNA sequences as markers for the synaptic connection between two neurons (Zador 2011). In others, the design builds on existing expertise with integrated circuit technology, applied at the dimensions of red blood cells.

The past decade also marked an essential shift in the perception of whole brain emulation and the possibility of substrate-independent minds. In my personal role, seeking the accomplishment of SIM, I was also dealing with the essential tasks of objective-oriented roadmapping and the development of research networks in 2000, but I was often confronted with the need to speak of these ideas with great care and to present them within the comfort zone of a traditional research interest. This was particularly true when speaking with leaders in neuroscience, computer science, and related fields such as the burgeoning fields of neural engineering and nanotechnology. Whole brain emulation was science fiction, beyond the horizon of feasible science and engineering. That is not true any more. Now, leading scientists and principal investigators, including Ed Boyden, Sebastian Seung, Ted Berger, and George Church, consider high resolution connectomics and efforts towards whole brain emulation to be serious and relevant research and technology development goals addressed in their laboratories.

Structural Connectomics and Functional Connectomics

In the brain, processing and memory are both distributed and involve very large numbers of components. The connectivity between those components is as important to the mental processing being carried out as the characteristic response functions of each individual component. This is the structure-function entanglement in neural processing. From a tool development perspective, it is tempting to focus primarily on the acquisition of one of those dimensions, either the detailed structure or the collection of component functions. In principle, that could be adequate. Theoretically, we should be able to look at the detailed morphology of neuronal cell bodies, their axonal and dendritic fibers, and the morphology of synapses where connections are made, and to identify the component functions from that as well. To make the necessary identification, categorization, and parameter tuning, we will need extensive libraries that correlate morphology with function. The mapping from morphology to function should also be injective (or one-to-one), so that there is no ambiguity about which of a number of possible functional components might match the same morphology. It is not yet clear if that is indeed the case, even though recent work (Bock et al. 2011; Briggman et al. 2011) has shown promising results. Another difficulty that appears if we rely exclusively on data obtained from structure is that it becomes very difficult to verify corrections that need to be made when there are data acquisition or reconstruction errors.

Similarly, it is in principle possible to deduce a functional connectivity map from a purely functional acquisition of brain data. The functional approach (as in all scientific modeling) picks a black box level at a resolution that is considered great enough to discern the functional mechanisms that cooperate to achieve functions of mind. An obvious example of a black box level is to consider each individual neuron (with all of its dendritic and axonal fiber) as a single component to be modeled. The approach is then to measure all discernible input to the black box and all discernible output (at least in the domains that are considered relevant, e.g., conductance equivalents). By observing enough of the input and output, we can derive transfer functions that represent what the component does. If we also observe how all of the components operate concurrently, then the ways in which processing at one component affects others may be deduced. That leads to a map of functional connectivity between the components.

Unfortunately, there is also a limitation to this approach, namely due to the completeness of observations that can be achieved. If the time during which measurements are taken is relatively small or does not involve a sufficiently thorough set of events observed, then it is possible to miss pairs of I/O that would indicate the presence of latent function. There are some ways to improve upon this by using patterns of stimulation in order to put each component through its paces, but then we run into the problem that the brain is plastic. Components may change their responses as a result of the exercises. Latent function may be better obtained from structural data acquisition.

Even if purely structural or purely functional data acquisition could provide all the necessary information for a whole brain emulation, then such a constraint would still carry a burden of risk that is better avoided from the perspective of sensible engineering. It seems unwise to construct an enormously complex emulation by carrying out a single-shot transformation. It is far better to turn it into a problem of successive partial transformations. For each of those, operational feedback allows for verification. For all of these reasons, we would prefer to be able to acquire data about both function and structure at the scope and resolution that are required for WBE. Today, we see that research and tool development in both domains is represented by efforts that we will here designate as either *structural connectomics* or *functional connectomics*.

Leaders in the field of *structural connectomics* include Ken Hayworth and Jeff Lichtman (also known for the Brainbow technique: Lichtman et al. 2008) at Harvard University. Hayworth and Lichtman are responsible for the development of the ATLUM, which is aimed at solving the problem of how to collect all of the necessary ultra-thin slices from a whole brain in a manner where subsequent imaging by electron microscopy could obtain unambiguous data at resolutions up to 5 nm over the entire volume. Winfried Denk (Max-Planck) and Sebastian Seung (MIT) popularized the search for the human connectome, but did not solve the issue of volume and quantity involved with whole brains. The Denk group has produced many significant collaborative results, such as representations and simulations based on reconstruction (Briggman et al. 2011; Bock et al. 2011). The laboratory of Bruce McCormick (now led by Yoonsuck Choe) took a slightly different approach to automated structural data collection from whole brains. They focused on light microscopy and built the KESM, which collects image data immediately through the diamond blade that is used to section a brain. Light microscopy limits the resolution that can be obtained, so that the technique is a useful precursor to tools required for WBE, even if it cannot see individual synapses.

Groups led by Anthony Zador and Ed Callaway have chosen an entirely different route to the acquisition of the full connectome, and are using a bio-tagging procedures. Zador's work involves the use of viral vectors to deliver unique DNA payloads to the pre- and post-synaptic neurons of each synaptic connection. After the payloads are delivered to the full set of neurons examined the cell bodies are extracted and DNA recovered from each. By identifying the specific DNA sequences found within it would be possible to find matching pairs of tags, which in effect act as pointers between pairs of connected neurons.

Ground-breaking work on *functional connectomics* includes work in the lab of George Church (Harvard), who is well known for his work in genomics, but now has a keen interest in developing high-resolution, large-scale acquisition and interfacing technology. The approach taken there involves work by Yael Maguire to develop measurement devices at the scale of red blood cells (about 8 micrometers in diameter). The technology is based on existing fabrication capabilities from the integrated circuit industry, builds on prior successful work embedding chips in cells (Gomez-Martinez et al. 2010), and adds to this RFID-inspired passive communication, and infrared signaling and power technology. Even before those tools reach their full potential, there are ongoing efforts in the Ed Boyden group to scale up multi-electrode arrays to thousands of recording channels that are integrated with light-guides for optogenetic stimulation. Such a stimulation-recording array would provide previously unobtainable feedback about mechanistic hypotheses that are relevant to WBE. Peter Passaro (University of Sussex) is working on a systematic automation scheme for research and data acquisition essential to WBE, and on suitable model conventions that build on work by Chris Eliasmith (University of Waterloo) (Eliasmith and Anderson 2003).

As in the case of structural connectomics, there are also alternative tool developments aimed at recording characteristic functional responses in all neurons, but that choose a biological implementation. They are a collection of designs being developed in collaboration between groups already listed above (Ed Boyden, George Church, Yael Maguire), as well as Konrad Kording, and Rebecca Weisinger and myself (Halcyon Molecular). This category of biological recording designs is collectively and tentatively identified as "molecular ticker-tape" approaches.

Structure-Function and Questions of Resolution and Scope

As we pointed out in the preceding paragraphs, both structure and function are important, and they are not entirely independent either. There are at present a few projects that are specifically investigating hypotheses that address the main two research questions for whole brain emulation, namely: (1) the question of the scope and resolution that are needed to acquire data and then produce an emulation that satisfies the objective of SIM, and (2) the question of structure-function interdependence, the procedural requirement that imposes, but also the benefits that can be obtained by, using one to infer or verify the other. Additionally, there is a range of projects under way that will supply valuable results applicable to WBE, even if the projects arose to meet other scientific or engineering goals.

An example of important research aimed directly at the objective of WBE is the effort by David Dalrymple (Harvard) to reconstruct the functional and subject-specific neuronal networks of the nematode *C. Elegans*. He is doing this to test one of the hypotheses with significant consequences for chosen methods in WBE: Can data acquisition and re-implementation result in an emulation that satisfies the objectives of WBE without needing to acquire data at the molecular level? The results may point to specific places where molecular-level information does need to be obtained. Or, if successful, we may immediately go on to hypotheses at the level of brains with predominantly spiking neurons and chemical synapses, such as in vertebrate brains. This is an example of a laudable systematic approach to hypothesis testing for the development of SIM.

Henry Markram, located at École Polytechnique Fédérale de Lausanne (EPFL), has publicly stated his aim of constructing a functional simulation of a whole cortex using the Blue Brain approach. As explained earlier, Blue Brain is based on model generation by stochastic sampling. This means that without using a tool such as the ATLUM to acquire and reconstruct in accordance with the structure and function in an individual brain, the Blue Brain Project will not develop a whole brain emulation in the truest sense. Even so, the large-scale model building methods, verification protocols, simulations, and hypothesis testing that result from Blue Brain will be extremely valuable for the development of substrate-independent minds.

The collaborative work published by Bock et al. (2011) and by Briggman et al. (2011) are outstanding examples of projects that generate results with useful insights about scope and resolution, as well as about structure-function. They showed for retina and neurons in the visual system that, in principle, it is possible to identify characteristics of function from morphology. Their protocols included methods of validating from functional recordings.

One more example to show how work in related disciplines such as neural engineer and brain-machine interfaces can produce results on a step-wise route towards SIM: Ted Berger (University of Southern California) is the first to develop a cognitive neural prosthetic. His prosthetic replacement chip for neuronal circuitry in hippocampal region CA3 is obviously still early-phase, and has small connection bandwidth and other limitations. Nevertheless, the work forces researchers to confront challenges of functional interfacing within core circuitry of the brain that are close analogues of the challenges involved in whole brain emulation.

SIM within our Life-Spans

The problem of achieving substrate-independent minds is one of solving several specific issues: Determining the scope and resolution of that which generates the experience of "being" that takes place within our minds, building tools that can acquire data at that scope and resolution, devising a re-implementation for satisfactory emulation with adequate input and output, and carrying out procedures that achieve the transfer (or "upload") in a manner that satisfies continuity.

It does not require a full understanding of our biology, but it does require that we consider carefully the limits of that which produces the experience of being. Accomplishing SIM is a problem that researchers in neuroscience and related fields can grasp and simplify into sensible granular parts. To our present knowledge, there are no aspects of the problem that lie beyond our physical understanding or beyond the ability to engineer solutions. As such, it is a feasible objective and one that can be dealt with through a hierarchy of projects and by the allocation of such resources as are needed to carry out the projects within the time-span desired. If that time-span is the span of a human life or a career then we should carry out project planning and resource allocation accordingly. It is possible.

Furthermore, many of the pieces of the puzzle that make up the set of projects to achieve SIM are already of great interest to neuroscience, to neuro-medicine, and to computer science. Acquisition of large-scale, high-resolution brain data is a hot topic and has spawned the new field of *connectomics*. Understanding the resolution and scope at which the brain operates is of great interest to researchers and developers of neural prostheses. And even the emulation of specific brain circuitry is the topic of recent grants and efforts in computational neuroscience. There is work being carried out on all of those pieces today. What SIM needs now is a roadmap that ties it all together along several promising paths, and that insures that attention is given to those key pieces of the puzzle that may not yet be receiving enough of it. Finally, we need to insure that the allocation of effort and resources is raised to the levels that make success a likelihood within the time-frame desired.

What is the Rationale for Investing in SIM Projects Now?

There is a larger context to consider. The development of SIM does not take place in isolation, nor does work on any other ambitious goal, from biological life-extension to artificial general intelligence. If SIM is not achieved by the time another intelligence appears that is competitive with ours in terms of its ability, performance, and adaptability, then – and without any hyperbole or sensationalism – it is quite possible that we may never have another chance to achieve it.

The possibility of SIM has in recent years finally become something that is technologically considered and taken seriously by leaders in neuroscience. As explained earlier, the time to the first successful SIM is related directly to the resources that are allocated to the effort. The projects involved are not demonstrably constrained by a need for sequential execution or long minimum durations of trials. By contrast, such constraints do appear quickly in other areas that try to address biological breakdown or maintenance, curing diseases and combating age-related problems.

An intensive program to achieve SIM is therefore possible, such that it minimizes the time to success and at the same time minimizes the existential risk posed by other technological developments that are taking place at this time. Given this opportunity, would you want to risk unnecessarily choosing a path where you may end up looking back only to realize that we simply did not try hard enough? SIM can be developed within the lifespan of the majority of humanity that is alive today.

References

Bock, Davi D., et al. (2011) "Network Anatomy and In Vivo Physiology of Visual Cortical Neurons." *Nature* 471, pp. 177–182.

Boyden, Edward S., Zhang, F., Bamberg, E., Nagel, G., and Deisseroth, K. (2005). "Millisecond-Timescale, Genetically Targeted Optical Control of Neural Activity." *Nature Neuroscience* 8/9, pp. 1263–1268.

Briggman, Kevin L., Helmstaedter, M., and Denk, W. (2011) "Wiring Specificity in the Direction-Selectivity Circuit of the Retina." *Nature* 471, pp. 183–188.

Eliasmith, Chris and Anderson, C.H. (2003) "Neural Engineering: Computation, Representation and Dynamics in Neurobiological Systems." Cambridge, MA: MIT Press.

Gomez-Martinez, R., Vazquez, P., Duch, M., Muriano, A., Pinacho, D., Sanvincens, N., Sanchez-Baeza, F., Boya, P., de la Rosa, E., Esteve, J., Suarez, T., and Plaza, J. (2010) "Intracellular Silicon Chips in Living Cells." *Small* 6/4, pp. 499–502.

Hayworth, Kenneth J. (2011) "Lossless Thick Sectioning of Plastic-Embedded Brain Tissue to Enable Parallelizing of SBFSEM and FIBSEM Imaging." High Resolution Circuit Reconstruction Conference, Janelia Farms, Ashburn, VA.

Hayworth, Kenneth J., Kasthuri, N., Hartwieg, E., and Lichtman, J.W. (2007) "Automating the Collection of Ultrathin Brain Sections for Electron Microscopic Volume Imaging." Program No. 534.6, 2007 Neuroscience Meeting, San Diego, CA.

Koene, Randal A. (2011a) "Pattern Survival Versus Gene Survival." KurzweilAI.net, February 11, 2011. http://www.kurzweilai.net/pattern-survival-versus-gene-survival.

Koene, Randal A. (2011b) "Achieving Substrate-Independent Minds: No, We Cannot 'Copy' Brains." KurzweilAI.net. August 24, 2011. http://www.kurzweilai.net/achieving-substrate-independent-minds-no-we-cannot-copy-brains.

Koene, Randal A. (2012) "Experimental Research in Whole Brain Emulation: The Need for Innovative In-Vivo Measurement Techniques." *International Journal of Machine Consciousness* special issue 4/1.

Koene, Randal A., Tijms, B., van Hees, P., Postma, F., de Ridder, S., Ramakers, G., van Pelt, J. and van Ooyen, A. (2009) "NETMORPH: A Framework for the Stochastic Generation of Large Scale Neuronal Networks with Realistic Neuron Morphologies." *Neuroinformatics* 7/3, pp. 195–210.

Lichtman, Jeff, Livet, J., and Sanes, J. (2008) "A Technicolour Approach to the Connectome." *Nature Reviews Neuroscience* 9/6, pp. 417–422.

Markram, Henry (2006) "The Blue Brain Project." *Nature Reviews Neuroscience* 7, 153–160.

McCormick, B. and Mayerich, D.M. (2004) "Three-Dimensional Imaging Using Knife-Edge Scanning Microscopy." Proceedings of the Microscopy and Micro-analysis Conference 2004, Savannah, GA.

Oberlaender, Marcel, de Kock, C.O.J., Bruno, R.M., Ramirez, A., Meyer, H.S., Dercksen, V.J., Helmstaedter, M., and Sakmann, B. (2011) "Cell Type-Specific Three-Dimensional Structure of Thalamocortical Circuits in a Column of Rat Vibrissal Cortex." *Cerebral Cortex* doi:10.1093/cercor/bhr317, pp. 1–17.

Sandberg, Anders and Bostrom, N. (2008) *Whole Brain Emulation: A Roadmap.* Oxford: Future of Humanity Institute, Oxford University.

Zador, Anthony (2011) "Sequencing the Connectome: A Fundamentally New Way of Determining the Brain's Wiring Diagram." Project Proposal, Paul G. Allen Foundation Awards Grants.

15

Uploading

Ralph C. Merkle

Your brain is a material object. The behavior of material objects is described by the laws of physics. The laws of physics can be modeled on a computer. Therefore, the behavior of your brain can be modeled on a computer. Q.E.D.

So why haven't we done it already?

Well, we'd need a fairly big computer. And we'd have to get a very detailed description of your brain. The only ways we know of getting *that* detailed a description are destructive. That means we'd have to take your brain apart. Most people most of the time object to this. Even if *you* don't object, the legal system would. Destructive analysis of someone's brain is viewed dimly by the courts. These minor objections could be circumvented by waiting until you're legally dead. At that point, the courts wouldn't object if you didn't object. And although brain function has usually (though not always) stopped by the time you're declared legally dead, the information should still be there for a while (though you'd probably lose short-term memory). When we power down the system we lose volatile memory, but non-volatile memory and the circuitry are still there.

Let's assume we've solved the legal hassles, and we're preparing to analyze your brain using the new, advanced Mark 7 Neural Analysis System. We've hooked up the Mark 7 to the Intel Pentadecium. The first question we might ask is: How much memory should we buy? How many bits does it take to describe your brain?

Your brain is made of atoms. Each atom has a location in three-space that we can represent with three coordinates: X, Y, and Z. Atoms are usually a few tenths of a nanometer apart. If we could record the position of each atom to within 0.01 nanometers, we would know its position accurately enough to know what chemicals it was a part of, what bonds it had formed, and so on. The brain is roughly 0.1 meters across, so 0.01 nanometers is about 1 part in 10^{10}: we need to

Originally published in *Extropy: The Journal of Transhumanist Thought* 11 (1993). Copyright © Max More.

The Transhumanist Reader: Classical and Contemporary Essays on the Science, Technology, and Philosophy of the Human Future, First Edition. Edited by Max More and Natasha Vita-More.
© 2013 John Wiley & Sons, Inc. Published 2013 by John Wiley & Sons, Inc.

know the position in each coordinate to within one part in 10 billion. A number of this size can be represented with about 33 bits. There are three coordinates, X, Y, and Z, so the position of an atom can be represented in 99 bits. An additional few bits are needed to store the type of the atom (whether hydrogen, oxygen, carbon, etc.), bringing the total to slightly over 100 bits.

With about 100 bits per atom we could certainly describe your brain as precisely as we'd need. (Purists might object that this does not take into account the positions of the electrons. While this is technically true, it's usually not hard in biological systems to infer the electronic structure if you have the coordinates of all the nuclei. We might wish to have a little more information, e.g., Na+, OH–, etc. With this additional ionization information our knowledge of the system would be essentially complete). Examining the published plots of the number of atoms required to store a bit of information as a function of the year, we find that somewhere between 2010 and 2020 we should be able to store one bit with one atom. If one atom in your brain is described by 100 bits, and each bit occupies one atom, then the memory required to hold a digital description of your brain accurate to the last atom would occupy about 100 times the size of your brain. The brain is somewhat over 1 liter, so it would require a computer memory with a volume of somewhat over 100 liters to encode the location of each and every atom in the brain in a digital format. There are somewhat over 10^{26} atoms in the brain, so our storage system needs to hold about 10^{28} bits.

For those readers who might view the feasibility of such a memory system with some doubt, recall that DNA requires roughly 16 atoms to store a bit of information (not including the water in which it floats). Your body, with 10^{10} bits per cell stored in DNA and 10^{14} cells, stores almost 10^{24} bits of information (and it's unlikely that you're an optimal memory storage device). We're assuming only a modest improvement in storage technology over DNA; and as we'll see, we don't actually need as much storage as we've computed here.

How Many Bits to Describe a Molecule?

While such a feat is remarkable, it is also much more than we need. Chemists usually think of atoms in groups, called molecules. For example, water is a molecule made of three atoms: an oxygen and two hydrogens. If we describe each atom separately, we will require 100 bits per atom, or 300 bits total. If, however, we give the position of the oxygen atom and give the orientation of the molecule, we need: 99 bits for the location of the oxygen atom plus perhaps 20 bits to describe the type of molecule ("water," in this case) and perhaps another 30 bits to give the orientation of the water molecule (10 bits for each of the three rotational axes). This means we can store the description of a water molecule in only 150 bits, instead of the 300 bits required to describe the three atoms separately. (The 20 bits used to describe the type of the molecule can describe up to 1,000,000 different molecules – more than are present in the brain.)

As the molecule we are describing gets larger and larger, the savings in storage get bigger and bigger. A whole protein molecule will still require only 150 bits to describe, even though it is made of thousands of atoms. The canonical position of every atom in the molecule is specified once the type of the molecule (which occupies a mere 20 bits) is given. A large molecule might adopt many configurations, so it might at first seem that we'd require many more bits to describe it. However, biological macromolecules typically assume one favored configuration rather than a random configuration, and it is this favored configuration that we will describe.

Describing the brain one atom at a time is much less compact than describing it in terms of one molecule at a time.

Do We Really Need to Describe Each Molecule?

While this reduces our storage requirements quite a bit, we could go much further. Instead of describing molecules, we could describe entire sub-cellular organelles. It seems excessive to describe a mitochondrion by describing each and every molecule in it. It would be sufficient simply to note the location and perhaps the size of the mitochondrion, for all mitochondria perform the same function: they produce energy for the cell. While there are indeed minor differences from mitochondrion to mitochondrion, these differences don't matter much and could reasonably be neglected.

If we're concerned about the behavior of the nervous system then worrying about the location of each mitochondrion seems excessive. We could describe an entire cell with only a general description of the function it performs: this nerve cell has synapses of a certain type with that other cell, it has a certain shape, and so on. If we assume there are 10^{15} synapses, and if we need (very roughly) 100 bits per synapse, this brings us down to 10^{17} bits. We could be yet more economical of storage: a group of cells in the retina might perform a "center surround" computation, so the entire group (including all their synapses and fine morphology) could be summarized in one succinct functional description.

How Many Bits Do We Really Need?

This kind of logic can be continued, but where does it stop? What is the most compact description which captures all the essential information? While many minor details of neural structure are irrelevant, our memories clearly matter. If we can't fully describe long-term memory we've gone too far.

How many bits does it take to hold human memory? Cherniak (1990) said: "On the usual assumption that the synapse is the necessary substrate of memory, supposing very roughly that (given anatomical and physiological 'noise') each synapse encodes about one binary bit of information, and a thousand synapses per neuron are available for this task: 10^{10} cortical neurons $\times 10^3$ synapses $= 10^{13}$ bits of arbitrary information (1.25 terabytes) that could be stored in the cerebral cortex." A problem with hardware-based estimates is that they have to make assumptions about how the information is stored. The brain is highly redundant and not completely understood: the mere fact that a great mass of synapses exists does not imply that they are in fact contributing to the memory capacity. This makes the work of Landauer (1986) very interesting for he has entirely avoided this hardware guessing game by measuring the actual functional capacity of human memory directly.

A Functional Estimate of Human Long-Term Memory Capacity

Landauer works at Bell Communications Research – closely affiliated with Bell Labs where the modern study of information theory was begun by C.E. Shannon to analyze the information-carrying capacity of telephone lines (a subject of great interest to a telephone company). Landauer naturally used these tools by viewing human memory as a novel "telephone line" that carries information from the past to the future. The capacity of this "telephone line" can be determined by measuring the information that goes in and the information that comes out – the great power of modern information theory can be applied.

Landauer reviewed and quantitatively analyzed experiments by himself and others in which people were asked to read text; look at pictures; hear words, short passages of music, sentences, and nonsense syllables. After delays ranging from minutes to days the subjects were then tested to determine how much they had retained. The tests were quite sensitive (they did not merely ask "What do you remember?"), often using true/false or multiple choice questions, in which even a vague memory of the material would increase the chances of making the correct choice. Often, the differential abilities of a group that had been exposed to the material and another group that had not been exposed to the material were used. The difference in the scores between the two groups was used to estimate the amount actually remembered (to control for the number of correct answers an intelligent human could guess without ever having seen the material). Because experiments by many different experimenters were summarized and analyzed, the results of the analysis are fairly robust; they are insensitive to fine details or specific conditions of one or another experiment. Finally, the amount remembered was divided by the time allotted to memorization to determine the number of bits remembered per second.

The remarkable result of this work was that human beings remembered very nearly two bits per second under *all* the experimental conditions. Visual, verbal, musical, or whatever – two bits per second. Continued over a lifetime, this rate of memorization would produce somewhat over 10^9 bits, or some hundreds of megabytes.

While this estimate is probably only accurate to within an order of magnitude, Landauer says "We need answers at this level of accuracy to think about such questions as: What sort of storage and retrieval capacities will computers need to mimic human performance? What sort of physical unit should we expect to constitute the elements of information storage in the brain: molecular parts, synaptic junctions, whole cells, or cell-circuits? What kinds of coding and storage methods are reasonable to postulate for the neural support of human capabilities? In modeling or mimicking human intelligence, what size of memory and what efficiencies of use should we imagine we are copying? How much would a robot need to know to match a person?"

Landauer's estimate is interesting because of its small size. While Landauer doesn't measure everything (he did not measure, for example, the bit rate in learning to ride a bicycle, nor does his estimate even consider the size of "working memory") his estimate of memory capacity suggests that the capabilities of the human brain are more approachable than we had thought.

How many bits do we need to satisfactorily describe your brain? We have quite a range: from 10^{28} to 10^9. If we assume we have to describe every neuron and every synapse (and every nerve impulse traveling along every neuron), we're probably safe in estimating something like 10^{18} bits. Those who object to this approximation can buy the more expensive High Fidelity system which keeps track of each and every atom. If people will buy gold-plated Monster Speaker cables...

How Much Computing Power?

Now that we have a rough idea of the information storage we'll need, how many operations a second will we need? How fast does the brain operate? While mips are appropriate for a PC, there are several measures we might use for the brain. We might count the number of synapses, estimate their average speed of operation, and so determine synapse operations per second. If there are roughly 10^{15} synapses operating at about 10 impulses/second (Kandel et al. 1991), we get roughly 10^{16} synapse operations per second.

A second approach is to estimate the computational power of the retina, and then multiply this estimate by the ratio of brain size to retinal size. The retina is relatively well understood so we can make a reasonable estimate of its computational power. The output of the retina – carried by the optic nerve – is primarily from retinal ganglion cells that perform "center surround" computations (or related computations of roughly similar complexity). If we assume that a typical center surround computation requires about 100 analog adds and is done about 100 times per second (Binford), then computation of the output of each ganglion cell requires about 10,000 analog adds per second. There are about 1,000,000 axons in the optic nerve (Kuffler et al. 1984: 21), so the retina as a whole performs about 10^{10} analog adds per second. There are about 10^8 nerve cells in the retina (1984: 26), and between 10^{10} and 10^{12} nerve cells in the brain (1984: 7), so the brain is roughly 100 to 10,000 times larger than the retina. By this logic, the brain should be able to do about 10^{12} to 10^{14} operations per second (in good agreement with the estimate of Moravec, who considers this approach in more detail [Moravec 1988: 57, 163]).

The Brain Uses Energy

A third approach is to measure the total energy used by the brain each second, and then determine the energy used for each "basic operation." Dividing the former by the latter gives the total number of basic operations per second. We need two pieces of information: the total energy consumed by the brain each second, and the energy used by a "basic operation."

The total energy consumption of the brain is about 25 watts (Kandel et al. 1991). Much of this is used either for "housekeeping" or is wasted; perhaps 10 watts is used for "useful computation."

Nerve Impulses Use Energy

Nerve impulses are carried by either myelinated or un-myelinated axons. Myelinated axons are wrapped in a fatty insulating myelin sheath, interrupted at intervals of about 1 millimeter exposing the axon. These interruptions are called "nodes of Ranvier." Propagation of a nerve impulse in a myelinated axon is from one node of Ranvier to the next – jumping over the insulated portion.

A nerve cell has a "resting potential" – the outside of the nerve cell is 0 volts (by definition), while the inside is about –60 millivolts. When a nerve impulse passes by, the internal voltage briefly rises above 0 volts because of an inrush of Na+ ions. The inrushing Na+ goes through special protein pores in the nerve cell membrane called "voltage activated sodium channels." They are normally closed, but when the nerve impulse comes by they open for about a millisecond and then spontaneously close again (Kandel et al. 1991).

The Energy of a Nerve Impulse

When a single voltage activated sodium channel opens, it has a conductance of about 15 picosiemens (Hille 1984). (A siemen is the reciprocal of an ohm, and is also called a "mho.") In myelinated nerve cells there are roughly 60,000 channels at each node of Ranvier (and nowhere else). The total charge that crosses the membrane at one node in one millisecond can thus be computed: about 5.4×10^{-11} coulombs (over 300 million ions per node). The energy dissipated is just the charge times the voltage, or 3.2×10^{-12} joules. If we view this 1-millimeter jump as a "basic operation" then we can easily compute the maximum number of such "Ranvier ops" the brain can perform each second: 3.1×10^{12}.

Although the details differ for unmyelinated nerve cells, the energy cost of traveling 1 millimeter is about the same.

To translate "Ranvier ops" (1-millimeter jumps) into synapse operations we must know the average distance between synapses, which is not normally given in neuroscience texts. We can estimate it: a human can recognize an image in about 100 milliseconds, which can take at most 100 one-millisecond synapse delays. A single signal probably travels 100 millimeters in that time (from the eye to the back of the brain, and then some). If it passes 100 synapses in 100 millimeters then it passes one synapse every millimeter – which means one "synapse operation" is about one "Ranvier operation."

If propagating a nerve impulse a distance of 1 millimeter requires about 3.2×10^{-12} joules and the total energy dissipated by the brain is about 10 watts, then nerve impulses in your brain can collectively travel at most 3.1×10^{12} millimeters per second. By estimating the distance between synapses we can in turn estimate how many synapse operations per second your brain can do. This estimate is three to four orders of magnitude smaller than an estimate based simply on counting synapses and multiplying by the average firing rate, and similar to an estimate based on functional estimates of retinal computational power. It seems reasonable to conclude that the human brain has a "raw" computational power towards the low end of the range between 10^{12} and 10^{16} "operations" per second.

We'll use the upper end of this range, 10^{16} operations a second.

Our Model Isn't Perfect

We have been glossing over a point: a computational model of a physical system will fail to precisely predict the behavior of that system down to the motion of the last electron for two reasons: quantum mechanics is fundamentally random in nature, and any computational model has an inherent limit to its precision. The former implies that we can at best predict the probable future course of events, not the actual future course of events. The latter is even worse – we cannot precisely predict even the probable course of future events. A good example of this second point is the weather – weather prediction more than a week or two into the future might well be inherently impossible given any error in the initial conditions or computations. Any error at all (rounding off to a mere million digits of accuracy) will eventually result in gross errors between the actual events and the events predicted by the computational model. The model predicts sunshine next Tuesday, and we get rain. This kind of error cannot be avoided.

We have been simplifying our computations even further by not bothering to compute the state of every atom, or even of every molecule. We've been operating at the level of synapses or higher, which introduces another sort of "noise" into the computation.

It's safe to conclude that any computational model of your brain will almost certainly deviate from the behavior of the original – eventually in some gross and detectable fashion. If you decide that it doesn't matter which of two courses of action to follow and allow yourself to decide on whim, then it seems plausible that some slight influence might cause a computational model of your brain to select the opposite course. But is this difference "significant"? Given that our model is highly accurate for short periods of time and that any deviations are either random or represent the accumulation of slight errors, does it matter that the behavior of the model and of the original eventually deviate in some gross and obvious fashion?

We can view this another way: your brain, as a physical system, is already subject to a variety of outside and essentially random influences caused by (among other things): temperature fluctuations; microwaves, light, and other electromagnetic radiation; cosmic rays; last night's dinner; a beer, etc. If the errors in our computational model are smaller than these influences do we really care about the difference? Is it "significant"? The human brain can and does continue to function reasonably well in the presence of gross perturbations (the death of many neurons, for example) yet this does not detract from our consciousness or life – I don't die even if tens of thousands of neurons do. In fact, I usually don't even notice the loss. A model of your brain that described the behavior of every synapse and nerve impulse, and did a reasonably accurate job at that level, would seem to capture everything that is essential to being "you."

Yet how can we tell? How will we judge the "accuracy" of our computational model? How can we say what is "significant" and what is "insignificant"? We might adopt a variation of the Turing test: if an external tester can't tell the difference, then there is no difference. But is the opinion of an external tester enough? How about your opinion? If you "feel" a difference, wouldn't this mean that the model was a "mere copy" and not really you?

Well, we could ask: "Hi! We've uploaded your brain into an Intel Pentadecium, how are you feeling?" "Absolutely top notch!" "Do you think you're not you?" "Nope, I'm me. And this simulated body is great!" "How's the orgy?" "Wonderful! Who worked on this software? I'd like to shake their hand, they've done a really great job! Uh, I hope you don't mind, but maybe I could talk with you a bit more after the party's over? I'm being distracted…"

The Ultimate in Experimental Evidence: Try it and See!

If everyone agrees that you're you, including you, and if behavioral tests can't show any difference, then is there any difference? Perhaps, but the grounds for objection are getting rather slim. If the changes that have been introduced by the uploading process are smaller than the behavioral changes introduced by (say) a beer, a night's sleep, or a cup of coffee, then it's getting rather difficult to argue that uploading has somehow destroyed the real you and substituted a "fake" you that just seems (by all objective measures) to be you.

Summary

Roughly, uploading will need a computer with a memory of about 10^{18} bits, able to do around 10^{16} "operations" a second. A computer of this capacity should fit comfortably into a cubic centimeter in the early twenty-first century.

It will also require the highly accurate analysis of your nervous system. This kind of analysis should also become feasible in the twenty-first century.

The biggest obstacle to uploading today is the primitive state of current technology and the unfortunate fact that our current hardware has an MTBF (Mean Time Between Failures) of

70 years. (I've already used up 41, how about you?) Even worse, actual failures occur unpredictably and the failure mode is catastrophic, resulting in complete erasure of all software. Bummer.

But if you can bridge the gap (it's only a few decades) then you've got it made. All you have to do is freeze your system state if a crash occurs and wait for the crash recovery technology to be developed. Fortunately, cryonic suspension services are available today which quite literally let you freeze your state. Which means if you can't stay alive and healthy until the technology is developed (and approved by the FDA, don't forget the regulatory delays!) you can be suspended until you can be uploaded.

And then you'll get to find out exactly how good that Roman Orgy simulation package really is.

References

Binford, Tom. Private communication.

Cherniak, Christopher (1990) "The Bounded Brain: Toward Quantitative Neuroanatomy." *Journal of Cognitive Neuroscience* 2/1, pp. 58–68.

Hille, Bertil (1984) *Ionic Channels of Excitable Membranes*. Sunderland, MA: Sinauer.

Kandel, Eric R., Schwartz, James H., and Jessell, Thomas M. (1991) *Principles of Neural Science*, 3rd edn. Amsterdam: Elsevier.

Kuffler, Stephen W., Nichols, John G., and Martin, A. Robert (1984) *From Neuron to Brain*, 2nd edn. Sunderland, MA: Sinauer.

Landauer, Thomas K. (1986) "How Much Do People Remember? Some Estimates of the Quantity of Learned Information in Long-term Memory." *Cognitive Science* 10, pp. 477–493.

Moravec, Hans (1988) *Mind Children*. Cambridge, MA: Harvard University Press.

Part IV

Core Technologies

To a greater degree than other philosophies of life, transhumanism's realization depends on continuing technological advancement. Current levels of technology are not sufficient to achieve the goals of extending the maximum human lifespan, enhancing our cognition, refining our emotions at a neurobiological level, expanding our civilization reliably beyond this planet, and so on. Part IV includes essays from renowned technological thinkers on some of the core technologies for converting radical transhumanist ideas into practical applications. Crucial advances can come from unexpected directions, but some of the technologies that have especially attracted interest in transhumanism are artificial intelligence (as already seen in Goertzel's essay in Part III), nanotechnology, biotechnology, computing, robotics, and brain-machine interfaces.

The "father of AI" and long-time transhumanist Marvin Minsky has written numerous essays and books on artificial intelligence, consciousness, and other topics of great relevance to the achievement of transhumanist goals. Since one intent of this book is to convey a historical sense of the development of transhumanism, we have chosen to publish not a formal essay but a typically opinionated talk by Minsky that conveys some of the flavor of transhumanist conference discussions in the mid-1990s. These conferences generated and developed ideas well outside the mainstream of the time – ideas that have increasingly become seriously discussed in today's mainstream. Here Minsky emphasizes differences in thinking between transhumanists and others; says why you want to live longer in order to be able to solve the hard problems; explains how Freud was one of the first to understand that the mind is not a unitary entity; the silliness of those who believe machines cannot be conscious; and why various approaches to machine intelligence are a bad idea.

Originally published in *Extropy: The Journal of Transhumanist Thought* 13 (1994). Copyright © Max More.

Roboticist Hans Moravec forms a picture of the cybernetic human mind in his 1992 essay "Pigs in Cyberspace." As machines become smarter, organizations of robots with increased intelligence could expand, occupy, and manipulate matter. Either humanity will have produced a worthy successor, or transcended inherited limitations and transformed itself into something quite new. Moravec suggests a virtual out-of-body experience as replacing the human biological body with a "brain in a vat" scenario, which has often been used to mean disembodiment. However, a person cannot exist without some form of physical system. Moravec's supposition actually proposes a cybermind, rather than a disembodiment, where cyberspace becomes what we might consider to be a new type of body. While Moravec's forecasts and future timeline are stimulating and always grand in scope, they might not necessarily reflect those of other transhumanists.

J. Storrs Hall, originator of the Utility Fog concept, examines the potential of nanoscale computing devices in this 1992 essay. Nanoscale devices are crucial for nanomedicine, for reengineering the body and brain, and for cleaning up the environment, among many other applications. Nanotechnological designs up to the present may or may not accurately describe the precise devices we will use in the future, but analyses like Hall's take us out of the limited perspective of today and usefully illuminate the true potential and limits of computing.

Evolutionary biologist and gerontologist Michael Rose argues in this new essay that biological aging is not inevitable. Rose outlines a new immortality strategy, based on his work in gerontology and evolutionary biology. Many transhumanists avoid the term "immortality," but Rose has a specific, grounded meaning in mind. First, he surveys how people now usually envision how biological immortality will be achieved. As revealed in fiction, the common view is that a simple technological fix will stop aging completely. This view is shared, says Rose, by molecular and cell biologists who imagine one or a few fundamental aging processes. He contrasts this view with his own "penicillin-like idea" about biological immortality, based on an evolutionary genetic view of aging. Rose concludes with some practical advice to stop aging earlier (including a paleolithic-based diet for people over 30 or 40), cautious supplementation and avoidance of most prescription drugs and, when available, taking advantage of methods for repair at the level of cultured tissues and other macroscopic structures. Rose's perspective is one of several competing views of aging tracked by transhumanists.

The final piece in Part IV consists of a dialogue between Ray Kurzweil and nanotechnology pioneer Eric Drexler. They discuss what it would take to achieve successful repair and revival of a fully functioning human brain from cryonics, with memories intact. They agree that despite the challenges, the brain's functions and memories can be represented surprisingly compactly, suggesting that successful repair and revival of the brain may be achievable.

16

Why Freud Was the First Good AI Theorist

Marvin Minsky

I usually shock people by telling them about all sorts of possible wonders of the future, but it is probably impossible to shock an Extropian. If I am talking to a general audience I usually explain to them that if it weren't for their bad habits and superstitions they could live forever. I was telling a small general audience that if we figured how the brain worked well enough so that we could make backup tapes – obviously nobody would go anywhere unless they had a recent backup, because you know what happens when you cross the street, then you could just reload it into another better body – and nobody seemed to be reacting to this in the way that they ought to. So I asked how many of them would like to live 500 years: 500 years isn't even immortality, it's just extended lifespan. About 15 percent of these 100 people thought this was a good idea but the others didn't. Various people said that it would get boring, and what would they do, and wouldn't they become a nuisance to others – that one was correct.

We live in a culture where people think death is sort of nice because it's like retirement or a vacation. I pursued this a little longer until I couldn't stand it any more. It turned out that none of them had any ambitions or goals except to get a better car, and after they got a very good car then they wouldn't care about anything.

How many of you don't want to live 500 years? [*Audience: "I want to live more."*] That's a problem: we live in a society in which people consider it a virtue to not be discontented with your lot and they believe in various kinds of gods and other sorts of creators.

I'm an atheist because I believe being an agnostic is really very bad for your mental health, and since it doesn't matter whether you're right or wrong anyway. I can't imagine a god that would care one way or the other in the first place, and even if there were one I can't see any reason why if he wrote a book of rules you would care. Just because the creator says "X" doesn't mean that there is any reason to obey it.

Originally published in *Extropy Online* (2002). Copyright © Max More.

The Transhumanist Reader: Classical and Contemporary Essays on the Science, Technology, and Philosophy of the Human Future, First Edition. Edited by Max More and Natasha Vita-More.
© 2013 John Wiley & Sons, Inc. Published 2013 by John Wiley & Sons, Inc.

But there is a much more serious problem: how come we're not immortal? If you look at the state of technology today, it's pretty good. We've learned a lot since the time of Kepler and Galileo, but a lot of stuff has happened in 400 years. Very little happened in the 1,500 or 2,000 years between Euclid and Galileo, so there was a big hiatus. I'm sure that most of us feel that it's only another 100 years until we have nanotechnology and downloading and immortality – some people like Moravec say that technically you could do it in 30 or 40 years – maybe it's 200, who cares, with cryonics it might not matter. The question is, if we're within a century or two of immortality – now I don't just want longevity, you want to live longer, but the reason you want to live longer is that there isn't enough time to learn to solve hard problems, it takes about 50 years to get good at anything these days and then everyone would have to start over so you want to be smarter and faster (maybe it doesn't matter if you're faster), but if you do understand how the brain works then you can improve it – and we're just dressed-up chimpanzees, and we have a long way to go.

Science has been sort of opposed by superstition. I turned on late-night television not long ago and there were three different psychic phone programs on our seven free stations (I don't have cable). You have these paid actors pretending to have had psychic experiences.

I get the feeling that things are worse than they were with respect to rampant superstition. A long time ago I read an article in the *New York Times Magazine* where somebody had wondered if things were getting worse. So they got a lot of historians: historians can prove anything they are paid to prove. It was a wonderful article where various historians had a very nice quote every hundred years or so, except for the dark ages they didn't have any in that period, in which somebody wise was saying how much stupider the children were than when he was a kid. If you collect those statements you can see a steady decline from the time of Aristotle – but the sampling technique isn't very good. It didn't have any such quotes between 300 and 1200, so that was sort of conspicuous.

Every now and then there is a centennial and I think the reason that there is this fake Freud title on my talk is that 1995 is the centennial of the first good book on structural psychology, namely Freud's *Interpretation of Dreams*, which came out in 1895. It's the first major work which discusses the mind as though there weren't a single little homunculus or mastermind in the middle of it pulling the strings.

When I was a kid I opened an encyclopedia and it showed this hollow head (it reminds me of Zardoz) and you see the eyes and there were little TV cameras (they weren't TV cameras when I was a kid, but the equivalent) and with microphones for the ears and all of this I/O stuff comes in and then there's a little guy sitting at the desk running things. So that's the single self idea that there's a "me" or a central agent in the middle of all this hardware, the "ghost in the machine."

Freud's book is the first one that I know of that says that in the mind there isn't a single thing there, there are at least three or four major systems. There is the common-sense reasoning system – later he wrote a book on the psychopathology of everyday life in which he tries and fails to account for how people do ordinary common-sense reasoning, but he recognizes that as a very hard problem. If you look at the later Freud a lot of people think that Freud must have studied emotions and emotional illnesses and disorders because that was the really hard and important problem, but Freud himself said the really hard thing to understand is how people do ordinary everyday non-neurotic reasoning.

The reason I suggested that he was a great AI researcher is that in trying to make this theory of how people's motivations worked in this period 1895 and a couple years thereafter, he wrote this long essay, some of which is lost, for the Project for Scientific Psychology. The project wasn't published until around 1950 by Carl Pribram, and it has little diagrams which are sort of neural network like, but more like the hydraulic motivation theory that later Nikolaas Tinbergen and Konrad Lorenz won the Nobel Prize for, this diagram that is the foundation of modern ecological theory.

One of Freud's ideas which was not popular in philosophy was that children think differently from adults and their learning to think. And there are a lot of different structures, there is an id which is a basic collection of instincts and the common-sense reasoning system: I think of it as a sandwich. His conception is that there are some problems to be solved, and reinforcement (Skinner-like) systems for learning how to get food and other basic needs, receptors for telling when you've succeeded, and so forth. Then there's parts of the mind that do reasoning and planning, which Freud had no idea of how they worked, and then there is this other structure which is constructed in the baby's mind by social mechanism called the superego, a piece of machinery that we have and other animals don't have so much of, which is a collection of rules or knowledge about what sort of person you want to be and what kinds of methods you're allowed to use for solving your problems. If you want your baby brother's toy you can get it by grabbing it away, only then there is a big fuss. The best thing of course is to kill the baby brother so that he can't come and take it back, but there is this mechanism through which you learn the values, the morals (Freud describes this in his later books, it's not so much in the *Interpretation of Dreams*), that there is some piece of machinery which he called the Oedipus Complex and interjection of the values of the attachment person.

I've been working on theories like that, there is one page in *Society of Mind* about the question of how that's done. But the point is that Freud is an important figure because he's the first one to consider that the mind is a big complicated kludge of different types of machinery which are specialized for different functions. If you look at the brain you find 400-odd different pieces of computer architecture with their own busses and somewhat different architecture. Nobody knows much about how any of those work yet but they're on the track. The idea that the brain is made of neurons and works largely by sending signals along the nerve fibers which are the connections between them is only from about 1890. The neuron doctrine, that the nerve cells are not a single organism, not a single thing but there are a lot of independent gadgets which do separate things and send signals that are informational rather than chemical and so forth, is only a hundred years old. In the pop psychology of the new age this is blurred and most people are entranced by the idea that if you feel bad or good it is because of some neurotransmitter or chemical. Chemicals aren't what make you feel good, the chemicals are just like other signals to the AND and OR complicated gates on the neurons. All chemicals are more or less equivalent. It's not in the nature of vitamin C that it's healthy, it's because it has some particular function among the 30-odd thousand metabolic pathways for doing very specific things.

If people want to live longer there were two ways: one is you can do physics and biology and chemistry and develop science, and by the time of Archimedes they were well on the way. Greek science wasn't bad; I just read Lucretius's book on optics and he has some half-baked theories of how you see and so forth. These theories are not very good but they could have been improved within a hundred years I think if the experimental science paradigm had taken root.

The other way was if you do various kinds of mumbo-jumbo then this great agent in the sky will come down and give you eternal life, in which case you could have an infinite number of sports cars. And so Pascal's wager: either you believe in God or you don't; if there is no God it can't do any harm to believe in him because he's not going to punish you because he doesn't exist; on the other hand if you don't believe in him and there is one then he'll be mad at you and you won't get eternal life. That argument convinced a lot of people that it didn't do any harm to believe in religion. But in fact it did them harm and it's what killed them all because if they had believed in science instead of religion 2,000 years ago we would all be immortal now. Pascal's wager was exactly wrong. Well I think it was exactly wrong because it's been a long time and I haven't seen anyone get eternal life.

There's been a wonderful spate of very well-selling books in the last four or five years: these are books proving by various kinds of really silly arguments, like Penrose, and Searle, proving that you can't be immortal and you can't do anything about your brain, you can't even understand it – because it doesn't work!

Searle has this elaborate argument to show that even if a machine did everything the same as you it couldn't understand what it's doing because it doesn't have something called intentionality which was a bogus concept invented by a philosopher named Brentano in 1876 or so. Intentionality is the thing that relates the idea of for example a Powerbook which is very abstract and only exists in the mental world somehow to the actual Powerbook over there. [*Audience member: "Platonic ideas?"*] I don't know if it's Platonic, I know Plato had the idea that there were ideas and that they were somehow related to the real things… but whatever Plato did didn't seem to lead to any good theories of psychology. Searle says that a machine can't really understand (this is something, for reasons I can't understand, he says that living tissue like brains have, but sticks and stones don't), and that's all there is to it. This is some irreducible property. If you read comp.ai.philosophy you will find people saying it's some magical trick which animates things that understand and things that don't understand don't have it. These people tend to think that you either understand or not, it's a very digital thing. There is no such thing as a little understanding any more than there is a little pregnancy or a little death. All of those superstitions are equally silly.

Then there is another fellow named Penrose who is really quite a good mathematical physicist. He had the same argument about why machines can't be conscious only his reasons are incredibly elaborate and silly. The main argument in his first book (I haven't read the second) has about 12 chapters and each one has a couple of wrong proofs of this. Penrose's method is that by giving enough false proofs then you can't help feeling that if there is a lot of smoke then there must be fire.

[*Audience question about robot COG*]

Robot COG is a hoax proposed by some professors at a lab at MIT. Their idea is that if you build a big machine out of computers and give it hands and eyes then eventually a very smart student will turn up who will program it to do something significant. The world has fallen in love with the work of Rod Brooks and his students on mini robots, even though as far as I can tell no interesting discoveries were made in the last seven or eight years of building these cute little things that crawl around, nothing that wasn't known already and nothing that you couldn't have found out in much less time by simulating them. It's a very serious disease that has spread all over the world. The best mini robots I've seen, at least a couple of years ago, were done right around here at USC. There's a group there that makes mini robots and they look at least as good as the MIT ones, but there is nothing that somebody who has built one can tell someone else that isn't obvious. As far as I can tell COG has no cognitive theory.

I can summarize my view of this skepticism by saying that it's another persistence of this religious idea that there is a magic understanding: there is a magic substance that's responsible for understanding and for consciousness, and that there's a deep secret here and in order to solve it we'll have to make some fundamental new discovery. In Searle's case he throws up his hands and says, "I don't know what the nature of this is," and in the case of Penrose there is desperate floundering around and he says, "Maybe it's got something to do with quantum coherency or something like that." Among Penrose's reasons is the idea that if a human mathematician thinks hard enough and goes into the right kind of trance then the mathematician can tell which statements about mathematics are true.

[*Question: "Was there ever a computer which tried to work out mathematical laws?"*]

There was Doug Lenat's project called AM which managed to start with rather little and discovered numbers; now it wasn't so hard for it to discover numbers because it had a function for the length of the list that it inherited from the underlying list. It fooled around with various hypotheses and discovered that some numbers were divisible by others and some weren't. It got interested in numbers that had only one divisor, and there weren't any except one, and numbers which had a large number of divisors. It didn't discover anything good about them, but it discovered that there were some numbers that had only two divisors and those were interesting. In fact it even discovered that there were certain numbers that had only three divisors and those are the perfect squares of primes. In the course of doing all this it had to do division and in fact there was an error in the division algorithm but it never hurt anything because Lenat's program wasn't proving things, it was just finding them out. He wrote another program called Eurisko some years later which discovered more stuff. In the case of AM the machine discovered quite a lot about arithmetic and then it slowed down and stopped discovering interesting things after that; no one ever understood why. Lenat and Brown wrote a paper on their theory of why it did so well and stopped working and I didn't agree with them. I wrote a paper which was published in *Byte* magazine of all places called "The Sparseness Hypothesis." I thought that the discovery of these arithmetic things was inevitable and it wasn't because they got just the right representation. If it ever discovered anything in an orderly way it would have to discover arithmetic early. This is my argument and if you want to read it you can look at my Web page, it will download it to you: it is all in ASCII so it only takes a few seconds (to download, not to read).

Let me talk about two things briefly like Bart Kosko: he had a way of explaining the hard part of each thing and then left an hour and a half explaining the details. How many different sentences did Bart use to tell you if you were smart enough maybe you could understand this, but he wasn't going to rub your nose in it? Every Kosko paragraph is suppressing a whole lecture.

Let's take understanding which is the basis of Searle's confusion. I have a rule that works both for Penrose and Searle which is, if it were written by a sophomore he would have gotten a B because there was some pretty good stuff. If he were a junior it would be a C, and so on. Searle has this Chinese room problem in which he talks about a machine that simulates something that people would say requires intelligence, but since the computer doesn't have any intelligence and the database doesn't have any understanding, it has to do with understanding sentences in a language you don't know. Searle's argument is that if you have a computer and a database, where the computer using the database can translate from Chinese to English then this must be a sham because since the computer processor is just flip-flops and whatever it is and certainly doesn't understand Chinese and since the database is just a bunch of data in a disk file, it can't understand Chinese then the combination can't understand it either and it's just making you think that it understands. So that's basically the Chinese argument and it's like saying that there can't be a car because it's just wheels and motors and stuff like that. That's why I guess I wouldn't give it a B if it were by a freshman after all. When you read the paper twice then you always increase the grade or decrease it because you suddenly realize that the student was better or worse than you thought.

What is understanding? It seems to me that the problem that has happened in psychology on the whole and even in artificial intelligence, is that they've missed the lesson that Freud taught us, and I'm not saying that I'm a great admirer about the next 40 years of his research on psycho-sexual theories and so forth. I read a lot of that once but it seems to me that by 1905 Freud had produced a whole bunch of AI-like ideas that should have been followed up, but people got more interested in his theories of emotions and neuroses.

Let's take this problem of how to make a machine that understands. When I was a little kid I read a book by Hendrick van Loon – he wrote children's books which were wonderful. In one of them there was a story about a little kid who was only learning by rote, and the teacher would explain that the Nile is the longest river in the world and he would ask Johnny, "Did you understand what I said?" and Johnny said, "Yes, the Nile is the longest river in the world" and later the teacher would ask, "What's the longest river in the world?" and Johnny couldn't answer that because he hadn't understood the sentence, he had just literally memorized it. So we know that there is such a thing as learning by rote and maybe that is what Searle is accusing machines of doing.

What is understanding? What I claim is that there isn't any such thing. There is no such thing as consciousness, there is no such thing as understanding and all of the trouble these people are having is because they've gotten trapped into using words that have become very popular for social reasons, it is very useful to say that this kid doesn't understand, meaning that his performance and versatility and ability to apply what he's supposed to learn isn't good enough and he's going to have to come back after school or repeat second grade… but of course that would interfere with his social development, so we can't do that… and blah, blah…

So what is there if there is no such thing as understanding? Here is a little paradox, it's the reason that everybody in the philosophy business has gotten trapped into hopeless nonsense. It's just what van Loon said: If you understand something exactly one way then you don't understand it at all. It's "physics envy" that has stopped the psychologists (that's a Freudian expression, I suppose). The physicists have been very successful at reducing things to be very simple and so they decided they would take the brain with its 400 different computers and explain that that there aren't 400 different ones, there is just one that is very simple and that's a terrible mistake. So what do I mean by, "if you understand something one way that you don't understand it at all?" Suppose you want it as a sentence and then you get another sentence which matches the other sentence's end in exactly the same way as your sentence begins, then there is an operation called chaining where you can splice out – when you say, "I wonder what the Nile is" then Johnny substitutes this other one and says, "It's the longest river in the world." So he understands it that one way and he can pass that test.

But what happens if you're in a room and you see a telephone, or you see a chair, an object, you wouldn't understand what the chair is if you only saw it one way. You might see it as four sticks (and there's a chapter on this in *Society of Mind* talking endlessly about a chair), but you see that thing as a structure there is a rigid horizontal platform, you know enough about sticks that somehow they hold the chair up. I don't understand how chairs work actually because there are no triangles in them, and it's amazing that they work at all. But you also understand it in a dozen other ways, you understand that the seat of the chair is this far off the floor and that is just about the same as the distance from your heels to your knees so it allows you to… your legs are independent from your hips, so it's comfortable and there's this back you can lean back on so that your vertebrae feel better and so forth. In other words, to understand a chair you have to know what a person feels like at different times, when you're tired and so forth, and you also know how much it costs, and a dozen different things.

That is what Searle was missing, there was no such thing as understanding but what there is, I think, in the brain, one of the things that happens in these 400 different computers is that there are probably 5 or 10 different ways to represent… whenever you learn something, you not only learn it, you learn it in different representations. I know what that chair is like in the visual sense, I know what it feels like, how stiff the materials are, I know what happens when I walk across the room in the dark and stub my toe on it, because there is a correlation between walking in the dark and not having shoes on. The point is that no one way will tell you much.

Now why is it good to represent things in several ways? I bet that in this part of the brain you are representing things in terms of long-range planning, in scripts, the way the great Roger Shank describes. In another part of the brain, maybe around the language area, you are representing things as trees of dependencies on very orderly structures. In other parts of the brain you are representing them as semantic networks which are not so well understood. Probably toward the back of the brain you are representing them in a sort of pictorial fashion, like when people are basically very bad at three dimensions, but you have little blotches of two dimensions and when you think of a chair you can think of how it looks from the front and from the side, and a little bit like this. So the reason why you can convince yourself that you can imagine the chair is because you have these many different ways of representing it.

And then you've got some ways of representing it that are the kind of neural nets that have become popular in the last few years, where you can recognize it when you see it but you don't have the slightest idea of how you do it. A lot of the knowledge in the brain is of this very useful and fast, but philosophically worthless knowledge because it's inarticulate, it's very hard… a lot of people like neural nets and I think I heard Bart talking about it today, that it's better than traditional statistical methods in many cases for getting a machine to learn to recognize patterns. On the other hand if the knowledge that you get is buried in the form of coefficients, of just numbers distributed through the structure, then you can't reason about it, and so I absolutely agree that fuzzy logic is much better than regular logic for almost all purposes except that if you could represent things in terms of regular logic with formal axioms then there is a slight chance that you'll be able to pull those out and manipulate them and get inferences that you can't get from knowledge buried in neural nets.

So one of the tragedies of AI is that everyone except for maybe a dozen people in the world have each made a choice and they say, "I'm going to build an intelligent machine representing knowledge in such-and-such a way," somebody else does it another way, each of them is a dead end because it can do a few things but it can't do the other things that Searle and Penrose and everybody else would agree a smart person does. So AI is full of these dead ends of single representations.

What I've tried to develop in the "Society of Mind" and in the new book is a different idea, and I think it corresponds a little to what Dan Dennett says, namely when you think about something you're always thinking about it in four or five different ways, all the time. It's not one rule-book that destroys the Searle structure. What's happening is that they're always breaking, if you think about something, if you're thinking about an image but all of a sudden you can't see it any more… if I describe a couple of triangles and they're tangent to a circle and I ask you what does the line between the centers of the two circles do, you can't answer it. If there are five or six things in a geometric figure then only one person in thousand can see that clearly, although everybody can see the circle and the triangle.

It's like a chess master who maybe sees pieces of the board that are about five by five but can understand the connections between them. According to Adrian de Grout, who wrote this great

PhD thesis on what it's like to be a Chess Grand Master, which he was, none of his friends who were Grand Masters could see a whole board but they never needed to, they could imagine fragments of it and they knew exactly how they were related by non-visual methods. For good chess players having a board is no help at all. It's just as easy to play blindfolded chess as non-blindfolded chess because whenever you make a move you construct a network of relationships and it's no use having them in sight because you're never thinking about the board as it is but how it will be in three moves. If I were to learn chess again I would do it without a board – when I'm downloaded and uploaded again I'll run that.

OK, so that's the point: there is no such thing as understanding, but the point is that when you're thinking about something you're doing it five different ways and I'll bet that every one second or two seconds one of them breaks, the other four go on, maybe two of them break and the other three go on, and then one of these things has repaired itself.

In my book I proposed it very vaguely, only a couple of people seem to understand what I was saying so I'm rewriting it. The idea is that there are things called paranoms which make sure that these different computers are proceeding independently but they're sort of locking in on the representation that the others are using. So that's what happening, there is no central process in you except really powerful trivial ones, the little central processes which say, "Boy, I've been working on this problem for ten minutes and I'm not getting anywhere. Let's go swimming – We're only a block from Santa Monica beach." I've been turning that agent off all day, every 15 or 20 minutes…

This mysterious thing called understanding, Brentano's intentionality, and this absolute atomic relation between an idea and the meaning is complete hogwash. You are a kludge and what you have is half a dozen really crummy connections between the representations and the other representations and the stuff coming in through your senses – and that's why nobody is going to understand it by using the physics approach. The same thing with Penrose who says, "I don't see any method by which a computer could be conscious, and so it must be…" – it's like the real reason why people think that Edward de Vere wrote Shakespeare is that they look at these plays and they say that nobody could write well enough to write these plays, so it must have been someone else!

Anyway, there is no such thing as consciousness either, so what is the phenomenon which drives Penrose up the wall? He says here's this thing, I know I have it, I know these other people have it, it's so wonderful it lets you feel and think and understand stuff but there is nothing in a computer that could have it so… and a great thing about physicists is that physicists make unified theories, there are two different phenomena and the best thing a physicist can do… well, the really best thing a physicist can do is prove somebody else's theory is wrong, but the next best thing is to take two things which are unrelated and to find a single theory to explain both. So as far as I can see Roger Penrose feels that he understands most things but he doesn't understand quantum gravity and he doesn't understand consciousness, so they must be the same. And that of course is the reason for religion, we don't understand how people work it out, we don't understand why they get sick and if we believe that people who are bad should be punished and we meet people who aren't punished, we wonder about that, and everybody has a million questions, and so the religious theory is: Oh, that's easy, there is just one answer and it's called God and if you really believe in this then you'll see how all questions can be answered. The usual answer is, at least the Catholic answer is: you ask them a hard one like why did so-and-so break their leg, and the answer is, "Well you should know by now that you can't understand the ways of God." So that's the unified theory. Speaking of skepticism, my favorite sentence which I actually heard once as I walked by this accident which had just happened and his mother said, "Thank God he didn't break both legs." That puts the whole thing in perspective.

I think consciousness is thirty-odd different things that we don't understand so we give them all the same name but the prominent one is that you know that you can see... here is a microphone, I can see the microphone... I don't have the foggiest idea how I see it but we know that there are all sorts of image processors in certain parts of the brain and that there are feature recognizers and this semantic thing so that I parse this into parts – here is this little round thing, and here is this cylindrical thing, and here is this goose-neck flexible thing – a tremendous amount of processing, probably using a hundred different bits of machinery. Vision involves a full third of the brain, nearly half. At least all these things are active, we don't know how it works. So you get information from the outer world through all of this stuff and we are all used to that and we talk about seeing and hearing. If you consider the chain of events that happens where the stuff goes through the various parts of the brain, there are a lot of things happening there before it gets to the language part of you that says, "I see the microphone."

There are parts of the brain that get their input not from the outside world but from other parts of the brain, and so when you're thinking about such-and-such, parts of your brain are thinking about this certain thing, there are other parts which are watching that part of the brain and remembering what that looks like. In other words there are parts of your brain that are taking pictures of the mental state of other parts of your brain and storing them in little caches, little temporary places.

Suppose that first that you think about what would it be like... suppose I wanted to change a light-bulb, imagine changing a light-bulb in one of those [*pointing to chandelier*]... well I can't reach it, so what should I do? I guess I could get that chair and put it on the table, so this is called imagining, then I'd stand on the chair and guess what, I still couldn't reach it. So that's not so good. Well, let's see, let me try another way: I could take this table and pick it up and put it on that table and then it would be about that high and now if I put that chair on it I could reach it. So I'll do that. Now, what did I do? I found two different solutions to the problem, I stored them both away and then I compared them. In the first case I reached just about this high, in the second case it was about three feet higher – that's better. So, I'm remembering what my mind did a minute ago.

If you take all of the things you heard about consciousness, I think most of them can be explained by various arrangements in which parts of the brain have some memories of what recently happened in other parts. Now you can't have an idea like that if you're like Skinner or Chomsky or anyone who is not in the Freudian line because the idea of different parts of your mind thinking different ways and storing things in buffers nobody had that kind of idea until the late 1950s. Computer science was the first way of talking that let you think about how complicated processes could go on. So, that's what's missing in these traditional philosophers like Penrose and Searle, they're still using the ordinary, naive ideas like understanding and consciousness.

I think in the next 40 or 50 years, if we're lucky, if people don't go on more and more bad fads like COG and like neural networks and so forth, but if we got a decent community of people to think about how to make things that manage several different representations instead of sticking to one. There is almost nobody thinking about how to build a kludge that can do the different things the mind can do.

Then we'll know enough to be able to look at brains and nanotechnology will come along so we'll get the wiring diagrams and we'll start to understand how the whole thing works even if cryonics does a lot of damage, once we understand how brains usually work we'll be able to look at these badly damaged frozen ones and figure out the connections and functions and eventually the multiple representations of various kinds of knowledge and if anyone wants to pay the bill you can reconstruct people and get back to work again. It won't cost much, of course, if you believe the nano-enthusiasts because once you build smart enough robots, they'll work for free, because they are smart and you've arranged their goals for them. Of course we're going to have the same problems with the smart machines that Drexler discusses when you make the self-reproducing dangerous nanotechnology devices. How do you build a system that is smart enough to evolve and think of new things but is somehow never inclined to go into business for itself?

In fact, how do we control the Extropians once they…

I think I've over-talked, but I'll be glad to start a fight with anyone who wants to.

17

Pigs in Cyberspace

Hans Moravec

Exploration and colonization of the universe await, but Earth-adapted biological humans are ill equipped to respond to the challenge. Machines have gone farther and seen more, limited though they presently are by insect-like behavioral inflexibility. As they become smarter over the coming decades, space will be theirs. Organizations of robots of ever-increasing intelligence and sensory and motor ability will expand and transform what they occupy, working with matter, space, and time. As they grow, a smaller and smaller fraction of their territory will be undeveloped frontier. Competitive success will depend more and more on using already available matter and space in ever more refined and useful forms. The process, analogous to the miniaturization that makes today's computers a trillion times more powerful than the mechanical calculators of the past, will gradually transform all activity from grossly physical homesteading of raw nature to minimum-energy quantum transactions of computation. The final frontier will be urbanized, ultimately into an arena where every bit of activity is a meaningful computation: the inhabited portion of the universe will transformed into a cyberspace.

Because it will use resources more efficiently, a mature cyberspace of the distant future will be effectively much bigger than the present physical universe. While only an infinitesimal fraction of existing matter and space is doing interesting work, in a well-developed cyberspace every bit will be part of a relevant computation or storing a useful datum. Over time, more compact and faster ways of using space and matter will be invented, and used to restructure the cyberspace, effectively increasing the amount of computational spacetime per unit of physical spacetime.

Computational speedups will affect the subjective experience of entities in the cyberspace in a paradoxical way. At first glimpse, there is no subjective effect, because everything, inside and

Edited transcript of a talk given at Extropy Institute's EXTRO-3 conference in San Jose, California, August 1997. Originally published in *Extropy: The Journal of Transhumanist Thought* 10 (1993), pp. 5–7. Copyright © Max More.

outside the individual, speeds up equally. But, more subtly, speedup produces an expansion of the cyber universe, because, as thought accelerates, more subjective time passes during the fixed (probably lightspeed) physical transit time of a message between a given pair of locations – so those fixed locations seem to grow farther apart. Also, as information storage is made continually more efficient through both denser utilization of matter and more efficient encodings, there will be increasingly more cyber-stuff between any two points. The effect may somewhat resemble the continuous-creation process in the old steady-state theory of the physical universe of Hoyle, Bondi, and Gold, where hydrogen atoms appear just fast enough throughout the expanding cosmos to maintain a constant density.

A quantum-mechanical entropy calculation by Bekenstein suggests that the ultimate amount of information that can be stored given the mass and volume of a hydrogen atom is about a mega-byte. But let's be conservative, and imagine that at some point in the future only "conventional" physics is in play, but every few atoms stores a useful bit. There are about 10^{56} atoms in the solar system. I estimate that a human brain-equivalent can be encoded in less than 10^{15} bits. If a body and surrounding environment takes a thousand times more storage in addition, a human, with immediate environment, might consume 10^{18} bits. An AI with equivalent intelligence could prob-ably get by with less, since it does without the body-simulation "life support" needed to keep a body-oriented human mind sane. So a city of a million human-scale inhabitants might be effi-ciently stored in 10^{24} bits. If the atoms of the solar system were cleverly rearranged so every 100 could represent a bit, then a single solar system could hold 10^{30} cities – far more than the number (10^{22}) of stars in the visible universe! Multiply that by 10^{11} stars in a galaxy, and one gets 10^{41} cities per galaxy. The visible universe, with 10^{11} galaxies, would then have room for 10^{51} cities – except that by the time intelligence has expanded that far, more efficient ways of using spacetime and encoding data would surely have been discovered, increasing the number much further.

Mind without Body?

Start with the concepts of telepresence and virtual reality. You wear a harness that, with optical, acoustical, mechanical and chemical devices, controls all that you sense, and measures all of your actions. Its machinery presents pictures to your eyes, sounds to your ears, pressures and temperatures to your skin, forces to your muscles, and even smells and tastes for the remaining senses. Telepresence results when the inputs and outputs of this harness connect to a distant machine that looks like a humanoid robot. The images from the robot's two camera eyes appear on your "eyeglass" viewscreens, and you hear through its ears, feel through its skin, and smell through its chemical sensors. When you move your head or body, the robot moves in exact synchrony. When you reach for an object seen in the viewscreens, the robot reaches for the object, and when it makes contact, your muscles and skin feel the resulting weight, shape, texture, and temperature. For most practical purposes you inhabit the robot's body – your sense of consciousness has migrated to the robot's location, in a true "out of body" experience.

Virtual reality retains the harness, but replaces the remote robot with a computer simulation of a body and its surroundings. When connected to a virtual reality, the location you seem to inhabit does not exist in the usual physical sense, rather you are in a kind of computer-generated dream. If the computer has access to data from the outside world, the simulation may contain some "real" items, for instance representations of other people connected via their own harnesses, or even views of the outside world, perhaps through simulated windows.

One might imagine a hybrid system where a virtual "central station" is surrounded by portals that open on to views of multiplereal locations. While in the station one inhabits a simulated body, but when one steps through a portal, the harness link is seamlessly switched from the simulation to a telepresence robot waiting at that location.

The technical challenges limit the availability, "fidelity," and affordability of telepresence and virtual reality systems today – in fact, they exist only in a few highly experimental demonstrations. But progress is being made, and it's possible to anticipate a time, a few decades hence, when people spend more time in remote and virtual realities than in their immediate surroundings, just as today most of us spend more time in artificial indoor surroundings than in the great outdoors. The remote bodies we will inhabit can be stronger, faster, and have better senses than our "home" body. In fact, as our home body ages and weakens, we might compensate by turning up some kind of "volume control." Eventually, we might wish to bypass our atrophied muscles and dimmed senses altogether, if neurobiology learns enough to connect our sensory and motor nerves directly to electronic interfaces. Then all the harness hardware could be discarded as obsolete, along with our sense organs and muscles, and indeed most of our body. There would be no "home" experiences to return to, but our remote and virtual existences would be better than ever.

The picture is that we are now is a "brain in a vat," sustained by life-support machinery, and connected by wonderful electronic links, at will, to a series of "rented" artificial bodies at remote locations, or to simulated bodies in artificial realities. But the brain is a biological machine not designed to function forever, even in an optimal physical environment. As it begins to malfunction, might we not choose to use the same advanced neurological electronics that make possible our links to the external world, to replace the gray matter as it begins to fail? Bit by bit our brain is replaced by electronic equivalents, which work at least as well, leaving our personality and thoughts clearer than ever. Eventually everything has been replaced by manufactured parts. No physical vestige of our original body or brain remains, but our thoughts and awareness continue. We will call this process, and other approaches with the same end result, the downloading of a human mind into a machine. After downloading, our personality is a pattern impressed on electronic hardware, and we may then find ways to move our minds to other similar hardware, just as a computer program and its data can be copied from processor to processor. So not only can our sense of awareness shift from place to place at the speed of communication, but the very components of our minds may ride on the same data channels. We might find ourselves distributed over many locations, one piece of our mind here, another piece there, and our sense of awareness at yet another place. Time becomes more flexible – when our mind resides in very fast hardware, one second of real time may provide a subjective year of thinking time, while a thousand years of real time spent on a passive storage medium may seem like no time at all. Can we then consider ourselves to be a mind without a body? Not quite.

A human totally deprived of bodily senses does not do well. After 12 hours in a sensory deprivation tank (where one floats in a body-temperature saline solution that produces almost no skin sensation, in total darkness and silence, with taste and smell and the sensations of breathing minimized) a subject will begin to hallucinate, as the mind, somewhat like a television tuned to a nonexistent channel, turns up the amplification, desperately looking for a signal, becoming ever less discriminating in the theories it offers to make sense of the random sensory hiss it receives. Even the most extreme telepresence and virtual reality scenarios we have presented avoid complete bodylessness by always providing the mind with a consistent sensory (and motor) image, obtained from an actual remote robot body, or from a computer simulation. In those scenarios, a person may sometimes exist without a physical body, but never without the illusion of having one.

But in our computers there are already many entities that resemble truly bodiless minds. A typical computer chess program knows nothing about physical chess pieces or chessboards, or about the staring eyes of its opponent or the bright lights of a tournament. Nor does it work with an internal simulation of those physical attributes. It reasons instead with a very efficient and compact mathematical representation of chess positions and moves. For the benefit of human players this internal representation is sometimes translated to a recognizable graphic on a computer screen, but such images mean nothing to the program that actually chooses the chess moves. For all practical purposes, the chess program's thoughts and sensations – its consciousness – is pure chess, with no taint of the physical, or any other, world. Much more than a human mind with a simulated body stored in a computer, a chess program is a mind without a body.

So now, imagine a future world where programs that do chess, mathematics, physics, engineering, art, business, or whatever have grown up to become at least as clever as the human mind. Imagine also that most of the inhabited universe has been converted to a computer network – a cyberspace – where such programs live, side by side with downloaded human minds and accompanying simulated human bodies. Suppose that all these entities make their living in something of a free market way, trading the products of their labor for the essentials of life – in this world memory space and computing cycles. Some entities do the equivalent of manual work, converting undeveloped parts of the universe into cyberspace, or improving the performance of existing patches, thus creating new wealth. Others work on physics or engineering problems whose solutions give the developers new and better ways to construct computing capacity. Some create programs that can become part of one's mental capacity. They trade their discoveries and inventions for more working space and time. There are entities that specialize as agents, collecting commissions in return for locating opportunities and negotiating deals for their clients. Others act as banks, storing and redistributing resources, buying and selling computing space, time, and information. Some we might class as artists, creating structures that don't obviously result in physical resources, but which, for idiosyncratic reasons, are deemed valuable by some customers, and are traded at prices that fluctuate for subjective reasons. Some entities in the cyberworld will fail to produce enough value to support their requirements for existence – these eventually shrink and disappear, or merge with other ventures. Others will succeed and grow. The closest present-day parallel is the growth, evolution, fragmentation, and consolidation of corporations, whose options are shaped primarily by their economic performance.

A human would likely fare poorly in such a cyberspace. Unlike the streamlined artificial intelligences that zip about, making discoveries and deals, reconfiguring themselves to efficiently handle the data that constitutes their interactions, a human mind would lumber about in a massively inappropriate body simulation, analogous to someone in a deep diving suit plodding along among a troupe of acrobatic dolphins. Every interaction with the data world would first have to be analogized as some recognizable quasi-physical entity: other programs might be presented as animals, plants, or demons, data items as books or treasure chests, accounting entries as coins or gold. Maintaining such fictions increases the cost of doing business, as does operating the mind machinery that reduces the physical simulations into mental abstractions in the downloaded human mind. Though a few humans may find a niche exploiting their baroque construction to produce human-flavored art, more may feel a great economic incentive to streamline their interface to the cyberspace.

The streamlining could begin with the elimination of the body-simulation along with the portions of the downloaded mind dedicated to interpreting sense-data. These would be replaced with simpler integrated programs that produced approximately the same net effect in one's consciousness. One would still view the cyberworld in terms of location, color, smell, faces, and so on, but only those details we actually notice would be represented. We would still be at a disadvantage compared with the true artificial intelligences, who interact with the cyberspace in ways optimized for their tasks. We might then be tempted to replace some of our innermost mental processes with more cyberspace-appropriate programs purchased from the AIs, and so, bit by bit, transform ourselves into something much like them. Ultimately our thinking procedures could be totally liberated from any traces of our original body, indeed of any body. But the bodiless mind that results, wonderful though it may be in its clarity of thought and breadth of understanding, could in no sense be considered any longer human.

So, one way or another, the immensities of cyberspace will be teeming with very unhuman disembodied superminds, engaged in affairs of the future that are to human concerns as ours are to those of bacteria. But, once in a long while, humans do think of bacteria, even particular individual bacteria seen in particular microscopes. Similarly, a cyberbeing may occasionally bring to mind a human event of the distant past. If a sufficiently powerful mind makes a sufficiently large effort, such recall could occur with great detail – call it high fidelity. With enough fidelity, the situation of a remembered person, along with all the minutiae of her body, her thoughts, and feelings, would be perfectly recreated in a kind of mental simulation: a cyberspace within a cyberspace where the person would be as alive as anywhere. Sometimes the recall might be historically accurate; in other circumstances it could be artistically enhanced: it depends on the purposes of the cybermind. An evolving cyberspace becomes effectively ever more capacious and long lasting, and so can support ever more minds of ever greater power. If these minds spend only an infinitesimal fraction of their energy contemplating the human past, their sheer power should ensure that eventually our entire history is replayed many times in many places, and in many variations. The very moment we are now experiencing may actually be (almost certainly is) such a distributed mental event, and most likely is a complete fabrication that never happened physically. Alas, there is no way to sort it out from our perspective: we can only wallow in the scenery.

18

Nanocomputers

J. Storrs Hall

If the price and performance figures for transportation technology had followed the same curves as those for computers for the past 50 years, you'd be able to buy a top-of-the-line luxury car for $10. What's more, its mileage would be such as to allow you to drive around the world on one gallon of gas. That would only take about half an hour since top speed would be in the neighborhood of 50,000 mph (twice earth's escape velocity).

Oh, yes, and it would seat 5,000 people.

Comparisons like this serve to point out just how radically computers have improved in cost, power consumption, speed, and memory capacity over the past half-century. Is it possible that we could see as much improvement again, and in less than another half-century? The answer appears to be yes.

At one time, people measured the technological sophistication of computers in "generations." There were vacuum tubes, discrete transistors, ICs, and finally large-scale integration. However, since the mid-1970s, the entire processing unit has increasingly come to be put on a single chip and called a "microprocessor." After these future advances have happened, today's microprocessors will look the way ENIAC does to us now. The then-extant computers need a different name; we'll refer to them as nanocomputers. "Micro" does exemplify at least the device size (on the order of a micron) and instruction speed (on the order of a microsecond) of the microprocessor. In at least one design, which we'll examine below, the nanometer and nanosecond are the appropriate measures instead.

Do we really need nanocomputers? After all, you have to be able to see the screen and press the keys even if the processor is microscopic. The answer to this question lies in realizing just how closely economics and technological constraints determine what computers are used for. In the mid-1960s, IBM sold a small computer for what was then the average price of a house. Today,

Originally published in *Extropy: The Journal of Transhumanist Thought* 13 (1994). Copyright © Max More.

The Transhumanist Reader: Classical and Contemporary Essays on the Science, Technology, and Philosophy of the Human Future, First Edition. Edited by Max More and Natasha Vita-More.
© 2013 John Wiley & Sons, Inc. Published 2013 by John Wiley & Sons, Inc.

single-chip micros of roughly the same computational power cost less than $5 and are used as controllers in toaster-ovens. Similarly, we can imagine putting a nanocomputer in each particle of pigment to implement "intelligent paint," or at each pixel location in an artificial retina to implement image-understanding algorithms.

This last is a point worth emphasizing. With today's processing technology, robots operating outside a rigid, tightly controlled environment are extremely expensive and running at the ragged edge of the state of the art. Even though current systems can, for example, drive in traffic at highway speeds, no one is going to replace truck drivers with them until their cost comes down by some orders of magnitude. Effective robotics depends on enough computational power to perform sensory perception; nanocomputers should make this cost-effective the way microcomputers did text processing.

Beyond providing robots with the processing power humans already have, there is the opportunity of extending those powers themselves. Nanocomputers represent enough power in little enough space that it would make sense to implant them in your head to extend your sensorium, augment your memory, sharpen your reasoning. As is slowly being understood in the world of existing computers, the interface to the human is easily the most computationally intensive task of all. Last but not least – in some sense, the most important application for nanocomputers – is as the controllers for nanomechanical devices. In particular, molecular assemblers will need nanocomputers to control them; and we will need assemblers to build nanocomputers. (In the jargon of nanotechnology, an "assembler" is a robot or other mechanical manipulator small enough to build objects using tools and building blocks that are individual molecules.)

What's a Nanocomputer?

Currently, the feature sizes in state-of-the-art VLSI fabrication are on the order of half a micron, i.e. 500 nanometers. In 15 years, using nothing more than a curve-fitting, trend-line prediction, this number will be somewhere in the neighborhood of 10 nanometers; would it be appropriate to refer to such a chip as a nanocomputer?

For the purposes of this essay, no. We want to talk about much more specific notions of future computing technology. First, we're expecting the thing to be built with atomic precision. This does *not* mean that there will be some robot arm that places one atom, then another, and so forth, until the whole computer is done. It means that the "design" of the computer specifies where each atom is to be. We expect the working parts (whether electrical or mechanical) to be essentially single molecules.

We can reasonably expect the switches, gates, or other embodiment of the logical elements to be on the order of a nanometer in size. (They may have to be further apart than that if electrical, due to electron tunneling.) In any case, it is quite reasonable to expect the entire computer to be smaller than a cubic micron, which contains a billion cubic nanometers.

Nanotechnology

The nanotechnology-assembler-nanocomputer dependence sounds like a self-referential loop, and it is. But many technologies are that way; machine tools make precision parts used in machine tools. Bootstrapping into a self-supporting technology is not a trivial problem, but it's not an impossible one either.

Another self-referential loop in nanotechnology is slightly more complicated. We would like assemblers to be self-reproducing. This would allow for nanocomputers and other nanotechnological products to be inexpensive, because each fixed initial investment would lead to an exponentially increasing number of nanomechanisms, rather than a linearly increasing number.

But how can a machine make a copy of itself? The problem is that while we can imagine, for example, a robot arm that can screw, bolt, solder, and weld enough to assemble a robot arm from parts, it needs a sequence of instructions to obey in this process. And there is more than one instruction per part. But the instructions must be embodied in some physical form, so to finish the process we need instructions to build the instructions, and so on, in an infinite regress. The answer to this seeming conundrum was given mathematically by John von Neumann, and at roughly the same time (the 1950s) was teased out of the naturally occurring self-reproducing machines we find all around us, living cells. It turns out to be the same answer in both cases.

First, design a machine that can build machines, like the robot arm above. (In a cell, there is such a thing, called a ribosome.) Next, we need another machine which is special-purpose, and does nothing but copy instructions. (In the cell it's called a replisome.) Finally, we need a set of instructions that includes directions for making both of the machines, plus whatever ancillary devices and general operating procedures may be needed. (In the cell, this is the DNA.) Now we read the instructions through the first machine, which makes all the new machinery necessary. Then we read it through the second machine, which makes a new set of instructions. And there's our whole new self-reproducing system, with no infinite regress.

General Computer Principles

When you get right down to it, a computer is just a device for changing information. You put in your input, and it gives you your output. If it's being used as the controller for anything, from a toaster to a robot, it gets its input from its sensors and gives its output to its motors, switches, solenoids, speakers, and what have you. Internally, the computer has a memory, which is used to store the information it's working on. Many functions, even so simple as a push-on, push-off lightswitch, need memory by definition. But the computer also uses memory to help break the job down to size, so as to be able to change the data it receives in little pieces, one at a time. The more memory you allow, and the smaller the pieces, the simpler the actual hardware can be.

There is a "folk theorem" in the computer world that the NAND gate is computationally universal. This is true in the sense that one can design any logic circuit using only NAND gates. However, something much more surprising is also true. Less than 10 years ago, Miles Murdocca, working at Bell Labs, showed (in an unpublished paper) how to build a universal computer using nothing but delay elements and *one single OR gate*. Just one. Not circuits using arbitrarily many of just one kind of gate.

Murdocca's computer works by driving the notion of a computer to its very barest of essentials. A computer is a memory and a device to change the information in the memory. Generally we add two more specifics: The information is encoded and changed under the rules of Boolean logic; and the changes happen in synchronized, discrete steps. To build a computer, then, we need some way to remember bits; some way to perform Boolean logic; and some way to clock the sequence of remember, perform, remember, perform, etc.

In computers from historical times to date, information has been encoded either as the position of a mechanical part, the voltage on a wire, or a combination (as in a relay-based computer). The major reason is that these are the easiest encodings to use in the logic part of the particular technology in question. It seems reasonable to expect to see these encodings at the nano level, for the same reasons.

Additional Constraints for Nanocomputers

About a year ago I had the occasion to design a nanocomputer using Eric Drexler's mechanical rod logic, which will be examined in detail later in this essay. As someone who was used to the size and speed constraints of electronics, I was in my glory with this new medium. I went wild, adding functionality, pipelining, multicomputing, the works. I could build a supercomputer beyond the wildest dreams of Cray, the size of a bacterium! What I *didn't* do was pay any attention to "this crazy reversible computing stuff."

Until I did the heat dissipation calculations. The problem is that there really is a fundamental physical limit involved in computation, but it represents an amount of energy so small (it's comparable to the thermal energy of one atom) that it is totally negligible in existing physical devices. But in a nanocomputer, it far outweighs all the other heat-producing mechanisms; in fact, my nanocomputer design had the same heat dissipation per unit volume as a low-grade explosive. Back to the drawing board...

Since the earliest electronic computers in the 1940s, energy dissipation per device has been declining exponentially with time. Device size has undergone a similar decline, with the result that overall dissipation per unit volume has been relatively constant (see the horizontal bar in Figure 18.1). Historically, the portion represented by the thermodynamic limit for irreversible operations was completely insignificant; it is still in the parts per million range. However, with densities and speeds in the expected range for nanocomputers, it is extremely significant. Thus nanocomputer designers will be forced to pay attention to reversibility.

Efficient computers, like efficient heat engines, must be as nearly reversible as possible. Rolf Landauer showed in a landmark paper (in 1961) that the characteristic irreversible operation in

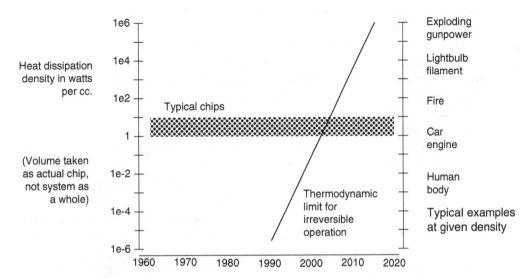

Figure 18.1   Heat dissipation vs its theoretical limit. Originally published in *Extropy* 13 (1994). Copyright © Max More.

computation is the erasure of a bit of information; the other operations can be carried out in principle reversibly and without the dissipation of energy. And as in heat engines, the reason reversibility matters is the Second Law of Thermodynamics, the law of entropy.

Entropy

The subject of entropy seems to give rise to more misconceptions and disagreements than any other scientific principle. Relativity and quantum mechanics have been similarly abused, but much of the abuse is in the form of extensions of the concepts that are frankly metaphorical. Relativity and quantum mechanics do not, in general, apply to the everyday world, but entropy does. When people use metaphorical extensions of entropy on phenomena that are governed by actual entropy, confusion occurs.

It's possible, on the other hand, to give a metaphorical explanation of entropy that is carefully rigged to give all the same answers as actual entropy. Here it is; but if you'd prefer to take my word for it that nanocomputers *must* be reversible, you can skip to the next section.

Let us suppose that we are going to have a computer simulation of some closed physical system. We can have as high an accuracy as we like, but the total amount of information, i.e. the number of bits in the computer's memory, is in the end some fixed finite number. Now since the physical system we're simulating is closed, there will be no input to the simulation once it is started.

Since there is a fixed number of bits, say K, there is a fixed number of possible descriptions of the system the simulation can ever possibly express, namely 2^K of them. Now by the first law of thermodynamics, conservation of energy, total energy in a closed system is constant. Thus we can pick all of the states with a given energy, and call them "allowable," and the rest are forbidden. The first law constrains the system to remain within the allowable subset of states but says no more about which states within that set the system will occupy.

There is another constraint, however, in the sense that the laws of physics are deterministic; given a state, there is a single successor state the system can occupy in the next instant of time. (In the real world, this is more complicated in two ways: Time and the state space are continuous, and quantum mechanics provides for multiple successor [and predecessor] states. However, the mathematical form of quantum mechanics [i.e. Hamiltonian transformations] gives it properties analogous to the model, so for perspicuity, we will stick with the discrete, deterministic model.) What is more, the laws are such that each state has not only a unique successor, but a unique predecessor.

Let's try to make this notion a little more intuitive. Each "state" in our computer simulation corresponds to some description of all the individual atoms in the physical system. For each atom, we know exactly where it is, exactly how fast it is going, exactly in what direction, etc. As we move forward in time, we can calculate all the electrical, gravitational, and, if we care, nuclear, forces on that atom due to all the other atoms, and compute just where it will be some tiny increment of time in the future. Clearly, to just the same degree of precision, we can calculate exactly where it must have been the same tiny amount of time in the past. The math of the physical laws allow you to simulate going backwards just as deterministically as you can simulate going forwards. So, suppose we have a simulation of a box which has a partition dividing it in half. There is some gas in one half, i.e. atoms bouncing around, and none in the other. Now suppose the partition disappears: the atoms that would have bounced off it will continue on into the empty half, which pretty soon won't be empty any more. The atoms will be distributed more or less evenly throughout the box.

What happens if we suddenly stop the simulation and run it backwards? In fact, each atom will retrace the exact path it took since the partition disappeared, and by the time the partition should reappear, the atoms will all be in the original half.

In reality, we don't see this happen. Remember that in our model there is a distinct causal chain of states from the state where the atoms are all spread out but about to move into half the box, to the state where they are actually in half the box. This means that the number of states from which the atoms are about to compress spontaneously (in some specific number of timesteps) is the same as the number of states in which they are all in one half of the box.

The important thing to remember is that the total energy (which is proportional to the sum of the squares of the velocities of the atoms) must be the same. If we used a simulated piston to push the atoms back into the original half, we would find a one-to-one mapping between spread-out states and compressed ones; but the compressed ones would be higher-energy states.

How many states are we talking about here? Well, suppose that all we know about any specific atom is which side of the box it is in, which we can represent with a single bit. If the box has just 100 atoms in it, there will be more than, 267,000,000,000,000,000,000,000,000,000 states in which the atoms are spread around evenly, and one state where they are all on one side. A similar ratio holds between the number of states (with full descriptions) where the atoms are spread out, and the subset of those states where they are about to pile over into one side.

We are now going to talk about entropy. In order to relate the simulation model of a physical system to the way physical scientists view physical systems, we'll use the term "microstate" to represent what we have been calling a state in the simulation, i.e. one specific configuration of the system where all the bits are known. We'll use "macrostate" to refer to what a physical scientist thinks about the system. This means knowing the temperature, pressure, mass, volume, chemical composition, physical shape, etc., but not knowing everything about every atom.

Clearly, there are lots of microstates in a macrostate. The log of the number of microstates in a given macrostate is the entropy of the macrostate. (Physical entropies are generally given as natural logs, but we will talk in terms of base 2 logs with the understanding that a scaling factor may be needed to translate back.) To put it more simply, the entropy of a given macrostate is the number of bits needed to specify which of its microstates the system is actually in.

With these definitions, the second law of thermodynamics is quite straightforward. If a proposed physical transformation maps a macrostate with a higher entropy into one with a lower entropy, we know it is impossible. Remember the causal chains of (micro)states: they can neither branch nor coalesce. Now suppose, at the beginning of some physical process, the system was in a macrostate with a trillion microstates; we have no idea which microstate, it could be any one of them. Therefore at the end of the process, it can still be in a trillion microstates, each at the end of a causal chain reaching back to the corresponding original microstate. Obviously, the system cannot be in any macrostate with fewer than a trillion microstates, i.e. with a lower entropy than that of the original macrostate.

Now suppose I have a beaker of water at a specific temperature and pressure. It has, according to a physicist or chemist, a specific entropy. But suppose I happen to know a little more about it, e.g. I have a map of the currents and vortices still flowing around in it from when it was stirred. There are a lot of the microstates that would be allowed from the simpler description, that I know the water is not really in. Isn't its entropy "really" lower? Who gets to say which is the "real" macrostate, whose size determines the "true" entropy of the system?

The answer is, that entropy isn't a property of the physical system at all, but a property of the description. After all, the real system is only in one single microstate! (Ignoring quantum mechanics.) This does sound a bit strange: Surely the "true" entropy of any system is then 0. And we should be able to induce a transformation from this system into any macrostate we like, even one with much lower entropy than that of the original macrostate of the system as conventionally measured. Let's consider the little box with the atoms of gas in it. The gas is evenly spread over through the box, a partition is placed, and there is a Maxwell's Demon with a door to let the atoms through selectively. But the demon isn't going to try anything fancy. We're going to assume that we know the exact position and velocity of each atom in advance, so we will be able to provide the demon with a control tape that tells him when to open and close the door *without observing the atoms at all*. In fact, this would work; the demon can herd all the atoms into one side without expending any energy.

Why doesn't this violate the second law? Well, let's count up the causal chains. The entropy problem in the first place is that there are many many fewer microstates in the final macrostate, namely with all the atoms on one side, than in the original, so that many original microstates must somehow map into a single final one. But with the demon at work, we can run the simulation backwards by running the demon backwards too; the sequence of door-opening and closing that got us to our particular final microstate is clearly enough information to determine which original microstate we started from. Thus the final state, *including the tape*, is still in a one-to-one mapping with the original state, and the second law is not violated.

The curious thing to note about this gedanken experiment is that the demon can compress the gas without expending energy; what he *cannot* do is erase the tape! This would leave the system with too few final states.

What happens if the demon starts with a blank tape, instead of one where the microstate of the system is already recorded? Can he measure the system on the fly? Again yes, but only if he writes his measurements on the tape. Again the critical point is that the data on the tape serves to make the number of possible final microstates as large as the number of possible original microstates.

In practice, of course, the way one would obtain the same result, i.e. moving the atoms into half the box, would be to use a piston to compress the gas and then bring it in contact with a heat sink and let it cool back to the original temperature. Energy, in the form of work, is put into the system in the first phase and leaves the system, in the form of heat, in the second phase. At the end of the process the system is the same as the demon left it but there is no tape full of information. Clearly there is some sense in which the dissipation of heat is equivalent to erasing the tape.

In terms of the simulation model, the demon directly removes one bit from the position description of each atom (storing it on the tape). The piston compression moves a bit from the position to the velocity description, and the cooling process removes that bit (storing it in the heat sink). The entropy of the gas decreases, and that of the heat sink increases.

Of course, dissipating heat is not the only way to erase a bit. Any process that "moves" entropy, i.e. decreasing it in one part of a system at the expense of another part, will do. For example, instead of increasing the temperature of a heat sink, we could have expanded its volume. Or disordered a set of initially aligned regions of magnetization (in other words, written the bits on a tape). Or any other physical process which would increase the amount of information necessary to identify the system's microstate. However, heat dissipation is probably the easiest of these mechanisms to maintain as a continuous process over long periods of time, and it is well understood and widely practiced.

A state-of-the-art processor, with 100,000 gates erasing a bit per gate per cycle, at 100 MHz, dissipates about 28 nanowatts due to entropy. (At room temperature. Each bit costs you the natural log of 2, times Boltzmann's constant, times the absolute temperature in Kelvins, joules of energy dissipation, which comes to about 2.87 maJ [milli-attoJoule, 10^{-21} Joules]). Since it actually dissipates 100 million times this much, or more, nobody cares. But with a trillion-fold decrease in volume and thousand-fold increase in speed, the nanocomputer is "a whole 'nother ball game." Thus there are two new design rules that the nanocomputer designer must adopt: (1) Erase as few bits as possible. (2) Eliminate entropy loss in operations that do not erase bits.

We eliminate entropy loss in logical operations by what is known as "logical reversibility." Suppose we have in our computer registers A and B, and an instruction ADD A,B that adds A to B. Now in ordinary computers that would be done by forming the sum A + B, erasing the previous contents of register B, and then storing the sum there. However, it isn't logically necessary to do this; since we can recreate the old value of B by subtracting A from the new value, no information has been lost, and thus it is possible to design a circuit that can perform ADD A,B *without* erasing any bits.

Addition has the property that its inputs and results are related in such a way that the result can replace one of the inputs with no loss of information. However, many useful, even necessary, functions don't have this property. We can still use those functions reversibly; the only trick needed is not to erase the inputs! Ultimately, of course, you have to get rid of the input in order to process the next one; but you can *always* erase the *output* without entropic cost if you've saved the input.

This leads to structures in reversible computation called "retractile cascades." Each of a series of (logical) circuits computes a function of the output of its predecessor. If the final output is erased first, and then the next-to-last, and so forth, the entire operation is reversible, and can be done (in theory!) without any energy dissipation. If we adopt these rules throughout our computer design, we can reduce the number of bits erased per cycle from around 100,000 to around 10.

Drexler's Mechanical Logic

K. Eric Drexler, "the father of nanotechnology," has designed and subjected to a thoroughgoing analysis, a *mechanical* logic for nanocomputers. A mechanical logic has the disadvantage of being slower than an electronic one, but has the major advantage that at the molecular level it is possible to design, and analyze the operation of, a mechanical logic with current molecular simulation software, and be reasonably certain that the design, if built, would work.

By the time we get around to actually building molecular computers, our analytical tools will be better than they are now, and what's more we'll be able to augment the simulations with physical experiments. So real nanocomputer designs won't have to be nearly so conservative as this one. In particular, they'll probably be electronic, and thus probably some orders of magnitude faster. But don't worry: this mechanical design is already plenty fast.

This formulation is sometimes called "rod logic" because instead of wires, it uses molecular-sized rods (e.g. a nanometer in diameter and from 10 to 100 nanometers long). Each rod represents a logic 0 or 1 by its position, sliding slightly along its length to make the transition. To do logic, the rods have knobs on them which may or may not be blocked by something, preventing the rod from changing state. The "something" is simply other knobs on other rods, which block or don't block the first rod, depending on their state (see Figure 18.2). The logic is clocked

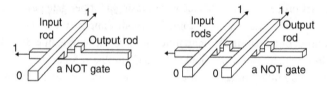

Figure 18.2   Rod logic. Originally published in *Extropy* 13 (1994). Copyright © Max More.

by pulling on rods through the equivalent of a spring, so that it moves unless blocked. (We can draw a workable parallel to transistors, which block or don't block a clock from changing the voltage on a wire, depending on the voltage of another wire.)

The rods move in a fixed, rigid housing structure which might be thought of as a hunk of diamond with appropriate channels cut out of it (although it wouldn't be built that way). The rods are supported along their entire length so the blocking does not place any bending stress on them. Any logic function is now simply constructed: for an AND gate, for example, take two input rods and place knobs so that they block the output rod when they are in the "0" position. The output rod will only be able to move to the "1" when both inputs are "1."

(Now that we can build a single gate, aren't we just about finished, by virtue of Murdocca's design? Well, we'd still need clocking and some mechanism to handle a delay-line memory; but more to the point the design produces a computer that is about a billion times slower than you could build with conventional logic designs!)

The motion of the rods is limited by the speed of sound (in diamond); but they are so short (e.g. one-tenth of a micron) that the switching times are still a tenth of a nanosecond. The speed of an entire nanocomputer of this kind of design will be limited by thermal noise and energy dissipation, which can produce enough variation in the shapes of the molecular parts to keep them from working right. Drexler gives a detailed analysis of the sources of such error in *Nanosystems* (Drexler 1992: ch. 12). The energy dissipated per switching operation is conservatively estimated at about 0.013 maJ.

This is less than 5 percent of the fundamental limit for bit destruction; as long, of course, as the gate in question doesn't destroy bits! Most of the logic design in a rod logic nanocomputer *must* be either conservative logic or retractile cascades. To demonstrate the difference, consider a NOT gate. One can implement a conservative NOT because it has an exact inverse (which happens to be itself). One could implement a conservative NOT in rod logic with a single gear meshing with racks on input and output rods. A retractile NOT, on the other hand, would be a single rod crossing with knobs preventing the output from moving to "1" if the input was "1." The "retractile" part is that the output must be let back down easy, in such a way that the energy stored in the spring is retrieved, before the input is reset for the next operation. If this is not done, e.g. if the input is released first, the output rod will return under force of its spring and the energy stored in the spring will be dissipated as heat. In order for this not to happen, the output rod must be returned first, and then the input may be.

One very powerful and widely used technique in logic design is called the PLA (programmed logic array). A PLA is readily designed in retractile cascade style; it also has a remarkably good match to the geometric constraints of the rod logic, which requires the input and output rods from any interaction to form a right angle. The PLA consists of three sets of rods: the inputs, the minterms, and the outputs (see Figure 18.3). First the input rods are moved, i.e. set to the input values. Then the minterm rods are pushed; some of them move and some don't depending on

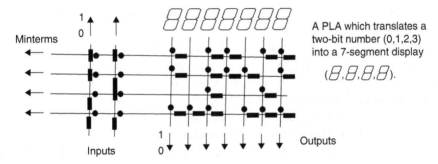

Figure 18.3   PLA. Originally published in *Extropy* 13 (1994). Copyright © Max More.

which inputs blocked them. In an electronic PLA each input is both fed directly into these interactions, and its negation is; this need not be done in the rod logic since its effect can be had by altering the position of the knobs. Sometimes the number of minterms can be reduced for the same reason. After the minterm rods are pushed, the output rods are pushed, and the appropriate value is encoded in which ones actually move. Now, the important thing in preserving reversibility (what makes this a retractile cascade) is that after this operation, first, the output rods must be let back down gently; then the minterms let back down gently; and finally the inputs can be released.

Notice that, in the figure, the input rods are at rest in the 0 position, while the output rods are at rest in the 1 position. (And in any given operation, exactly one of the minterm rods will slide to the left.)

PLA's can implement any logic function necessary in a computer, although there are more efficient circuits for some of them that are commonly used instead. More crucial, however, to a full grasp of the mechanisms of a nanocomputer, is memory.

Registers and Memory

Memory is a problem; if we follow the rules for conservative or retractile reversible logic, memory is impossible to implement. This is because any memory with a "write" function erases bits *by definition*.

In Drexler's rod-logic design, all the bit-erasing functionality is concentrated in the registers. The register design is fairly complex, to keep the energy dissipated in this process near its theoretical minimum.

The main problem is that for a physical system to retain one of two states reliably, which is what you want in a memory, there must be a potential barrier between the states that is significantly higher than kT, or thermal fluctuations will be sufficient to flip the bit at random. But in simple implementations, the height of the barrier determines how much energy is lost when the system changes state.

Consider an ordinary light switch. When you flip it, there's a spring that resists your finger until the halfway point, and then it snaps into place, dissipating all the energy you put into it as heat, vibration, and sound. (A "silent" switch is worse, since it dissipates by friction and you have to push all the way across.) The weaker the spring, and the more likely that some vibration will flip the switch when you didn't intend it. The trick is to have some way to change the strength of the spring (or to have the effect of doing so).

In Figure 18.4, there is a simplified version of Drexler's register. The bit it contains is reflected in the position of the shaded ball. (In the real design it's more complicated so that the value can be read!) (a) and (b) show the register when it contains 0 and 1 respectively. In (c), the barrier has been lowered and the ball is free to wander freely between both positions; this stage increases entropy. In (d), the register is reset to 0. The similarity to compressing a gas-filled cylinder is apparent; this is where $\ln(2)\, kT$ joules of work are converted into heat. Now to write the next bit, the input rod (on the right) is either extended (a 1, see (f)) or not (a 0, see (e)) and then the barrier raised. Finally, the spring rod (on the left) is retracted to get back to (a) or (b). If a 1 was written, the input rod did work to compress the ball into the spring, but that energy can be retrieved when the spring rod is retracted. The mechanisms to do this are just the same as in the logic portions, e.g. having the rods mechanically coupled to a flywheel.

Registers like this which are going to be used to erase bits will tend to be located near heat sinks or coolant ducts; bit erasure is the largest component of power dissipation in the rod logic design. Memory can be implemented as lots of registers; registers occupy about 40 cubic nanometers per bit. Thus about 3 megabytes' worth of registers fill a cubic micron. One would probably use register memory for cache, and use a mechanical tape system for main storage, however. The "tape" would be a long carbon chain with side groups that differed enough to be 1s and 0s. Since the whole computer is mechanical, the difference in speeds is not as bad as macroscopic tapes on electronic computers. Such a tape system might have a density in the neighborhood of a gigabyte per cubic micron. Access times for using a tape as a random access memory consist almost entirely of latency; if the length of individual tapes is kept to under 100 kbytes, this is in the 10s of microseconds.

Motors

In order to drive all this mechanical logic we need a motor of some kind; Drexler has designed an electric motor which is nothing short of amazing. (Clearly this is of import well beyond computers.) The reason is that the scaling laws for power density are in our favor as we go down toward the nanometer realm. At macroscopic sizes, almost all electric motors are electromagnetic; at nano scales, they will be electrostatic. The motor is essentially a van de Graff generator run in reverse (but it works just fine as a generator, as do some macroscopic electric motors). The power density of the motor is over $10^{15}\ \mathrm{W/m^3}$; this corresponds to packing the power of a fanjet from a 747 into a cubic centimeter. (It's not clear what you'd do with it if you did, though!)

Ultimately, the ability to make small, powerful motors is going to be more important for nanorobots than nanocomputers per se. The speed advantage of electronics over mechanical logic is almost certain to drive the descent into nanocomputer design.

Other Logics for Nanocomputers

Before going into other extensions of conventional digital logic, there is another form of nanocomputer that may appear earlier for technological reasons. That's the molecular biocomputer.

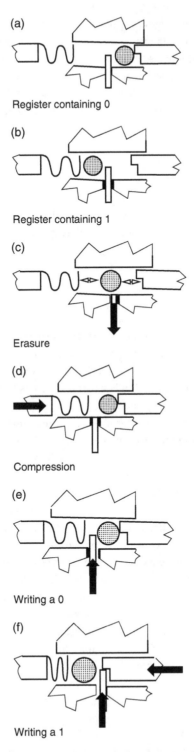

(a)

Register containing 0

(b)

Register containing 1

(c)

Erasure

(d)

Compression

(e)

Writing a 0

(f)

Writing a 1

Figure 18.4   Register operation. Originally published in *Extropy* 13 (1994). Copyright © Max More.

Imagine that a DNA molecule is a tape, upon which is written 2 bits of information per base pair (the DNA molecule is a long string of adenine-thymine and guanine-cytosine pairs). Imagine, in particular, this to be the tape of a Turing machine, which is represented by some humongous clump of special-purpose enzymes that reads the "tape," changes state, replaces a base pair with a new one, and slides up and down the "tape." If one could design the enzyme clump using conventional molecular biology techniques (and each of the individual functions it needs to do are done somewhere, somehow, by some natural enzyme) you'd have a molecular computer.

Other Mechanical Logics

Now, back to mechanical logic. Most macroscopic mechanical logic in the past has typically been based on rods that turned instead of sliding. It's reasonable to assume that similar designs could be implemented at the nano scale.

Electronic Logic

It's clear that quantum mechanics allows for mechanisms that capture a single electron and holds it reliably in one place. After all, that's what an atom is. Individual electrons doing specific, well-defined things under the laws of quantum mechanics, is what happens in typical chemical reactions. Clearly there is no basic physical law that prevents us from building nanocomputers that handle electrons as individual objects.

What is not so clear is how, specifically, they will work. Quantum mechanics is computationally very expensive to simulate, and intuitively harder to understand, than the essentially "physical object" models used in mechanical nanotechnology designs thus far. Indeed, the designs are typically larger and slower than they would have to be in reality, simply to avoid having to confront the analysis of quantum effects.

Ultimately, however, nanotechnologists will be "quantum mechanics." Computers based on quantum effects will be even smaller, more efficient, and much faster than mechanical ones of the type presented above. They will use much the same logical structure: it's quite possible to design retractile cascades even in conventional transistors (where it's an extension of techniques called "dry switching" in power electronics and "hot clocks" in VLSI design).

There are schemes, with some mathematical plausibility, to harness quantum state superposition for implicit parallel processing. In my humble opinion, these will require some conceptual breakthrough (or at the very least, significant experimental clarification) about the phenomenon of the collapse of the Schroedinger wave function before they can be harnessed by a buildable device. Keep your fingers crossed!

Conclusion

Beyond certain rapidly approaching limits of size and speed, any computer must use logical reversibility to limit bit destruction. This is particularly true of nanocomputers with molecular-scale components, which if designed according to standard current-day irreversible techniques, explode.

We can design nanocomputers today which we are virtually certain would work if constructed. They use mechanical parts that are more than 1 atom but less than 10 atoms across in a typical short dimension. The parts move at rates of up to 10 billion times per second; processors built that way could be expected to run at rates of 1,000 MIPS. Such a processor, and a megabyte of very fast memory, would fit in a cubic micron (the size of a bacterium). A gigabyte of somewhat slower memory would fit in another cubic micron. A pile of ten thousand such computers would be just large enough to see with the naked eye.

Reference

Drexler, K. Eric (1992) *Nanosystems: Molecular Machinery, Manufacturing, and Computation*, New York: Wiley Interscience.

Further Reading

Hennessy, J.L. and Patterson, D.A. (1990) *Computer Architecture: A Quantitative Approach*. San Mateo, CA: Morgan Kaufmann.
Leff, Harvey S. and Rex, Andrew F., eds. (1990) *Maxwell's Demon: Entropy, Information, Computing*. Princeton, NJ: Princeton University Press. See particularly papers by Landauer and Bennett.
Proceedings of the Physics of Computation Workshop, Dallas (October 1993). IEEE Press. See particularly papers by Merkle, Hall, and Koller.
Watson, J.D., Hopkins, N.H., Roberts, J.W. Steitz, J.A., and Weiner, A.M. (1987) *Molecular Biology of the Gene*, 4th edn. Menlo Park, CA: Benjamin/Cummings.

19

Immortalist Fictions and Strategies

Michael R. Rose

Introduction: Something Like Penicillin for Immortality

I have worked in the field of aging research for 35 years, as of this writing. Over that time, most academics who work in the area have become convinced that great strides have been made in solving the scientific problem of aging. Thus these researchers and their fan-base of journalists, novelists, and bloggers have become steadily more excited about the prospects for intervening in the process. If 30 years ago few were willing to talk about the prospects of greatly extending human lifespan, it is now much more common. I started writing about this prospect in 1984 in "The Evolutionary Route to Methuselah" (Rose 1984). At that time, my boldness attracted headlines and radio interviewers from around the world. Now the basic idea has become commonplace, virtually an internet advertising-copy cliché for the promotion of nutritional supplements that can be bought online, to say nothing of the excellent agit-prop for ending aging supplied by the relentless Aubrey de Grey over the last few years.

The single best warrant for such chatter has been the creation of laboratory animals with greatly extended lifespans. I was one of the first to achieve this feat, back in the 1970s, but many more have since. Now there is nothing unusual about labs that have some kind of Methuselah flies or Methuselah worms or Methuselah mice. You can read about them all over the Internet. Biologists have created these beasts using a variety of methods: experimental evolution, random and directed mutation, as well as diet. Contrary to most scientific opinion in 1976, there are no absolute barriers to greatly extending the lifespans of animals in laboratories.

Recall the example of bacteria being killed by the fungus *Penicillium* in Alexander Fleming's 1928 laboratory cultures leading to the widespread use of penicillin in the 1950s. This is one of better-known folk-tales of biomedical research. The laboratory manipulation of aging has thus

The Transhumanist Reader: Classical and Contemporary Essays on the Science, Technology, and Philosophy of the Human Future, First Edition. Edited by Max More and Natasha Vita-More.
© 2013 John Wiley & Sons, Inc. Published 2013 by John Wiley & Sons, Inc.

naturally led many, especially those in the transhumanist (H+) and immortalist movement, to the hope that we could soon achieve similar things for human aging.

About 15 years ago, I became interested in the scientific problem of biological immortality, and it has since been the chief focus of my research. Recently my closest colleagues on this project and I have published a book summarizing our work on this project (Mueller et al. 2011). While working on a draft of the manuscript, I stumbled upon a penicillin-like idea that has given me a very different view of the prospects for significantly slowing human aging, and indeed the prospects for starting to move toward biological immortality for a significant number of people now alive. I will endeavor to share this idea here.

But before I do so, I will try to put this proposal within the larger context of how people now generally envision how biological immortality will be achieved. Such visions are then compared with the available science concerning biological immortality. Then I give my latest thinking about the practical prospects for biological immortality, particularly for those now alive, including my penicillin-like idea.

Immortality in Fiction

First, a confession. There are no words for how tired I have become over decades of having the scientific problem of biological aging, and particularly my own work on it, widely misunderstood. Over hundreds of interviews, only a minority of journalists I have spoken with have understood what I am talking about. Some of the very best get it. For example, Jonathan Weiner's *Long for this World* (Weiner 2010) isn't too far off. Like most journalists writing about the evolution of aging, he tends to think more about trade-offs than Hamilton's forces of natural selection, though the latter are the real keys to the control of aging. Still, reading Weiner's book on immortality gives the reader at least a vague sense of the biological and technological issues in play.

But more relief for my aggravation has been supplied recently by works of fiction. *The Postmortal* (Magary 2011) puts the central scientific issue in stark terms. For his novel is premised on a technology which perfectly embodies the scientific vision that I expressly reject, while directly rejecting my scientific vision. This works extremely well as a plot device, and I recommend that everyone reading these words should follow up by reading Magary's novel.

In the novel, a fictional scientist called Graham Otto manages to engineer biological immortality in laboratory fruit flies. Actually he does so accidentally, when he is using fruit fly genetic engineering to test out strategies for changing hair color. He injects a particular genetic construct into some flies and finds that they stop aging. Completely. The character says, "But none of the flies I injected with the vector dropped. Ever. They just kept flying around." Then he tries the same genetic vector on mammals, such as his pet dog, and they too stop aging. Naturally, humans are next, and the world is never the same again.

In the chapter in the novel titled "A Little Bit of Bloodshed Now or a Lot Later On," this is expressly contrasted with the following scientific view:

> Up until Otto's serendipitous mistake, it was assumed that biological aging was controlled by hundreds, if not thousands, of separate genetic proteins found in the body – proteins that worked in concert to determine the rate of aging across various parts of an animal. (From the fictitious article, "The Man Who Conquered Death," by Mike Dermott.)

Put in headline language, the plot-device for the novel assumes that the cell biological view of aging as a product of a small number of key pathways is correct, while further assuming that the evolutionary genetic view of aging is incorrect.

This happens all the time in science fiction. In Bob Shaw's *One Million Tomorrows* (1970), there is a simple treatment that sustains health indefinitely, with the portentous side-effect of rendering males utterly impotent. Plot hi-jinks ensue, because all the biologically immortal women then compete for the attention of the males who continue to be able to have sex, and thus continue aging. Fortunately, we now have Viagra, so presumably Shaw should update his novel. In Aldous Huxley's far more literary 1939 novel *After Many a Summer Dies the Swan*, the consumption of raw carp guts gives immortality, though aging continues. Science fiction thrives on technological magic bullets. So does cell biology, which has much in common with science fiction, as I will explain shortly.

Interestingly, Robert A. Heinlein's 1958 *Methuselah's Children* has much longer-lived humans first achieved by selective breeding among those from the long-lived Howard families, an analog of one of the ways I have done it. (See my 2005 popular science book *The Long Tomorrow* or the hard-core *Methuselah Flies* [Passanati et al. 2004].) So science fiction doesn't always have to be simple-minded, it seems.

In his 2011 novel *2030*, Albert Brooks imagines a ridiculously easy cure for cancer transforming the life expectancy of a near-future United States. Not as apocalyptic as the complete cure for aging in *The Postmortal*, the Brooks novel is nonetheless rather dystopian. Personally, I think that the dystopian strains of both novels are overblown. Humankind has already managed to cope with great extensions in average lifespan over the last 150 years, and like Sonia Arrison (see *100 Plus* [2011]) I don't think that anything that could happen with aging in the real world would pose insuperable difficulties for anyone but the most rabid defenders of universal retirement at the age of 65. But still, dystopian novels are always worth reading for their evocation of possible, though not necessarily likely, adverse side-effects.

In any case, what most of these novels show is the infatuation the reading public has with simple technological fixes that stop aging completely. And this they have in common with molecular and cell biologists, who variously imagine one, a handful, or perhaps as many as seven fundamental aging processes. By an interesting coincidence, these cell-molecular biologists generally conclude that the bit of the cell's machinery which they work on is the key to aging.

Some discussion as to why actual scientists and "bioengineers" might imagine aging could be so simple is needed. There is tremendous historical precedent, for one thing. Starting with the great Aristotle, continuing with Francis Bacon in the seventeenth century, and the early Nobel Prize Laureate Elie Metchnikoff, many rather bright men have supposed that there is a simple physiological process driving the pathophysiological complexity of aging. More recently, the brilliant Leo Szilard and Leslie Orgel tried their hand at proposing such simple unitary physiological causes for aging in the 1950s and 1960s.

Scientists like Alex Comfort, John Maynard Smith, and myself have made it a practice to take down these theories using laboratory experiments designed as falsifications for their claims of scientific sufficiency. (Read, for examples, Comfort 1979.) We usually do that by showing that perturbing the hypothesized machinery for aging either has no effect or only a minor one. As I explain at length in my 1991 book, *Evolutionary Biology of Aging*, it is not that the single-bullet theories of aging are all entirely irrelevant. It is just that there are in fact many such bullets, all "targeted" on later ages by the declining forces of natural selection. Evolutionary biologists like George C. Williams, William Hamilton, and Maynard Smith have been making this point based on evolutionary theory for decades. But over the last year or so, we have shown this directly using genome-wide technologies (Rose et al. 2010; Burke et al. 2010; Rose and Burke 2011). We now know *definitively* that the Graham Otto version of the genetics of aging is not correct. Exactly the view which *The Postmortal* contradicts turns out to be correct.

Yet belief in magic bullets for aging persists, even among otherwise respectable biologists and technologists. Leaving aside historical precedent, I think that there is a simple law of human nature which explains their difficulty with the evolutionary genetic view, which is best credited as Upton Sinclair's saying: "It is difficult to get a man to understand something, when his salary depends upon his not understanding it!" As the cell and molecular biologists who work on aging are not good at doing evolutionary biology, it is not likely that they are going to accept that evolutionary biologists (1) have solved the scientific problem of aging, (2) can easily manipulate aging using experimental evolution, and (3) have far greater understanding of the technological constraints on transforming aging than any cell biologist. For them to think otherwise would mean that they couldn't get their grants funded, get their start-up companies funded, publish articles, or receive tenure. Plus they have the great advantage of popular wisdom being entirely on their side, and in this respect they have much in common with the Aristotelian proponents of the geocentric theory of astrophysics.

Now it is not that the cell biologists can't point to experiments which seem to fit their views, as is common in natural science. (After all, the Earth's Moon does indeed have a geocentric orbit.) Good colleagues of mine like Robert Reis are able to produce nematode worms that live ten times longer than their unmutated controls, if they use ingenious genetic and environmental manipulation. But nematodes have well-developed physiological machinery for sustaining states of metabolic arrest, in which they can survive for very long periods of drought or starvation. The available evidence suggests that such capacities can be genetically altered for the purpose of keeping adult nematodes alive for remarkably long periods. But such mutants have greatly reduced reproduction, and reduced competitive ability. The Methuselah mice that have been produced by mutation are miniaturized, and lack the ability to sustain their body temperature unaided by a normal "nurse" mouse. They are so deficient in competitive ability that normal mice kill them unless the miniatures are protected. A simple way of describing this pattern is to realize that these laboratory monstrosities have extended lifespan, but impaired "healthspan." They last longer, but do so in exchange for "living" less. Similar results can be achieved by castrating Pacific salmon or deflowering soybean. There is even evidence that castrating adult men increases their lifespan by a significant amount.

One final novel is relevant here: *Limitless*, originally published in 2001by Alan Glynn as *The Dark Fields* (Glynn 2001). If you saw the 2011 film *Limitless*, the novel will make interesting reading, for the film culminates with the Bradley Cooper protagonist's transformation into a kind of superhuman thanks to a benign variant of an amphetamine-like pharmaceutical, NZT-48. Just like "The Cure" in *The Postmortal*, some biochemist is able to gift humanity with a cost-free enhancement in the film. But the book is very different. For the book instead tells a story based on a super-amphetamine, called MDT-48, as the plot-hinge. Like Adderall, MDT-48 is addictive, and causes major side-effects, including severe insomnia and sudden death.

If the cell biologists ever do find a single "anti-aging" drug that increases human lifespan substantially, evolutionary biologists predict that it will have huge adverse side-effects. Interestingly, there is evidence in fruit flies that lithium has both such effects (Matsagas et al.

2009): it increases lifespan at low doses, but reproduction and competitive success are impaired, as was observed in the nematode mutants with greatly extended lifespans. That is, healthspan is impaired, even as lifespan is extended. Lithium is a highly toxic substance, which can kill if serum levels rise abruptly, and its long-term use at lower therapeutic doses is associated with chronic sedation, neuropathy, tremor, and weight gain. Not a reasonable trade-off for a few years of extra life, although that may depend on your personal preferences.

Science of Biological Immortality

Before turning to my recent penicillin-like idea, let me list some important scientific findings about biological immortality that might help prepare the reader for changing their own life.

1. There are animals alive today that undergo little or no aging. The best characterized are coelenterates, particularly the *Hydra* cultures studied by Daniel Martinez (1998). All such non-aging animals are fissile, with relatively symmetrical division as the chief means of reproduction. It is under such conditions that evolutionary biologists predict that aging will not evolve. Thus there is no cell or molecular biological barrier that prevents evolution from achieving biological immortality. Indeed, the existence of such animals should lead anyone to question the assumption among many cell and molecular biologists that some inherent feature of biochemistry, molecular biology, or cell biology necessitates aging.

2. Biologically immortal animals can still die from accident, infection, or mutation. They do not, however, show the eventually rapid increases in adult death rates under good conditions shown by animals that do age. That is the difference between biological immortality and the mythological immortality of Greek gods or virtuous Christians after death.

3. In cohorts of species that undergo protracted aging, very good conditions in laboratories, zoos, or medically treated populations sometimes allow some individuals to achieve a post-aging immortal phase. During this "late life" phase, mortality rates plateau. For example, it is only because human mortality rates plateau after the age of 90 years that so many humans have survived from 100 to 110. If the acceleration in mortality rates that occurs between the ages of 30 and 80 continued without remit, virtually no one would live past the age of 105 in a population of less than 10 billion.

4. As we explain in great detail in our book *Does Aging Stop?* (Mueller et al. 2011), evolutionary theory can explain why aging stops. It happens because the forces of natural selection eventually fall to such low levels that evolution no longer distinguishes among later ages in its neglect of survival at such ages. These words are hard to wrap one's mind around, because this effect is not intuitive. It was only discovered by the kind of numerical simulations that we present in *Does Aging Stop?*

5. Unlike the repeatedly refuted cell biological theories of aging, evolutionary theories of aging and biological immortality have been repeatedly corroborated in strong-inference experiments. We predict *in advance* how specific experimental manipulations will change patterns of aging. These predictions have then been clearly corroborated in large-scale replicated experiments with laboratory animals. Put crudely, evolutionists have scientifically solved the intellectual problems of aging and biological immortality. Naturally, thanks to patterns of human nature epitomized by Sinclair's Saying, cell and molecular biologists either fail to understand the scientific situation or somehow overlook it.

Technological Prospects for Near-Term Human Biological Immortality

So, if I have sufficiently disabused you of the cell-molecular-biology fictions of Magary or de Grey, what advice do evolutionary biologists have to offer for indefinitely evading the Grim Reaper?

Well, this evolutionary biologist would like to offer you a three-point plan: (1) stop your aging earlier; (2) preferentially take those supplements and medications that preserve overall health; and (3) seek repair at the level of cultured tissues and other macroscopic structures. Off we go.

1. Stop aging earlier

Since your aging is expected to stop if you live long enough, an important question to think about is, how can I get my aging to stop earlier? This is where my penicillin-like idea comes in.

One of the bigger anomalies for evolutionary thinking about aging is the great health benefits of adopting "paleo" diets and lifestyles, which more and more people seem to be doing. (Full disclosure: it has worked for me and those of my friends who have tried it.) There are any number of relatively propagandistic books about this. Some examples are *The Paleo Diet* (Cordain 2002), *The New Evolution Diet* (de Vany 2011), and *The Primal Blueprint* (Sisson 2009). But there are also some very good medical data showing the benefits of adopting pre-agricultural regimens, much of it being collected or cited in Staffan Lindeberg's *Food and Western Disease* (2010).

As we point out in *Does Aging Stop?*, this is anomalous from the standpoint of the results of experimental evolution (see Garland and Rose 2009), which show that only about a hundred generations or so are enough to achieve quite substantial adaptation to a novel environment in outbred sexual species like ourselves. Since most Eurasian populations have been agricultural for at least 5,000 years, or around 200 human generations, we should be well-adapted to agricultural lifestyles. And indeed the health and athletic performance of people under 30 years of age, when on agricultural diets, suggest that they are indeed adapted to the agricultural lifestyle.

So why have so many obtained health benefits from adopting paleo diets and lifestyles? This anomaly led me to a key insight. The declining forces of natural selection don't just lead to aging in all non-fissile animal species. They also scale the evolutionary response to an environmental change with adult age. One or two hundred generations of living agriculturally were enough to adapt young people to that way of life. But not enough to adapt older people from those same populations. At later ages, we are still not sufficiently reconstructed by evolution to thrive on diets that predominantly feature foods derived from grasses (grains, rice, corn) or milk (milk, cheese, yogurt, cream).

This suggests that the benefits of a switch to paleo diets and lifestyles will accrue primarily at later adult ages, at least among adults from long-agricultural populations. (Individuals from populations that have only recently adopted agriculture should avoid agricultural foods and activity patterns at all ages.) It further suggests the possibility that our aging might stop earlier if we make this switch, particularly because the demography under our ancestral hunter-gatherer conditions probably favored an earlier transition from aging to late-life mortality plateaus. This is all explained in scientific detail in the book *Does Aging Stop?* and somewhat gently at the free website 55theses.org. At the website, my webmaster Rob Paterson has elicited particularly anodyne statements from me, suitable for consumption by the scientifically more virginal.

But the upshot of all that material is simple at the prescriptive level: adopt a paleo diet and lifestyle after the age of 40 years. Your aging should then be partially reversed and slowed. Depending on your ancestry, it should come to a stop much earlier, between the ages of 55 and 75, perhaps.

2.   Use supplements and medications carefully

With your aging slowed or even stopped, you have to be careful about the supplements, medications, and recreational drugs that you use. The problem is that there are almost always toxic effects with high or chronic dosing of such substances. This is true even for such seemingly benign substances as Vitamins A, C, and E. Alcohol in moderation has been associated with some health benefits, particularly for cardiovascular disease. But it is both acutely and chronically toxic at high levels of intake.

Since molecular and cell biologists are singularly ill-equipped to make predictions about the long-term health effects of substances that have striking benefits for isolated cells or proteins, their advice about useful supplementation is to be systematically distrusted. Thus a vast number of widely consumed non-prescription substances (1) probably don't have the whole-organism benefits that this type of biologist blithely extrapolates; (2) are highly likely to have adverse side-effects; or (3) chiefly have value as placebos. There are ways to develop beneficial candidate supplements, as I have described in an earlier publication (Rose et al. 2010). But no one has yet implemented this research program properly, to my knowledge. In any case, a good nutrigenomic strategy for developing anti-aging supplements should start with a relatively healthy paleo-lifestyle population, which has already slowed or stopped its aging.

Finally, and most regrettably, most prescription medications have significant side-effects when used chronically. I have already given the example of lithium. But the Matsagas et al. (2009) study which I cited earlier suggests that valproate might have even worse side-effects, when used chronically. This is NOT an argument for the abandonment of medications that might well be keeping the patients who receive them alive. But it is an argument for great care about the chronic use of medications that do not clearly serve to sustain vital functions, medications like Botox, for example.

The recent explosion of genome-wide "omic" technologies offers the prospect of radically improving pharmaceutical development. In particular, such technologies are wholly disabusing most objective biologists of the notion that our physiology reduces to a relatively simple set of pathways that can be understood using the conventional theories and experiments of twentieth-century cell or molecular biology. With detailed information about the extensively radiating effects of candidate medications, it should be possible to move toward the development of more benign medications. These would be medications that do *not* impair overall healthspan as they treat specific acute medical problems, unlike many of the medications that are now available.

3.   When available and needed, get tissue repair

The thinking of cell and molecular biologists about aging is scientifically infirm, but they are developing some great repair technologies. Contrary to fictions put about by proponents of SENS and other cell-molecular technologies, they are very far from understanding how to re-engineer the molecular biology of individual cells so as to reverse or stop aging. But this doesn't mean that they won't be able to find ways to achieve tissue repair.

The reason for this technological disparity is that we are very far from being able to figure out exactly how cells work, just as we are very far from being able to figure out how the whole human body works when it is healthy. Both are underlain by extremely complex webs of causation, replete with extensive feedbacks, redundancy, and nonlinear effects, built by evolution fine-tuning thousands of genes. So trying to re-engineer either cells or entire bodies is well beyond our present scientific capacity.

Where we *have* made progress is in getting our cells to proliferate and to differentiate outside of the human body. In doing so, cell biologists take advantage of controls over proliferation and differentiation *that evolution has already built*. Tweaking these a bit so as to produce simple types of healthy tissue is a reasonable project. Indeed, significant progress is already being made with the development of replacement tissues for muscle, bone, and skin. It isn't necessary to master all of the causal network underlying cardiovascular disease to replace dead or diseased heart muscle. Literally patching a heart using cardiac muscle grown in tissue culture can be a useful form of repair. Likewise, for skin, corneas, and other relatively simple tissues, growing autologous replacement tissues *ex vivo* offers the prospect of useful tissue-level repair of the aging human body.

Thus repair at the tissue level will be an area where significant progress will be made. This is the more likely route toward making our bodies indefinitely repairable objects, as opposed to the protein and intracellular types of repair favored in the SENS program of de Grey (see de Grey and Rae 2007). The latter strategy presumes that we know vastly more about how cells and organisms age than we do in fact. The former strategy is based on the technological premise that we can make our best progress by exploiting as much of what evolution has already built as possible, improving on it only in the most straightforward ways.

Fictitious Technology vs Actual Technology

Conventional science fiction in the Western tradition has long featured fanciful stories of space exploration. Well before Jules Verne, in the eighteenth century Giacomo Casanova wrote fiction about a trip to the Moon. Such science fiction continued up until the 1950s, before the Apollo mission rendered such works otiose by actually accomplishing the feat. Notably, the technological details of the works of fiction were characteristically ridiculous compared to the actual technologies used. In particular, fictional technologies are always far easier, far less arduous, compared to the actual technologies which accomplish the feat around which the fictions revolve.

Thus we have the simple genetic vector of *The Postmortal*, the Pepto-Bismol-looking pink liquid of the 1992 film *Death Becomes Her*, and the repair of the Seven Deadly Sins of SENS. All these fictitious technologies are fairly straightforward, especially if they are explained by the silver-tongued. Indeed, this was the scam that the Taoists and alchemists used to attract the support of their patrons over the last two millennia, that and the conversion of base metals to gold.

But actual technological feats take a vast amount of work. Getting to the Moon and achieving nuclear transmutation were both quite difficult. Of material significance is that achieving these technological feats required the efforts of a wide range of physical scientists. Building biologically immortal humans will likewise take a great deal of work, for there are extremely complex evolutionary genetic networks underpinning still more complex networks of interacting gene products, which in turn generate hundreds of different kinds of cells, all of which establish, constrain, and mold human patterns of aging. Toward the end of this century, we will have largely defeated aging, and human biological immortality will be as normal as treating pathogens with antibiotics and antivirals is now. People will still die of aging-related diseases, but only after living extremely long healthspans. More perhaps will die of accident, homicide, suicide, or infection by that time. Much of twenty-first-century biology will have to be orchestrated toward service of this goal, with evolutionary biology playing the conductor's role.

Biological immortality certainly won't be achieved easily or abruptly, which is one reason why we have relatively little to fear with respect to its effects on society. The effective defeat of contagious disease in the latter part of the twentieth century came a century after Pasteur properly established the germ theory of disease. The evolutionary theory of aging is now adequately established, both mathematically and experimentally. A long struggle against the recalcitrant medical establishment and the entrenched cytogerontologists lies before us. They have the money, power, and prestige. All the evolutionists have is scientific truth.

I think many of you know how this is going to play out.

References

Arrison, Sonia (2011) *100 Plus: How the Coming Age of Longevity Will Change Everything, from Careers and Relationships to Family and Faith*. New York: Basic Books.

Burke, Molly K., et al. (2010) "Genome-Wide Analysis of a Long-Term Evolution Experiment with *Drosophila.*" *Nature* 467, pp. 587–590.

Comfort, Alex (1979) *The Biology of Senescence*, 3rd edn. New York: Elsevier North Holland, Inc.

Cordain, Loren. (2002) *The Paleo Diet*. New York: Wiley.

de Grey, Aubrey and Rae, M. (2007) *Ending Aging*. New York: St. Martin's Griffin.

de Vany, Arthur (2011) *The New Evolution Diet*. New York: Rodale.

Garland, Theodore Jr. and Michael R., eds. (2009) *Experimental Evolution*. Berkeley: University of California Press.

Glynn, Alan (2001) *The Dark Fields*. New York: Little, Brown and Company.

Lindeberg, Staffan E. (2010) *Food and Western Disease: Health and Nutrition from an Evolutionary Perspective*. New York: Wiley-Blackwell.

Magary, Drew (2011) *The Postmortal*. London: Penguin Books.

Martinez, Daniel E. (1998) "Mortality Patterns Suggest a Lack of Senescence in Hydra." *Experimental Gerontology* 33, pp. 217–225.

Matsagas, Kennedy, et al. (2009) "Long-Term Functional Side-Effects of Stimulants and Sedatives in *Drosophila melanogaster.*" *PLoS One* 4(8), e6578.

Mueller, Laurence D., Rauser, Casandra L., and Michael R. (2011) *Does Aging Stop?* New York: Oxford University Press.

Passanati, Hardip B., Rose, Michael R., and Matos, Margarida (2005) *Methuselah Flies: A Case Study in the Evolution of Aging*. Singapore: World Scientific Publishing.

Rose, Michael R. (1984) "The Evolutionary Route to Methuselah," *New Scientist*, July 26.

Rose, Michael R. (1991) *Evolutionary Biology of Aging*. New York: Oxford University Press.

Rose, Michael R. (2005) *The Long Tomorrow: How Advances in Evolutionary Biology Can Help Us Postpone Aging*. New York: Oxford University Press.

Rose, Michael R., et al. (2010) "Evolutionary Nutrigenomics." In G.M. Fahy et al., eds., *The Future of Aging: Pathways to Human Life Extension*. Berlin: Springer.

Rose, Michael R. and Burke, Molly K. (2011) "Genomic Croesus: Experimental Evolutionary Genetics of Aging." *Experimental Gerontology* 46, pp. 397–403.

Sisson, Mark (2009) *The Primal Blueprint*. Malibu: Primal Nutrition.

Weiner, Jonathan (2010) *Long for this World: The Strange Science of Immortality*. New York: HarperCollins.

20

Dialogue between Ray Kurzweil
and Eric Drexler

What would it take to achieve successful cryonics reanimation of a fully functioning human brain, with memories intact? A conversation at the Alcor Conference on Extreme Life Extension between Ray Kurzweil and Eric Drexler sparked an email discussion (November 23, 2002) of this question. They agreed that, despite the challenges, the brain's functions and memories can be represented surprisingly compactly, suggesting that successful reanimation of the brain may be achievable.

Ray Kurzweil. Eric, I greatly enjoyed our brief opportunity to share ideas (difficulty of adding bits to quantum computing, cryonics reanimation, etc.). Also, it was exciting to hear your insightful perspective on the field you founded, now that it's gone – from what was regarded in the mainstream anyway as beyond-the-fringe speculation – to, well, mainstream science and engineering.

I had a few questions and/or comments (depending on whether I'm understanding what you said correctly). Your lecture had a very high idea density, so I may have misheard some details.

With regard to cryonics reanimation, I fully agree with you that preserving structure (i.e., information) is the key requirement, that it is not necessary to preserve cellular functionality. I have every confidence that nanobots will be able to go in and fix every cell, indeed every little machine in every cell. The key is to preserve the information. And I'll also grant that we could lose some of the information; after all, we lose some information every day of our lives anyway. But the primary information needs to be preserved. So we need to ask, what are the types of information required?

One is to identify the neuron cells, including their type. This is the easiest requirement. Unless the cryonics process has made a complete mess of things, the cells should be identifiable. By the time reanimation is feasible, we will fully understand the types of neurons and be

Originally published in *Extropy Online* (2002). Copyright © Max More.

able to readily identify them from the slightest clues. These neurons (or their equivalents) could then all be reconstructed.

The second requirement is the interconnections. This morphology is one key aspect of our knowledge and experience. We know that the brain is continually adding and pruning connections; it's a primary aspect of its learning and self-organizing principle of operation. The interconnections are much finer than the neurons themselves (for example, with current brain-imaging techniques, we can typically see the neurons but we do not yet clearly see the interneuronal connections). Again, I believe it's likely that this can be preserved, provided that the vitrification has been done quickly enough. It would not be necessary that the connections be functional or even fully evident, as long as it can be inferred where they were. And it would be okay if some fraction were not identifiable.

It's the third requirement that concerns me; the neurotransmitter concentrations, which are contained in structures that are finer yet than the interneuronal connections. These are, in my view, also critical aspects of the brain's learning process. We see the analogue of the neurotransmitter concentrations in the simplified neural net models that I use routinely in my pattern recognition work, The learning of the net is reflected in the connection weights as well as the connection topology (some neural net methods allow for self-organization of the topology, some do not, but all provide for self-organization of the weights). Without the weights, the net has no competence.

If the very-fine-resolution neurotransmitter concentrations are not identifiable, the downside is not equivalent to merely an amnesia patient who has lost his memory of his name, profession, family members, etc. Our learning, reflected as it is in both interneuronal connection topology and neurotransmitter concentration patterns, underlies knowledge that is far broader than these routine forms of memory, including our "knowledge" of language, how to think, how to recognize objects, how to eat, how to walk and perform all of our skills, etc. Loss of this information would result in a brain with no competence at all. It would be worse than a newborn's brain, which is at least designed to begin reorganizing itself. A brain with the connections intact but none of the neurotransmitter concentrations would have no competence of any kind and a connection pattern that would be too specific to relearn all of these skills and basic knowledge.

It's not clear whether the current vitrification-preservation process maintains this vital type of information. We could readily conduct an experiment to find out. We could vitrify the brain of a mouse and then do a destructive scan while still vitrified to see if the neurotransmitter concentrations are still evident. We could also confirm that the connections are evident as well.

The type of long-term memory that an amnesia patient has lost is just one type of knowledge in the brain. At the deepest level, the brain's self-organizing paradigm underlies our knowledge and all competency that we have gained since our fetal days (even prior to birth).

As a second issue, you said something about it being sufficient to just have preserved the big toe or the nose to reconstruct the brain. I'm not sure what you meant by that. Clearly none of the brain structure is revealed by body parts outside the brain. The only conceivable way one could restore a brain from the toe would be from the genome, which one can discover from any cell. And indeed, one could grow a brain from the genome. This would be, however, a fetal brain, which is a genetic clone of the original person, equivalent to an identical twin (displaced in time). One could even provide a learning and maturing experience for this brain in which the usual 20 odd years were sped up to 20 days or less, but this would still be just a biological clone, not the original person.

Finally, you said (if I heard you correctly) that the amount of information in the brain (presumably needed for reanimation) is about 1 gigabyte. My own estimates are quite different. It is true that genetic information is very low, although as I discussed above, genetic information is not at all sufficient to recreate a person. The genome has about 0.8 gigabytes of information. There is massive redundancy, however. For example, the sequence "ALU" is repeated 300,000 times. If one compresses the genome using standard data compression to remove redundancy, estimates are that one can achieve about 30 to 1 lossless compression, which brings us down to about 25 megabytes. About half of that comprises the brain, or about 12 megabytes. That's the initial design plan.

If we consider the amount of information in a mature human brain, however, we have about 10^{11} neurons with 10^3 average fan-out of connections, for an estimated total of 10^{14} connections. For each connection, we need to specify (i) the neurons that this connection is connected to, (ii) some information about its pathway as the pathway affects analog aspects of its electro-chemical information processing, and (iii) the neurotransmitter concentrations in associated synapses. If we estimate about 10^2 bytes of information to encode these details (which may be low), we have 10^{16} bytes, considerably more than the 10^9 bytes that you mentioned.

One might ask: How do we get from 10^7 bytes that specify the brain in the genome to 10^{16} bytes in the mature brain? This is not hard to understand, since we do this type of meaningful data expansion routinely in our self-organizing software paradigms. For example, a genetic algorithm can be efficiently coded, but in turn creates data far greater in size than itself using a stochastic process, which in turn self-organizes in response to a complex environment (the problem space). The result of this process is meaningful information far greater than the original program. We know that this is exactly how the creation of the brain works. The genome specifies initially semi-random interneuronal connection wiring patterns in specific regions of the brain (random within certain constraints and rules), and these patterns (along with the neurotransmitter-concentration levels) then undergo their own internal evolutionary process to self-organize to reflect the interactions of that person with their experiences and environment.

That is how we get from 10^7 bytes of brain specification in the genome to 10^{16} bytes of information in a mature brain. I think 109 bytes is a significant underestimate of the amount of information required to reanimate a mature human brain.

I'd be interested in your own reflections on these thoughts. with my best wishes,

Eric Drexler. Ray – Thanks for your comments and questions. Our thinking seems closely parallel on most points.

Regarding neurotransmitters, I think it is best to focus not on the molecules themselves and their concentrations, but rather on the machinery that synthesizes, transports, releases, senses, and recycles them. The state of this machinery must closely track long-term functional changes (i.e., long-term memory or LTM), and much of this machinery is an integral part of synaptic structure.

Regarding my toe-based reconstruction scenario [creating a brain from a bit of tissue containing intact DNA – Ed.], this is indeed no better than genetically based reconstruction together with loading of more or less default skills and memories – corresponding to a peculiar but profound state of amnesia. My point was merely that even this worst-case outcome is still what modern medicine would label a success: the patient walks out the door in good health. (Note that neurosurgeons seldom ask whether the patient who walks out is "the same patient" as the one who walked in.) Most of us wouldn't look forward to such an outcome, of course, and we expect much better when suspension occurs under good conditions.

Information-theoretic content of long-term memory

Regarding the information content of the brain, both the input and output data sets for reconstruction must indeed be vastly larger than a gigabyte, for the reasons you outline. The lower number [10^9] corresponds to an estimate of the information-theoretic content of human long term memory found (according to Marvin Minsky) by researchers at Bell Labs. They tried various methods to get information into and out of human LTM, and couldn't find learning rates above a few bits per second. Integrated over a lifespan, this yields the above number. If this is so, it suggests that information storage in the brain is indeed massively redundant, perhaps for powerful function-enabling reasons. (Identifying redundancy this way, of course, gives no hint of how to construct a compression and decompression algorithm.)

Best wishes, with thanks for all you've done. P.S. A Google search yields a discussion of the Bell Labs result by, yes, Ralph Merkle.

Ray Kurzweil. Okay, I think we're converging on some commonality.

On the neurotransmitter concentration level issue, you wrote: "Regarding neurotransmitters, I think it is best to focus not on the molecules themselves and their concentrations, but rather on the machinery that synthesizes, transports, releases, senses, and recycles them. The state of this machinery must closely track long-term functional changes (i.e. LTM), and much of this machinery is an integral part of synaptic structure."

I would compare the "machinery" to any other memory machinery. If we have the design for a bit of memory in a DRAM system, then we basically know the mechanics for the other bits. It is true that in the brain there are hundreds of different mechanisms that we could call memory, but each of these mechanisms is repeated many millions of times. This machinery, however, is not something we would need to infer from the preserved brain of a suspended patient. By the time reanimation is feasible, we will have long since reverse-engineered these basic mechanisms of the human brain, and thus would know them all. What we do need specifically for a particular patient is the state of that person's memory (again, memory referring to all skills). The state of my memory is not the same as that of someone else, so that is the whole point of preserving my brain.

And that state is contained in at least two forms: the interneuronal connection patterns (which we know is part of how the brain retains knowledge and is not a fixed structure) and the neurotransmitter concentration levels in the approximately 10^{14} synapses.

My concern is that this memory state information (particularly the neurotransmitter concentration levels) may not be retained by current methods. However, this is testable right now. We don't have to wait 40 to 50 years to find this out. I think it should be a high priority to do this experiment on a mouse brain as I suggested above (for animal lovers, we could use a sick mouse).

You appear to be alluding to a somewhat different approach, which is to extract the "LTM," which is likely to be a far more compact structure than the thousands of trillions of bytes represented by the connection and neurotransmitter patterns (CNP). As I discuss below, I agree that the LTM is far more compact. However, we are not extracting an efficient LTM during cryopreservation, so the only way to obtain it during cryo reanimation would be to retain its inefficient representation in the CNP.

You bring up some interesting and important issues when you wrote, "Regarding my toe-based reconstruction scenario, this is indeed no better than genetically-based reconstruction together with loading of more or less default skills and memories – corresponding to a peculiar but profound state of amnesia. My point was merely that even this worst-case outcome is still what modern medicine would label a success: the patient walks out the door in good health."

I agree that this would be feasible by the time reanimation is feasible. The means for "loading" these "default skills and memories" is likely to be along the lines that I described above, to use "a learning and maturing experience for this brain in which the usual 20 odd years were sped up to 20 days or less." Since the human brain as currently designed does not allow for explicit "loading" of memories and skills, these attributes need to be gained from experience using the brain's self-organizing approach. Thus we would have to use this type of experience-based approach. Nevertheless, the result you describe could be achieved. We could even include in these "loaded" (or learned) "skills and memories," the memory of having been the original person who was cryonically suspended, including having made the decision to be suspended, having become ill, and so on.

False reanimation

And this process would indeed appear to be a successful reanimation. The doctors would point to the "reanimated' patient as the proof in the pudding. Interviews of this patient would reveal that he was very happy with the process, delighted that he made the decision to be cryonically suspended, grateful to Alcor and the doctors for their successful reanimation of him, and so on.

But this would be a false reanimation. This is clearly not the same person that was suspended. His "memories" of having made the decision to be suspended four or five decades earlier would be false memories. Given the technology available at this time, it would be feasible to create entirely new humans from a genetic code and an experience / learning loading program (which simulates the learning in a much higher speed substrate to create a design for the new person). So creating a new person would not be unusual. So all this process has accomplished is to create an entirely new person who happens to share the genetic code with the person who was originally suspended. It's not the same person.

One might ask, "Who cares?" Well no one would care except for the originally suspended person. And he, after all, is not around to care. But as we look to cryonic suspension as a means towards providing a "second chance," we should care now about this potential scenario.

It brings up an issue which I have been concerned with, which is "false" reanimations.

Now one could even raise this issue (of a false reanimation) if the reanimated person does have the exact CNP of the original. One could take the philosophical position that this is still a different person. An argument for that is that once this technology is feasible, you could scan my CNP (perhaps while I'm sleeping) and create a CNP-identical copy of me. If you then come to me in the morning and say "good news, Ray, we successfully created your precise CNP-exact copy, we won't be needing your old body and brain anymore," I may beg to differ. I would wish the new Ray well, but feel that he's a different person. After all, I would still be here.

So even if I'm not still here, by the force of this thought experiment, he's still a different person. As you and I discussed at the reception, if we are using the preserved person as a data repository, then it would be feasible to create more than one "reanimated" person. If they can't all be the original person, then perhaps none of them are.

However, you might say that this argument is a subtle philosophical one, and that, after all, our actual particles are changing all the time anyway. But the scenario you described of creating a new person with the same genetic code, but with a very different CNP created through a learning simulation, is not just a matter of a subtle philosophical argument. This is clearly a different person. We have examples of this today in the case of identical twins. No one would say to an identical twin, "we don't need you anymore because, after all, we still have your twin."

I would regard this scenario of a "false" reanimation as one of the potential failure modes of cryonics.

Reverse-engineering the brain

Finally, on the issue of the LTM (long-term memory), I think this is a good point and an interesting perspective. I agree that an efficient implementation of the knowledge in a human brain (and I am referring here to knowledge in the broadest sense as not just classical long-term memory, but all of our skills and competencies) would be far more compact that the 10^{16} bytes I have estimated for its actual implementation.

As we understand biological mechanisms in a variety of domains, we find that we can redesign them (as we reverse engineer their functionality) with about 10^6 greater efficiency. Although biological evolution was remarkable in its ingenuity, it did get stuck in particular paradigms.

It's actually not permanently stuck in that its method of getting unstuck is to have one of its products, homo sapiens, discover and redesign these mechanisms.

We can point to several good examples of this comparison of our human engineered mechanisms to biological ones. One good example is Rob Freitas' design for robotic blood cells, which are many orders of magnitude more efficient than their biological counterparts.

Another example is the reverse engineering of the human auditory system by Lloyd Watts and his colleagues. They have found that implementing the algorithms in software from the reverse engineering of specific brain regions requires about a factor of 10^6 less computation than the theoretical potential of the brain regions being emulated.

Another good example is the extraordinarily slow computing speed of the interneuronal connections, which have about a 5 millisecond reset time. Today's conventional electronic circuits are already 100 million (10^8) times faster. Three-dimensional molecular circuits (e.g., nanotube-based circuitry) would be at least 10^9 times faster. Thus if we built a human brain equivalent with the same number of simulated neurons and connections (not just simulating the human brain with a smaller number of units that are operating at higher speeds), the resulting nanotube-based brain would operate at least 10^9 times faster than its biological counterpart.

Some of the inefficiency of the encoding of information in the human brain has a positive utility in that memory appears to have some holographic properties (meaningful information being distributed through a region), and this helps protect the information. It explains the usually gradual (as opposed to catastrophic) degradation of human memory and skill. But most of the inefficiency is not useful holographic encoding, but just this inherent inefficiency of biological mechanisms. My own estimate of this factor is around 10^6, which would reduce the LTM from my estimate of 10^{16} for the actual implementation to around 10^{10} for an efficient representation, but that is close enough to your and Minsky's estimate of 10^9.

However, as you point out, we don't know the compression/decompression algorithm, and are not in any event preserving this efficient representation of the LTM with the suspended patients. So we do need to preserve the inefficient representation.

With deep appreciation for your own contributions.

Eric Drexler. With respect to inferring memory state, the neurotransmitter-handling machinery in a synapse differs profoundly from the circuit structure in a DRAM cell. Memory cells in a chip are all functionally identical, each able to store and report different data from millisecond to millisecond; synapses in a brain are structurally diverse, and their differences encode relatively stable information. Charge stored in a DRAIVI cell varies without changes in its stable structure; long-term neurotransmitter levels in a synapse vary as a result of changes in its stable structure. The quantities of different enzymes, transport molecules, and so forth, determine the neurotransmitter properties relevant to LTM, hence neurotransmitter levels per se needn't be preserved.

My discussion of the apparent information-theoretic size of human LTM wasn't intended to suggest that such a compressed representation can or should be extracted from the detailed data describing brain structures. I expect that any restoration process will work with these far larger and more detailed data sets, without any great degree of intermediate compression. Nonetheless, the apparently huge gap between the essential mental information to be preserved and the vastly more detailed structural information is reassuring – and suggests that false reanimation, while possible, shouldn't be expected when suspension occurs under good conditions. (Current medical practice has analogous problems of false life-saving, but these don't define the field.)

Ray Kurzweil. I'd like to thank you for an engaging dialogue. I think we've converged to a pretty close common vision of these future scenarios. Your point is well taken that human memory (for all of its purposes), to the extent that it involves the neurotransmitters, is likely to be redundantly encoded. I agree that differences in the levels of certain molecules are likely to be also reflected in other differences, including structural differences. Most biological mechanisms that we do understand tend to have redundant information storage (although not all; some single-bit changes in the DNA can be catastrophic). I would point out, however, that we don't yet understand the synaptic structures sufficiently to be fully confident that the differences in neurotransmitter levels that we need (for reanimation) are all redundantly indicated by structural changes. However, all of this can be tested with today's technology, and I would suggest that this would be worthwhile.

I also agree that "the apparently huge gap between the essential mental information to be preserved and the vastly more detailed structural information is reassuring." This is one example in which the inefficiency of biology is helpful.

Eric Drexler. Thank you, Ray. I agree that we've found good agreement, and I also enjoyed the interchange.

Part V

Engines of Life
Identity and Beyond Death

One point on which all transhumanists agree – and one that distinguishes transhumanism from humanism and other philosophies of life – is the view that it is both possible and desirable to scientifically overcome biological aging and death. In an important sense, the quest to bring the aging process under control and to push back death ever farther is central to transhumanism. The possibilities opened up by greater intelligence, wisdom, wellbeing, and physical capabilities will be severely limited if aging continues to cause us to wither and perish within a handful of decades.

The desirability of indefinitely extending our lifespan – essentially making death a matter of choice – seems obvious to transhumanists. To almost everyone else, it's far from obvious and typically seen as a frightening, unnatural, or at least an impossible idea. Interestingly, even the many millions who believe in an indefinite life *after* death through religious and spiritual processes rail against the quest to achieve superlongevity here in the world we experience and know exists. Critics of life extension invariably exhume a few of the same arguments over and over again. Among these are the overpopulation, resources, boredom, and meaninglessness arguments.

The essays in Part V address varied aspects and implications of radically extended lifespans. Aubrey de Grey critically analyses pro-mortality arguments by leading critics Leon Kass and William Hurlbut. Despite disagreeing with Kass's conclusion, de Grey has a degree of sympathy for basing moral judgments on feelings. However, thinking about those feelings critically should lead to the view that life is good and death is bad and the more life the better, so long as we and those we care about remain healthy. De Grey is less sympathetic to Hurlbut's insistence that one's life has a natural length and that if lengthened, like a symphony, would be ruined.

While the transhumanist goal of defeating the inevitability of death is clear, the time it might take to achieve it is not. Even if the radical extension of human life spans is achievable, it may

The Transhumanist Reader: Classical and Contemporary Essays on the Science, Technology, and Philosophy of the Human Future, First Edition. Edited by Max More and Natasha Vita-More.
© 2013 John Wiley & Sons, Inc. Published 2013 by John Wiley & Sons, Inc.

come too late for many or all of us now living. Is there a plausible solution – a way to bridge the gap? Today, when a person collapses with a life-threatening condition, we transport them in an emergency vehicle across space to a location where more advanced medical technology is available. The future will be a place of far more advanced medical technology than today. Just as today's medicine can save and even revive those who would once have been considered dead, future medical capabilities might revive and repair today's fatal conditions. If only we could have an ambulance ride through time to those advanced capabilities.

Medical physicist and cryobiologist Brian Wowk argues in his "Medical Time Travel" that this may indeed be possible. Today's practice of cryopreservation (or "cryonics") involves preserving people immediately after declaration of legal death then maintaining them in an unchanging state for as long as it will take to deliver them into a future able to repair biological damage and revive them. Although legally and clinically dead, the people undergoing this "medical time travel" are (under good conditions) in essentially the same condition as patients undergoing open heart surgery. They are not dead in any final sense.

The more closely one looks at the concept of death, the more evident it becomes that historical criteria are flawed. Although cryopreservation cannot yet be reversed, death has not occurred unless biochemistry becomes *irreversibly* damaged. A crucial insight is that irreversibility depends on the level of technology. This realization is one reason transhumanist discussions so frequently turn to philosophical issues of personal identity – the conditions under which an individual can be said to continue in existence, to survive. Another reason is that longer lives coupled with physiological, cognitive, and emotional enhancements mean that we will undergo unprecedented degrees of change over time. How should we rethink our notions of personal identity and survival under these scenarios? Sociologist and bioethicist James Hughes surveys the most favored transhumanist views on this topic, including the "patternist" or "information-theoretic" theories, in "Transhumanism and Personal Identity."

Preventing biological aging and reversing and reviving us biologically is not the only possible path to radically extended lives. In Part III, Merkle and Koene argued that personal survival might be secured by transferring one's personality onto a non-biological platform. In Giulio Prisco's "Transcendent Engineering", this idea is taken to greater lengths and given a spiritual or religious spin that many transhumanists will dislike. Prisco uses "religion" here in a way that captures some of the transcendental goals of major religions while entirely rejecting the supernatural and anti-rational aspects that many of us consider essential to true religions. Contrary to "mainstream transhumanism" Prisco embraces parallels between transhumanism and spirituality or religion. He considers the future technological possibilities for resurrection of the dead by means of uploading, and of synthetic, non-physical realities in which we and the resurrected dead may live.

21

The Curate's Egg of Anti-Anti-Aging Bioethics

Aubrey de Grey

As a leader of the crusade to defeat aging, working to demonstrate both its feasibility and its desirability, I am often seen as an implacable opponent of all arguments that defend aging and criticize this crusade. This is an oversimplification. In short, even though my conclusion is unequivocally that this crusade is not only morally justified but is the single most urgent imperative for humanity, I nonetheless feel that some of the ideas put forward by others in their process of reaching the contrary view are worthy of serious analysis. Here I discuss these, as well as some ideas that I feel are much less well-founded.

Leon Kass held, for several years recently, the distinction of being by far the most politically influential bioethicist on the planet. He got there not only by having a particularly good way with words, but also by having a message whose content resonated with the public, including certain elected representatives. And it resonated for good reason, in my view: Kass really has talked a lot of sense, even when that sense has led to (in my view) nonsense later on. The topic of defeating aging is a particularly stark example of this. In fact, the areas on which I think he is right are so key to the arguments involved that I feel he is genuinely susceptible to persuasion of the merits of extreme life extension, albeit not of many other aspects of modern or anticipated biomedical modifications of our natural lives. It is seldom effective to overstate one's disagreements, nor to overlook one's areas of agreement, with someone whose views one would like to alter – and Kass's influence has been so great that even a softening of his opposition to such work would have considerable policy consequences.

The most straightforward way to explain what I like about Kass's views on life extension is to refer not to their most high-profile exposition, the chapter "Ageless Bodies" from the President's Council report (2003), but rather to two of Kass's earlier publications. The first of these is an essay titled "The Wisdom of Repugnance," which first appeared in the journal *The New Republic* (Kass 1997). This essay was not about life extension but about human reproductive cloning, and

The Transhumanist Reader: Classical and Contemporary Essays on the Science, Technology, and Philosophy of the Human Future, First Edition. Edited by Max More and Natasha Vita-More.
© 2013 John Wiley & Sons, Inc. Published 2013 by John Wiley & Sons, Inc.

needless to say I find its thrust flawed in many ways which I will not enumerate here. But the pivotal passage in the essay, from which its title is drawn, starts like this:

> "Offensive." "Grotesque." "Revolting." "Repugnant." "Repulsive." These are the words most com-
> monly heard regarding the prospect of human cloning. Such reactions come both from the man or
> woman in the street and from the intellectuals, from believers and atheists, from humanists and
> scientists. Even Dolly's creator has said he "would find it offensive" to clone a human being. ...
>
> Revulsion is not an argument; and some of yesterday's repugnances are today calmly accepted –
> though, one must add, not always for the better. In crucial cases, however, repugnance is the
> emotional expression of deep wisdom, beyond reason's power fully to articulate it. Can anyone
> really give an argument fully adequate to the horror which is father-daughter incest (even with
> consent), or having sex with animals, or mutilating a corpse, or eating human flesh, or even just
> (just!) raping or murdering another human being? Would anybody's failure to give full rational
> justification for his or her revulsion at these practices make that revulsion ethically suspect? Not
> at all. On the contrary, we are suspicious of those who think that they can rationalize away our
> horror, say, by trying to explain the enormity of incest with arguments only about the genetic risks
> of inbreeding.

A common reaction to this passage, and to others like it, has been that it amounts to capitula-tion: that Kass is conceding that he has no articulable argument for his view, and thus that his view is irrational, the sort of view that only the uneducated masses are entitled to hold, and hence invalid. I feel that such a reaction is incorrect and misses the entirely correct point that Kass is making. In short, I think he is right that ethics is ultimately more about instinct than about logic. Morality is not absolute but relative – relative to what one already "knows" to be "right." On discussing this with a philosopher recently, I was entertained to discover that my position here has a name – I am apparently a non-cognitivist. So are most of us, I claim, and we have no need to be ashamed of it. Kass misuses this insight, however: a hint of how appears in the above passage. Some activities that used to be repugnant to most people are now largely agreed to be unexceptionable: homosexuality, for example. This is a case where what is repug-nant to us now is the fact that we so recently felt that repugnance! Kass dodges this by describing those cases in which our attitudes have not changed as "crucial" – but he conspicuously omits any discussion of what makes these cases crucial, leaving as his only criterion the circular obser-vation that they have not changed.

If our moral instinct is self-defining, how can it change? I think the answer is clear, though perhaps surprising: we apply the scientific method to it. Our non-acceptance of homosexuality was progressively seen to be inconsistent with other, even more deeply held, aspects of our sense of right and wrong, such as the right to do what one likes that does not harm others; this bears a rather clear similarity to the emergence of relativity and the quantum theory from the increas-ingly awkward internal inconsistency of classical physics with respect to (for example) whether light is made of waves or particles.

This way of looking at the evolution of morality also illuminates the opposite transition, the emergence of popular repugnance at something that was once accepted. Kass largely avoids such cases (he makes no mention of slavery, for example), but not entirely: he does mention murder. I need not review how recently it was that those of European descent, when colonizing distant lands, freely massacred indigenous populations: we all know our history all too well. Here too, we came to appreciate the inconsistency of such attitudes with others that we found more central to our ethical code, and having done so we have set aside our misguided ways.

What can such history tell us about the future of morality, and in particular about what we will think in future of the desirability of aging? It tells us a great deal. The other earlier publication by Kass to which I referred above is "L'Chaim and its Limits: why not immortality?", first published in 2001 in *First Things*. This article is clear, at first:

> How much longer life is a blessing for an individual? Ignoring now the possible harms flowing back to individuals from adverse social consequences, how much more life is good for us as individuals, other things being equal? How much more life do we want, assuming it to be healthy and vigorous? Assuming that it were up to us to set the human lifespan, where would or should we set the limit and why?
>
> The simple answer is that no limit should be set. Life is good, and death is bad. Therefore, the more life the better, provided, of course, that we remain fit and our friends do, too.
>
> This answer has the virtues of clarity and honesty.

Indeed it does and those are virtues not lightly dismissed. How, then, does Kass proceed? As follows:

> But most public advocates of conquering aging deny any such greediness. They hope not for immortality, but for something reasonable – just a few more years.

Huh? How can one possibly suggest that the statements of "most public advocates" – people who are simply following the maxim of only going as far as their audience might be willing to follow them – bear on the ethics of the situation? But reassurance is swift, because this is not the end of Kass's argument: indeed, he continues by stating cogently that these statements are a self-deception and that we do not, in fact, feel any limits on how long we want to live while still healthy. He then proceeds to the many societal difficulties that the availability of an indefinite lifespan might bring, which were repeated in "Ageless Bodies" (Kass 2003) and with which readers are thus familiar enough to make their repetition here unnecessary. However, he is also perfectly candid in regard to the paltry force of his argument: he peppers it with statements such as "I know I won't persuade many people to my position" and "To praise mortality must seem to be madness."

This, not his resort to emotional justification for a moral position, is where Kass capitulates. For what is the source of this distaste for death that is so profound that Kass openly concedes that he will not appreciably diminish it? It is none other than that same wisdom of repugnance upon which his entire argument pivots and which I find rings so true. Death is, quite simply, repugnant, however much the slowness of most people's physical and cognitive decline may allow us to come to terms with it in advance. The fellow-countrymen of the mass-murdering pioneers of the New World, sitting at home and hearing patchily of such events, doubtless felt some mild discomfort at them but felt that it was ultimately the natural order of things in a generally brutal world, still rife with wars between wealthy nations. It took an advance in our understanding of how to live together, and a consequently greater appreciation of the value of all human life, to open our eyes to the horror of such activity and bring it to an end. Quite simply, we became civilized enough to resolve the stark internal inconsistency of our moral position. We are still becoming more civilized today; shortly we will, at long last, arrive at the collective realization that death of the old is as barbaric as death of the ethnically unfamiliar. Those who defend our current amorality in this regard will be consigned to the same dark corners of history as those who defended ethnic "cleansing" in centuries past. Even to suggest that the value of a life varies with how long it has already been lived, as Arthur Caplan has (see Glaser 2004), will (shortly? I hope so!) be seen as an indefensibly ageist stance.

What about other opponents of the crusade against aging? William Hurlbut was a founding member of the President's Council on Bioethics that Kass led. Though generally regarded as a supporter of Kass, Dr. Hurlbut has demonstrated great sincerity and creativity in the quest to identify ways to bridge society's differences in relation to bioethical issues; prominent among these has been his promotion of "altered nuclear transfer" (ANT), a possible method for creating immunologically matched embryonic stem cells without destroying bona fide embryos (Hurlbut 2005). (I also proposed a method for this, which may be ethically more unambiguous than ANT [de Grey 2004].) A number of Hurlbut's statements merit discussion.

An argument that I find particularly weak appears often in Hurlbut's output on this topic: the comparison of life to a symphony. The idea that one's life has a natural length, in the same way that the quality of a symphony might be diminished if it were doubled in length, makes the unstated (and decidedly implausible) assumption that at the end of a symphony one will never want to listen to another symphony! There is indeed a persuasive case that certain activities that one might engage in for a few decades (such as a career) should not be extended but instead repeated in novel forms, after retraining and adult education, but that says nothing about how many careers one should have in a lifetime. And surely it is not the biological changes currently associated with aging, but rather our cognitive features – ones that can be repeated in varied form indefinitely – that define the meaning of one's life. Otherwise, what meaning can there be in the greater part of adulthood while one's physical function is essentially unchanging?

Hurlbut has also made a statement that encapsulates the bioconservative fallacy as I see it. He asserts that he is "not convinced" that life extension would be good for us – and leaves it at that. He thus insinuates, without quite saying, that we should adopt the precautionary principle with regard to life extension and avoid developing it because we are uncertain whether it will benefit mankind. But this is utterly without justification. In what other context would we regard an action (or inaction) that hastens someone's death as the safer option? Even in the tragic case of Terry Schiavo a commentator not generally noted for his progressive views – President Bush – stated that it is best to "err on the side of life." Yet those who doubt the benefits of life extension argue that condemning 100,000 people every day to an unnecessarily (as it will eventually be) early death on the basis of their age is a policy that needs no more justification than an uncertainty regarding whether life extension will be good for us.

In responding to the suggestion that Kass's "wisdom of repugnance" actually constitutes a strong argument for life extension, Hurlbut has noted that "Young children love their grandparents. They don't find them repulsive. They see in them the beauty of the generative spirit, of the nurturing mind." But this fails to address the actual question: Would those children be happier or sadder if their grandparents were not only wise and loving but also youthful?

Hurlbut's reluctance to confront the true issues is also revealed in his attitude to the question whether he is against extended lives per se or only against an abrupt extension of life expectancy. He has responded by saying that he regards extreme life extension as "biologically unlikely." Well, if it is so unlikely, why did the President's Council devote 15 percent of their "Beyond Therapy" report to it?

Similarly, when asked whether we have the right to deny future generations the opportunity to live much longer than people currently can, Hurlbut claims that other biomedical goals are more important. What on earth does that have to do with a question of human rights?

I hope these brief remarks will serve to stimulate debate on the views held by Dr. Hurlbut and other similarly influential thinkers concerning the postponement of aging.

References

de Grey, Aubrey D.N.J. (2004) "Inter-Species Therapeutic Cloning: The Looming Problem of Mitochondrial DNA and Two Possible Solutions." *Rejuvenation Res* 7/2, pp. 95–98.

Glaser, Vicki P. (2004) "Personal Profile: An Interview with Arthur Caplan." *Rejuvenation Res* 7/2, pp. 148–153.

Hurlbut, William B. (2005) "Altered Nuclear Transfer as a Morally Acceptable Means for the Procurement of Human Embryonic Stem Cells." *National Catholic Bioethics Quarterly* 5/1, pp. 145–151.

Kass, Leon R. (1997) "The Wisdom of Repugnance." *New Republic* (June 2), pp. 17–26.

Kass, Leon R. (2001) "L'Chaim and Its Limits: Why Not Immortality?" *First Things* 113, pp. 17–24.

Kass, Leon R. (2003) "Ageless Bodies, Happy Souls." *The New Atlantis* (Spring).

President's Council on Bioethics (2003) *Beyond Therapy: Biotechnology and the Pursuit of Happiness.* http://bioethics.georgetown.edu/pcbe/reports/beyondtherapy/beyond_therapy_final_webcorrected.pdf.

Further Reading

Arking, Robert (2004) "Meeting Report. A New Age for Aging? Ethical Questions, Scientific Insights, and Societal Outcomes." *Rejuvenation Res* 7/1, pp. 53–60.

de Grey, Aubrey D.N.J. (2004) "Leon Kass: Quite Substantially Right." *Rejuvenation Res* 7/2, pp. 89–91.

de Grey, Aubrey D.N.J. (2004) "Three Self-Evident Life-Extension Truths." *Rejuvenation Res* 7/3, pp. 165–167.

de Grey, Aubrey D.N.J. (2004) "Aging, Childlessness, or Overpopulation: The Future's Right to Choose." *Rejuvenation Res* 7/4, pp. 237–238.

Glaser, Vicky P. (2005) "An Interview with William B. Hurlbut." *Rejuvenation Res* 8/2, 110–122.

White, Ronald F. (2004) "Review of Overall C. 'Aging, Death, and Human Longevity: A Philosophical Inquiry.'" *Rejuvenation Res* 7/4, pp. 261–262.

22

Medical Time Travel

Brian Wowk

Time travel is a solved problem. Einstein showed that if you travel in a spaceship for months at speeds close to the speed of light, you can return to earth centuries in the future. Unfortunately for would-be time travelers, such spacecraft will not be available until centuries in the future.

Rather than Einstein, nature relies on Arrhenius to achieve time travel. The Arrhenius equation of chemistry describes how chemical reactions slow down as temperature is reduced. Since life is chemistry, life itself slows down at cooler temperatures. Hibernating animals use this principle to time travel from summer to summer, skipping winters when food is scarce.

Medicine already uses this kind of biological time travel. When transplantable organs such as hearts or kidneys are removed from donors, the organs begin dying as soon as their blood supply stops. Removed organs have only minutes to live. However with special preservation solutions and cooling in ice, organs can be moved across hours of time and thousands of miles to waiting recipients. Cold slows chemical processes that would otherwise be quickly fatal.

Can whole people travel through time like preserved organs? Remarkably, the answer seems to be yes. Although it is seldom done, medicine sometimes does preserve people like organs awaiting transplant. Some surgeries on major blood vessels of the heart or brain can only be done if blood circulation through the entire body is stopped (Aebert et al. 1998; Ehrlich et al. 1995). Stopped blood circulation would ordinarily be fatal within 5 minutes, but cooling to +16°C (60°F) allows the human body to remain alive in a "turned off" state for up to 60 minutes (Rosenthal 1990). With special blood substitutes and further cooling to a temperature of 0°C (32°F), life without heartbeat or circulation can be extended as much as three hours (Haneda et al. 1986). Although there is currently no surgical use for circulatory arrest of several hours

The Transhumanist Reader: Classical and Contemporary Essays on the Science, Technology, and Philosophy of the Human Future, First Edition. Edited by Max More and Natasha Vita-More.
© 2013 John Wiley & Sons, Inc. Published 2013 by John Wiley & Sons, Inc.

(Greenberg 1997), it may be used in the future to permit surgical repair of wounds before blood circulation is restored after severe trauma (Bellamy et al. 1996).

While some biological processes are merely slowed by deep cooling, others are completely stopped. Brain activity is an important example. Brain electrical activity usually ceases at temperatures below +18°C (64°F), and disappears completely in all cases as freezing temperatures are approached (Stecker et al. 2001). Yet these temperatures can still be survived. In fact, not only can the brain survive being turned off, surgeons often use drugs to force the brain to turn off when temperature alone doesn't do the trick (Rung et al. 1991). They do this because if the brain is active when blood circulation is stopped, vital energy stores can become depleted, later causing death. This reminds us that death is not when life turns off. Death is when the chemistry of life becomes irreversibly damaged.

Specialized surgeries are not the only cases in which the brain can stop working and later start again. Simple cardiac arrest (stopping of the heart) at normal body temperature also causes brain electrical activity to stop within 40 seconds (Lind et al. 1975). Yet the heart can remain stopped for several times this long with no lasting harm. Anesthetic drugs, such as barbiturates, can flatten EEG (brain electrical activity) readings for many hours while still permitting later recovery (Bird and Plum 1968). This prolonged drug-induced elimination of brain activity is sometimes used as a treatment for head injuries (Toyama 1993). Patients do not emerge from these comas as blank slates. Evidently human beings don't require continuous operation like computer chips. Brains store long-term memories in physical structures, not fleeting electrical patterns.

Perhaps the most extreme example of brains completely stopping and later starting again are the experiments of Isamu Suda reported in the journal *Nature* and elsewhere (Suda et al. 1966; Suda et al. 1974). Suda showed recovery of EEG activity in cat brains resuscitated with warm blood after frozen storage at –20°C (–4°F) for up to seven years.

Reversible experiments in which all electrical activity stops, and chemistry comes to a virtual halt, disprove the nineteenth-century belief that there is a "spark of life" inside living things. Life is chemistry. When the chemistry of life is adequately preserved, so is life. When the chemistry of a human mind is adequately preserved, so is the person.

Suda's frozen cat brains deteriorated with time. Brains thawed after five days showed EEG patterns almost identical to EEGs obtained before freezing. However brains thawed after seven years showed greatly slowed activity. At a temperature of –20°C, liquid water still exists in a concentrated solution between ice crystals. Chemical deterioration still slowly occurs in this cold liquid.

Preserving the chemistry of life for unlimited periods of time requires cooling below –130°C (–200°F) (Mazur 1984). Below this temperature, any remaining unfrozen liquid between ice crystals undergoes a "glass transition." Molecules become stuck to their neighbors with weak hydrogen bonds. Instead of wandering about, molecules just vibrate in one place. Without freely moving molecules, all chemistry stops.

For living cells to survive this process, chemicals called cryoprotectants must be added. Cryoprotectants, such as glycerol, are small molecules that freely penetrate inside cells and limit the percentage of water that converts into ice during cooling. This allows cells to survive freezing by remaining in isolated pockets of unfrozen solution between ice crystals (Mazur 1984). Below the glass transition temperature, molecules inside these pockets lock into place, and cells remain preserved inside the glassy water-cryoprotectant mixture between ice crystals.

This approach for preserving individual cells by freezing was first demonstrated half a century ago (Polge et al. 1949). It is now used routinely for many different cell types, including human embryos. Preserving organized tissue by freezing has proven to be more difficult. While isolated cells can accommodate as much as 80 percent of the water around them turning into ice, organs are much less forgiving because there is no room between cells for ice to grow (Fahy et al. 1987). Suda's cat brains survived freezing because the relatively warm temperature of –20°C allowed modest quantities of glycerol to keep ice formation between cells within tolerable limits.

In 1984 cryobiologist Greg Fahy proposed a new approach to the problem of complex tissue preservation at low temperature (Fahy et al. 1984). Instead of freezing, Fahy proposed loading tissue with so much cryoprotectant that ice formation would be completely prevented at all temperatures. Below the glass transition temperature, entire organs would become a glassy solid (a solid with the molecular structure of a liquid), free of any damage from ice. This process was called "vitrification." Preservation by vitrification, first demonstrated for embryos (Rall and Fahy 1985), has now been successfully applied to many different cell types and tissues of increasing complexity. In 2000, reversible vitrification of transplantable blood vessels was demonstrated (Song et al. 2000).

New breakthroughs in reducing the toxicity of vitrification solutions (Fahy, Wowk, Wu, and Painter 2004), and in adding synthetic ice-blocking molecules (Wowk et al. 2000; Wowk and Fahy 2002), continue to push the field forward. In 2004, successful transplantation of rabbit kidneys after cooling to a temperature of –50°C (–58°F) was reported (Fahy, Wowk, Wu, Fan, et al. 2004). These kidneys were prevented from freezing by replacing more than half of the water inside them with vitrification chemicals. Amazingly, organs can survive this extreme treatment if the chemicals are introduced and removed quickly at low temperature.

Reversible vitrification of major organs is a reasonable prospect within this decade. What about vitrification of whole animals? This is a much more difficult problem. Some organs, such as the kidney and brain, are privileged organs for vitrification because of their high blood flow rate. This allows vitrification chemicals to enter and leave them quickly before there are toxic effects. Most other tissues would not survive the long chemical exposure time required to absorb a sufficient concentration to prevent freezing.

It is useful to distinguish between reversible vitrification and morphological vitrification. Reversible vitrification is vitrification in which tissue recovers from the vitrification process in a viable state. Morphological vitrification is vitrification in which tissue is preserved without freezing, with good structural preservation, but in which key enzymes or other biomolecules are damaged by the vitrification chemicals. Morphological vitrification of a kidney was photographically demonstrated in Fahy's original vitrification paper (Fahy et al. 1984), but 20 years later reversible kidney vitrification is still being pursued.

Given this background, what are the prospects of reversibly vitrifying a whole human being? It's theoretically possible, but the prospects are still distant. Morphological vitrification of most organs and tissues in the body may now be possible, but moving from morphological vitrification to reversible vitrification will require fundamental new knowledge of mechanisms of cryoprotectant toxicity, and means to intervene in those mechanisms.

If reversible vitrification of humans is developed in future decades, what would be the application of this "suspended animation?" Space travel is sometimes suggested as an application, but time travel – specifically, medical time travel – seems more likely to be the primary application. People, especially young people dying of diseases expected to be treatable in future years, would be most motivated to try new suspended animation technologies. Governments would probably not even allow anyone but dying people to undergo such an extreme process, especially in the early days. Applications like space travel would come much later.

Medical time travel, by definition, involves technological anticipation. Sometimes this anticipation goes beyond just cures for disease. After all, if people are cryopreserved in anticipation of future cures, what about future cures for imperfections of the preservation process itself? As the medical prospect of reversible suspended animation draws nearer, the temptation to cut this corner will become stronger. In fact, some people are already cutting this corner very wide.

In 1964, with the science of cryobiology still in its infancy, Robert Ettinger proposed freezing recently deceased persons until science could resuscitate them (Ettinger 1964). The proposal assumed that fatal injury/illness, the early stages of clinical death, and crude preservation would all be reversible in the future. Even aging was to be reversed. This proposal was made in absence of any detailed knowledge of the effects of stopped blood flow or freezing on the human body. The proposal later came to be known as "cryonics."

Cryonics was clever in that it circumvented legal obstacles to cryopreserving people by operating on the other side of the legal dividing line of death. However, 40 years later, as measured by the number people involved and the scientific acceptance of the field, cryonics remains a fringe practice. Why? Probably because by operating as it does, cryonics is perceived as interment rather than medicine. One organization, the Cryonics Institute, is even licensed as a cemetery. It advertises that its services are delivered by professional morticians (as if this is an endorsement?). Dictionaries now define cryonics as "freezing a dead human." Is it any wonder that cryonics is unpopular? It is a failure by definition!

Is this view biologically justified? In the 1980s another cryonics organization, the Alcor Life Extension Foundation, adopted a different approach to cryonics. Under the leadership of cardiothoracic surgery researcher Jerry Leaf and dialysis technician Mike Darwin Alcor brought methods of modern medicine into cryonics. Alcor sought to validate each step of their cryopreservation process as reversible, beginning with life support provided immediately after cardiac arrest, and continuing through hours of circulation with blood replacement solutions. Leaf and Darwin showed that large animals could be successfully recovered after several hours at near-freezing temperatures under conditions similar to those in the first hours of real cryonics cases (see *Alcor's Pioneering Total Body Washout Experiments*). Blood gas measurements and clinical chemistries obtained in real cryonics cases further demonstrated that application of life-support techniques (mechanical CPR and heart-lung machines) could keep cryonics subjects biologically alive even in a state of cardiac arrest and legal death (Darwin 1996).

This leaves cryonics today in an interesting situation. It is stigmatized as something that cannot work because the subjects are legally deceased. Yet under ideal conditions the subjects are apparently alive by all measurable criteria, except heartbeat. They are biologically the same as patients undergoing open heart surgery, legal labels notwithstanding. The cryopreservation phase of cryonics is of course not yet reversible. But cryonicists would argue that this does not imply death either because death only happens when biochemistry becomes irreversibly damaged, and "irreversibility" is technology-dependent.

To clarify these issues, cryonicists have proposed the "information-theoretic criterion" for death (Merkle 1992). According to this criterion, you are not dead when life stops (we already know that from clinical medicine), you are not dead when biochemistry is damaged, you are only dead when biochemistry is so badly damaged that no technology, not even molecular nanotechnology (Drexler 1986), could restore normal biochemistry with your memories intact. By this criterion, someone who suffered cardiac arrest days ago in the wilderness is really dead. Someone who suffered only a few minutes of cardiac arrest and cryoprotectant toxicity during morphological vitrification may not be.

Whether one accepts this information-theoretic criterion or not, the modern cryonics practice of using life support equipment to resuscitate the brain after legal death raises important issues. Among them is the scientific issue that cryonics cannot be dismissed simply by calling its subjects "dead." Two minutes of cardiac arrest followed by restoration of blood circulation does not a skeleton make. There should be a rule that no one be allowed to say "dead" when discussing cryonics. It is usually a slur that communicates nothing scientific.

Whether cryonics can work depends on biological details of cerebral ischemic injury (brain injury during stopped blood flow), cryopreservation injury, and anticipated future technology. There is much published literature on cerebral ischemia, and a small but growing body of writing on relevant future technologies (Darwin 1977; Drexler 1986; Donaldson 1988; Freitas 1999, 2003). There is, however, very little information on the quality of preservation achieved with cryonics (Alcor staff 1984; Darwin et al. 1995). It would seem logical to look to cryobiologists for this information.

Cryobiologists, professional scientists that study the effect of cold on living things, decided long ago that they didn't want their field associated with cryonics (Darwin 1991). The Society for Cryobiology bylaws even provides for the expulsion of members that practice or promote "freezing deceased persons." The result has been the polarization of cryobiologists into either outspoken contempt or silence concerning cryonics. The contempt camp typically speaks of cryonics as if it hasn't changed in 40 years. The silent camp doesn't comment on the subject, and usually follows a "don't ask, don't tell" policy about cryonics sympathizers among them. This political environment, plus the fact that most cryobiologists work outside the specialty of organ cryopreservation, makes obtaining informed cryobiological information about cryonics very difficult.

The most important cryobiological fact of cryonics (other than its current irreversibility) is that cryoprotectant chemicals can be successfully circulated through most of the major organs of the body if blood clots are not present. We can conclude this by simply considering that everything now known about long-term preservation of individual organs was learned by removing and treating those organs under conditions similar to ideal cryonics cases. It is generally observed that the quality of cell structure preservation (as revealed by light and electron microscopy) is very poor when there is no cryoprotectant, but steadily improves as the concentration of cryoprotectant is increased (provided toxicity thresholds are not exceeded). Recent years have seen a trend toward using higher cryoprotectant concentrations in cryonics, yielding structural preservation that is impressively similar to unfrozen tissue (Darwin et al. 1995).

Somewhere between freezing, morphological vitrification, reversible vitrification of the central nervous system, and reversible vitrification of whole people, there is technology that will lead medicine to take the idea of medical time travel seriously within this century. Whether what is now called cryonics will eventually become that technology remains to be seen. It will depend on whether cryonicists can manage to outgrow the stigma attached to their field, and develop methods that are validated by more biological feedback and less hand waving. It may also depend on whether critics of cryonics can manage to engage in more substantive discussion and less name calling. The ultimate feasibility of medical time travel is a question of science, not rhetoric.

References

Aebert, H., Brawanski, A., Philipp, A., Behr, R., Ullrich, O.W., Keyl, C., and Birnbaum, D.E. (1998) "Deep Hypothermia and Circulatory Arrest for Surgery of Complex Intracranial Aneurysms." *European Journal of Cardiothoracic Surgery* 13, pp. 223–229.

Alcor staff (1984) "Histological Study of a Temporarily Cryopreserved Human." *Cryonics* (November), pp. 13–32.

Alcor's Pioneering Total Body Washout Experiments. Alcor Life Extension Foundation http://www.alcor.org/Library/html/tbw.html.

Bellamy, R., Safar, P., Tisherman, S.A., Basford, R., Bruttig, S.P., Capone, A., Dubick, M.A., Ernster, L., Hattler, B.G. Jr., Hochachka, P., Klain, M., Kochanek, P.M., Kofke, W.A., Lancaster, J.R., McGowan, F.X. Jr., Oeltgen, P.R., Severinghaus, J.W., Taylor, M.J., and Zar, H. (1996) "Suspended Animation for Delayed Resuscitation." *Critical Care Medicine* 24, pp. S24–47.

Bird, Thomas D. and Plum, Fred (1968) "Recovery from Barbiturate Overdose Coma with a Prolonged Isoelectric Electroencephalogram." *Neurology* 18, pp. 456–460.

Darwin, Michael G. (1977) "The Anabolocyte: A Biological Approach to Repairing Cryoinjury." *Life Extension Magazine* (July/August), pp. 80–3.

Darwin, Michael G. (1991) "Cold War: The Conflict Between Cryonicists and Cryobiologists." *Cryonics* (June, July, August).

Darwin, Michael G. (1996) "Cryopreservation of CryoCare Patient #C-2150." *Biopreservation Tech Briefs* 18.

Darwin, M., Russell, R., Wood, L., and Wood, C. (1995) "Effect of Human Cryopreservation Protocol on the Ultrastructure of the Canine Brain." *Biopreservation Tech Briefs* 16.

Donaldson, Thomas (1988) "24th Century Medicine." *Analog Science Fiction/Science Fact* (September).

Drexler, K. Eric (1986) *Engines of Creation*, 1st edn. New York: Anchor Press/Doubleday.

Drexler, K. Eric (1981) "Molecular Engineering: An Approach to the Development of General Capabilities for Molecular Manipulation." *Proceedings of the National Academy of Sciences* 78, pp. 5275–5278.

Ehrlich, M., Grabenwoger, M., Simon, P., Laufer, G., Wolner, E., and Havel, M. (1995) "Surgical Treatment of Type A Aortic Dissections: Results with Profound Hypothermia and Circulatory Arrest." *Texas Heart Institute Journal* 22, pp. 250–253.

Ettinger, Robert Chester Wilson (1964) *The Prospect of Immortality*, 1st edn. New York: Doubleday.

Fahy, Gregory M., Levy, D.I., and Ali, S.E. (1987) "Some Emerging Principles Underlying the Physical Properties, Biological Actions, and Utility of Vitrification Solutions." *Cryobiology* 24, pp. 196–213.

Fahy, Gregory M., MacFarlane, D.R., Angell, C.A., Meryman, H.T. (1984) "Vitrification as an Approach to Cryopreservation." *Cryobiology* 21, pp. 407–426.

Fahy, Gregory M., Wowk, Brian, Wu, J., and Paynter, S. (2004) "Improved Vitrification Solutions Based on the Predictability of Vitrification Solution Toxicity." *Cryobiology* 48, pp. 22–35.

Fahy, Gregory M., Wu, J., Phan, J., Rasch, C., Chang, A., and Zendejas, E. (2004) "Cryopreservation of Organs by Vitrification: Perspectives and Recent Advances." *Cryobiology* 48, pp. 157–178.

Freitas, Robert A. (1999) *Nanomedicine*, vol. 1: *Basic Capabilities*, 1st edn. Georgetown, TX: Landes Bioscience.

Freitas, Robert A. (2003) *Nanomedicine*, vol. 2A: *Biocompatibility*, 1st edn. Georgetown, TX: Landes Bioscience.

Greenberg, Mark S. (1997) "General Technical Considerations of Aneurysm Surgery." In *Handbook of Neurosurgery*, 4th edn. New York: Thieme.

Haneda, Kiyoshi, Thomas, Robert, Sands, M.P., Breazeale, D.G., and Dillard, D.H. (1986) "Whole Body Protection During Three Hours of Total Circulatory Arrest: An Experimental Study." *Cryobiology* 23, pp. 483–494.

Lind, Bjorn, Snyder, J., Kampschulte, S., and Safar, P. (1975) "A Review of Total Brain Ischaemia Models in Dogs and Original Experiments on Clamping the Aorta." *Resuscitation* 4, pp. 19–31.

Mazur, Peter (1984) "Freezing of Living Cells: Mechanisms and Implications." *American Journal of Physiology* 247, pp. C125–142.

Merkle, Ralph C. (1992) "The Technical Feasibility of Cryonics." *Medical Hypotheses* 39, pp. 6–16.

Polge, C., Smith, A., Parkes, A.S. (1949) "Revival of Spermatozoa after Vitrification and Dehydration at Low Temperatures." *Nature* 164, p. 666.

Rall, William F. and Fahy, Gregory M. (1985) "Ice-Free Cryopreservation of Mouse Embryos at −196 Degrees C by Vitrification." *Nature* 313, pp. 573–575.

Rosenthal, Elisabeth (1990) "Suspended Animation: Surgery's Frontier." *New York Times* (November 13).

Rung, George W., Wickey, G. Scott, Myers, J.L., Salus, J.E., Hensley, F.A. Jr., and Martin, D.E. (1991) "Thiopental as an Adjunct to Hypothermia for EEG Suppression in Infants Prior to Circulatory Arrest." *Journal of Cardiothoracic and Vascular Anesthesia* 5, pp. 337–342.

Song, Ying C., Khirabadi, Bijan S., Lightfoot, F., Brockbank, K.G., and Taylor, M.J. (2000) "Vitreous Cryopreservation Maintains the Function of Vascular Grafts." *Nature Biotechnology* 18, pp. 296–299.

Stecker, Mark M., Cheung, Albert T., Pochettino, A., Kent, G.P., Patterson, T., Weiss, S.J., and Bavaria, J.E. (2001) "Deep Hypothermic Circulatory Arrest: I. Effects of Cooling on Electroencephalogram and Evoked Potentials." *Annals of Thoracic Surgery* 71, pp. 14–21.

Suda, Isamu, Kito, K., and Adachi, C. (1966) "Viability of Long Term Frozen Cat Brain in Vitro." *Nature* 212, pp. 268–270.

Suda, Isamu, Kito, K., and Adachi C. (1974) "Bioelectric Discharges of Isolated Cat Brain after Revival from Years of Frozen Storage." *Brain Research* 70, pp. 527–531.

Toyama, Takeko (1993) "Barbiturate Coma." In Jonathan Greenberg, ed., *Handbook of Head and Spine Trauma*. New York: Marcel Dekker, pp. 230–233.

Wowk, Brian and Fahy, Gregory M. (2002) "Inhibition of Bacterial Ice Nucleation by Polyglycerol Polymers." *Cryobiology* 44, pp. 14–23.

Wowk, Brian, Leitl, Eugen, Rasch, Christopher M., Mesbah-Karimi, Nooshin, Harris, Steven B., and Fahy, Gregory M. (2000) "Vitrification Enhancement by Synthetic Ice Blocking Agents." *Cryobiology* 40, pp. 228–236.

23

Transhumanism and Personal Identity

James Hughes

Enlightenment values are built around the presumption of an independent rational self, citizen, consumer, and pursuer of self-interest. Even the authoritarian and communitarian variants of the Enlightenment presumed the existence of autonomous individuals, simply arguing for greater weight to be given to their collective interests. Since Hume, however, radical Enlightenment empiricists have called into question the existence of a discrete, persistent self. Today neuroscientific reductionism has contributed to the rejection of an essentialist model of personal identity. Contemporary transhumanism has yet to grapple with the radical consequences of the erosion of liberal individualism on their projects of individually chosen enhancement and longevity. Most transhumanists still reflect an essentialist idea of personal identity, even as they embrace projects of radical cognitive enhancement that would change every constituent element of consciousness. Transhumanists need to grapple with how their projects and ethics would change if personal identity is an arbitrary, malleable fiction.

Personal Identity and the Enlightenment

The Enlightenment thinkers attempted to move past the idea of human nature as being defined by God-given immortal souls inhabiting flesh, to the view that we are rational minds emerging out of and transforming nature. For John Locke, for instance, an immaterial and supernatural soul was not a necessary explanation for the self. He proposed that it was within God's power to create matter that could think, and that it is our capacity to think which makes us persons. By setting aside the immaterial soul as the basis of identity, however, there was a problem with the identity of a person at the resurrection of souls at the Last Judgment. If consciousness resides in the flesh, and the reconstituted body at the end of things has none of the stuff of the original

The Transhumanist Reader: Classical and Contemporary Essays on the Science, Technology, and Philosophy of the Human Future, First Edition. Edited by Max More and Natasha Vita-More.
© 2013 John Wiley & Sons, Inc. Published 2013 by John Wiley & Sons, Inc.

body, then how could it be the same person? Because the mind in that flesh would remember its previous self. For Locke memory connected one's present self to one's past, and was therefore the basis of personal identity.

> to find wherein personal Identity consists, we must consider what Person stands for; which, I think, is a thinking intelligent Being, that has reason and reflection, and can consider itself as itself, the same thinking thing in different times and places… (Locke 1689)

Remarkably Locke also considers the problem of the splitting of personal identity through the example that consciousness might reside in a severed finger, and suggests that both the body and the finger could then have their own personhood. But the limb that had a continuous subjective identity is what is crucial for "in this personal identity is founded all the right and justice of reward and punishment." Thinking that we are the same person over the time was essential for moral accountability. We have to believe that we are the same person who acted justly or wrongly in the past, and will be punished or rewarded in the future.

But the further investigation of the nature of memory and consciousness almost immediately began to erode this idea of personal identity. Fifty years after Locke, David Hume's dissection of the self takes the new materialism and empiricism in a more radical direction. In Hume's analysis our belief that anything had an enduring substance was a perceptual illusion. In his *Treatise on Human Nature* he applies this skepticism to personal identity, and argues that the self is also an illusion created by the contiguity of sense perceptions and thoughts. The self is merely a "a bundle or collection of different perceptions which succeed one another with an inconceivable rapidity and are in perpetual flux and movement" (Hume 1739). While for Locke memory was the core of personal identity, knitting together past and present self, for Hume memory was what created the illusion that there was some kind of continuity between past and present mental states.

Hume did not pursue the conclusion his view of the self might have for moral accountability or political theory, and for understandable reasons. Locke's materialist psychology proposed that we had real, substantial selves grounded in our memory, and that these selves had interests that we could know and pursue. But Hume's rejection of personal identity was incompatible with the Enlightenment project of building a new society of rational individuals pursuing self-interest through democracy and market exchange. If we are as confused about the very nature of our selves as Hume proposed, it calls into question a society founded on the equality of citizens, morally accountable persons, and individual rights, and would instead validate benevolent despotism towards collective goods.

Humean skepticism about personal identity also was, and remains, deeply anti-intuitive. Almost all human beings are fairly certain of their personal identity over time. The spread of liberal individualism, along with market economies, liberal political regimes, and expanding realms of individual choice have only made the intuitive belief in the continuous self, whether rooted in an assumed supernatural substance or simply materialism, even stronger.

The contradiction between the Enlightenment's concept of Lockean selfhood, foundational to liberal individualism, and the Humean empiricist recognition that the self is a fiction lay dormant until the twentieth century when neuroscience, another product of the Enlightenment, revived the debate. As neuroscientists collected accounts of patients with lesions and degenerative diseases they began to create an empirical model of the ways that the brain creates the ongoing narrative of the self, and illustrate just how malleable and fragile that narrative is. Multiple personality disorders are simply an extreme of the fractured tumult of desires and self-images in all brains, validating Hume's claim that our personalities are more like parliaments than monarchs. Patients with severed corpus callosums can have their left hemispheres pursue goals separate from and contradictory to those being pursued by the right hemispheres. As Thomas Metzinger has documented so brilliantly in his 2009 *The Ego Tunnel: The Science of the Mind and the Myth of the Self*, neuroscience shows that the "self-y" feeling is simply a useful heuristic that our minds create, without any underlying reality (see also Noe 2009).

Similarly, behavioral economists have carried out a deconstruction of the idea of the rational, utility-maximizing individual, showing that our preferences are not autonomous or coherent, and that our behavior is generally irrational. For instance Daniel Kahneman's work on the experiencing versus the remembered self shows that our memories of our lives are fictional narratives that bear little relationship to our actual moment-to-moment experience (Redelmeier et al. 2003).

Moral and political theorists have been slow to respond to this erosion of the core assumptions of Western thought. One of the few exceptions is the Oxford philosopher Derek Parfit, whose landmark 1986 *Reasons and Persons* argued a Humean account of personal identity, but connecting it to a utilitarian moral theory. For Parfit there is no substantial self, only correlations between our mental states at any two times, and that correlation declines over time. The self exists only insofar as an entity like England exists – it has a physical history and on top of that an evolving set of cultural groups and political institutions. But any attempt to definitely say that England began at a particular time and constitutes a specific set of people and institutions would simply be an arbitrary fiction.

For Parfit the moral and political upshot of our declining relationship to all future versions of our selves is that we have a corresponding interest in the welfare of all other future persons. At some point our future selves are likely to be so dissimilar from our current selves that we are better off acting in the interest of all 80-year-olds instead of simply our own. Of course even critics who accepted a declining self-similarity over time have scoffed at the possibility that an individual would ever bear as much similarity to other future persons as to the future person in their body.

With that cue, the transhumanist project of cognitive and biological enhancement enters the equation and proposes not only many more years over which the ties of personal identity could attenuate, but radical changes to desire, memory, cognition, and identity which will fundamentally challenge our presumptions about the self.

Enhancement, Transhumanism and Personal Identity

Transhumanism has inherited many ideological contradictions from Enlightenment philosophy (Hughes 2010). These include the conflict between atheism and the belief that intelligence could become godlike, or between teleological techno-optimism and the rationalist acknowledgment that the future is uncertain. The conflict between the Lockean and Humean views of the self is another Enlightenment contradiction working away within transhumanism. But the personal identity conundrum is perhaps more exclusive to transhumanism than the other intra-Enlightenment debates since it is precisely the prospect of radical neuroscience that has made the erasure of the illusion of personal identity so tangible.

Nick Bostrom acknowledged the problem of personal identity for transhumanism:

Many philosophers who have studied the problem think that at least under some conditions, an upload of your brain would be you. A widely accepted position is that you survive so long as certain information patterns are conserved, such as your memories, values, attitudes, and emotional dispositions, and so long as there is causal continuity so that earlier stages of yourself help determine later stages of yourself. ... These problems are being intensely studied by contemporary analytic philosophers, and although some progress has been made, e.g. in Derek Parfit's work on personal identity, they have still not been resolved to general satisfaction.

In her 2009 essay "Future Minds: Transhumanism, Cognitive Enhancement and the Nature of Persons" Susan Schneider cites Ray Kurzweil's 2005 parsing of the personal identity debate into four positions:

1. **The ego theory** – a person's nature is her soul or nonphysical mind, and this mind or soul can survive the death of the body.
2. **The psychological continuity theory** – you are essentially your memories and ability to reflect on yourself (Locke) and, more generally, your overall psychological configuration, what Kurzweil referred to as your "pattern."
3. **Materialism** – you are essentially the material that you are made out of – what Kurzweil referred to as "the ordered and chaotic collection of molecules that make up my body and brain."
4. **The no self view** – there is no metaphysical category of person. The "I" is a grammatical fiction (Nietzsche). There are bundles of impressions but no underlying self (Hume). There is no survival because there is no person (Buddha, Parfit).

(Schneider 2009)

In *The Singularity is Near* (2005), Kurzweil advocates for position 2, which has been dubbed "Patternism," and this is the dominant view among transhumanists in general. Patternism permits radical changes to the body and brain so long as the sense of continuity, the memory of a flow of mental states leading to the present, is maintained. Even something as radical as the recording of a personality in a brain and its reinstantiation in a computer would count as personal identity if the mind in the computer remembered the process leading to the change and identified with the prior biological person.

One philosopher who defends the variant of the patternist view in great depth is Max More.[1] More wrote his doctoral thesis on Derek Parfit's personal identity arguments and their implications for radical human enhancement. Although largely arguing that his view is consistent with Parfit's anti-essentialism, in the end More (1995) argued that so long as the radically transformed person was consistent with, or a fulfillment of, the values of the prior person, then personal identity had been maintained. More specifically argues against a focus on continuity of memory as important for identity. For More's "transformationalist" account values are the core of identity for most of us. On the other hand:

This is not true for everyone ... Some persons lack a strong core of values. These persons would give up their identity through transforming ... Those who value self-transformation strongly can undergo more changes in other characteristics while maintaining identity. (More 1995)

In other words, the pattern that determines personal identity is one of strongly held values, especially the value of self-transformation, and those without these strong values are at great risk of losing personal identity as they undergo enhancement.

Mark Walker (2008) also grapples with the personal identity objection to cognitive enhancement and adopts an implicitly patternist view. Walker says that since radical changes might violate personal continuity the path from humanness to "godlike" posthumanity should be gradual.

If we must accept gradualism then the worst consequence is that it seems to slow down the process whereby one might become a posthuman, it does not prohibit it. In terms of the neural surgery experiment, we might imagine that if too many neurons are added to your brain at once you will cease to exist, but if neurons are gradually added your identity will be preserved. Accepting this means that I could not demand as a right to be upgraded to a posthuman overnight, but I could consistently demand as "my right" the right to a number of small interventions that would eventually lead to me becoming a posthuman.

… we may be able to autonomously determine our identity through the exercise of technology on our biology. In fact this would be a higher expression of our autonomy than we can achieve today. (Walker 2008)

Both More and Walker concede that some enhancements would break personal identity by breaking the continuity of the personality pattern. But both believe, unlike many bioconservative critics, that personal continuity is nonetheless possible.

Schneider (2009) suggests, however, that the transhumanists' patternist theories are inadequate to establish the continuity of personal identity after radical cognitive enhancements or uploading. Transhumanist enhancement scenarios propose radical malleability in memory, values, and all other elements of the "pattern." Transhumanists also accept the plausibility, even inevitability, of multiple copies of personalities which would all feel identity with the prior original person. While most transhumanists don't see the multiplication of selves as problematic, it is usually considered incompatible with the assumed transitive unity of identity over time. If there can be more than one You, do you really exist in the first place? She concludes by asking:

what is it that ultimately grounds your decision to enhance or not enhance if not that it will somehow improve who you are? Are you perhaps merely planning for the well-being of your closest continuent? (Schneider 2009)

Schneider does not address the fact that there are transhumanists, such as myself, who have taken the position that the self is an illusion (Hughes 2001, 2005). I have argued that radical longevity and cognitive enhancement will push liberal democratic society to adopt post-liberal individualist moral, legal, and political frameworks that do not assume personal identity, although what the contours of such frameworks might be I cannot say. It is hard to discern, however, what meaning "liberty, equality, and fraternity" would have without the convenient fiction of autonomous individuals as citizens.

Parfit's no-self utilitarianism, in which only the interests of all future persons, and not one's own personal identity, are taken into account, is one such possibility. It would then be possible to argue that even though personal identity is a fiction, the good of the collective future person would be improved by maintaining the fiction of personal identity in life and law. This is similar to the debate over free will and legal culpability in the light of neuroscience; even if neuroscience demolishes the idea that any criminal truly chooses a criminal act, social utility will be greater if we pretend that individuals have moral choice and are accountable for their actions.

Many other accommodations to the erosion of personal identity can be imagined, however, from efforts to use neurotechnologies to create a rigid and secure personal invariability, to their use to replace individual identity with completely collective identity (e.g. "the Borg"). The erosion may come about without any coercion; the selective suppression of the brain mechanisms that create the illusion of the self, such as proprioception, will likely be attractive targets for people exploring neurotechnologies for therapeutic and recreational reasons. Experiences previously accessible only to yogis, such as body boundlessness, empathic unity with others, or absorptive concentration, will likely become commonplace. The recording of memory and experience will also enable the sharing of memory and experience with others, which many will want as a means to closeness, evangelism, or simply vanity. How much of someone else's life would one need to remember before it called into question one's own identity? By experimentally modifying our values and desires we could become people we wouldn't have wanted to be previously, from amoral to supermoral.

Bostrom seems to have this kind of development in mind in his 2001 essay "Existential Risks." After discussing natural and technological threats that could wipe humanity out, he addresses the threat of "shrieks" and "whimpers," futures in which our descendants still exist but not in forms which have maintained some essential continuity with who we are today. In 2004 he proposed a shriek scenario that might result from voluntary use of enhancement in the pursuit of capitalist competition.

> We can thus imagine a technologically highly advanced society, containing many sorts of complex structures, some of which are much smarter and more intricate than anything that exists today, in which there would nevertheless be a complete absence of any type of being whose welfare has moral significance. In a sense, this would be an uninhabited society. All the kinds of being that we care even remotely about would have vanished … the catastrophe would be that such a world would not contain even the right kind of machines, i.e. ones that are conscious and whose welfare matters. (Bostrom 2004)

In other words, if we adopt a personal identity theory in regards the human project then some forms of post-personal identity societies might also be societies that no longer represent the human project. But then, the critique of identity essentialism probably applies at the level of society even more clearly than for individuals. If there is no real self and no real humanity then we are left with the question of whether we want to collectively pretend that we do exist, and if so, to what ends?

Note

1   Notably, More is recognized as the founder of modern transhumanism and, in particular, developed the transhumanist philosophy of Extropy as one school of transhumanist thought.

References

Bostrom, Nick (2001) "Existential Risks: Analyzing Human Extinction Scenarios and Related Hazards." *Journal of Evolution and Technology* 9/1.
Bostrom, Nick (2004) "The Future of Human Evolution." In Charles Tandy, ed., *Death and Anti-Death: Two Hundred Years After Kant, Fifty Years After Turing*. Palo Alto, CA: Ria University Press, pp. 339–371.
Hughes, James (2001) "The Future of Death: Cryonics and the Telos of Liberal Individualism." *Journal of Evolution and Technology* 6/1.
Hughes, James (2005) "The Illusiveness of Immortality," In C. Tandy, ed., *Death and Anti-Death*, vol. 3: *Fifty Years after Einstein, One Hundred Fifty Years after Kierkegaard* New York: Ingram.
Hughes, James (2010) "Contradictions from the Enlightenment Roots of Transhumanism." *Journal of Medicine and Philosophy* 35/6, pp. 622–640.

Humanity + (2003) Transhumanist FAQ. http://humanityplus.org/philosophy/transhumanist-faq/.

Hume, David (1739) *A Treatise of Human Nature*. Book I: *Of the Understanding*. Part IV: *Of the Skeptical and Other Systems Of Philosophy*. Section VI: *Of Personal Identity*. http://www.gutenberg.org/files/4705/4705-h/4705-h.htm.

Kurzweil, R. (2005) *The Singularity Is Near: When Humans Transcend Biology*. New York: Viking.

Locke, John (1689) *Essay Concerning Human Understanding*. http://oregonstate.edu/instruct/phl302/texts/locke/locke1/Essay_contents.html.

Metzinger, Thomas (2009) *The Ego Tunnel: The Science of the Mind and the Myth of the Self*. New York: Basic Books.

More, Max (1995) *The Diachronic Self: Identity, Continuity, Transformation*. Ann Arbor, MI: A Bell & Howell Company. http://www.maxmore.com/disscont.htm.

Noe, Alva (2009) *Out of Our Heads: Why You Are Not Your Brain, and Other Lessons from the Biology of Consciousness*. New York: Hill & Wang.

Parfit, Derek (1986) *Reasons and Persons*. Oxford: Oxford University Press.

Redelmeier, D.A., Katz, J., and Kahneman, D. (2003) "Memories of Colonoscopy: A Randomized Trial." *Pain* 104, pp. 187–194.

Schneider, Susan (2009) "Future Minds: Transhumanism, Cognitive Enhancement and the Nature of Persons." In Vardit Ravitsky, Autumn Fiester, and Arthur L. Caplan, eds., *The Penn Center Guide to Bioethics*. New York: Springer, pp. 844–856.

Walker, Mark (2008) "Cognitive Enhancement and the Identity Objection." *Journal of Evolution and Technology* 18/1, pp. 108–115. http://jetpress.org/v18/walker.htm.

24

Transcendent Engineering

Giulio Prisco

In "Engineering Transcendence" (Prisco 2004) I argued that science may someday develop the capability to resurrect the dead and build (and/or become) God(s), and proposed to base a "transhumanist[1] religion" on this idea. I also argued that the ultra-rationalist, aseptic engineering language dear to most technophiles does not seem able to have an emotional impact on the majority of other people. This means that "traditional" technologically based ideas about the future might remain confined to a very small minority of the technically oriented.[2]

Evolutionary biologist Richard Dawkins, in a recent interview in the *New York Times* (Powell 2011), said "it's highly plausible that in the universe there are God-like creatures." Further, in his book *The God Delusion*, Dawkins wrote:

> "[T]here are very probably alien civilizations that are superhuman, to the point of being god-like in ways that exceed anything a theologian could possibly imagine. … As Arthur C. Clarke put it, in his Third Law: "Any sufficiently advanced technology is indistinguishable from magic."
>
> In what sense would they be superhuman but not supernatural? In a very important sense, which goes to the heart of this book. The crucial difference between gods and god-like extraterrestrials lies not in their properties but in their provenance. Entities that are complex enough to be intelligent are products of an evolutionary process. No matter how god-like they may seem when we encounter them, they didn't start that way. Science fiction authors … have even suggested (and I cannot think how to disprove it) that we live in a computer simulation, set up by some vastly superior civilization. But the simulators themselves would have to come from somewhere. The laws of probability forbid all notions of their spontaneously appearing without simpler antecedents. They probably owe their existence to a (perhaps unfamiliar) version of Darwinian evolution … (Dawkins 2006)

Dawkins' position is similar to the perception I value: Dawkins rejects the "supernatural," but he acknowledges no limit to the evolution of civilizations in the physical universe and their

The Transhumanist Reader: Classical and Contemporary Essays on the Science, Technology, and Philosophy of the Human Future, First Edition. Edited by Max More and Natasha Vita-More.
© 2013 John Wiley & Sons, Inc. Published 2013 by John Wiley & Sons, Inc.

technologies, and he is open to the possibility of civilizations (perhaps including our own) attaining God-like powers at a certain point in their evolution. Yet his attitude may be criticized by some of his "New Atheist"[3] followers as too accommodating toward religion. I often find New Atheists' "New Bigotry" annoying, and using the ideas of their Commander-in-Chief in support of my own gives me a certain perverse pleasure.

I.   Cornerstones of Transcendent Engineering

The cornerstones of the transcendent engineering spirituality or "religion" include:

Mind uploading

Someday it will be possible to transfer entire personalities from their original biological brain to more durable and powerful engineered substrates.

I am persuaded that the ultimate realization of the dream of achieving an indefinite lifespan, with vastly enhanced cognitive abilities, lies in leaving biology behind and moving to a new, post-biological, cybernetic phase of our evolution. Mind uploading, the transfer of a human mind, memories, personality and "self" (whatever "self" is) to new high-performance substrates is the ultimate technology for immortality. Therefore I have always been interested in mind uploading and I consider it as the "Holy Grail" of transhumanism: let our minds break free of our biological brains and bodies, and we will be free to roam the universe and grow beyond limits as "software angels."

Once we develop the technology to transfer human minds to computer systems, uploaded minds will have many different post-biological embodiment options to interact with the rest of the world. Some uploads will choose to live in robotic bodies or synthetic biological bodies similar to our current bodies, but with vastly enhanced capabilities. For example, those who want to explore space will be able to choose rugged bodies able to endure the conditions of space. Other uploads will choose to live as pure software without a permanent physical body.

I am persuaded that, within a few decades, we will develop operational technologies for destructively scanning biological brains in such a way as to retain enough information for future re-instantiation of the mind. Of course, non-destructive scanning would be much better, but experts disagree on its possible timeline, and even feasibility in principle. I prefer to keep an open mind and, since non-destructive, very high resolution brain scanning seems feasible in principle (that is, it is compatible with the laws of physics and so it is just another engineering problem), I tend to think it will be achieved sooner or later.

Another possibility is the Bainbridge–Rothblatt "soft" approach: we can create a "lifelogging" database with blogs, pictures, videos, answers to personality tests, etc. (see the CybeRev and LifeNaut projects of Martine Rothblatt [Rothblatt 2009]), hoping that some future AI technology may be able to merge the information in the database with suitable "human firmware" (me-program) and bring it to life. I think this approach is basically feasible in principle, but needs data transfer rates from brain to computer storage much faster than we can achieve today (Vita-More 2010).

Time-scanning

Someday it will be possible to acquire very detailed information from the past. Once time-scanning is available, we will be able to resurrect people from the past by "copying them to the future" via mind uploading. Note: time-scanning is not time travel, and it is free from the "paradoxes" of time travel. Time-scanning is just a form of archaeology – uncovering the past by means of available evidence and records. Of course the very high-definition form of time-scanning proposed here is orders of magnitude more powerful and sophisticated than archeology as we know it, but the concept is the same.

Time-scanning is often called "Quantum Archeology", based on the possibility that the best technologies for time-scanning may be based on weird quantum effects such as past-to-future entanglement; no one really knows, so I prefer using a less specific term.

In *The Physics of Immortality* (1994) Frank Tipler describes how future intelligent beings may steer the gravitational collapse of the universe (the so-called Big Crunch) in such a way as to have unlimited subjective time, energy, and computational power available before reaching the final singularity (Omega Point). Having done so, they may wish to restore to consciousness all sentient beings of the past, perhaps through a "brute force" computational emulation of the past history of the universe. After death we may wake up in a simulated environment with many of the features assigned to the afterlife by the major religions.

Since Tipler's "Heaven" where we will be resurrected is a simulated world, his is a special case of the synthetic realities scenario, which identifies the civilization running the simulation: they are our descendants at the end of time, with perhaps only a couple of seconds of objective time left, but an infinite span of subjective time and computing power.

Tipler proposed a specific and detailed Omega Point theory, which has attracted a lot of criticism. But critics miss the point: perhaps Leonardo's aircraft sketches would not have been able to fly (the knowledge needed to design a flying machine was just not available at his time), but this does not lessen the value of Leonardo's insight that a device conceptually similar to his own sketches would someday fly. Similarly, we do not know enough physics and mathematics to assess specific Omega Point theories, but this does not lessen the value of Tipler's insight: someday science and technology may resurrect the dead.

Science fiction writers proposed some of the most suggestive time-scanning and resurrection scenarios. In *The Light of Other Days*, Sir Arthur C. Clarke and Stephen Baxter imagine a near-future world profoundly transformed by the invention of a "Wormcam": a remote viewing device that permits scanning any location at any time, including in the past, by using micro wormholes naturally embedded with high density in the fabric of space-time (every space-time pixel is connected with every other space-time pixel). Soon engineers are able resurrect the dead:

> It was possible now to look back into time and read off a complete DNA sequence from any moment in an individual's life. And it was possible to download a copy of that person's mind and, by putting the two together, regenerated body and downloaded mind, to restore her ... We live on Mars, the moons of the outer planets, and we're heading for the stars. There have even been experiments to download human minds into the quantum foam ... We intend to restore all human souls, back to the beginning of the species. We intend to put right the past, to defeat the awful tragedy of death in a universe that may last tens of billions of years. (Clarke and Baxter 2000)

Synthetic realities

Someday it will be possible to build artificial realities inhabited by sentient life. Perhaps future humans will live in synthetic realities. Perhaps we will wake up in a synthetic reality after having been copied to the future. Or... perhaps we are already there.

The "intelligence" of simulated characters (NPC) in computer games is still light years behind real intelligence. However, I am persuaded that real, self-aware AI of human and higher level will be achieved someday, perhaps by the computer gaming industry itself, and perhaps in the next couple of decades. Then, computer games will contain sentient, intelligent persons like you and I.

If computer game characters can be intelligent and sentient, perhaps we are sentient and intelligent computer game characters. Do we live in a computer simulation? This is a frequent discussion topic in transhumanist interest groups. Who is running the simulation? Perhaps unknowable aliens in another level of reality have invented our world and us. A frequent assumption is that future humans run our reality as a historically accurate simulation of their past (our present).

Within a 1992 essay entitled, "Pigs in Cyberspace", Hans Moravec formulated (in modern terms) the idea of our reality as a simulation:

> An evolving cyberspace becomes effectively ever more capacious and long lasting, and so can support ever more minds of ever greater power. If these minds spend only an infinitesimal fraction of their energy contemplating the human past, their sheer power should ensure that eventually our entire history is replayed many times in many places, and in many variations. The very moment we are now experiencing may actually be (almost certainly is) such a distributed mental event, and most likely is a complete fabrication that never happened physically. (Moravec 1992)

By "almost certainly is" Moravec refers to the idea that observers living in simulated realities may vastly outnumber observers living in original physical realities.

If those who live in a simulated reality can themselves simulate lower-level realities, perhaps upper-case Reality is nothing more than an infinite cascade of realities simulated within higher-level realities (dreams within dreams, or turtles all the way down). This may well be the simplest explanation of the world, since assuming an infinite regress permits doing without a "base reality" which generates all other realities.

II.   Two Possibilities of Resurrection

Transcendent engineering offers not one, but two possibilities of resurrection: We may be copied to the future by our descendants by using time-scanning and mind uploading; or, we may already be living in a synthetic reality and the system admins may make a backup copy of interesting patterns every now and then. Hope in resurrection is, I believe, a necessary component of any effective alternative to traditional spiritualities.

If we live in a synthetic reality, then in a certain sense we cannot even rule out the supernatural, or miracles. The simulators, the system admins, cannot violate their laws of physics, but they can violate our laws of physics if they want. It seems that the supernatural, which we have kicked out of the back door of superstition, may come back through the main door of science.

A computer able to simulate a reality as complex as ours, inhabited by conscious observers, must be much more complex and powerful than any computer that we can imagine today, and it would likely be fully self-aware. So if we are living in a simulation, the computational system simulating our reality is not a what, but a who. Not an inanimate machine, but a thinking and feeling person, orders of magnitude smarter and more complex than us. We don't live in a mere machine, but in a Transcendent Mind. The last chapter of Hans Moravec's *Robot – Mere Machine to Transcendent Mind* (1999) has a fascinating preview of super-intelligent, human–AI hybrids spreading to the universe as "Mind Fire" and holding entire simulated realities in their vast minds.

Berkeley thought that the reality we perceive, and ourselves in it, exist in the mind of "that supreme and wise Spirit, in whom we live, move, and have our being": God. In other words, we are thoughts in the Mind of God. It is easy to see that Berkeley and Moravec say very similar things, each in the language of his philosophy and age.

Apparently, there is an important difference between Berkeley and Moravec: As an eighteenth-century Christian and a representative of the Church, Berkeley believed in supernatural phenomena, in principle not understandable by science, while Moravec, as a modern engineer, believes reality is fully understandable and explainable by science. Future engineers within the framework of future science will develop Moravec's simulated realities. If our reality is a simulation, everything in our universe can be understood in terms of the physical laws of the higher-level reality in which it is simulated.

But… this does not mean that it must always be understandable in terms of our own physical laws: Moravec's simulation cosmology may contain supernatural phenomena, because the reality engineers up there may choose to violate the rules of the game. Yes, as Dawkins says they are creatures naturally evolved in their physical universe and they cannot violate their physics (Dawkins 2006), but they can violate ours if they want.

Make this simple experiment: Run a Game of Life program, choose an initial pattern, and let it evolve for a while. Now, stop the program, flip a cell, and resume the program. You have just performed a miracle: something that goes against the physical laws (the simple cellular automata evolution rules of Life) of the lower-level reality that you are simulating. Of course the Game of Life is too simple to contain conscious observers, but hypothetical observers within the game would observe an event that cannot be understood in terms of the physical laws of their universe. A miracle.

Berkeley and Moravec are not only saying similar things, they are saying the same thing using different wording. Moravec's "Transcendent Mind" is, by definition, omnipotent (all powerful), omniscient (all knowing), and omnipresent (always and everywhere present) in the simulated reality He thinks. He is Berkeley's "supreme and wise Spirit, in whom we live, move, and have our being," a God. Perhaps the Mind hears our prayers, and sometimes answers them with a miracle; including the greatest miracle, resurrection.

According to our best scientific understanding, it seems that the dead stay dead, but if we live in a simulation, the Mind can copy us before we die and paste us in a new, perhaps better, simulation.

III.   Conclusion

I am the first to admit that this is a mythology and not a scientific theory. I believe it is a mythology compatible with rationality and the scientific worldview. Modern science says that reality, at a fundamental level, is much weirder than our simple, intuitive models, and lets us glimpse at vague and veiled shadows of wonderful things in heaven and earth. If anything, I am persuaded that reality may be much weirder than mythology.

Many transhumanists with an ultra-rationalist approach have a very hard time considering parallels between transhumanism, spirituality, and/or religion. Good interpretations of religion have done great good to many people, and following William James (1896) I think a modern transhumanist religion, with religion's contemplation of transcendence and hope in personal resurrection, but without its bigotry and intolerance, can be a powerfully positive force in the life of a person, which is what really matters.

I often call this transhumanist mythology "The Turing Church" (Goertzel 2011), to emphasize the key role of substrate-independent mentality. The Turing Church is not an organization, but a meta-organization, mailing list, and online meeting point for spiritually oriented transhumanists. The Turing Church's mythology does not make a great difference in practice: we still live in a difficult and dangerous world, cancer still kills, we still age and die, there are still wars and atrocities, and billions of persons are still hungry, powerless, sick, and unhappy. Contemplating the cosmic visions of the Turing Church gives me a sense of wonder and a sense of hope in a beautiful future... if only we can build it. It also gives me more motivation, energy, and drive to try to give a small contribution toward making our world a better place.

Ultra-rationalist "bureaucrats of philosophy" usually dismiss "hippie new-age attitudes", but we should not forget that the hippie new-age attitude of the 1960s shaped the Internet technology revolution (R.U. Sirius 2006). Perhaps we had the right attitude in the beautiful, visionary anti-authoritarian 1960s, and we should recover it to shape new transhumanist technology revolutions. My experience with new-agers is that, yes, they are easily deluded or scammed, and yes, they move from a guru to a new guru and from crystals to pyramids, but they are intellectually and spiritually alive, perhaps more alive and awake than others; seekers of something beautiful that they cannot define. I look forward to new approaches bridging the gap between the 1960s and the 2010s, cosmic visions and technology, spirituality and transhumanism.

I concluded "Engineering Transcendence" with a call to arms: "I would support developing a strong, religious formulation of transhumanism as a front-end for those who need one." Some quasi-religious interpretations of transhumanism have been developed, as outlined above, and documented by Robert Geraci in his book Apocalyptic AI (Geraci 2010).

Geraci defines Apocalyptic AI as a modern cultural and religious trend originating in the popular science press:

> Popular science authors in robotics and artificial intelligence have become the most influential spokespeople for apocalyptic theology in the Western world ... Apocalyptic AI advocates promise that in the very near future technological progress will allow us to build supremely intelligent machines and to copy our own minds into machines so that we can live forever in a virtual realm of cyberspace ... Ultimately, the promises of Apocalyptic AI are almost identical to those of Jewish and Christian apocalyptic traditions. Should they come true, the world will be, once again, a place of magic.

According to Geraci, Apocalyptic AI is a religion: a religion based on science, without deities and supernatural phenomena, but with the apocalyptic promises of religions. And he thinks that, while the Apocalyptic AI religion has a powerful but often hidden presence in our culture, the transhumanist community embraces it openly and explicitly. Transhumanism is first defined as "a new religious movement", and throughout the book Geraci continues to see it as a modern religion.

I prefer not to define transhumanism as a spiritual endeavor or a religion; first because it wouldn't be correct, and second because I don't want to lose all my transhumanist friends. What all transhumanists have in common is the conviction that using advanced technologies to radically change the human condition is both feasible and desirable. Within this broad definition there are many possible interpretations of transhumanism, and one of these interpretations is the Turing Church mythology, or Apocalyptic AI.

Notes

1   Transhumanism – often abbreviated as *H*+ or *h*+, is an international intellectual and cultural movement that affirms the possibility and desirability of fundamentally transforming the human condition by developing and making widely available technologies to eliminate aging and to greatly enhance human intellectual, physical, and psychological capacities. http://en.wikipedia.org/wiki/Transhumanist (accessed October 5, 2011).
2   "Engineering Transcendence" is a blog covering spirituality. This blog was not received enthusiastically by most transhumanists, but it was by some transhumanists and spiritually minded individuals.
3   The term "New Atheism" is the name given to a movement among some early twenty-first-century atheist writers who have advocated the view that "religion should not simply be tolerated but should be countered, criticized, and exposed by rational argument wherever its influence arises" (Hooper 2006). New Atheists argue that recent scientific advances require a negative bias or attitude about religion and spirituality. The movement is most often associated with Richard Dawkins, Daniel C. Dennett, Sam Harris, Christopher Hitchens, and Victor J. Stenger.

References

Clarke, Arthur C. and Baxter, Stephen (2000) *The Light of Other Days*. New York: Tor. http://en.wikipedia. org/wiki/The_Light_of_Other_Days (accessed October 5, 2011).

Dawkins, Richard (2006) *The God Delusion*. New York: Houghton Mifflin. http://books.google.com/books/ about/The_God_Delusion.html?id=yq1xDpicghkC (accessed October 5, 2011).

Geraci, Robert (2010) *Apocalyptic AI: Visions of Heaven in Robotics, Artificial Intelligence, and Virtual Reality*. New York: Oxford University Press. http://www.oup.com/us/catalog/general/subject/ReligionTheology/ SociologyofReligion/?view=usa&ci=9780195393026 (accessed October 5, 2011).

Goertzel, Ben (2011) *Technological Transcendence: An Interview with Giulio Prisco*. http://hplusmagazine. com/2011/02/08/technological-transcendence-an-interview-with-giulio-prisco/ (accessed October 5, 2011).

Hooper, Simon (2006) "The Rise of the New Atheists". CNN. http://articles.cnn.com/2006-11-08/world/ atheism.feature_1_new-atheists-new-atheism-religion?_s=PM:WORLD (reviewed October 28, 2011).

James, William (1896) "The Will to Believe: An Address to the Philosophical Clubs of Yale and Brown Universities." http://educ.jmu.edu//~omearawm/ph101willtobelieve.html. (accessed October 5, 2011).

Moravec, Hans (1992) "Pigs in Cyberspace." *Extropy* 10 (January). http://www.primitivism.com/pigs.htm (accessed October 5, 2011).

Moravec, Hans (1999) *Robot –Mere Machine to Transcendent Mind*. New York: Oxford University Press. http://www.frc.ri.cmu.edu/~hpm/book97/index.html (accessed October 5, 2011).

Powell, Michael (2011) "A Knack for Bashing Orthodoxy." *New York Times*. http://www.nytimes. com/2011/09/20/science/20dawkins.html (accessed October 5, 2011).

Prisco, Giulio (2004) "Engineering Transcendence." http://giulioprisco.blogspot.com/2006/12/engineer- ingtranscendence.html.

Rothblatt, Martine (2009) "Mindfiles, Mindware and Mindclones." http://mindclones.blogspot.com/ (accessed October 5, 2011).

R.U. Sirius (2006) *How the Sixties Shaped the Personal Computer Revolution, in True Mutations*. http://boing- boing.net/2007/02/13/ru_sirius_true_mutat.html (accessed October 5, 2011).

Tipler, Frank (1994) *The Physics of Immortality: Modern Cosmology, God, and the Resurrection of the Dead*. First Anchor: New York. http://129.81.170.14/~tipler/physicsofimmortality.htm (accessed October 5, 2011).

Vita-More, Natasha (2010) *MIND and MAN: Getting Mental with Giulio Prisco*. http://hplusmagazine. com/2010/09/12/mind-and-man-getting-mental-giulio-prisco/ (accessed October 5, 2011).

Part VI

Enhanced Decision-Making

The kinds of changes to the human condition envisioned and recommended by transhumanists clearly have massive implications. Transhumanists recognize the potential downsides as well as the upsides of these technologically mediated changes. The emerging new choices only add to the range, complexity, and difficulty of choices revolving around technology. Our human brains did not evolve to process such decisions effectively. That is why, in addition to pursuing the neurological and computational aspects of cognitive enhancement (discussed in Part III on the Cognitive Sphere), transhumanists have a strong interest in alternative means for improving our decision-making processes. This interest includes paying close attention to the decision sciences, cognitive and behavioral psychology, and diverse frameworks for structured decision-making and forecasting.

Will we achieve posthuman wisdom and arrive at optimal decisions simply by becoming more intelligent and accessing more facts? Unfortunately not. If intelligence and knowledge acquired through education and fact-finding were sufficient, we would expect doubts about well-established scientific theories to fade away when more information is provided. This "deficit model" of science communication has been found wanting in several studies. Additional information can actually polarize views further and lead to a hardening of beliefs as we filter information through our existing perspectives. These discouraging results are not the whole picture. The essays in this section show how better tools and perspectives can improve our decision-making – a crucial task in a world where technology becomes ever more potent, for better or worse. This section includes three domains of thought that explore thinking processes and issues through the lenses of economics, applied philosophy, and electronic hyperlink theory.

Robin Hanson's "Idea Futures" was an early explication of a mechanism that has since come to be known as "decision markets." These markets harness the "wisdom of crowds" to improve decision-making and forecasting accuracy. Subsequent work has shown how decision markets

The Transhumanist Reader: Classical and Contemporary Essays on the Science, Technology, and Philosophy of the Human Future, First Edition. Edited by Max More and Natasha Vita-More.
© 2013 John Wiley & Sons, Inc. Published 2013 by John Wiley & Sons, Inc.

typically yield results more accurate than those from the best experts in areas as diverse as predicting sales of printer supplies and box-office take for movies in their first days of release.

Max More's Proactionary Principle was designed as a replacement for the precautionary principle – an overly simple and biased rule for making decisions in the presence of significant risk, especially in the context of technological and environment issues. More diagnoses severe shortcomings in the "precautionary principle" and offers in its place a more comprehensive, structured, and balanced decision-making and risk-assessment tool.

In their 1994 essay, Mark Miller and co-authors explain how electronic media, as exemplified by the Xanadu project, could enable societies to make better decisions. Written during the very early days of the Web, this essay forms a historical observation of the use of hyperlinks, emergent properties, "transclusion," historical trails, detectors, permissions, and reputation-based filtering.

25

Idea Futures
Encouraging an Honest Consensus

Robin Hanson

Introduction

Are you fascinated by some basic questions about science, technology, and our future? Questions like: Is cryonics technically feasible? When will nano-assemblers be feasible and how quickly will resulting changes come? Does a larger population help or hinder the world environment and economy? Will uploading be possible, and if so when? When can I live in space? Where will I be able to live free from tyranny? When will AIs be bucking for my job? Is there intelligent life beyond earth? If you are like most *Extropy* readers, such questions matter to you.

Now how do we, as a society, go about answering such questions? People who have an appropriate background, and who are interested enough in a particular question, can research that subject in depth themselves, and come to a considered opinion. And people who happen to know, respect, and trust such a person can simply take those opinions as their own, avoiding all the hard work. But what is everyone else to do, people whose actions often implicitly depend on such questions?

In practice, people usually defer to larger social institutions on most questions, institutions which combine and evaluate contributions from many specialists, and which offer apparent institutional consensus estimates on many different questions. These consensuses may be uncertain and temporary, and individuals may prefer to combine the results of several institutions, but the basic need for such estimates remains.

For example, popular media chose what they consider to be ranges of reasonable and noteworthy opinions on noteworthy issues for presentation. Peer-reviewed academic journals

Originally published in *Extropy* 8 (1992). Copyright © Max More.

and societies offer more detailed, though less accessible, consensuses about which opinions are reasonable and in favor. Government agencies often try to form and act on such consensuses, as the United States EPA does for pesticide health risks. And there are many other such consensus institutions, such as opinion polls.

How well do these institutions work? How many of us are confident that, when a technical controversy arises, a widely visible consensus will quickly emerge representing society's honest best estimate on the issue, reflecting the relevant insights of the best relevant experts? Or that those with foresight will eventually be rewarded for advocating positions which later become accepted?

People who have little contact with an existing social institution, or who have a position of power within it, may feel things are basically okay. But those "in the trenches" typically voice more skepticism. Your opinion on the trustworthiness of newspapers probably changed for the worse the last time you read about an event in which you were personally involved. Since subjects like cryonics and nanotechnology have often been unfairly treated by most current institutions, I expect at least a few *Extropy* readers to be dissatisfied with such institutions.

Skeptics about current institutions are not typically focused on methods, often the center of philosophical discussions, but on incentives. Skeptics see too many rewards for bias, and too few for honesty and care, and so distrust official statements. People often promote beliefs which serve their self-interest, and try to appear more confident, original, and knowledgeable than they are. People don't correct for standard human biases (Kahneman and Tversky 1982), such as wishful thinking, overconfidence, and belief fixation. They massage evidence, suppress criticism, and just plain lie. Fashion, eloquence, and politics often dominate expert consensus. Rewards often go to those whose ideas are popular now, rather than those who are later proved correct (Tullock 1966). Paid advocates distort the consensus we perceive by using raw media exposure, bribes, and by exploiting human biases (Cialdini 1988). An honest consensus of relevant experts is often lost from public view.

Box 25.1   Some Controversial Claims

- By 2030, the greenhouse effect and other causes will have raised the average world sea levels by 1 meter.
- Cold fusion of deuterium in palladium can produce over 10 watts/cc. net power at STP.
- By the time we have surveyed our galaxy in the infrared to the 25th magnitude, there will not be any evidence of another technological civilization in our galaxy.
- By the time world GNP is four times the 1990 level, 1,000 people will have physically lived in space over 90 percent of the time for the previous seven years.
- By the year 2000, over 20,000 people in the U.S. will commute to work in Vertical Take-Off and Landing (VTOL) aircraft they park in their garage and drive down the street.
- The rest mass of the electron neutrino is greater than .01 eV in ordinary space.
- If labor-saving device X were widely used in industry Y, industry employment five years later would be less.
- Death-bed confessions or other evidence will eventually show that person X was murdered.

Many existing social institutions, such as investigative reporting, due process, public debates, and peer review, claim to address these problems. But there is room for improvement. To improve the way ideas evolve, many people try to reform existing social institutions, and a few try to invent new ones (Linstone and Turoff 1975; Kantrowitz 1977; Hanson 1988). In this essay I suggest a new social institution, called "idea futures," which can create a visible expert consensus with clear incentives for honest contribution.

Concept

Idea Futures is intended to aid the evolution of a wide range of ideas, from public policy to the nature of the universe, and in particular should be able to help us predict and understand our future. The basic concept is to combine two phenomena, convergence and markets, and so make "a futures market in ideas." Let me explain.

Disagreement is rarely as fundamental as it seems. In the long run, beliefs often converge. For example, in science the steady accumulation of evidence eventually settles most debates. We take the advice of experts, indicating that we think we would come to believe what they believe, if only we were to study what they have studied. Randomly selected juries usually reach a unanimous verdict, even more often than seems rational. Theory (Seidenfeld 1990) and experiment (Linstone and Turoff 1975) indicate that the people's beliefs should and do converge. In sum, we generally trust in a convergence of human judgment. If people wait long enough for evidence to surface and then take enough effort to study and debate a specific enough claim, they often come to agree. When the people are reasonable, knowledgeable, and detached enough, and when they avoid subjects like religion, they usually agree. When such a group is diverse and independent enough, we believe we would probably also agree.

Markets are a way to create a consensus about the value of an ownable item, i.e., the "price." Futures markets are a way to create an immediate consensus about future consensus. For example, a market in corn creates a price in corn, so that most buyers pay about that price. A futures market in corn creates a futures price, which is an immediate estimate of what the actual price of corn will be in, say, nine months. Traders have clear incentives to make honest contributions to the consensus; you "put your money where your mouth is." A trader who believes the future price will be higher than the market indicates buys, and in so doing raises the consensus price. Those who are right make money from those who are wrong.

Of course markets have limitations. Ideally, items to value should be of wide interest, exclusively ownable, cheaply transferable, and have many identical copies. How can we apply this to ideas? By creating coupons whose value depends on whether an idea is validated. For example, a coupon which says "Exchangeable for $1 should a person land on Mars by 2020" is a direct tie between an idea, people on Mars, and money, a well-known unit of incentive. Such coupons can be thought of metaphorically as futures, and more literally as bets, a metaphor often used to describe both investments and science.

If convergence creates a future consensus in ideas, and if futures markets can create an immediate and honest consensus about a future consensus, then futures markets might be able to create an immediate and honest consensus in ideas. If the market price for a "$1 if person on Mars" coupon were 23¢, then that would typically represent a consensus that there was about a 23 percent chance of this happening. Anyone could express their opinion on the subject by trading coupons, or could just read the "market odds" to see the best present estimate. This market consensus would compare favorably to other methods of forming perceived consensus, such as by advertising, opinion polls, or elite committees. An idea futures consensus could be simultaneously open, egalitarian, universal, expert, honest, self-consistent, and cheap.

A mature idea futures market could offer coupons on many claims about the future of technology and society. The consensus prices would give a consistent set of probabilities for various possible future events, and conditional probabilities for some events given others. Investors there should be as diverse as investors are elsewhere, with a mix of short-term and long-term focuses, large investment houses and daring do-it-yourself individuals, each contributing their specialized knowledge about an issue or the connection between two issues to the total consensus.

Like cryonics, idea futures is another way to take advantage now of the fact that the future should be rich with power and knowledge. We create good incentives now by letting the future settle our bets.

To make the whole idea more vivid let us consider a simple (fictional) scenario.

Scenario

Pat Thgisni was not a model student. A knack for making experiments work is probably what got him into graduate school – it certainly wasn't his grades. Worse, he was unkempt and had a disturbing habit of bending people's ears with one harebrained idea after another. Definitely not one of the rising stars of the University of Toledo Physics Department.

In his second year, 1992, Pat hit upon his best idea yet, "superscattering." If a neutrino could scatter off all the nuclei in a crystal at once, the interaction could be a billion times more powerful, perhaps allowing neutrino telescopes (Weber 1988). Pat showed his calculations to Professor Ezra Puccuts, a local and renowned neutrino expert, though rusty on scattering. Professor Puccuts explained to Pat that a similar idea had occurred to him, but he had found it conflicted with an accepted formula. Such a negative conclusion wasn't worth a publication.

Pat persisted, however, bringing out his pages of calculations. After 10 minutes of going through the first page, and finding three glaring, though irrelevant, math errors, Professor Puccuts lost his patience. "I do not have the time to correct your math for you," he declared, and shut the door. Over the next few months Pat redid his calculations several times, but Professor Puccuts was not interested and other professors referred Pat back to him. Pat submitted his work for publication anyway, and then waited; he did not have the $100K he figured it would cost to do an experiment.

That Christmas in LA, Pat told the story to his family. His brother Al, a sports fanatic, suggested that Pat dare them to make a bet. Before Pat could object, Al described how idea futures were revolutionizing the oil industry, and were a new way for the little guy to contribute to the world of ideas. After a few more drinks, Pat saw the light.

Pat wrote up a precise statement of his claim, and then stopped by the idea futures mart in Las Vegas [Actually, science bets are illegal in Nevada.] on his way back to Toledo. He paid $100 to have a reputable judging group decide if it was precise enough for them to judge in 2013 (which it was), $20 to the Bank of Vegas so they would issue coupons on it, and another $20 to have a computer market set up. Finally, he funded an automated market maker with $200 in seed capital, and set the initial market odds at 30 percent. Back at the university, Pat set his computer up to track the market, and then spread the word, causing an epidemic of giggles. One of

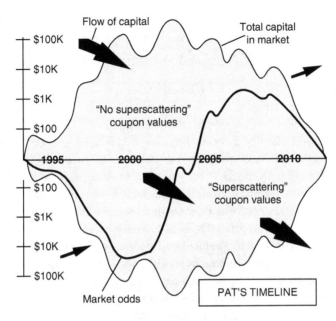

Figure 25.1   "Pat's Timeline." Originally published in *Extropy* 8 (1992). Copyright © Max More.

Professor Puccuts' smirking students agreed to put up $20 against him, and a half-dozen other students joined in, mostly at $2 each.

It worked like this. While Pat bought coupons which said "$1 if superscattering" from the market maker for around 30¢, the other students bought "$1 if no superscattering" coupons from the market maker for around 70¢. Whoever was right in the end would make money on the deal, receiving the $1 plus 7 percent interest per year, compounded. Every time Pat bought a coupon the market odds went up, and every time the other students bought the odds went down. The market maker got these coupons from the bank, who would sell the pair of coupons "$1 if superscattering" and "$1 if no superscattering" to anyone for $1 a pair. The bank made money on transaction charges, and risked nothing because exactly one of the pair would be worth $1 (plus interest) in the end. The bank also bought such pairs back for $1, allowing people to sell coupons back to the market maker. Many students took advantage of this feature in the next few weeks, as some professors made it clear they were not amused.

In 1995, Pat earned an early PhD. Like most students, he could not find an academic position and went to work in industry. A year later he finally published his superscattering article in a vanity journal. Over the years, Pat had tried to follow the literature to see if anyone else had the same idea, but without success. Meanwhile bets slowly trickled in, with the odds hovering around 15 percent. In 1997 the market told Pat of another bettor, in Peru, who made a number of publicly declared purchases, or "public bets," of superscattering coupons. The Peruvian had also published on the idea, but in an obscure Peruvian journal. Someone else created a market on whether there would be a compact neutrino telescope, which became popular with amateur astronomy clubs. Certain traders even specialized in keeping these two markets in rough correspondence. By 1998, the total value of all coupons out on superscattering, the "market capital," reached $8K.

That year an aide to Nevada Senator Sue Toshgib, member of the Senate Committee on High Tech, noticed the high odds for neutrino telescopes, and traced it to Pat's claim. Sue saw an opportunity to push Nevada's fledgling idea futures industry, and made an issue of the fact that the markets had apparently discovered a number of potential new technologies. For example, she said, if there was a 15 percent chance of superscattering, why wasn't this possibility being pursued in the labs?

Wheels turned, but Professor Puccuts' technical explanations did not satisfy Senator Toshgib. Federal funding agencies wanted to avoid a confrontation, but also wanted to protect their turf from every senator's whim. So they prodded the administration of the University of Toledo to quietly make a few bets with university overhead funds. This infusion of capital overwhelmed what Pat and a few others could scrape up. The odds fell to 2 percent, and the issue was dropped.

But the $100K now in the game raised the interest of a few experienced speculators looking for an angle. They hired a few grad students to try the superscattering calculations, and the odds crept up to 6 percent over the next year. About the time the university realized there might be no limit to the capital required to keep the odds down, Professor Puccuts published a paper showing why superscattering was impossible. The hired grad students were intimidated, and the odds fell to 1 percent. Six months later a student from across the hall over heard Professor Puccuts mention that an equation in his paper was an ad hoc approximation. So he re-tried the calculation, and got a rather different result. He told his old professor, Professor Yikkul, and they jointly wrote a paper. As rumors spread, the market odds shot to 20 percent.

In 2001 the first experiment was started. The odds fluctuated under the influence of some false rumors, and some experimenters' friends made extra income by trading before the experimental results were revealed. In 2005 the market odds were at 70 percent, and by 2008 the issue seemed pretty much settled, with the market odds at 98 percent. Pat, who had doggedly stuck with superscattering, sold his coupons to reap a total profit of $700K on his $20K investment (which was all his spouse would let him risk). This profit came from selling "$1 if superscattering" coupons for 98¢, after buying them for as little as 1¢, and from the 7 percent interest the Bank of Vegas had agreed to pay on the money it held. Just before the coupons were to be judged in 2013, the last traders sold their coupons to avoid paying a judging fee. The market was closed down and the judges were never needed.

Pat was still not offered an academic position, as Professor Yikkul became the celebrated discoverer of superscattering. So Pat started a new market, to be judged by a detailed historical study in 30 years, on who was the first discoverer of superscattering. Certain universities vowed to let professors defend their own ideas. Professor Puccuts, who never bet any of his own money, still has tenure.

Scope

Mechanisms like idea futures have been used for a long time to create consensus about corn prices, stock dividends, life expectancy, marine accident risks, horse races, and football games. So clearly it can work for some topics. But the vision offered here is to make much wider use of such mechanisms. Some areas of science and technology seem similar enough to horse races to suggest betting will work there also, but what about everything else?

There are a number of parameters which indicate when a claim will be more difficult to handle, including the time and expense required to resolve a claim, the probability it will never be resolved, the strength of emotions on the issue, the lopsidedness of the odds, and the scarcity of interested traders. The procedures described below are intended to allow idea futures to handle as many claims as possible. I hope to make the case for wide applicability plausible enough to inspire interest and experiments.

Procedures

In idea futures markets people would exchange coupons. Each coupon is issued by a bank, and specifies a judging organization who will decide the issue "beyond a reasonable doubt." Coupons have the basic form "$X if A," where A is a claim and $X is a "conditional value." A claim includes a sentence, such as those in Box 25.1, "Some Controversial Claims," and any clarifications on word meanings. The claim part of a coupon also specifies who will judge the claim, a judging date, and any declarations about the decision criteria or process to be used. There can be many coupons on the same claim, each to be judged by different judges on different judging dates.

Coupons also specify a total judging fee and a maximum percentage judging fee. The judging fee is obtained by reducing the face value of each coupon in the market on the judging date by whatever percentage is necessary given the total market capital. If this would violate the maximum percentage judging fee, then the banks must try to create enough market capital by gambling the existing capital in an "audit lottery." If the coupons win the lottery, enough capital is created to support judging, and coupon face values are increased. If not, coupons are worthless and judging is not needed.

The judging fee creates an incentive to "settle out of court" by selling before the judging date, as happened in Pat's superscattering market. Audit lotteries preserve incentives for honest evaluation even when an issue is of only limited interest and very expensive to judge (Polinsky 1983), such as whether your daughter would make a good doctor, if only someone would pay her way through medical school. Pat specified that an audit lottery be used, if necessary, to fund the historical study on who discovered superscattering.

Judge's verdicts should be "beyond a reasonable doubt" and are expressed as percentages to be paid off to each side. Judges have additional incentives to be careful if they agree to spend some fraction of their judging fee to keep the market price of an "appeals" coupon near that of their verdict. Appeals coupons are on the same claim, but judged much later by independent judges with a much larger budget.

If there is not yet enough evidence or funding to decide a question, judges may be allowed to postpone judging to a new date with a new, perhaps larger, judging fee. They could in the process offer some clarification of the question, and would use up some portion of the max percentage judging fee to pay for their trouble. Markets can also be set up so that if no decision can be agreed on, judges can declare "all bets are off."

The conditional value part of a coupon, the $X, specifies a standard investment instrument, such as a stock, bond, or mutual fund, and gives specifics like amount, date of purchase, interest rate, etc. There should be a liquid market in such instruments, so that it is always clear what the equivalent cash value is. In the superscattering example, bonds issued by the Bank of Vegas paying 7 percent interest were used. There can be coupons with different investment instruments for each claim and judge combination described above. By building on standard investments, an idea futures investor can expect a better rate of return than he could get with any standard investment alone.

Banks are long-lived financial institutions trusted to properly report judging fees. A bank's main function is to split and join coupons. For example, the claim "True" can be split into "A" and "not A." Imagine giving a bank one share of General Motors (GM) stock. The bank would see this as a "1 GM share stock if True" coupon and exchange it for the coupon pair "1 GM share if A" and "1 GM share if not A." The bank would hold on to the pair and if A wins, give the 1 GM share to any holder of a "1 GM share if A" coupon. While the bank held the 1 GM share betting stakes, the wealth it represents would, we hope, be put to productive use by GM. An "A" coupon can be further split into "A and B" and "A and not B." Using certain combinations of such coupons, one can bet on the conditional probability of "B given A" and be insensitive to the verdict on A.

Each type of coupon must have at least one public market for trading coupons. Preferably, such markets will be continuous bid/ask markets allowing anyone to post or take offers via computer. A single computer could implement thousands of low-activity markets.

To increase liquidity and reduce price fluctuations and spreads, anyone can fund automated market makers (Black 1971), computer programs always available for trading. A simple market maker algorithm exists which can function indefinitely and not be cheated by clever combinations of traders (see Math Appendix). The degree of price smoothing it provides depends on the amount of sacrificial cash it starts with. This provides a way to subsidize a market, as does offering to pay part of the judging fee. Pat funded such a market maker to promote trading in his market.

If the odds on different claims are inconsistent, i.e., do not adhere to the standard axioms of probability, then arbitrageurs can make money by buying or selling "Dutch books" (Debus 1970). This profit comes at no risk if the final verdicts can be trusted to be consistent. Therefore arbitrage activity should keep the total social consensus roughly self-consistent.

Other market innovations, such as options, baskets, and hedges, allow investors to specialize in details they think they know about and ignore other issues. Options allow bets on price volatility, independent of the way the price moves. Baskets allow one to ignore differences; one can buy a basket of all types of coupons on a certain claim, and ignore differences in judges, investment instruments, etc. Hedges allow bets on price differences, such as when investors kept the odds on superscattering and compact neutrino telescopes in rough correspondence. For

---

Box 25.2   Idea Futures Home Version

1. Choose a claim like "I will win this hand of stud poker."
2. Get a pencil, and some chips. Let red chips be "$10 if claim," blue chips be "$10 if not claim," and something else be money.
3. Give each person $100.
4. At any time players may buy or sell pairs of red and blue chips for $10.
5. Place the pencil across the bar below between 5 and 6 on the CLAIM side. This means the market maker will sell one red chip for $6 or buy it for $5.
6. Whoever yells first, such as "buy red for 6," can trade one chip at the offered price. The pencil then immediately moves in that direction, such as to 6–7. Repeat till market settles.
7. Reveal new information, like the next card, and repeat step 6.
8. If the claim was right in the end, reds are worth $10, blue $0. If wrong, blue is $10, red $0. Have fun!

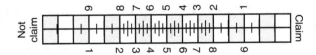

Figure 25.2 "Claim/Not Claim." Originally published in *Extropy* 8 (1992). Copyright © Max More.

example, one could correct for the human bias of overconfidence by betting that on average the odds are not as extreme as the market odds.

While Pat had to risk a substantial portion of his wealth on one question, a more typical scenario would include larger private research labs whose salaried employees have a direct investment in many questions.

Idea futures markets could be integrated with one or more publishing media or "registries." People could make "public bets," where they buy a coupon for a claim, write a statement of support, and commit to having registries reveal both of these at a pre-specified date. Track records could be compiled from such information and used as reputation scores. People with high scores could become investment advisors, making a public bet with each piece of advice. An advanced publishing medium (Hanson 1988) would allow anyone to post evidence and arguments and link them to the disputed claim.

Advantages

Idea futures offers many possible advantages. A visible consensus would immediately form on a wide range of hotly debated issues. This consensus would be relatively universal, expert, honest, self-consistent, and cheap. Such a consistent consensus might allow society as a whole to approach the level of rational consistency that is now only expected of individuals.

The market consensus could carry social weight, serving as a coordination point for thousands of independent conversations. In each discussion, the market odds on an issue could be assumed as the default unless specific arguments were presented to the contrary. Dissenters could be given the time-honored challenge to "put up or shut up." In the same tradition, those willing to put themselves on the line would be given due respect and attention. I have observed that the challenge of a bet makes people noticeably more cautious about what exactly they are claiming.

As debates become settled, they would leave a trail of agreed-upon statements. These could be used to counter bogus statements, often made by those ignorant of solid expert consensus. Visionaries like Pat would have a new way to try to convince others of a revolutionary claim; they could throw all available capital into bets. If this were enough to change the market odds, they could point to these odds in arguments. If not, they would at least expect to make a healthy profit, and gain social credit for being serious. True cranks would end up subsidizing leveler heads.

The social weight of consensus could help damp many presently distorting biases. It would be harder for popular media to create consensus by sheer repetition of a claim; they would have to convince those willing to bet. A sincere public relations campaign could make a public bet, but an insincere one would know it was throwing money away. And an insincere attempt to throw enough money away to change the market odds runs the risk of the word getting out and the market ending right back where it started. Finally, hedge bettors can correct for standard biases in individual judgment.

Individuals would have clear monetary incentives to be honest and careful in contributing to the market consensus. If the odds you believe are different enough from the market odds, you believe you will on average make money, even more than with a standard investment like a stock index fund. And compared to stocks, idea future bets are precise and modular. In stock bets one must usually bet on a combination of ideas, such as the company's product, marketing strategy, production techniques, etc. In idea futures you can bet on exactly the issue you think you know something about.

It might be fun! Imagine a page in the newspaper like the stock page, showing this week's odds on controversial issues. Imagine coming home from an enlightening discussion to change your investments. Imagine reading something you disagreed with, and stopping for a minute to make a bet against it. The knowledge you created while reading would be directly useful to society and yourself, instead of thrown away as is usual now.

Non-scientists could have a direct, even if small, influence and personal stake in science to heighten their interest, like the amateur astronomy clubs in the story of Pat. Amateur trading would induce scientific research by traders seeking an edge, subsidize professionals who can better predict, and might even fund research by judges. Savings would be encouraged and research would be directed more at issues of general interest. Capital and hence intellectual effort would flow to markets where there is broad interest, strong disagreement, and relevant data obtainable for a modest effort or a short wait.

Idea futures markets create information, combining what individuals know. A market with more capital will probably have better information, as people will see there is more to win by figuring out the answer. By subsidizing a market you can pay to create information, though you won't get exclusive access. This might be a better way for government to fund scientific research, instead of the usual grant-giving approach (Hanson 1990). In fact, governments might use odds from subsidized markets as factual input for government decisions. We could all have our say about whether projected usage would justify a new mass transit system, or whether a death was suspicious enough to justify an autopsy. Schools might even admit students based on the market odds of candidates getting a high GPA if they attend.

Idea futures can also provide insurance. A risky business venture based on a new technology might bet against that technology to reduce total risk. Idea futures can be a foundation for reputation systems, providing another way to encourage experts to give honest advice, and allow other experts to disagree. Idea futures offers all these benefits without requiring any coercion or taxation. Unlike patents, it requires no international enforcement or litigation about the origins of an idea.

Criticisms

By now you probably have in mind at least one objection to idea futures, and will not be entirely comfortable with it until this objection is addressed. Longer papers on this subject (Hanson 1990) consist largely of detailed responses to such objections. Space limitations preclude such detail here so Box 25.3, "A Few Concerns about Ideas Futures," just gives a list of some issues addressed in those papers.

Box 25.3   A Few Concerns about Idea Futures

Isn't gambling illegal? Isn't betting a useless zero-sum game? Does anyone ever bet this way? What about compulsive gambling? Is there enough interest in science questions? Will these markets be too thin? Doesn't betting only work for clear-cut questions like horse races? How often do beliefs really converge? What if beliefs never converge? What do convergent beliefs have to do with truth? What about badly worded claims? Can't wrong ideas still be useful? What if the fine print differs from the summary? What about sucker bets? Don't science questions resolve too slowly? Why should I trust the judges? Won't judging cost too much? Won't wealthy people have too much influence? Won't the market be dominated by fools? Won't advertising manipulate opinion? Aren't markets full of cheats and thieves? What about insider trading? What about "moral hazard"? What about incentives to start false rumors? What about incentives to keep information secret? Won't an apparent consensus create a crowd mentality? Will the new incentives slow or stop convergence? Won't different claim wordings, judges, and base assets confuse the consensus? Won't the consensus reflect risk preferences as well as beliefs? Won't betting challenges discourage creativity? What's the point of a "consensus" that people disagree with? Isn't it better for people to argue out their own disputes? Won't this have the same problems as patents? Wouldn't anonymous trading screw up reputation statistics? If this is so great, why hasn't it happened already? Won't greed sully the pure pursuit of ideas? Does a few dollars of compensation in the end really help a rejected visionary? Doesn't this presume there is some absolute truth? Won't convergence be culturally relative? Isn't consistency unhealthy? Doesn't organized crime take over anything having to do with gambling? What about libel and national security? What about "Nuclear war will destroy 90 percent of the world by 2020"? Won't different claim wordings, judges, and investment instruments fragment the market? Why should verdicts be consistent with one another? Won't judges be reluctant to contradict the market? What if the probabilities get very small? Why not do without judges?

Related Work

In Bayesian decision theory, an agent's degree of belief in A is often defined to be the price they would be willing to pay for a "$1 if A" coupon (De Finetti 1976). Idea futures just applies this definition to a society as a whole to find our consensus degree of belief. In the presence of a market, agents appear to agree (Kadane and Winkler 1988).

As was mentioned before, there are markets similar to idea futures in commodities, finance, insurance, and sports betting. Science and technology bets are frequently made between individuals (Hall 1989; Tierney 1991; *Wall Street Journal* 1989), as they have been through history (Debus 1970). The idea of betting on a wide range of legislative and technological issues is raised in science fiction (Brunner 1975; Verne 1872), and scattered proposals (Fairley et al. 1984; Hofstee 1984; Leamer 1986; Zeckhauser and Viscusi 1990) have been made to formalize bets in science.

Business schools widely use such markets to teach MBA students about markets (Forsythe et al. 1990). In economic theory, the coupons I have been describing are called "contingent assets," and are often used as a foundation in analyzing financial investments (Sharpe 1985) and the effect of uncertainty (Laffont 1989). Ideally, there would be a "complete market," with assets contingent on every possible state of the world. In reality markets are not complete, and various sorts of "market failure" are traced to this fact.

Incompleteness is usually (Hirshleifer 1971) explained as due to judging difficulties, finite transaction costs, and market thinness. In fact, these authors are often unaware that such markets are almost universally prohibited by anti-gambling laws, as joint-stock companies, life insurance, and commodity futures (Rose 1986) were prohibited before special interests managed to obtain exemptions. Though unevenly enforced, such laws prohibit public science bets between strangers in all of the US and in most of the world.

Only Great Britain, to my knowledge, allows such bets, and then only for the last three decades. English bookmakers perceive little demand for science bets, and so take them mainly to induce popular articles mentioning the going odds on unusual subjects (Sharpe 1990). This publicity brings in new clients, who may then switch to the "real" betting on sports. Because of this, bookies prefer small bets on subjects "in good taste" that anyone can understand, like UFOs, Yetis, and Moon landings. They avoid subjects that seem too esoteric for the general public, like the recent "cold fusion" claims, and subjects that won't very clearly resolve themselves, as a judging industry has not yet evolved.

Bookmakers traditionally prefer to set prices and stick to them, rather than setting up markets, letting prices fluctuate, and playing market maker. Because of this, they are usually unwilling to offer bets on claims where they do not know how to estimate the odds, and few bookies have advanced science educations. As a result, they mainly take safe bets, siding with the scientific establishment against "crazy" outside theories, which doesn't help the image problem betting has in many quarters. One cannot even subscribe to a publication listing the going prices on science questions. It should be possible to improve on this.

An Appeal

Idea futures is mainly just a curiosity to most people, even those convinced of its feasibility and desirability. It would require substantial effort to implement, and in some sense is a trivially obvious idea, given the appropriate theoretical background. I think the only people who might actually be willing to work to make it happen are people who are particularly unhappy with current methods of forming and communicating scientific consensus, and how those methods have treated issues dear to them. People perhaps like *Extropy* readers, sympathetic to markets and subjects, like cryonics and uploading, which current consensus institutions deal poorly with. I fear it will require more effort than I alone can muster to make it real. It may well be that if you don't do it, no one will; what do you say?

There are many options for pursuing idea futures. I have worked to gain the attention of "science policy" academics (Hanson 1993), and idea futures will soon be a known, if oddball, suggested alternative mechanism for science funding. I have mostly developed a board game and to a lesser extent an email reputation game. Legal research is probably the most important task, but it is on hold for a lack of funds.

Conclusion

I have argued that futures markets in ideas could help the evolution of ideas by creating a visible consensus of relevant experts, and better incentives for honesty and care when making contributions. Idea futures might offer these and many other benefits cheaply and without coercion. Though some problems remain, it seems worth further study.

I leave the reader with this challenge: Can you think of a question where (1) you think the answer will eventually become clear, or would with enough study, and (2) you think you disagree with some generally perceived majority opinion? If so, imagine creating a market in that claim and then making a few trades.

Math Appendix

Variables

$P(A)$ = Market probability of A
$J(A)$ = Judge's verdict probability of A
$\$X$ = An investment with a current market value of X dollars.
C = Total value of distributed coupons on a claim
F = Total budget available for judging
f = Maximum percentage judging fee

Identities

$\$X$ = "$\$X$ if True"
"($\$X$ if A) if B" = "$\$X$ if (A and B)"

Exchanges

(These remain valid if change $\$X$ to "$\$X$ if A," or multiply all $ by a constant)
Split/Join: $1 < - >$ "$1 if B," "$1 if not B"
Trading on A: $\$P(A) < - >$ "$1 if A"
On A given B: $\$P(A \text{ given } B) < - >$ "$\$P$ if not B," "$1 if B and A"
Cash in with Judges: "$1 if A" $- > \$J(A)$ "$1 if not A" $- > \$(1 - J(A))$

Dutch book example

If $P(A) + P(\text{not } A) < 1$, then can buy "$1 if A" and "$1 if not A" for less than $1, sell the pair to the bank for
  $1, and make a profit.

Judging fees

1) If $f{*}C > = F$, pay $\$F$ to judges, reduce coupon values $\$X - > \$X{*}(1-(F/C))$
2) If $f{*}C = 0$, no judging happens
3) If $0 < f{*}C < F$, Take C and play a lottery: With probability $C{*}f/F$, increase value of coupons $\$X - > \$X{*}F/(C{*}f)$ and do 1) Otherwise $\$X - > \$0$ and do 2)

Market maker algorithm (see Box 25.2)

Choose a function M(i) from integers to [0,1] such that M(i) > M(i + 1), M(0) = 1/2.
Choose a transaction quantity Q.
Market starts at j = 0.
Offer "$Q if A" - > $(Q*M(j)) and if taken j - > j + 1 Offer "$Q if A" < - $(Q*M(j + 1)) and if taken j - > j–1
If M(i) = 1/(1 + exp(i/k)), total loss < ~ $Q*k/2.

References

Black, Fischer (1971) "Towards a Fully Automated Exchange." *Financial Analyst Journal* (July and November).

Brunner, John (1975) *The Shockwave Rider*. New York: Harper & Row.

Cialdini, Robert B. (1988) *Influence, Science and Practice*. Boston: Scott, Foresman & Co.

De Finetti, Bruno (1976) "Probability: Beware of Falsifications." In H. Kyburg and H. Smokler, eds., *Studies in Subjective Probability*. New York: Robert Krieger (1980), pp. 192–224.

Debus, Allen G. (1970) *Science and Education in the Seventeenth Century*. London: MacDonald.

Fairley, William, Meyer, Michael B., and Chernick, Paul L. (1984) "Insurance Market Assessment of Technological Risk." *Procedures of the Society for Risk Analysis International Workshop on Uncertainty in Risk Assessment, Risk Management, and Decision Making* (September 30), pp. 89–102.

Forsythe, Robert, Nelson, Forrest D., Neumann, George R., and Wright, Jack (1990) "The Explanation and Prediction of Presidential Elections: A Market Alternative to Polls." *Economics Working Paper*, (April 12), pp. 90–111. University of Iowa, Iowa City.

Hall, S. (1989) "Professor Thorne's Time Machine." *California* (October), pp. 68–77.

Hanson, Robin (1988) "Toward Hypertext Publishing, Issues and Choices in Database Design." *ACM SIGIR Forum* 22/1–2 (Winter).

Hanson, Robin (1990) "Could Gambling Save Science? Encouraging an Honest Consensus." *Procedures of the Eighth International Conference on Risk and Gambling* (London, July).

Hanson, Robin (1993) "Comment on the Scientific Status of Econometrics." *Social Epistemology* 7/3, pp. 255–256.

Hirshleifer, Jack (1971) "The Private and Social Value of Information and the Reward to Inventive Activity." *American Economics Review* 61/4 (September), pp. 561–574.

Hofstee, Willem K.B. (1984) "Methodological Decision Rules As Research Policies: A Betting Reconstruction of Empirical Research." *Acta Psychologica* 56, pp. 93–109.

Kadane, Joseph B., and Winkler, Robert L. (1988) "Separating Probability Elicitation from Utilities." *Journal of the American Statistical Association* 83/402 (June), Theory and Methods, pp. 357–363.

Kahneman, Daniel. and Tversky, Amos, eds. (1982) *Judgment under Uncertainty: Heuristics and Biases*. New York: Cambridge University Press.

Kantrowitz, Arthur (1977) "The Science Court Experiment: Criticisms and Responses." *Bulletin of the Atomic Scientists* (April), pp. 44–50.

Laffont, Jean-Jacques (1989) *The Economics of Uncertainty and Information*. Cambridge, MA: MIT Press.

Leamer, Edward (1986) "Bid-Ask Spreads For Subjective Probabilities." In P. Goel and A. Zellner, eds., *Bayesian Inference and Decision Techniques*. Amsterdam: Elsevier, pp. 217–232.

Linstone, Harold A. and Turoff, Murray, eds. (1975) *The Delphi Method*. London: Addison-Wesley.

Polinsky, A. Mitchell (1983) *An Introduction to Law and Economics*. Boston: Little, Brown.

Rose, I. Nelson (1986) *Gambling and the Law*. Hollywood: Gambling Times Incorporated.

Seidenfeld, T. (1990) "Two Perspectives on Consensus for (Bayesian) Inference and Decisions." In H. Kyburg et al., eds., *Knowledge Representation and Defeasible Reasoning*. Boston: Kluwer Academic Press, pp. 267–286.

Sharpe, G. (1990) Phone conversations. William Hill Ltd. 19 Valentine Place, London SE1 8QH (July).

Sharpe, William (1985) *Investments*, 3rd edn. Upper Saddle River, NJ: Prentice Hall.

Tierney, John (1991) "A Bet On Planet Earth." *Reader's Digest* (March), pp. 61–64.

Tullock, Gordon (1966) *The Organization of Inquiry*. Durham, NC: Duke University Press.

Verne, Jules (1872) *Around the World in Eighty Days*. London.

Wall Street Journal (1989) "Fusion Fuss Is Turning Scientists into Gamblers." (April 18).

Weber, Joseph (1988) "Apparent Observation of Abnormally Large Coherent Scattering Cross Sections Using keV and MeV Range Antineutrinos, and Solar Neutrinos." *Physical Review D* 38/1 (July 1).

Zeckhauser, Richard and Viscusi, W. Kip (1990) "Risk Within Reason." *Science* 248 (May 4), pp. 559–564.

Further Reading

Drexler, K.E. (1986) *Engines of Creation*. New York: Doubleday.

26

The Proactionary Principle
Optimizing Technological Outcomes

Max More

In the past, it was possible to approach transhumanism as primarily involving philosophical discussion and technological speculation. While transhumanist goals such as radical life extension, uploading, and cognitive, sensory, and physical enhancement were speculative they were also considered scientifically feasible, even if the technologies to achieve those goals appeared remote. Other than an overall advocacy of progress, early transhumanism therefore had few resources or implications for action. Since little action was called for, no one needed to worry much about how to make the best decisions.

Nevertheless, the question remained: How could we make more than peripheral progress on these goals while we yet lacked tools smart, small, and subtle enough to engineer and redesign away our basic human limits? However, as expected, our tools and knowledge have progressed. We have decoded the human genome and our ability to identify our personal genetic variations continues to improve rapidly even as the cost of doing so plummets. Scientists have advanced our knowledge of proteomics and other biological complexities, and the workings of the brain. Despite being described as a failure, artificial intelligence has made considerable progress, at least in numerous specialized domains. At the same time, we see the convergence of biotechnology and nanotechnology, improvements in prosthetics, and growing success in restoring senses.

As their core ideas about radical life extension and human enhancement have spread and become more influential, transhumanists have felt less need for mere envisioning and advocacy and have shifted the emphasis to implementation and to careful consideration of costs and benefits. At the same time, some transhumanists have become excessively focused on hypothetical risks and apocalyptic imaginings. In contrast, the Proactionary Principle is motivated by the need to make wise decisions about the development and deployment of new technologies *and* by the crucial need to protect technological experimentation and progress.

The Transhumanist Reader: Classical and Contemporary Essays on the Science, Technology, and Philosophy of the Human Future, First Edition. Edited by Max More and Natasha Vita-More.
© 2013 John Wiley & Sons, Inc. Published 2013 by John Wiley & Sons, Inc.

I should note that the Proactionary Principle applies to all complex decisions involving technology, not just those with obvious relevance to transhumanist concerns. In other words, it is not a transhumanist-specific decision method. In the present context, though, the Principle is offered as a guide to address problems effectively and wisely, considering concerns, answering objections, and developing solutions and strategies – for both personal and group decisions.

The Origin of the Proactionary Principle

The Proactionary Principle emerged out of a critical discussion of the well-known precautionary principle that developed in Europe and has been used in the United States and elsewhere as a type of model for dealing with change. The precautionary principle comes in many forms, but one well-known version was presented by Soren Holm and John Harris in *Nature* magazine in 1999 and states:

> When an activity raises threats of serious or irreversible harm to human health or the environment, precautionary measures that prevent the possibility of harm shall be taken even if the causal link between the activity and the possible harm has not been proven or the causal link is weak and the harm is unlikely to occur.

Because of this principle's inadequacy and its placing the burden of proof exclusively on new technologies, it became apparent that a different decision model was needed. Extropy Institute created the Vital Progress (VP) Summit in 2004 to address this gap. The VP Summit participants saw the fatal weaknesses riddling the precautionary principle. Not least among these is its strong bias toward the status quo and against the technological progress so vital to the continued survival and wellbeing of humanity. Participants in understood that we need to develop and deploy new technologies to feed billions more people over the coming decades, to counter natural threats – from pathogens to environmental changes – and to alleviate human suffering from disease, damage, and the ravages of aging. We recognized the need to formulate an alternative, more sophisticated principle incorporating more extensive and accurate assessment of options while protecting our fundamental responsibility and liberty to experiment and innovate.

With input from some of those at the Summit, I developed the Proactionary Principle to structure decision-making as effectively as possible. The Principle urges all parties to actively take into account all the consequences of an activity – good as well as bad – while apportioning precautionary measures to the real threats we face. In addition, to do all this while appreciating the crucial role played by technological innovation and humanity's evolving ability to adapt to and remedy any undesirable side-effects.

The Wisdom of Structure

The human brain did not evolve to make complex decisions. The challenges of early human life did not equip us for the choices of modern, technological life. We learned to use cognitive short-cuts. These worked well most of the time in simple environments but often fail us in more nuanced circumstances. Many of these shortcuts and heuristics are now labeled as "cognitive biases." Organizational biases can magnify these cognitive biases. Unfortunately, merely knowing what these biases are is not enough to avoid falling prey to them. If we are to pursue transhumanism while maximizing the benefits and minimizing the risks of potent technologies, our thinking needs to be structured.

By structuring the decision process appropriately, we can minimize these biases and other typical decision-making weaknesses, while enhancing our abilities to create options and intelligently choose from among them. Intelligent structuring of decision-making:

- Reduces individual cognitive bias and strengthens objectivity by controlling unstructured judgment and unfounded inputs and by managing group dynamics with a systematic framework. Structuring can systematically check for biases and standard kinds of errors, as well as making conditions more conducive to objectivity.
- Improves decision accuracy by specifying methods and inputs. Even the most objective decision-makers will go wrong if they use unreliable tools and poor-quality information.
- Raises the quality of each step of the decision process by drawing systematically on the best available knowledge about analyzing, evaluating, creating, and deciding.
- Enhances convergent, analytical capabilities by helping to make sense of complex problems and by focusing attention in the right way on each element of the analysis.
- Enhances divergent thinking and the generation of alternatives.
- Minimizes both excessively risky and excessively conservative judgments by systematically comparing elements of the decision and by critically integrating diverse perspectives.
- Reduces risk by finding and evaluating more threats.
- Contributes to organizational transparency.

Structural wisdom comes not only from the fact of structuring itself, but also from structuring in a way that relies on the best methods, models, tools, and procedures available. Structural wisdom is all about guiding our decision-making by the smartest possible methods. The Proactionary Principle embodies the wisdom of structure. The precautionary principle does not.

The Failure of the Precautionary Principle

The version of the precautionary principle from the 1988 Wingspread Statement says:

> When an activity raises threats of harm to the environment or human health, precautionary measures should be taken even if some cause and effect relationships are not fully established scientifically.

Like the previously mentioned version – and all versions – this one calls for restrictive measures even in the absence of firm evidence of harmful effects. Notice that there is no call for a balanced, comprehensive, or objective assessment of both risks and benefits. The principle enshrines caution as the prime and only value. Caution, like suspicion or anger or confidence, enjoys a legitimate place in our toolbox of responses. However, it cannot serve by itself as a comprehensive, judicious, rational basis for making decisions about technological and environmental concerns. We get into trouble only when we elevate caution and cautionary measures to the status of an absolute principle – when we endow them with a crude veto power over all other values and over the use of maximum intelligence and creativity.

There's a simple but telling way to appreciate the threat to progress and human wellbeing posed by the precautionary principle: Take a look back at the scientific and technological achievements of the past, then ask: "Would these advances have been sanctioned or prohibited by the precautionary principle?" It is hard to think of a single significant advance that a literal application of this principle would not have blocked. Certainly, it would have prohibited the development and use of airplanes, aspirin, CAT scans, chlorine, all drugs, all forms of energy production, knives, and penicillin (which was toxic to guinea pigs). Taken literally, it would stop all progress. (And if we do not take it literally, how can it guide our decisions?) It has to be applied selectively and inconsistently – and this makes it dangerous.

This leads us to the *paradox of the precautionary principle*: The principle endangers us by trying too hard to safeguard us. It tries "too hard" by being obsessively preoccupied with a *single* value – safety. By focusing us on safety to an excessive degree, the principle distracts policymakers and the public from other dangers other than the one initially under consideration. The more confident we are in the principle, and the more enthusiastically we apply it, the greater the hazard to our health and our standard of living. The principle ends up *causing* harm by diverting attention, financial resources, public health resources, time, and research effort from more urgent and weighty risks.

Even worse, in practice this rule assumes that new prohibitions or regulations will result in no harm to human health or the environment. Unfortunately, well-intended interventions into complex systems invariably have unintended consequences. Only by closely examining possible ramifications can we determine whether or not the intervention is likely to make us better off. By single-mindedly enforcing the tyranny of safety, this principle can only distract decision-makers from such an examination.

Environmental and technological activism that wields the precautionary principle, whether explicitly or implicitly, raises clear threats of harm to human health and wellbeing. If we apply the principle to itself, we arrive at the corollary to the Paradox of the Precautionary Principle:

> According to the principle, since the principle itself is dangerous, we should take precautionary measures to prevent the use of the precautionary principle.

The severity of the precautionary principle's threat certainly does not imply that we should take *no* actions to safeguard human health or the environment. Nor does it imply that we must achieve full scientific certainty (or its nearest real-world equivalent) before taking action. It *does* imply that we should keep our attention focused on established and highly probable risks, rather than on hypothetical and inflated risks. It also implies an obligation to assess the likely costs of enforcing precautionary restrictions on human activities. Clearly, we need a better way to assess potential threats to humans and the environment – and the consequences of our responses. In order to develop a suitable alternative, we first need to appreciate the full extent of flaws in the precautionary approach.

Failure of objectivity. Any decision procedure adequate for handling the complexities of technological and environmental risks affecting multiple parties must be objective. Objectivity here means "following a structured, explicit procedure informed by the relevant fields of knowledge." Those fields include risk analysis, economics, the psychology of decision making, and verified forecasting methods. In the absence of a well-designed, structured procedure, assessment and decision making will be distorted by cognitive and interest-based biases, emotional reactions, ungrounded public perceptions and pressures from lobbyists, and popular but unreliable approaches to analysis and forecasting. The precautionary principle does nothing to ensure that decision makers use reliable, objective procedures.

Distracts from greater threats. The precautionary principle distracts citizens and policymakers from established, major threats to health. The heavy emphasis on taking precautionary measures for any proposed danger, no matter how speculative, draws attention away from any comparative assessment of risks and costs. The principle embodies the imperative to eliminate all risk from some proposed source, ignoring the background level of risk, and ignoring other sources of risk that may be more deserving of action. We should apply our limited resources first to major risks that we *know* are real, not merely hypothetical. The principle errs in focusing on future technological harms that *might* occur, while ignoring natural risks that are *actually* occurring.

Vague and unclear. Interpretation of the principle is open to extreme variability. Once given a specific interpretation, the principle is simple. Simplicity is appealing and can be a virtue – so long as it does not come at the expense of adequacy. The precautionary principle is *too* simple. In versions that mention "irreversible harm," no account is given of irreversibility. A claim of irreversibility may be false and, even if true, irreversible changes may not be substantial. The principle lacks clarity also because it leaves us without any guidance in the many cases where resulting harm arrives along with benefits. The principle leaves us in the dark as to *how* we should go about preventing harm. As we have seen, precautionary measures can themselves be harmful and costly.

Lack of comprehensiveness. Any procedure that claims to be both rational and equitable in assessing the desirability of restrictions on productive human activity must take into account the interests of all affected parties with legitimate claims. It must consider all reasonable alternative actions, including no action. It should not ignore the benefits of the activity in question, and the costs and risks of the restrictions, regulations, or prohibitions. Decision-makers should carefully consider not only concentrated and immediate effects, but also widely distributed and follow-on effects. Officials and activists who use the principle routinely inadvertently or deliberately ignore costs and side-effects of regulations and prohibitions, as well as the potential benefits of a technology, both in the near term and as it might develop over time.

Inappropriate burden of proof. The precautionary principle illegitimately shifts the burden of proof ("reverse onus") by requiring innovators and producers to prove their innocence when anyone raises "threats of harm." Activists enjoy a favored status since they can raise the prospect of precautionary measures with no more evidence than their fearful imagination. All they need to show is that a *possibility* of harm exists. No, not even this. All they need to show is that questions have been raised about the possibility of harm. Inventors and producers must then devote effort and resources to answering those questions.

To add to the fear-inducing power and chilling effect of the reverse onus, activists and regulators who invoke the precautionary principle invariably assume a *worst-case scenario*. By imagining the proposed technology or endeavor primarily in a worst-case scenario – while assuming that *preventing* action will have no disastrous consequences – the adherents of the principle immediately tilt the playing field in their favor. By combining reverse onus and catastrophic scenario-spinning, precautionists guarantee that managing *perceptions* of risk becomes more influential in policymaking than the reality of risk.

Failure to accommodate tradeoffs. One consequence (often intentional) of shifting the burden of proof is the inability of the principle to handle tradeoffs between harm to humans and to the environment. Since unaltered nature is implicitly an absolute value in the principle, no tradeoffs are to be allowed. The precautionary principle is all about avoiding possible harm – and human-caused harm, and primarily harm to the environment – rather than respecting a wider set of values.

This absolutist, univalued approach conflicts with the more balanced approach to risk and harm derived from common law. Common law holds us liable for injuries we cause, with liability increasing along with foreseeable risk. By contrast, the precautionary principle bypasses liability and acts like a preliminary injunction – but without the involvement of a court. By doing this, the precautionary principle denies individuals and communities the freedom to make tradeoffs in the way recognized by common-law approaches to risk and harm. No other values are admitted as a reason not to pursue extreme precaution.

Asymmetrical. Environmental activists – heavy users of the precautionary principle – usually target human-caused effects while giving the destructive aspects of "nature" a free ride. Yet nature itself brings with it a risk of harms such as infection, hunger, famine, and environmental disruption. The precautionary principle inherently favors nature and the status quo over humanity and progress, while routinely ignoring the potential benefits of technology and innovation. It fails to treat natural and human threats on the same basis. The principle does not account for the fact that the risks created by technological stagnation are at least as real as those of technological advancement.

Vulnerability to corruption. The inconsistent, discriminatory nature of precautionary regulations puts a kink in the rule of law. By giving regulators the power to insist on any degree of testing they choose, the precautionary principle opens up opportunities for corruption – undue influence, unfair targeting, and regulatory capture. It is the principle's vagueness, inconsistency, and arbitrariness that appeal to regulators who enjoy expanding their powers and wielding them selectively. An increase in corruption and arbitrary regulatory power is further ensured by making precaution and prevention the *default* assumption.

The precautionary principle cripples the technologies that can create our future because it prevents us from learning by experimenting. By halting activity, the principle reduces learning and reinforces uncertainty. As Ingo Potrykus, emeritus professor of Plant Sciences at the Swiss Federal Institute of Technology, and the inventor of Golden Rice, said: "The application of the precautionary principle in science is in itself basically anti-science. Science explores the unknown, and therefore can *a priori* not predict the outcome."

The Proactionary Principle

Scientific and technological experimentation and advance need protecting. Certainly, we should be careful and thoughtful about *how* we progress, but we must never forget that advance is vital and not inevitable. The precautionary principle and its ilk have been wielded as a means of blocking technological and economic development in general. In many other cases, entrenched interests have used it selectively to ward off new technologies that might threaten their position. Some technophiles may shrug this off, believing technological progress to be inevitable.

Apart from the general and specific enemies of change, however, we should recognize the tendency for societies to become increasingly cautious, bureaucratic, and sclerotic. Recently, several prominent friends of progress have argued that progress in many fields has slowed greatly compared to that of about a century ago, and that we may even be in the midst of a Great

Stagnation. Computer technology may continue on an exponential path of cost-performance improvement, but where are the cures for major diseases? Where are the hypersonic jets? What happened to our rising standard of living? Even if progress *is* inevitable over long periods of time, it certainly is not over a period of years and decades, which is long enough to make the difference between life and death for those of us alive today.

Curiously, others believe that, while technology is advancing rapidly and perhaps exponentially and that this is typically a good thing, it could also lead to our extinction. Extinction could come in the form of a super-intelligent artificial intelligence that does away with human beings; it could be runaway self-replicating nanomachines; or it could be engineered viruses that combine extreme infectiousness with extreme virulence. We should discuss these and other extinction risks – including those not caused by human activity, such as asteroid strikes, massive tsunamis, and gamma ray bursters – but we should not be obsessive over them to the extent that we join the supporters of the precautionary principle. Stopping progress to eliminate risk is itself risky. If certain groups will try to develop superbugs, we had better develop even faster and more powerful means to identifying and defeating them. Extinction risks, like other technological risks, point to the need for combining vigorous technological advance and wise decision-making. That is what the Proactionary Principle aims to provide.

At the center of the Proactionary Principle we find a commitment to scientific inquiry and discovery, technological innovation, and the application of science and technology to the improvement of the human condition. In a time where so many wallow in a culture of fear, the Principle champions the vigorous use of our uniquely human capabilities to improve ourselves and the world – to progress rather than regress, to advance extropy rather than to bow to entropy.

In embodying the wisdom of structure, the Principle guides decision-makers to look at many options and to consider the range of people likely to be affected. It helps decision-makers to take a *balanced* view of opportunities and risks. But let's not confuse this with being middle-of-the-road.

Preamble to the Proactionary Principle

The freedom to innovate technologically and to engage in new forms of productive activity is valuable to humanity and essential to our future. The burden of proof therefore belongs to those who propose measures to restrict new technologies. All proposed measures should be closely scrutinized. Rather than moving forward hesitantly, this means boldly stepping ahead while being mindful of where we put our feet.

A wise, balanced decision procedure will necessarily be more complex than the seductive simplicity of the precautionary principle. The exact wording of the Principle matters less than the ideas it embodies. The Principle is an inclusive, structured process for maximizing technological progress for human benefit while heightening awareness of potential side-effects and risks. In its briefest form, it says:

Progress should not bow to fear, but should proceed with eyes wide open.

More flatly stated:

Protect the freedom to innovate and progress while thinking and planning intelligently for collateral effects.

Expanded to make room for some specifics:

Encourage innovation that is bold and proactive; manage innovation for maximum human benefit; think about innovation comprehensively, objectively, and with balance.

We can call this "the" Proactionary Principle so long as we realize that the underlying Principle is less like a soundbite than a set of nested Chinese boxes or Russian babushka dolls. If we pry open the lid of this introductory-level version of the Principle, we will discover five component principles or "Pro-Actions" lying within. And for each principle, numerous best-practice tools can be deployed. Since this is an overview, not a field guide, I will not discuss any of those tools and techniques.

Here are the five component principles or Pro-Actions that comprise the Proactionary Principle:

- Be Objective and Comprehensive
- Prioritize Natural and Human Risks
- Embrace Diverse Input
- Make Response and Restitution Proportionate
- Revisit and Revise

Be Objective and Comprehensive

Big, complex decisions deserve to be tackled using a process that is objective, structured, comprehensive, and explicit. This means evaluating risks and generating alternatives and forecasts according to available science, not emotionally shaped perceptions, using the most well validated and effective methods available. Rather than reflexively huddling in committees, decision-makers should use the rich and growing body of knowledge about evidence-based methods for generating options, forecasting, and deciding. Objectivity can be improved by consistently using, for example, the devil's advocate procedure, reference-class forecasting, structured argumentation templates, and by using auditing procedures such as review panels. Different kinds of decisions and forecasts require different tools of anticipation and decision. Choosing from among a wide range of techniques will product better results.

Wise decisions will not emerge if options are limited to the obvious or politically popular. Consider all reasonable alternative actions, including no action. Estimate the opportunities lost by abandoning a technology, and take into account the costs and risks of substituting other credible options. When making these estimates, use systems thinking to carefully consider not only concentrated and immediate effects, but also widely distributed and follow-on effects, as well as the interaction of the factor under consideration with other factors. The greater the uncertainty and the less stable the situation, the less justification there is for major policy changes.

Prioritize Natural and Human Risks

Avoiding all risks is not possible. They must be assessed and compared. The fact that a risk or threat is "natural" should not give it any special status. Technological risks should be treated the same way as natural risks. Avoid underweighting natural risks and overweighting human-technological risks. Inaction can bring harm as well as action. Actions to reduce risks always incur costs and come at the expense of tackling other risks. Therefore, give priority to: reducing immediate threats over remote threats; addressing known and proven threats to human health and environmental quality over hypothetical risks; more certain over less certain threats; irreversible or persistent impacts over transient impacts; proposals that are more likely to be accomplished with the available resources; and to measures with the greatest payoff for resources invested.

Embrace Diverse Input

Take into account the interests of all potentially affected parties, and keep the process open to input from those parties or their legitimate representatives. Recognize and respect the diversity of values among people, as well as the different weights they place on shared values. Whenever feasible, enable people to make reasonable, informed tradeoffs according to their own values. Rather than banning a technology or technological product for everyone, provide information and appropriate warnings. Besides, prohibition rarely works. When it does, it abolishes the benefits of technologies. Limited experiments may be better than universal prohibition. Technologies that cause harm can often be put to different uses or applied in new, safer ways. (A drug that causes birth defects may be tremendously beneficial in people who aren't pregnant women. A pesticide may be just as beneficial and far less harmful when applied more precisely.)

Make Response and Restitution Proportionate

Consider restrictive protective measures only if the potential negative impact of an activity has both significant probability and severity. In such cases, if the activity also generates benefits, discount the impacts according to the feasibility of adapting to the adverse effects. If measures to limit technologies do appear justified, ensure that the extent of those measures is proportionate to the extent of the probable effects, and that the measures are applied as narrowly as possible while being effective. When harm has already occurred, the costs of those harms should be internalized as much as reasonably possible, such as by holding liable the producer of the technology (or the user, if they are responsible). Those responsible for harm should make restitution swiftly.

Revisit and Revise

When checking on our original decisions and the reasoning behind them, it's not good enough to rely on memory. We too readily revise our memories to fit later events. Getting in the habit of tracking assumptions, forecasts, and decisions and comparing them to actual outcomes enables an organization to learn from its mistakes. In some cases, this kind of assessment can be done continuously, improving the gains made in "learning by doing." In the case of new technologies and technological products – even when they have been thoroughly tested initially – organizations should continue to track them, especially when undesirable direct side-effects are likely (as in the case of drugs and complex software systems). Tracking technologies increasingly can help us regard daily use of technologies as continuing large-scale experiments.

All complex technological and economic decisions could be improved by applying the Proactionary Principle and its five Pro-Actions. For very large-scale policy decisions that affect millions of people and billions of dollars, we can work through the Pro-Actions in detail, bringing to bear the full panoply of tools and techniques. For simpler personal and organizational decisions, we can quickly think through the Pro-Actions to remind ourselves of considerations that might otherwise escape us unnoticed. As transhumanists, we will face decisions about using new technologies for ourselves, whether to recommend them to friends and family, and whether and in what context to advocate for them. At all these levels, the Proactionary Principle can provide guidance while protecting the imperative to progress.

27

The Open Society and Its Media

Mark S. Miller

with E. Dean Tribble, Ravi Pandya, and Marc Stiegler

Electronic media present tremendous opportunities for improving the nature of society. I will address how discourse affects society, and how changes in media may improve societal discourse. Then I will describe the Xanadu[1] system, and how it was built to achieve these goals.

Improving Society

Improving society is a difficult task. More generally, improving complex systems is a difficult task. If you cannot figure out which way is up, see if you can figure out which way is down. Doug Engelbart, back in the early 1960s, wanted to explain to people why interactive systems would make a significant difference to their lives, and to their ability to express ideas. The origin on the axis is what people were doing at the time – writing with pencil and paper. When he found himself unable to communicate to people how much better things could be, he contrasted their current experiences with how much *worse* things could be. He tied a pencil to a brick, handed it to people and said, "Okay, now write." People found it very difficult. The unwieldy nature of the tool interfered with their ability to express ideas. With the pencil and brick for contrast, he effectively asked two questions: "What made the difference?" and "How can we move further in the other direction?" (Engelbart 1962). This experiment showed people how important their tools and their media were to their effectiveness, and helped them start to see the next brick to remove.

Karl Marx performed a similar experiment on society over the course of most of this [the twentieth] century. Karl Marx tied a very large brick to a very large pencil and the last few years have revealed the result to be far worse than the even his harshest critics imagined (Popper

Originally published in *Extropy: The Journal of Transhumanist Thought* 12 (1994). Copyright © Max More.

The Transhumanist Reader: Classical and Contemporary Essays on the Science, Technology, and Philosophy of the Human Future, First Edition. Edited by Max More and Natasha Vita-More.
© 2013 John Wiley & Sons, Inc. Published 2013 by John Wiley & Sons, Inc.

1950). What made the difference between the societies? Two important elements were open markets and open media. How can we move farther in the other direction? In this presentation, I will be addressing the nature of open media, how they differ from closed media, and how social hypertext systems can enhance the advantages of those media. Applying information technologies to the further opening of markets is left as a mission for the reader.

Media Matter

Media matter, because it is in media that the knowledge of society evolves. The health of the process by which that knowledge evolves is critical to the way society changes. Karl Popper, the epistemologist, had the insight that knowledge evolves by a process of variation, replication, and selection, much as biology does. "Variation of knowledge" is what we call "conjecture" – hypothesis formation, tossing new ideas out there. "Replication of knowledge" is the spread of ideas through publication and conversation. "Selection of knowledge" is the discrediting of conjectures through the process of criticism.[2] The ability of our knowledge to progress over time depends on an ongoing process of criticism, and criticism of criticism. The ideas that survive the critical process tend, in general, to be better than those that do not.

In closed societies, when arguments cannot be spoken, hard truths cannot be figured out. When people cannot openly criticize, cannot openly defend against criticism, or cannot openly propose ideas that conflict with the official truths, then they are left with mistrust and cynicism as their only defense. This leads to the simple heuristic of assuming the official truth is always wrong. For example, because *science* was promoted by the Soviet propaganda machine, pseudo-science is on the rise in Russia. Because anti-Nazism was promoted by the East German propaganda machine, Neo-Nazism is on the rise in East Germany. The official truth is neither always right nor always wrong. Society needs a more sophisticated process for judging claims.

Our society does have open media. Are we in the best of all possible worlds? Are our media good enough? Can they be made significantly better? Among our media, TV is so bad that it is a joke. Only slogan-sized ideas can be expressed. We prize the quality of discourse in our books and journals, but critical discussions in them are only loosely connected. Starting from the expression of an idea, it is hard to find articles that criticize that idea. When arguments cannot be found and navigated, the next harder truths *still* cannot be figured out.

Xanadu

I rejoined Xanadu in 1988 largely because of fear about the dangers of nanotechnology, coupled with incredible excitement about the promises of nanotechnology. In looking at the dangers, I saw that none of us individually is clever enough to figure out how to solve those problems. The only hope that I saw in 1988 – I no longer believe it is the only hope – is that by creating better media for the process of societal discourse and societal decision-making, we stand a much better chance of surviving the dangers posed by new technologies, so that we may live to enjoy their benefits.

I am about to go through the elements of the hypertext system we built. Xanadu has frequently been called Golden Vaporware, and many people have wondered whether this is a never-ending project. One of the things I want to emphasize when I go through all of these features is that I am only referring to the features that are now running in the software. We planned on and anticipate other features, some of which will be mentioned in the *future plans* discussion, but the body of this presentation will only cover what is implemented and running.

First, I will discuss the four fundamental features – links, transclusion, versioning, and detectors. Marc Stiegler will then present an example using them. Then I will describe the remaining four features – permissions, reputation-based filtering, multimedia, and external transclusion, followed by some concluding remarks.

Links

Hypertext links are directly inspired by literary practice. Literature has many different kinds of links connecting documents into a vast web. Textual examples of these links include bibliographical references, marginal notes, quotation, footnotes, and Post-it notes.

We propose to build engines of citation, so that people can navigate this vast web of literature at the click of a mouse. Most computer text systems are predicated on a misconception that the meaning of a document is represented purely or primarily by its content. Documents are not islands. Conventional computer text systems put their effort into the appearance of individual documents. My experience in reading documents (especially reading a literature with which I am not familiar) is that it is difficult to understand documents without their context. A context helps answer questions such as "What were the ongoing controversies that the author had in mind?" "What views was he supporting or attacking?" "What attacks was he guarding against?" We must understand this whole web of connections in order to understand the documents we are reading. The Xanadu system is built to provide as much support for this contextual information as for content.

With the ability to follow the links in this vast web of documents, is it not easy to get lost? How does one stay oriented? One answer to these questions is *guides*, a new kind of document that provides an orienting view together with links into the existing literature. I expect guides to come largely from people making their own organizing views of a literature and then cleaning them up for publication, so others may benefit from their work.

Hyperlinks

Because "nanotechnology" is now used by many to mean any technology approaching the nanometer scale, we have been forced to retreat to the term "molecular nanotechnology." Hypertext terminology has gone through a drift similar to nanotech terminology. The Xanadu project is the one that coined the term "hypertext" and originated the notion of the hypertext "link." However, because the term *link* has come to be viewed as something much less capable than what we meant by it, we are now calling it the *hyperlink*. The distinction between the link and the hyperlink is crucial for supporting active criticism in open media.

Hyperlinks are fine-grained, bidirectional, and extrinsic. Frequently, an argument is not with a document or chapter as a whole. It is with a particular point that someone made at a particular place in the text. For example, someone refers to the fourth law of thermodynamics, and someone else writes a criticism saying there is no fourth law of thermodynamics, linking it to the original. The fine-grained property allows the link to designate the particular piece of text with which one is taking issue. Bidirectionality enables readers of the original document to find the criticism, enabling them to exercise fine-grained skepticism, and to constantly ask themselves, "What is the best argument against the thing I am reading *right now*?" and then, "What is the best argument against that, in turn?" Links provided by other hypertext systems generally have been only in the forward direction, enabling a reader to find those documents *referenced by* a given document. However, to find criticism, the reader must find the documents that *refer to* the document they are reading.

Extrinsic linking is the ability to link into a document without editing it. Several other systems support the creation of links that are fine-grained at the targeted end, but these others do so only by modifying both source and *target* documents.[3] Critics normally will not have the ability to modify the documents they are criticizing. They could spin off their own version into which they attach these links, but then other readers *still* cannot find these criticisms from the original documents.

Part of what we mean by "open media" is that everyone who is connected to the system can read what they are permitted to read, can write new things, and can make them accessible for others to read. This includes making links to anything that they have read, so that anyone else who reads the original can find the material that has been linked to it. All readers of the system are potential authors. We can think of this process as *active reading*. Frequently, people make marginal notes to themselves. This is a medium in which readers can share such things with each other. When much writing is commentary about other text, the commented-on text is the best rendezvous point for the authors and readers of commentary to find each other.

Emergent Properties

This kind of accessible criticism can provide for decentralized consumer reports. When people post on the system documents that are either products or descriptions of products, customers of those products can post criticisms of them. What did they think of using them? This commentary can guide the purchasing decisions of others.[4]

A particular capability we are used to in conversation (one that is almost impossible to successfully attain using paper-based literature) is hearing the absence of a good response to an argument. A reader not only can see what the most compelling arguments are against some statement, but also see when there are none, or when all the seemingly compelling arguments have been successfully refuted. Such absences are quite obvious in conversation. Electronic media can make these absences obvious as well, but in a context where the absence will be much more telling, because the missing argument could have come from a much larger audience over a more extended period of time.

Other hypertext systems with their unidirectional links reproduce the asymmetry present in our paper-based media – it is much easier to find something that a document cites than it is to find those documents that cite a given document. One of the effects of this asymmetry in paper media is the pathological division of scholarly fields into disjoint "schools." Instead of healthy intellectual engagement, debate, and cross-fertilization of ideas, we see a process of increasing inability to communicate between schools, and more preaching to the converted within a school. The terrible irony of attempting scholarship with unidirectional links is that *the very attempt to engage in healthy debate across schools accelerates the pathological division process*. How does this occur?

Let us consider two schools within a discipline. Generally, students within a school see the documents supporting the positions of that school. The students also see criticisms of documents in the other school. Intellectually eager and honest students, seeking to know both sides, occasionally will follow these criticism links forward. The result is that they will see the parts of the other school's literature that is *most soundly criticized* by their own school, immunizing them more and more against the foreign ideas. With bidirectional links, these students can also find the greatest challenges to their own school. Bidirectional links also enable them to find the *most telling criticisms* of the ideas they are inclined to accept.

Transclusion

Before there were modem economies, there were many little villages, each with their own little manufacturers having to go through a large amount of the production process themselves. These economies were, therefore, much less productive. An individual baker or shoemaker, for example, would reproduce the same kind of work that was being reproduced in many other villages, and would have to fashion a shoe, not quite from raw materials, but without intermediate goods. In extended economies, people can build on one another's work, and there can be a finer-grained division of labor and knowledge, with better specialization.

Now, with respect to literature, authors are frequently faced with the task of re-explaining and restating background material that has been explained well elsewhere. If you could just borrow that material, those existing good explanations, and incorporate them (with automatic credit where due), your efforts could be spent stating what is new. We introduce the concept of *transclusion* to separate the arrangement of a document from its content. There is an underlying shared pool of contents, and all documents are just arrangements of pieces from that pool. [For example, imagining] three circled appearances of the same text are actually just one piece of text in the underlying shared pool of contents, and it just happens to appear in three different arrangements which constitute three different documents. We refer to the three documents as *transcluding* that piece of text. The separation of content and arrangement also leads to good support for incremental editing. Different versions of a document are just different arrangements of mostly shared content.

This is more than just a hack to avoid the storage cost of making separate copies. Hyperlinks are linked to the content, not to a span in an arrangement. Therefore, when someone writes a criticism of content as it appears in one arrangement, that criticism is visible for the same content as it appears in all other arrangements, including arrangements that were made before the criticism was attached. The normal incremental editing process of a single document is analogous to *evolution by point mutation*. The ability to transclude text from other documents allows the analog of sexual recombination. Were links visible only from the arrangement into which they were made, both variation processes would destroy selection pressures by leaving criticisms behind.

Remembering the Past: Historical Trails

As you are editing, an *historical trail* gets left behind – breadcrumbs in history space. The historical trail is simply a sequential arrangement of the successive arrangements of contents. This is yet another kind of context important for understanding. "Things are the way they are because they got that way" (Weinberg 1985).

Understanding *how* they got that way often aids our understanding of what *they are*.

Preparing for the Future: Detectors

In addition to looking into the past, one also reads a literature knowing it will be changing. How can one keep up? To keep track of what is happening, to keep up with changes, we introduce *detectors*. One can post a *revision detector* to find out when things are edited, when new versions of something appear, and then one can use *version compare* to find out how they are different. With version compare, one can engage in *differential reading* – reading just the differences between the current version and the version most recently read.

Link detectors are a way of finding out when new links are made to existing material. Let us say that you published something, and you want to find out when others post comments on it. You would like to be informed of comments, but you do not want to have to go back and constantly recheck all the things that you have written, so you post a link detector on all the things that you have written, as well as on other documents on which you are interested in seeing further comments. You want to see what people will say about them. As new comments are posted on those documents, you are continually informed.

Email is just the special case where you establish a canonical point in the literature, for each person – a place others link to in order to send that person a message. That person simply has a link detector there saying, "Show me all new things that are attached to *here*." This generalizes to treating any shared point of interest in the literature as, in some sense, a "mailbox," or a "meeting room" for further conversation or conferencing about a topic. Canonical documents become meeting places. Should two disjoint discussions about the same topic spontaneously form in two places, anyone who notices can just make a link between them. The link detectors of each community will then inform them of the existence of the other.

At this point, I will shift over [to the work of] Mark Stiegler and Dean Tribble, who demonstrate, using the Xanadu software, an example involving exactly the elements discussed so far.

The WidgetPerfect Saga

This is a tongue-in-cheek story about how a hypertext system was able to save several thousand jobs. One special characteristic about this story is that it is a story from the year 1997.[5] It is a story about one of the events that took place at the company – most of you have heard of it – called WidgetPerfect. WidgetPerfect is the second largest manufacturer of widgets in the world, second only to their big competitor, Microwidget. The people at WidgetPerfect in the year 1997 had identified a really significant opportunity in the upcoming expanding environment of widget components technology.

They were developing the world's first fully modular widget. They had a team working on it. Dan Tribble was in charge of the preparation of the marketing materials for the modular widget. Ruth was in charge of the technical work team, and John was in charge of the budget and finance, as well as all the costing. At this point, the modular widget was in prototype stage when a very unfortunate thing happened. Microwidget, the big competitor, came out with a partially modular widget, hitting the marketplace first with an inferior product. It was technically inferior, but nonetheless it was in the marketplace first.

Dan was examining this Microwidget, partially modular widget, and it was overall inferior. Nonetheless, it had one really striking improved feature. It had a funculator made out of titanalum, whereas the fully modular widget that was being developed by Ruth only had a duralum funculator. This was an important improvement for certain key market sectors. Even though the partially modular widget did not have anything comparable to a thermoplastic coupler or a hypervelocity rotator, they had to make a change.

So, Dan created a new document in the marketing requirements describing this titanalum funculator. He attached a link to the part of the technical plan that specifically referred to the duralum funculator in the current plan. He made that a new requirement.

Now, Dan knew that in order to get anything to happen with improving the widget prototype, he would have to talk to Ruth. He was reaching for the telephone to call Ruth when Boeing, the largest purchaser of widgets in the world, called him about a $15 million widget order. He got distracted with this purchase, and he never quite got around to calling Ruth.

We have good news. Ruth, knowing that the success of her technical design depended on her being able to respond promptly to new requirements, had attached a link detector to her technical plan. This link detector would be constantly watching for new links of the link-type *requirement* to be attached. When Dan attached the new requirement to the duralum funculator, Ruth's link detector went off. Ruth was alerted. She followed the link detector out to the link, followed the link back to the new requirement, saw what the required change was, and modified the technical plan to reflect the use of a titanalum funculator.

Well, this was all very fine, except for an additional problem. As I think everyone here knows, titanalum is considerably more expensive than duralum, and so this had some significant effect on the manufacturing cost. Ruth knew that this would have an impact on the budget, and she was reaching for the telephone to call John when smoke started billowing from the laboratory where the prototype of the modular widget was being manufactured. She ran off to deal with the emergency and never quite got around to calling John.

We have good news. John, knowing the success of his budget was completely dependent on his responding to modifications to the technical plan, had attached a revision detector to the technical plan and this detector was constantly watching for updates. So, when the technical plan was indeed updated, John's revision detector went off. He followed the revision detector up to the technical plan, used the hypertextual version compare capabilities based on the transclusion relations, compared the new version of the plan to the old, and found that the change was deleting duralum and replacing it with titanalum. He then went back into the budget and updated the budget documents to reflect the increased costs caused by the use of titanalum.

As a consequence of this, the modular widget program was completed on time with a fully adequate specification. It was a completely superior product. It blew Microwidget off the face of the Earth. As a consequence, thousands of jobs at WidgetPerfect were saved.

Permissions

A social system, to a large extent, is a system of rights and responsibilities. Xanadu has an extensive permission system called the *club* system, intended to deal with some of these issues. Bob has sent it as a mail message to various people in a blind carbon copy ("bcc") relationship. Alice and Chuck are both members of the *bcc* club of people who have permission to read this document. Bob, though, is the only member who can read or edit the *bcc* club. If this were a *cc* list, Bob would still be the only person who could edit it, but it would be self-reading. Everybody who was a member of such a *cc* club could see who else was a member of that same club.

This demonstrates a principled answer to permissions *meta-issues* – one can distinguish between who can read a document, who can read the list of people who can read a document, and who can read that list, out to any desired degree of distinction (and similarly for the editing dimension). However, infinite regress and needless complexity are avoided by using clubs that are self-reading or self-editing (or both) whenever further distinction is currently not necessary. Should such distinction later become necessary, it can always be introduced by someone with appropriate edit permission to the club in question. Users only grow meta-levels on an as-needed basis.

Our permission system also supports the notion of *accountability*. All actions in the system are taken *by someone*. When you look at information in the system, you see some identity attached to the actions taken on the information. There are no official truths. There is only who said what, and the structure of the system reflects that.

Reputation-Based Filtering

One of the potential pitfalls of an open hypertext system is the junk problem. The ability to find good commentary and criticism will be especially important when reading very important documents, but it is precisely on *these* documents that one expects to be inundated with tons of worthless or irrelevant links. Without a filtering mechanism, it would be on exactly the documents for which one most needs good commentary that the provision of commentary would be most useless. For example, imagine how many links there would be onto the First Amendment to the Constitution.

Links can be *endorsed* as worth reading by various readers. However, no one may endorse with the identity of another. Different endorsers will establish varying reputations with different readers, much as with movie reviewers. Readers can filter their views of links into a document both by *who* endorsed as well as by link-type. When even this mechanism gives too coarse an answer, one can rely on documents such as a hypothetical *Guide to the Citations to the Bill of Rights*, endorsed by a reputable publishing house. This very same link-filtering ability is also what allows one to find such guides in the presence of a swamp of links.

Hypertext + Multimedia = Hypermedia

Increasingly, ideas are being expressed in media other than text, and increasingly, computers are used to handle these other media. We usually refer to *hypertext* because text is the most important case and the clearest example. However, nothing I have presented, none of the things you have seen the system do, is in any way specific to text, or even to media that have linear flow to them. It all applies equally well to a variety of other media (such as sound, engineering drawings, Postscript images, and compressed video). In all cases, one can make fine-grained links, edits, transclusions, and version compares (even if the data is block-compressed or block-encrypted). Although the implementation has some optimizations targeted at text, in no way does the *architecture* make any special cases for text. Documents can, of course, be composite arrangements in which several media are mixed together.

External Transclusion

No software system is an island. We do not imagine that once the product is available, everyone will instantly take all information to which they want access and transfer it into Xanadu. We have to coexist with many other systems for many good reasons.

We handle that with *external transclusion*. Our documents are able to transclude into arrangements that are within the system. These, in turn, are able to represent transclusions of materials that are stored elsewhere. By perceiving other systems through the window of Xanadu, you can see those other systems as if all those documents were within the Xanadu system. Through Xanadu, I could follow a link from a WAIS document into a Lexis document, even though neither system has any notion that such a link even exists. It is not just that the Xanadu system is not an island that we have to coexist with everything else; it is that through Xanadu, *those* systems are able to coexist with each other in a way they are unable to now, making *them* into non-islands.

Conclusions

When we started building the system, we were thinking purely in terms of paper-based literature – of writing. What we have built is something that has many of the best aspects of both writing and conversation. Many of the aspects of each are complementary. Many virtues of conversation make up for flaws in writing and vice versa. We found ourselves building a system that supports the dynamic give-and-take of conversation, and the persistence and thoughtfulness of literature.

Our status is that we currently have a working, portable server. It has some bugs in it, including some performance bugs, but we are working on it. However, all the features that I talked about so far, work. We are continuing ahead with the effort on both the server and the front end. The front end is in a preliminary stage. We consider it adequate to show that the server is real, and to exercise its features. We plan to do a much better front end. The protocol between the front end and the server is very stable, and has been stable for a long time now. Our plans are to get investors, and to finish both the front end and the server. The target for our first product is small to medium-sized workgroups within companies that have a large body of documents they need to be managing and evolving.

Our first product lacks one major feature. We provide hypertext because documents are not islands. We make the system interpersonal because people are not islands. We provide for the transparent windowing into other systems because no product is an island. However, for the moment, each server is still an island with respect to the other servers, and so each workgroup is also an island. We have designed the system so that, soon after first product, we will be able to weave all the servers together into a transparent distributed system. When you follow a link from one document to another, if the other document is not here but in some server in Tokyo, it will be transparently fetched for you, and the only thing you will notice is that following that link took longer.

For any media to radically improve the process of opinion formation in society, we believe it *needs* features equivalent to fine-grained, bidirectional, extrinsic, filtered links. These links must not get lost when the documents to which they are attached change. Issues of authority, privacy, and responsibility must be handled in a robust and secure fashion. Open entry of readers and editors is crucial for open discussion. Open entry of server providers is less obvious, but equally important, in order to make centralized control impossible. We will be providing support for people who want to do online services based on our software. All of this is necessary to achieve our open electronic publishing dream. In so doing, we hope to improve the quality of public debate, in order to obtain the benefits of the open society yet again.

Notes

We thank the whole extended Xanadu team for having struggled together for many years on a project that has been at least as much a cause as a business. We thank Eric Drexler for exploring the relationship of hypertext publishing to evolutionary epistemology (Drexler 1991). We thank Anita Shreve for extensive help in editing this presentation.

1   The Xanadu trademark has since become the sole property of Ted Nelson.
2   Karl Popper originally proposed that selection proceeds by a process of refutation. See Popper 1959. His student, William Bartley, generalized this to criticism. See Bartley 1962.
3   Examples include World Wide Web *anchors*, Microsoft Word *bookmarks*, Lotus Notes, and Folio Views *Popup text*.
4   The use of bidirectional links for decentralized consumer reports is already happening on the American Information Exchange.
5   This essay was written well before 1997, thus the fictitious *tongue-in-cheek* story is actually a hypothetical scenario about electronic media.

References

Bartley, William W. III (1962) *The Retreat to Commitment*. Chicago: Open Court Publishing.
Drexler, K. Eric (1991) "Hypertext Publishing and the Evolution of Knowledge." *Social Intelligence* 1/2.
Engelbart, Douglas C. (1962) "Augmenting Human Intellect: A Conceptual Framework." *SRI Project* 3578 (October).
Popper, Karl R. (1950) *The Open Society and its Enemies*. Princeton, N.J.: Princeton University Press.
Popper, Karl R. (1959) *The Logic of Scientific Discovery*. New York: Harper & Row.
Weinberg, Gerald M. (1985) *The Secrets of Consulting*. New York: Dorset House Publishing.

Part VII

Biopolitics and Policy

In the late 1980s and early 1990s, the emphasis of transhumanism was primarily on exploring technological possibilities and supporting the feasibility and desirability of technological transformation. As far more people have come to accept the plausibility of the core technologies that interest transhumanists – often referred to as NBIC (nano-bio-info-cogno technologies) – the original emphasis has shifted. Currently, much more thought is devoted to exploring the potential downsides to the core technologies of today and tomorrow, and how best to avoid negative impacts through strategy and sometimes by regulating them. At the same time, a new but more sophisticated advocacy has developed to engage in discussions and debates with bioconservatives and other participants in biopolitical debates. Seven essays in Part VII delve into crucial aspects of biopolitical discussions.

In "Performance Enhancement and Legal Theory", law professor Michael Shapiro clarifies some of the major ethical and policy issues concerning performance enhancement in sports, games, and contests. Shapiro explains "moral category" arguments such as arguments from nature, arguments from identity, from merit, and from external influence, and argues that there are serious problems in distinguishing disorder from augmentation models. This matters because some people have argued in favor of allowing treatments for disorders while prohibiting them for augmentations that are otherwise similar in nature.

Philosopher Andy Miah casts a critical eye on Donna Haraway's concept of the "cyborg" and Francis Fukuyama's views on "posthumanism." Miah argues that the technoprogressive pursuit of biological transgressions can enrich individual and collective human life, while also permitting societies to attend to any social injustices that might arise through such behavior. Miah concludes with a full articulation of the concept of "biocultural capital," which conveys a general, transhumanist justification for human enhancement.

The Transhumanist Reader: Classical and Contemporary Essays on the Science, Technology, and Philosophy of the Human Future, First Edition. Edited by Max More and Natasha Vita-More.
© 2013 John Wiley & Sons, Inc. Published 2013 by John Wiley & Sons, Inc.

Biophysicist Gregory Stock, author of several books on biotechnology and our future, and a participant in Extropy Institute's Biotech Futures conference in 1999, has examined in depth genetic engineering as a crucial technology for the biological path to transhumanist goals. (Others emphasize pathways based on information technology or nanotechnology.) In an excerpt from his 2002 book, *Redesigning Humans: Our Inevitable Genetic Future*, Stock asks whether there must be a battle over the use of technologies such as germline manipulation and in-depth embryo diagnosis. Stock contends that the discussion about human enhancement is not about medical safety, the wellbeing of children, or protecting the human gene pool; it's really about "about what it means to be human, about our vision of the human future." That is why critics like Leon Kass, formerly on the President's Council for Bioethics, urges "the wisdom of repugnance" more than he relies on specific, fact-based arguments.

Transgendered entrepreneur and inventor Martine Rothblatt looks at morphological freedom from a transgender perspective. Rothblatt looks ahead to a time when we may be able to separate our minds from our biological bodies by merging a "mindfile" of our neural connections with "mindware," allowing us to exist as software that could run on hardware of our choice. Rothblatt discusses the sex of an avatar, the option of operating multiple bodies, and why claims for transhuman civil rights may be based in part on increasing legal recognition of claims for transgender civil rights. In both cases, we seek to transcend an unchosen biological form in favor of recognizing the status of all conscious life.

Critics of transhumanist goals have sometimes claimed that the technologies that enable human physical and intellectual enhancement undermine virtue. Prolific author Ronald Bailey argues that enhancements will better enable people to flourish, that enhancements will not dissolve whatever existential crisis people feel, and that enhancements will enable people to become more virtuous. People should be free to refuse enhancements for themselves but should accord others the liberty to adopt them. While there will inevitably be resulting issues to deal with, Bailey argues that social concerns over an "enhancement divide" are largely illusory, and that we already have at hand the social "technology" that will enable the enhanced and the unenhanced to dwell together peacefully.

In a piece that effectively complements the Sandberg contribution, Patrick D. Hopkins considers the problems that may arise if we put the question of enhancement in terms of rights. Although rights language does have theoretical problems, such language plays a powerful role in the moral and legal landscape. But if transhumanists are to engage in talks of rights, they should understand the relative strengths and weaknesses of basing rights on appeals to autonomy, interests, and natural law. He finds the appeal to autonomy to be the weakest strategy. Appeals to interests – those things widely recognized as valuable, worthwhile, and even necessary for a life worth having had – and to the values of natural law – life, health, knowledge, and sociability – help show that enhancements can be noble and worthy and not unnatural or alien to human nature.

Professor Wrye Sententia considers the role of brain privacy, autonomy, and choice in relation to technological advances concerning the brain. She examines the legal implications of restricting cognitive liberty and ethical grounds for individual autonomy over the use and scope of technology. Cognitive liberty asserts the right to cognitive self-design: to cognitive enhancement, brain privacy, autonomy, and choice in relation to existing pharmacology, as well as anticipated technologies expected to be capable of modifying the brain.

Performance Enhancement and Legal Theory
An Interview with Professor Michael H. Shapiro

Which performance enhancement technologies do you think will raise the most interesting or problematic legal and ethical issues?

Some technologies emerging from the research being done now will, at least at first, be used within a disorder model. Let me comment on disorder models and the meaning of "enhancement." The terms "enhancement" and "augmentation"[1] are problematic – not meaningless, but hard to interpret. You can set up the problem in the following way: There are lots of things that we do to improve our situations that don't seem troublesome to most people. The prime example is placing these processes within a justificatory model based on remedying disorder, trauma, or the like. We don't think of these procedures as enhancement because they target (in theory) only disorders, injuries, and defects and (again in theory) generate only the improvement resulting from cure or palliation. Models are, roughly, abstract guides to action or evaluation or analysis generally. A disorder model has axioms of the form: If P has disease X, then P may (should? must?) use therapy Z to rectify the situation. This account leaves out various qualifications we can ignore for a time. We don't have to deal with whether the person can be forced to be treated – although it will turn out to be very interesting to consider whether some persons entrusted with complex tasks in either the public or private sectors can be required to accept technological enhancement in order to remain on the job. Of course, when readers of *Extropy* think about enhancement, they're certainly not confining themselves to matters of controlling disorder – they may not even think of the latter as true enhancement, although remedying diseases and injuries generally leaves one better able to perform than while ill. Also, we generally view traditional minor forms of enhancement (like caffeine) as part of a baseline that defines acceptability. Sometimes history serves to ratify practices that might be questioned on some theory. (Treating forms of attention deficit disorder with stimulants is, in theory, within the disorder model.)

In an article I wrote on performance enhancement in the *Southern California Law Review* in 1991, I started off with some examples to illustrate the distinction between enhancement and therapy. Kirk Gibson used cortisone for a bad knee and hit a home run that helped win the opening game of the 1988 World Series for the Dodgers. On the other hand, in the same year, Ben Johnson ran in the Olympics but was found to have taken steroids. This was not for medical purposes, however, and the Olympic officials nullified his victory.

The Transhumanist Reader: Classical and Contemporary Essays on the Science, Technology, and Philosophy of the Human Future, First Edition. Edited by Max More and Natasha Vita-More.
© 2013 John Wiley & Sons, Inc. Published 2013 by John Wiley & Sons, Inc.

But there are situations that are somewhat more ambiguous, and this is reflected in the law: the steroid problem in athletic competition inspired some statutes. They were meant to deal with these two primary justificatory models – disorder and augmentation. For example, in Florida, there's a statute that says: "Prescribing, ordering, dispensing, administering, supplying, selling, or giving growth hormones, testosterone or its analogs, human chorionic gonadotropin (HCG), or other hormones for the purpose of muscle building or to enhance athletic performance [are grounds for professional discipline]. For the purposes of this subsection, the term 'muscle building' does not include the treatment of injured muscle. A prescription written for the drug products listed above may be dispensed by the pharmacist with the presumption that the prescription is for legitimate medical use."[2]

Well, of course, one puzzle is that if you treat injured muscle, or fix broken bones, or give cortisone for a bad knee, you're improving performance, but you should still get a "therapeutic exemption."[3] But, you might say, it's bringing a person up to a previous baseline, so it's natural. These substances have dual uses, of course, and their effects and purposes may be hard to separate. What if the therapy takes you past your personal baseline – or even beyond assumed human limits?

Some argue that nature has some kind of moral force linked to it. But what you're doing when you give athletes steroids – or enhancers to anyone – is to try to raise them above their natural baseline.

But suppose someone with a lot of athletic talent is born with a predisposition for chronic arthritis and finally is given cortisone as an adult. This person never had a prior "normal" baseline. The most you can say is that there is a rough ideal normal baseline – that is, normal to the human species – that the person has always fallen short of. It's still a disorder model that's invoked to treat the arthritis, and the fact that it's "baseline" for that person doesn't suggest that treatment is questionable.

What about people who take caffeine for headaches? If I take commercial acetaminophen (Tylenol), which contains caffeine for additional pain control, it may improve my performance *both* by relieving the headache and by the stimulant effect. Sometimes musical performers will use beta blockers to keep their hands from trembling or to steady their voices. Substances which are generally thought to be performance *dampers* in some contexts may be performance enhancers in others. For example, people who are in rifle competitions might want to drink an alcoholic beverage.[4] It can reduce their tremors and calm them down. So, you have to sort out exactly what is being done for what purpose and consider what system of justification we're talking about – and whether that justifying model *should* make any difference.

The last point should be stressed. The very reason for distinguishing disorder from augmentation models is seriously in question, quite apart from the expectable difficulty of drawing boundaries between them.

To focus more on your question about legal and ethical issues, here are some examples: Think about human growth hormone [HGH]. There are people with diseases of the pituitary who are extremely short. I think many would agree that it's okay to give them human growth hormone – maybe even obligatory – provided we satisfy ourselves about the costs, which have to be weighed against the benefits. (The normative risks include the implied put-down of short stature.) We can leave aside for the time being the question of the child's current preferences.

But what about other persons who have no pathology underlying their short stature? Suppose you're a child predicted simply to be at the low end of what seems like normal variation in the bell curve of height. You'll just be very short – say, an adult male who's less than five feet tall – and you'll have trouble reaching the gas pedal on a car, people will be bumping into or falling over you, you won't get dates, and perhaps you won't advance in your career. What do we say here? You can try to view this situation under a "handicap" model instead of a disorder model – that is, the person is considered operationally impaired compared to the species norm, questions of disorder aside. But perhaps this is just evacuating the disease model, replacing it with an augmentation model in order to get to the species baseline, though not necessarily rising above it. In any case, why are only the disordered the only acceptable candidates for medical treatment with HGH? And why can't they go past the baseline?

One difficulty in condemning enhancement is that we all accept it in some form – even technological – as part of our shifting baseline of what's normal and acceptable. For example: I was going down the hall near my office and one of our visiting professors was walking in my direction. He had a cup of coffee in each hand. I said, "*Two* cups of coffee?" And he said, "Gotta be sharp!" But historically few people worry about caffeine use – side-effects aside – except in specific situations like athletic competition, though there is increasing grumbling about it.[5] There's no disorder model at work (treatment of headache, narcolepsy, etc., aside), but the augmentation is fairly modest.[6]

In the case of performance enhancement in sports, games, and contests – we might call admission to universities contests – I've divided up the analysis into several overlapping dimensions, which apply both to physical and mental enhancement. They are all morally freighted. There are *rigid moral category* arguments based on certain ill-defined concepts that misleadingly *appear* (to some) to be well defined – but they aren't – and purport to tell you in an algorithmic way what you can and can't do – but they don't. They include "nature" or "nature's gifts," "identity," and the "internal/external" contrast. The reason I have these moral category arguments set up like this is that they are often used in a ham-fisted, formalistic way. They are a partially reified and partially distorted subset of moral argument generally, but of course not distinct from such argument. The contrast here is not between using moral and nonmoral considerations, but between using moral concepts rationally as opposed to fashioning them into highly abstract and functionally inflexible moral categories of judgment. But, to emphasize, all moral category arguments, sound or ham-fisted or not, are moral arguments. Arguments resting on "frozen" moral categories are only particular forms of moral argument. Many of them overlap; some may be extensionally equivalent. For example, the loss of the sense of "gift" or "givenness" may be a trope for arguments from nature, or from Gods' Bounty. They may also suggest a kind of moral risk aversion: messing with What Is portends moral culpability – as well as moral heroism – for what we might do as trait (or even species) Creators. Such expanded realms of choice are novel in many respects, and they entail expanded realms of personal moral responsibility – a fearful and oppressive prospect for some, a grand opportunity for others. But the anti-enhancement argument based on giftedness[7] collides with the *Imago Dei* framework: we implement God's will by accepting creative powers based on the idea that humanity was created in the image of God.

So, the moral category arguments include overlapping sub-arguments, such as arguments from nature, arguments from identity, from merit, and from external influence. The natural/unnatural distinction generally lacks decisive power here. Nature may often thought to be morally weighted, but this moral weight, if any, is pretty attenuated. Still, you can often take what is natural – assuming you can define it at all – as a default guide to something that works; it can *sometimes* serve as a useful starting point.[8] But the presumption that it is a good guide to rectitude is often overcome: it's not natural to take antibiotics, for example. What people mean by "natural" or "unnatural" I think is whether or not it conforms to what has become part of the normal baseline for human beings – such as wearing clothes. We call it "natural" because it's traditional, useful, largely harmless, and seems instinct with surviving in nature. In this sense, it's natural for us to put clothes on, but obviously it's unnatural in some other, narrower sense. It is instructive to compare the different senses. I'll say some more about moral category arguments later.

There are also arguments based upon *harm and coercion*. Of course these are also moral arguments and make for legal arguments too. They appear to be somewhat less fixed and the arguments are often made in a less formalistic way than in the domain of more rigid forms of moral category. They gain some additional force where the technology is very risky – but of course traditional training, not to mention the sport itself, can be risky too. It's not always clear what the incremental risk is when – or if – the technology is used properly.

Next there are analytic paths I call *competitive coherence* arguments, whether concerning sports or other contests or games. People will say things like: "You cannot have performance enhancement in contests because it defeats the entire purpose of the game." In some forms these arguments make no sense because they circularly assume that enhancement is prohibited. But our question is whether there *ought* to be prohibition or constraint in the first place. The real issue concerns the situation where there is no prohibition, but competitors might be required to disclose what they're using. Without such disclosure, you'd have a different kind of game that you might not want, but it wouldn't (necessarily) be *incoherent*. "Breaking the rules" might not even be cheating (and so would be "within the rules," in a different sense of "the rules"), given how the game is defined and actually *performed*. We *expect* deliberate fouling in basketball, for example, and many expect irreparable actions inconsistent with "the rules," as in baseball.[9]

Finally, I invoke a set of arguments called *normative-systemic* arguments – they might be called social or institutional arguments – which seem to me to be the only arguments that make any sense, when part of a larger moral argument. But they aren't overwhelming either.

Suppose, for example, you have a performance enhancement technology that is extremely risky. There was a poll taken – how credible I can't tell – reported in Reuters in 1988, in which Olympic athletes were asked something like: "If you knew you could take this drug and you knew it would guarantee you a gold medal but would kill you five years later, would you take it?" Supposedly half of them said yes, but who knows whether they'd actually do it when confronted with it? Taking polls may be necessary to catch a glimmer of supposed facts, but they may not give you a firm grip on them.[10]

Now, here's a thought experiment to illustrate the argument: I have an 8-year-old and a 4-year-old. Do I want them to think it's okay to make that deal? Is it that important to get a gold medal, at the price of dying at an early age? That exchange seems to me to be bizarre – but of course I've never been an elite athlete with a chance for glory. Under *some* moral theories, including even autonomy theories, it would be wrong to take such risks; *future* autonomy would be totally shut down. Still, if some people already have this gold-medal-but-die-early preference, there are autonomy-based reasons for letting them go ahead with it, although there are counter-arguments from a variety of moral frameworks. But the question here is: can and should we control the acquisition of these risk-taking preferences in the first place? That sort of dangerous – even lethal – behavior will look to many like an assault on the value of life. And people – including children-people – learn from what they see. Athletic competitions may be particularly effective social learning mechanisms: "Everything I needed to know in life I learned from baseball" – that sort of thing.

So this is an individual and social norm-learning argument – and social norms have massive influence on thought and behavior. The spectacle of an open practice in which people take enormous risks with their health or their life in order to get a prize tends to reinforce value systems that may be acceptable in a society if a few people have them (say, the military class or a few with "the right stuff") but not if many do. It may be OK on a broader scale in a more complete warrior state (Sparta?), but not here. If external observers came down from another galactic quadrant, how would they measure the value we assign to life under a win-and-die system? But these are mixed empirical and moral questions that are hard to answer. And in any case, current enhancement techniques usually won't kill you if used properly.

Another argument from social learning is that if you perceive performance enhancement as producing a return disproportionate to your efforts, then it conveys the idea of getting something for nothing. It promotes a sort of welfare ethic: one should expect (at least partially) huge unearned benefits. But the prospect of huge and unearned gains is, in the case of steroids and most *current* enhancers, quite mistaken; one doesn't take a pill and immediately swell up and attain the strength and speed necessary to lift the continental shelf or at least win the decathlon. If people *do* see it this way, however, they see competitors getting something for nothing, which weakens values of diligence, fortitude, and so on. *We learn from what we see, and if we see it wrong, we still see it and learn (the wrong thing) from it.*

But current enhancers don't seem to actually work that way. It just means everybody just has to push harder. The other guy is going to be using it too!
Yeah, that's right. If everybody used it, of course, and if it improved everyone by the same absolute increment, you would be shifting the bell-shaped curve to the right. This won't be precisely true in fact, but it's a useful approximation in trying to model possible futures.[11] You would be improving absolute performance levels but, in many cases, not relative ones. In theory, no one's positional advantage would change. This is a major point, rarely made by anyone, never mind sports writers. The nature of the contest might change, of course, with significantly enhanced performance across the board. Some might, in response, want to change the rules of the game (e.g., a larger playing field). In any case, widespread performance enhancement might even make people more diligent and move them to try harder – generally considered a good thing – if only to avoid loss of relative position. And it's hard to see, if the same people keep on winning and losing, how you're getting an inappropriate reinforcement of something for nothing. True, absolute performance would seem to be heightened, suggested disproportionate returns. But the idea that you can get more bang for the buck might be far more reinforced if people were cheating and you knew they were cheating but you didn't know who. Detection mechanisms are quite imperfect and might always be so. This sort of thing is important in contests such as getting admitted to universities – SATs, etc., or applying for jobs or licenses – where performance enhancement bans or regulations would be sought to maintain a "level playing field" (not an entirely clear concept, but we can't cover everything here). Of course, if enhancements are banned and some people cheat, then the contest is unfair, at least going by the books.

These "by the books" and related cheating issues suggest the more comprehensive competitive coherence argument I mentioned earlier, which forms the weakest argument against enhancement. It trades on a misunderstanding. If you want to define what a sport or a game is, you have to consider not only the canonical definition in the rule book, but also how the game is actually played.[12] You could consider – and I'm going to use the term "cheating" in a paradoxical sense – constructing games based on seeing who can cheat the best. (But if it's an understood part of the game, can it be cheating?) Sports teams, during a game or even at practice, try to make sure that no one's spying on them. There have been a few scandals in which the supposed cheaters got caught.[13] Well, you could construct a not-really-cheating cheating game embracing such practices, whether explicitly or silently. You could have a comprehensive contest in which you not only play football but you spy, do psychological warfare, kidnap the opposing quarterback, and so on. Some may think this is unfair. But you could construct a game where those are the rules applying to everyone. You can even throw in an assumption that the ability and resources to cheat are fairly evenly distributed. Why don't we have games *defined* like this – at least at present? Games like this are internally coherent, but, not surprisingly, people may think they promote adverse individual and community-wide learning – and so do not cohere with the larger normative system. After all, you don't want kids in high school to play football and think it's okay to kidnap and kill the opposing quarterback. (Maybe this sort of thing is OK for training Sardaukar in Frank Herbert's *Dune* (1965). I certainly don't want to live in a society like that. But we're not quite there yet.

In a less fanciful situation, however, if you permit performance enhancement but require disclosure, the game is clearly not internally incoherent, and not obviously incoherent with basic social norms. The terms "cheating" and "preserving a level playing field" are largely pointless descriptors here.

Some of the authors in *the Journal of the Philosophy of Sport*[14] protest that if you allow steroids and certain other enhancers then what you are doing is not really testing talent, effort, skill, or diligence. What you are testing is how the body reacts to a certain chemical, or to some other technology. This is unpersuasive because, first, you could also argue that with traditional training, what we are testing is how one's body responds to lifting heavy objects, going on special diets, or training generally. We're testing arbitrary differences among persons, like variations in the genome. Second, even the capacity to try hard is affected, though not decisively, by genetics. I'm pretty clumsy. Should I protest: Why am I being judged against somebody else who's got better body control, better anti-clumsy genes, or is, by her nature, more driven to overcome limitations? Does that make any more sense than objecting that you're simply being tested to see how your system reacts to steroids?

I'm skipping over assessing the coherence of using what might be called supplements and implements – for example, better track shoes and running tracks – even better clothing, such as swimsuits.[15] There are also devices that form part of a contest's definitional core – poles in vaulting, autos in auto racing. Better poles are a kind of performance booster, but not an enhancer. If they were electromechanically contrived to allow people to jump forty feet, we'd have a different – but not incoherent – game. So you can see, again, that the concept of performance enhancement isn't entirely clear.

Could you explain a bit more about moral category arguments?

OK, back to moral category arguments – they overlap – for a bit. Performance enhancement sometimes gets people to thinking about questions like: are we sure just *who* is performing? There was a paragraph by H.L.A. Hart in an article that he wrote in the *Harvard Law Review* in 1958 in which he imagined a world in which we all changed traits constantly in ways that, on any theory, seem to involve a change of identity – or the absence of stable identity. Say you took a pill and it increased your mental and physical abilities enormously. (This is akin to what happened when the earth passed out of a longstanding cognitive dampening field in Poul Anderson's *Brain Wave* (1954). In such circumstances what does it even mean to say that someone won a contest? These questions suggest a world in which performance enhancement alters identity in such a way that it's very hard either to get a grip on what the game or the sport is, or who or what won it. Such "contests" wouldn't track our current notions of winning and losing, or our ideas of merit or desert. The main moral categories here are identity and merit.

But as things are now, it's very difficult to see how any current performance enhancement agents compromise identity (unless someone trivially identifies identity with whatever characterizes you as a given instant). We can anticipate technologies in the next generation, such as drugs that act like steroids but don't have serious adverse effects. Suppose performance enhancement with these drugs were accepted and regulated. There would be no identity crisis here. There wasn't even that serious an identity crisis with the Mentats in Frank Herbert's *Dune* novels: they all enhanced their mental abilities with the spice and were viewed as persons with continuing identities. But there are contexts in which we might not even care that much about identity – say, enhanced scientists finding cancer cures. (But what do we do when Nobel Prize time comes around?) Mentats were used as tools (probably not *mere* tools) to defend the feudal houses in the Dune setting; their identities, from that standpoint, were of limited importance. Putting it that way suggests an objectification argument against enhancement – part of another moral category: technological modification will, it is argued, reduce our value as separate, free persons to that of things for mere use as means.[16] I can't elaborate on that here. In most contexts, the argument is not powerful, but carries some weight where there are significant emotional and financial investments, as in germ line augmentation, because of incentives toward intrusive implementation. But one can easily imagine a reduced-humanity world, as in the *Spartacus: Blood and Sand* TV series pitting slaves against each other in combat.

Of course, there are many merit-recognition problems apart from the complexities induced by enhancement. Who gets credit for winning a football game? The team, the quarterback, the coach, the trainer, Mom and Dad, God? It's an interesting question, but not one to agonize over. In general, there's nothing unintelligible about dividing up credit, as long as you specify, if possible, what the credit is for. The problem of course is more vividly presented with technological enhancement. Who gets the credit for the enhanced performance of a person modified by germ line engineering? We have already genetically engineered larger mice by incorporating rat growth hormone genes into mice embryos. If germ line engineering produces a tall person who succeeds in the NBA, to whom do we give credit? The basketball player himself, the person who engineered the genes, the parents who decided to do this? The answer is yes to all – but credit *for what*? Still, we ask that very question with or without enhancement. Who gets credit for Yao Ming? Some have claimed that he came to be as a result of careful planning – a form of positive eugenics? – by China, whose parents had been "drafted" into the sports system. They nurtured him, he was trained by Chinese basketball, and by the Houston Rockets.[17] Lots of input there.

Hovering over all these issues – and strongly linked to them – are access-distribution problems. (I'm moving beyond your moral category question here.) It's one thing to complain that not everyone can get a Rolls-Royce. But if you could generate major changes in mental and physical ability only through very expensive technological applications, you may sharply and irreversibly increase social *partitioning* to the point of true "lock-in." Perhaps this is a form of "market failure" (economists may object to this description) arising from the risk of expanded unbridgeable stratifications. One couldn't simply say, "Talent will out and the smart have open futures," because talent and smartness are themselves for sale and only the wealthy (possibly but not necessarily talented) can afford them. Enhancement technologies aren't free, and future development and economies of scale may still leave them beyond the means of many persons. Whatever the conceptual difficulties in doing so, we think of these technologies as affecting merit attributes, which themselves are the bases for distributions: they are resource-attractors, and acceleratingly so, so the incremental role of merit diminishes. Compare compound interest, and objects that gain further gravitational power through continuing gravitational accretion of mass. If you're very smart, you might deserve some rewards more than other persons do. But when these commodities are themselves mechanisms to (in a loose sense) "enhance merit" itself – well, Who merits merit?, as I asked in a 1974 *Southern California Law Review* article.

I add a last point to this truncated discussion of distributional issues. There are those who downplay their importance, insisting that main point of analyzing enhancement is the threshold propriety of use.[18] This is quite overstated. Distributional issues cannot rightly be assumed away: the threshold propriety and the distributional issues, while distinct, are linked, conceptually and morally. Distribution is a critical issue not only in using technologies but in deciding whether to go ahead with developing them at all; the Matthew Effect is no small matter here.[19] If we decide that enhancement is tolerable, permissible, good, or even obligatory when distribution is not at issue, distributional effects – such as drastically exacerbated and irreversible social stratification – may render the moral price of enhancement unacceptable in some eyes, on some theories. *If the partition-ing is linked to race, ethnicity, gender, religion or other problematic classifications, the price may be that much higher.* Some might find it more acceptable if the distribution were required to benefit the worst off in some defined ways.[20] And even if enhancement is generally unacceptable, *it will occur*, and distributional issues may remain significant moral issues even when we deal with illicit goods.

What are the moral and public policy consequences of recognizing this inevitability of enhancement?

The apparent inevitability of enhancement generates serious moral and policy issues. One pos-sibility is that there is simply no *acceptable* way to stop enhancement. The parallel to the war on drugs is obvious. I suppose we could avoid an enhancement regime by installing a fully surveil-lant and otherwise intrusive prohibition and enforcement system, and even then it would be imperfect. The "least worst" option is to find some way, in athletics, education, the workplace ... to install acceptable enhancement systems. In real life, we will never tolerate total market free-dom, either because of clear market failures or situations that seem morally akin to them. In athletics, for example, even those calling for the removal of flat bans on enhancement concede that they will have to make room for systems to promote medical safety and promote access. (Black markets are more dangerous to health.) They will, one hopes, not be anywhere near as intrusive and morally questionable as I think the current regime is.

Difficulties in formulating distributional criteria for access to education and employment are compounded because there is, in principle, no determinately sound and complete system for selecting the traits to be used in forming different kinds of persons. Nozick's "genetic supermar-ket"[21] (in theory not limited to genetics) avoids the problem of centralized decisions, but pro-vides no guidance for individual choice for conscientious decision-makers who seek sound criteria. The "procedural solution" is often fairly empty (as in "Let's settle this through conversa-tion"; what does one converse about?). But the market is not a general solution across the board, although it is an indispensable starting point, if autonomy is a prime value.

In any event, we are bound to look for the least worst system, even if we can't discover or implement the best.

Finally, enhancement obviously impacts our basic values, which vary, in this domain, from con-gruence with each other to near-total conflict in assessing enhancement situations. Any practices that involve collisions between liberty, on the one hand, and its externalities and effects on equality in its various forms, on the other, will call forth government action. In turn, this will raise consti-tutional claims – because the constitution, expressly and by fair implication, embeds (at a high level of abstraction, to be sure) our basic moral values: autonomy, fairness, justice, equality, and social welfare or utility. But discussing the constitutional aspects of enhancement is for another time.

Notes

This is a modified, updated version of *Performance Enhancement and Legal Theory: An Interview with Prof. Michael H. Shapiro*, by Max More, *Extropy: The Journal of Transhumanist Thought* 17, H2 (1996). It is not an exact transcription of the interview.

1   Unless otherwise indicated, freestanding occurrences of "enhancement" and "augmentation" refer to signi-ficant technological modifications of performance capacities, whether on living beings or via the germ line.
2   Fla. Stat. Ann. § 458.331(ee) (Westlaw 2011) See Florida Statute: http://www.leg.state.fl.us/statutes/index.cfm?App_mode=Display_Statute&Search_String=&URL=0400-0499/0458/Sections/0458.331.html.

3   See also *Therapeutic Use Exemptions*, World Anti-Doping Agency, http://www.wada-ama.org/ (June 7, 2010).

4   Alcohol and beta-blockers are generally disallowed in official competition ("in-competition" only). See generally the *World Anti-Doping Code, The 2010 Prohibited List: International Standard*, §§P1, P2. "In-competition" apparently refers to testing at the time of the event, not at other times. See World Anti-Doping Agency, *World Anti-Doping Code*, §4.2.

5   See generally Cakic 2009 (discussing various drugs, including caffeine).

6   But note that caffeine is no longer a prohibited substance under World Anti-Doping Agency (WADA). *The World Anti-Doping Code, The 2010 Prohibited List: International Standard*.

7   See Sandel 2007: 85.

8   Others have made this point, and still others have disputed it. For example, compare Bostrom and Sandberg (2009) with Powell (2010).

9   It may seem odd, but it is not incoherent to celebrate baseball as a game of skill combined with "random" actions inconsistent with what are usually thought of as "the rules." Recall Armando Galarraga's officially ruined perfect game. Robert Wright (2010): "It's sad that Galarraga won't ever have what is rightfully his – so sad that some people are now saying baseball should do what pro football does: review close plays via video and reverse bad calls. Please, no. Bringing justice to baseball would defeat the whole point of the game." What could "rightfully his" mean on this theory?

10 See generally Sokol 1986: "Prior to the 1984 Olympic Games in Los Angeles, a survey of top U.S. athletes was taken. They were asked: If a drug were available that would guarantee a gold medal in L.A., but also meant certain death in five years, would they take the magic pill? 'Fifty-five per cent of those surveyed said "yes" and that is frightening,' says Geoff Gowan, president of the Coaching Association of Canada." (Found on Lexis.)

11 This interpersonal variation might be viewed as depending on differences in natural or acquired "aptitudes" for responding to technological enhancement. Merit "preserved"?

12 True, the rule book may be perverse. Suppose the rules contain a meta-rule specifying that errors in applying the rule by umpires/referees can never be corrected, thus structuring a game in part defined by random or even intentional errors. This seems close to the truth in some contests.

13 See generally PatsFans.com (2010): "Falcons Say Signal Stealing Part of Football..."

14 See Robert 2007.

15 There was a flap over using newly marketed swimsuits in official swimming events. See *New York Times* 2009.

16 This derives from the second formulation of Kant's Categorical Imperative. One translation: "Act in such a way that you always treat humanity, whether in your own person or in the person of any other, never simply as a means but always at the same time as an end" (Hill 1992: 38–39).

17 For a report on his background, see generally Time Asia, *The Creation of Yao Ming*, adapted from Lamar 2005. http://www.time.com/time/magazine/article/0,9171,1126765,00.html.

18 A similar point is made by Christine Overall (see Overall 2009: 327, 331–332). But cf. Arthur L. Caplan (2009: 199–200) (preferring to separate distributional issues from the merits of the technological improvement process).

19 Merton 1968: 159 See also Matthew 25:14–30. "For unto every one that hath shall be given, and he shall have abundance: But from him that hath not shall be taken away even that which he hath."

20 Note Rawls' "difference principle" in this connection (Rawls 1999: 87).

21 Nozick 1974: 315 n.*. See generally Glover 1984.

References

Anderson, Poul (1954) *Brain Wave*. New York: Ballantine Books.

Bostrom, Nick and Sandberg, Anders (2009) "The Wisdom of Nature: An Evolutionary Heuristic for Human Enhancement." In Julian Savulescu and Nick Bostrom, eds., *Human Enhancement*. Oxford: Oxford University Press, pp. 375–416.

Cakic, Vince (2009) "Smart Drugs for Cognitive Enhancement: Ethical and Pragmatic Considerations in the Era of Cosmetic Neurology." *Journal of Medical Ethics* 35 (October 29), pp. 611–615.

Caplan, Arthur L. (2009) "Good, Better, or Best." In Julian Savulescu and Nick Bostrom, eds., *Human Enhancement*. Oxford: Oxford University Press, pp. 199–209.

Glover, Jonathan (1984) *What Sort of People Should There Be?* New York: Penguin.

Hart, Herbert L.A. (1958) "Positivism and the Separation of Law and Morals." *Harvard Law Review* 71, pp. 593–622.

Herbert, Frank (1965) *Dune*. New York: Ace Books.

Hill, Thomas E. Jr. (1992) *Dignity and Practical Reason in Kant's Moral Theory*. Ithaca, NY: Cornell University Press.

Lamar, Brook (2005) *Operation Yao Ming*. Harmondsworth: Penguin Books.

Merton, Robert K. (1968) "The Matthew Effect in Science." *Science* 56.

New York Times (2009) "Performance-Enhancing Swimsuits." Editorial. (July 30).

Robert Nozick (1974) *Anarchy, State, and Utopia*. New York: Basic Books.

Overall, Christine (2009) "Life-Enhancement Technologies: The Significance of Social Category Membership." In Julian Savulescu and Nick Bostrom, eds., *Human Enhancement*. Oxford: Oxford University Press.

PatsFans.com (2010) "Falcons Say Signal Stealing Part of Football ..." (June 8). http://www.patsfans.com/new-england-patriots/messageboard/10/60827-falcons-say-signal-stealing-part-football.html.

Powell, Russell (2010) "What's the Harm? An Evolutionary Theoretical Critique of the Precautionary Principle." *Kennedy Institute of Ethics Journal* 20/2 (June), pp. 181–206.

Rawls, John (1999) *A Theory of Justice*, rev. edn. Cambridge, MA: Belknap Press of Harvard University Press.

Sandel, Michael J. (2007) *The Case against Perfection: Ethics in the Age of Genetic Engineering*. Cambridge, MA: Harvard University Press.

Simon, Robert L. (2007) "Good Competition and Drug-Enhanced Performance." Reprinted from the *Journal of the Philosophy of Sport* in William J. Morgan, ed., *Ethics in Sport*, 2nd edn. Champaign, IL: Human Kinetics, pp. 245–251.

Sokol, Al (1986) "U.S. Athletes Would Die for Olympic Gold Medal." *Toronto Star* (November 20, Thursday, final edition, sports section), p. H12.

Wright, Robert (2010) "Perfectly Unfair." *New York Times*, June 8.

Publications by Michael Shapiro in this Area

1974: "Who Merits Merit? Some Problems in Distributive Justice Posed by the New Biology." *Southern California Law Review* 48, pp. 318–370.

1991: "The Technology of Perfection: Performance Enhancement and the Control of Attributes." *Southern California Law Review* 65, p. 11.

1989: "The Technology of Success." [remarks on physical and mental performance enhancement] *L.A. Daily Journal* [county legal newspaper] January 17, p. 7, col. 1.

1989: "The Genetics of Perfection." *L.A. Daily Journal* [county legal newspaper] March 8, p. 7, col. 1.

2002: "Does Technological Enhancement of Human Traits Threaten Human Equality and Democracy?" *San Diego Law Review* 39, p. 769.

2003: with Roy G. Spece, Jr., Rebecca Dresser, and Ellen Wright Clayton, *Bioethics and Law: Cases, Materials and Problems*, 2nd edn. St. Paul: Thomson/West.

2005: "The Identity of Identity: Moral and Legal Aspects of Technological Self-Transformation." *Journal of Social Philosophy & Policy* 22/2, pp. 308–373. Reprinted in Ellen Frankel Paul et al., eds., *Personal Identity, Social Philosophy and Policy* 22. Cambridge: Cambridge University Press, 2006.

29

Justifying Human Enhancement
The Accumulation of Biocultural Capital

Andy Miah

There are various aspects of the debate on human enhancements that frustrate the possibility of reaching consensus on their value, and I will focus on two of the more crucial obstacles: (a) the need to rationalize medical resources and (b) the concern that such use would be the first step on a "slippery slope" to some undesirable end. Respectively, the decision to permit unfettered access to enhancements relies on being able to devote resources to such modifications and attending to the concern that such access would not lead to the collapse of healthcare or generally making society worse off. These societal questions, I suggest, have a higher priority than personal moral decisions about whether or not it is wise to seek enhancement, though I will go on to suggest how they are related. Moreover, I argue that these moral debates should be the immediate focus of transhumanist debate. I will argue for the similarities between the pursuit of technology for enhancement and health maintenance by presenting the concept of *biocultural capital*. This broadly describes how humanity ought to treat the emerging era of superhuman enhancement, while retaining a focus on utilizing technology to address fundamental human needs.

Rationalizing Medical Interventions on a Slippery Slope

Arguments against human enhancements often refer to the proper goals of medicine as an explanation for why enhancements would be, at best, secondary priorities for the medical profession compared with alleviating suffering. Moreover, to the extent that healthcare will always be saturated with primary obligations to alleviate suffering, then this view would lead one to conclude that there is no place within healthcare for enhancement, at least not until all primary needs have been addressed. Such a view derives in part from the need to *rationalize* resources within healthcare and for priorities to be set, in an attempt to distribute resources in a

The Transhumanist Reader: Classical and Contemporary Essays on the Science, Technology, and Philosophy of the Human Future, First Edition. Edited by Max More and Natasha Vita-More.

way that aligns with broad commitments to social justice. In short, the system attempts to give priority to the most vulnerable people.

When comparing human enhancements with human repair, the ability to make moral distinctions about whether some treatments are more deserving than others is also challenging (see Miah 2008a, 2011). One may attempt to draw a line between the alleviation of suffering (therapy) and the pursuit of happiness (enhancement), but this neat separation quickly disappears when scrutinizing what we aspire to when undertaking a medical intervention. While suffering may seem to be paramount, there are different degrees of suffering and all of them may be worthy of attention. Thus, there may be a good reason to permit someone to have cosmetic surgery to improve their mental health and an equally good reason to treat someone for a leg that is broken through undertaking some risky activity.

Moreover, the importance of making such a distinction on the basis of concerns about social justice – perhaps by deciding that the alleviation of some suffering is a higher priority than others – disappears in an environment where such services are not dependent on public funds, or where there is a clear governmental commitment towards supporting an expansive notion of health and wellbeing. For instance, in the Netherlands cosmetic dental work is offered through the state system, which is not the case in many other countries. On this basis, the justification for limiting medical interventions to just the alleviation of suffering, becomes less meaningful, since healthcare should aspire to promoting general improvements in wellbeing, of which enhancements are a part. For instance, consider a ballerina who seeks body sculpting in order to make her a more graceful dancer, or the fashion model who seeks cosmetic surgery for the sake of his career. While one might call into question the social norms that legitimize and valorize such practices, these are not persuasive reasons to forbid access to such technologies and, one may argue, their need is sincere and crucial to the individual's wellbeing.

A second dimension of the therapy-enhancement problem involves the so-called *slippery slope argument* in its various guises.[1] This argument dictates that one might reasonably withhold access to A (desirable), where it is likely or inevitable that such freedom will lead to circumstance B (undesirable). A common and contemporary example where this argument becomes apparent is in the context of genetic selection, which is already used for sex-related disorders within the United Kingdom. However, the line has been drawn between such avoidance of suffering through genetic dysfunction and *family balancing* where a couple may seek selection in order to ensure that they have a boy or a girl (Human Fertilisation and Embryology Authority 2003).

However, the slippery slope argument in this case would suggest that allowing access to sex-selection for family balancing (A), would lead to an acceptance of creating designer babies where it becomes a moral and legal entitlement to select embryos on the basis of a range of characteristics, such as height, hair color, and so on (B). In this case, withholding access to A is justified by the slippery slope argument, on the basis that it would lead to circumstance B, which is wholly undesirable. In this case, the slippery slope mediates between two kinds of enhancing cases – genetically selecting sex for family balancing and genetically selecting for other characteristics.

Yet similar arguments have even been made in relation to limiting access to certain kinds of *therapeutic* intervention – such as gene therapy – on the basis that their use would lead to an undesirable freedom to enhance. For instance, within the field of nanotechnology, experimental research is still searching for treatments for a range of life-threatening or debilitating conditions, such as Parkinson's disease. While Deep Brain Stimulation has made considerable progress, there is still a need to solve the problem of how to power miniature devices, which currently require a wire to go from the brain to a battery located in the patient's chest. The insertion of a remote, nano-sized device into the brain could provide a long-term solution to such conditions. However, some have argued against the introduction of permanent devices into the brain – on the basis of a slippery slope argument – suggesting that it could lead to a situation where such devices are used to alter a range of behavioral characteristics, such as affecting eating patterns or for undertaking social surveillance, which may be against an individual's best interest.

There are various forms to the slippery slope argument and the persuasiveness of each varies. Appeals to this argument are not limited to matters of human enhancement, and it has become a feature of many bioethical debates, from the use of contraceptives to concerns about euthanasia. However, its persuasiveness relies on the assumed or implied inadequacy of regulative structures to ensure that the limits of application are clearly applied.

A final problem with making an ethical distinction between therapy and enhancement concerns the way in which medical interventions work. For some time, medical science has approached healthcare by giving primacy to the principle of prevention before cure. Yet a similar principle may require to be employed in order to optimize and expand the resilience and capabilities of people; in short, to enhance them. On this basis, the distinction between therapy and enhancement becomes redundant, since preventing many illnesses will involve treating a patient *before* they are diagnosed with an illness and before they are considered to be suffering in a way that warrants medical intervention. Moreover, with successful treatment, the condition is perhaps unlikely to occur at all. The implications of this become apparent when considering age-related illnesses such as Parkinson's or Alzheimer's. In these cases, early intervention to prevent such conditions materializing may ensure that the condition does not arise at all. On this basis, one may claim that the person has been enhanced by increasing their resilience to a debilitating condition, yet the terminology of how to judge such an intervention is value-laden. For instance, while the effect of such early intervention would be to dramatically increase the individual's *healthspan* – increasing the duration in life for which one can expect to enjoy good health – there is also a concomitant extension of *lifespan* that is likely to ensue. After all, the preventive intervention will have eliminated the debilitating condition that otherwise would have ended a person's life prematurely.

This example reveals how transhumanist aspirations may be rooted in quite elementary principles of medical practice today. On this basis, the pursuit of treating age-related illnesses is both an extension of our pursuit of health and a pursuit of human enhancement in the strongest possible terms. Moreover, such an example is one of many ways in which people undertake early, pre-symptomatic interventions to protect against their natural biological vulnerabilities. More familiar interventions include inoculations for children, or fluoride in tap water, which have similar preventive functions.

These examples are useful when trying to situate the often abstract concept of enhancement. They describe a lifestyle whereby people may enjoy a degree of health that would be both unachievable were it not for enhancement and an alteration to what we regard to be species-typical functioning for a person at any given age.[2] The question arising from this is whether such forms of increasing resilience are more like those forms of medical intervention that respond to its "proper role" or whether they transcend such obligations. As suggested, medical practice has engaged with preventive techniques for many years, so it seems closer to what medicine already does, but the crucial point I wish to make is that many forms of enhancement will be just like this. By progressively ensuring that people do not fall victim to otherwise debilitating conditions, people will find themselves enhanced for life and increasingly capable.

While radical in terms of how it would affect humanity, this form of transhumanism is more modest than others, which may imply cultivating capabilities that are completely unfamiliar to the human species, such as the capacity of flight or breathing underwater. Yet, it is also among the most realistic and immediate ways in which transhumanist ideals are already changing humanity (Vita-More 2010). One of the main criticisms of this emerging era is the way in which it may commodify life, the focus of the next section.

Life as a Commodity

If one acknowledges the merit of systematically reinforcing human biology so it is optimized to flourish – while accepting that one cannot expect certainty of bringing about such conditions – then what objections might there be to such a system? Francis Fukuyama's (2002) primary concern is the commercial character of such a system of healthcare. He argues that such commercialization will lead inevitably to the commodification of life and this will diminish human flourishing, notably through it bringing about an impoverished view of human dignity. In response, I will seek to explain how the freedom to pursue commercial enhancements may be justified on the basis of what I call the accumulation of biocultural capital. However, first, it is necessary to clarify what kind of commercial transaction would ensue from commodifying life.

The treatment of human enhancements as commercial products is apparent in a range of literature that has discussed the emergence of biotechnologies. One of the more eloquent articulations of this scenario arises in Robert Nozick's (1974) concept of the "genetic supermarket." Nozick's metaphor imagines a set of circumstances where we can choose our genes, as we may choose food in a supermarket. The metaphor helpfully conveys the range of alternatives that may be available to people in such a period, yet it also implies a world where human characteristics are treated in the way we treat other commercial products, rather than with the respect we might hope.

After all, it is apparent within law that life is afforded greater privileges and protections than non-living matter and this has something to do with the relative moral status of such entities. To this end, there is a long-standing social recognition of the idea that life should be protected from excessive commercialization. In part, this is why there are laws to regulate the trafficking of organs along with their donation and other such practices that imply the shifting of biological matter from one person to another or into a system that may seek to commercialize such matter, as for biobanks or laboratories seeking to patent treatments. Thus, the prospect of commercializing life or even choices about life – such as the procreative technology of sex selection – provokes an intuitive protectionism, or, at least, a requirement of high standards of vigilance over the conduct of such industries which seek to trade in such business. Yet it is useful to scrutinize the precise objections that arise in response to such enterprises, as they relate directly to the value of promoting a culture of human enhancements.

There are both individual and societal risks associated with the commercialized provision of health products and treatments. For instance, commercial organ donation may diminish the value of the "gift relationship," where donation constitutes an act of altruism that would be corrupted by the introduction of a financial exchange.[3] Of course, the large numbers of patients who continue to wait for donor organs may offset the loss of such altruistic behavior. Alternatively, commercialization may lead to a situation where people who are financially vulnerable undertake such transactions in order to improve their life circumstances, which may be exploitative in a number of ways.

Despite these strong views about commodification, the premise that commercial transactions must be inherently wrong is at odds with how many people define value in their lives via the consumption of products. While capitalism and consumption may have a bad reputation, it is true also that acts of consumption are acts of differentiation, both collective and individual. People establish their sense of identity and belonging through the consumption of various devices – ideas, products, and so on. While it may also be true that the market determines the terms of this individuation, the variance that it provides seems, for many people at least, to be sufficient so as to enable the feeling of free agency.

Equally, to suggest that the medical industries are presently empty of consumerist tendencies, even before they give way to enhancement, is clearly false. From the international trade of pharmaceuticals to online sales of Viagra, health, illness, and medical treatments are inextricable from global consumer markets. While these examples might require us to stop short of talking about *life* as commodified – since they are products that affect aspects of our biology – other examples such as surrogacy or paid organ/egg donation reveals how commercial transactions are a growing part of established medical practice.[4] In this sense, the value of life has always been treated in some sense as a commodity; we are simply disagreeing about how much of life should be commodified. Moreover, biotechnology now forces us to consider who owns the commodity, which parts of life are commodified, and the means through which societies might regulate such commodification.

Accepting that aspects of life can be treated as a commodity need not mean endorsing the view that life is valuable *only* as a commodity or that its principal value is commercial. A more pressing concern is whether governments would be able to regulate a market of human biology in a way that protects these additional ways in which it should be respected. If one examines the egg and sperm auctioning site RonsAngels.com, a range of characteristics that it exhibits are reasonable grounds to support the concern about how a free market for biological products might transform the values of healthcare. In this site, clients bid for the sperm and ova of donors, which they can then utilize to procreate. While these details alone are likely to raise considerable ethical concerns, this particular instance of commercialized human biology is made even more complicated by the fact that the donors seem to be participants in Ron Harris' pornographic film industry, thus bringing an uncomfortable proximity between two kinds of social enterprise: health and pornography.

One may presume from RonsAngels.com that a society where human enhancements are readily available would look quite similar. However, it remains to be seen whether many such practices would remain under the scrutiny of present-day healthcare professions, or whether they would resemble some other commercial industry such as retail fashion perhaps. Regardless, I argue that the pursuit of human enhancements may be seen as an extension of our pursuit of *cultural capital*, which is a precondition of developed societies. More specifically, I describe human enhancements as forms of *biocultural capital*, which are becoming integral to how people aspire to improve their lives.

The Accumulation of Biocultural Capital

The term "biocultural capital" extends from the French social theorist Pierre Bourdieu's concept of "cultural capital," which is usefully articulated by Rojek:

> The term "cultural capital" refers to the knowledge of and skills in the discursive realm relating to society, the arts, leisure, sport, science, politics and all the other elements recognised as "culture" in society at large. (1995: 68)

By extension, I claim that biocultural capital refers to the various ways in which biotechnologies and the body/mind modification sciences are providing tools through which people can alter themselves to more adequately pursue their life goals. The modified definition does overlap with some of Bourdieu's thoughts, as he considers the role of the body in this accumulation of cultural capital, and even discusses the body as an unfinished product. As Shilling (1993: 128) notes,

> [Bourdieu] displays a clear interest in the unfinishedness of the body, and maintains a more comprehensive view of the materiality of human embodiment than those theorists who focus exclusively on language, consciousness, or even the body as flesh. Bourdieu recognises that acts of labour are required to turn bodies into social entities and that these acts influence how people develop and hold the physical shape of their bodies, and learn how to present their bodies through styles of walk, talk and dress. Far from being natural, these represent highly skilled and socially differentiated accomplishments which start to be learned early in childhood. As it develops, the body bears the indisputable imprint of the individual's social class.

While Bourdieu does not discuss the role that biological modifications might play in this accumulation, this concept of unfinishedness offers close conceptual ties to the language of trans- and post-humanisms that surround debates about human enhancements. Bourdieu's concept makes a number of important distinctions between types of cultural capital, though of particular use is his expression of *symbolic* and *embodied* cultural capital. These attributes inform my development of the notion of *biocultural capital*. However, some modifications to his terms are necessary, since human enhancements are ambiguously placed in relation to some aspects of Bourdieu's thesis. For instance, could one discuss the consumption of a drug that improves attention-span as an "act of labour", given that the labor required may be quite minor? Indeed, anti-enhancement advocates may argue that such an undertaking is troubling precisely because it implies no labor on the part of the individual – and as such is a quick fix that undermines the importance of human will and struggle in the achievement of certain goals.

In part, this is why it is necessary to modify Bourdieu's thesis to encompass the concept of *biocultural capital*, since his original conception does not distinguish explicitly between labors of the *will* and what I would call labors of *biological adaptation*. For, while ingesting a pill might not imply labor of a kind that implies will or determinism, such as that involved in exercising to lose weight, it does require a physiological adaptation to occur and this can also be conceived of as "labor." A good example of such labor may be the need to endure side-effects associated with a medical treatment or muscle soreness after exercise. Thus, as technology develops, our experience of labor is also transformed. A further modification relates to the claim that Bourdieu's concept of cultural capital is class-based. While the specific responses to this vary – from the suggestion that access to cultural capital is entirely socially stratified to the possibility that class is no longer a helpful concept – my conceptualization of biocultural capital draws attention to the way in which adoption of technologies straddles class divides, and this is likely to be true also of biological enhancements. Indeed, the consumption of cosmetic surgery provides some evidence of this, though it is, of course, sometimes a technology that requires considerable financial investment.

The concept of biocultural capital also acknowledges the *absence* of many enhancement practices within society. Thus, human enhancements remain either only prospective modifications for most people, or modifications that will yield benefits only if other technological developments come to pass. For instance, human cryonic suspension involves participants purchasing a prospective enhancement – the capacity to be brought back to life at some time in the future. Unless revival is made possible, this undertaking will have been a fruitless exercise. To this end, access to human enhancements is experienced predominantly via the consumption of biopolitics; i.e. it is a consumption of ideas and of possibilities.

When considering the ethics of accumulating biocultural capital, Bourdieu's "labor" does not distinguish between more or less worthy forms of capital. Nevertheless, Rojek (1995: 68) notes that Bourdieu *is* interested in "how society evaluates this cultural capital through visible and tacit systems of reward and punishment." Such systems may provide some basis for discerning normative judgments about enhancements, but as for other forms of cultural capital, it would be facile to claim that one form of enhancement is more worthwhile than another, in the same sense that we would not claim art to be more worthwhile than music. The argument from biocultural capital refutes the rejection of such distinctions on moral grounds, largely because decisions to undertake human enhancements constitute appeals to an aesthetic standard (which Bourdieu describes as "taste"). To elaborate, a suitable comparison might arise in the context of aesthetic appreciation more generally. Thus, the request for a moral justification for human enhancements is rather like asking what value accrues from having heard a Bob Dylan song, or having strolled around a Frank Gehry building. This is not to equate listening to music with invasive biological alterations; clearly there are important differences in terms of the commitment required to experience each. However, to the extent that each conveys a particular form of taste, they are similar.

Such occurrences, along with the desire to experience them, cannot be explained via some precise moral framework of general utility. Instead, through the consumption of these ideas and procedures, via the desire to expose ourselves to them, we enter into a transaction whereby the expectation for benefit is not preconceived or, at most, where there exists only a strong sense of the positive value that could arise from the exposure. In short, human enhancements are no guarantee of their leading to an improved life, but they provide the opportunity to choose one's future, rather than to leave it to chance. In sum, the strongest value claim that one can make in relation to body modifications is conceptually no different from the value claim one might make about reading a book or watching a movie. There is no objective, absolute benefit that will arise from either action, only a general sense in which the experience will enrich our lives. In any case, to expect certainty of benefit is too great a burden to place on the value of human enhancement, as we typically do not deem it necessary to justify our lifestyles before pursuing them.

A final point to note in relation to my concept of "biocultural capital" involves the use of term "biocultural" and some recent literature in which this concept is articulated. While I have used it thus far to discuss biological modifications as objects of consumption, there is a dual intention to my use of this term. The word "biocultural" is increasingly being used to articulate the middle ground between liberal and conservative approaches to human enhancement and the convergence of philosophical and cultural engagements around such practices. Smith and Morra's (2006) book, *From a Posthuman Present to a Biocultural Future* engages a diverse range of related topics from debates about the meanings associated with disability and prosthesis (Sobchack 2006), to the fetishization of amputation (Smith 2006). They use "biocultural" to describe and critique fundamental concepts within medicine – such as "health" – in contrast to "biomedical." In particular, the term draws attention to the importance of cultural conditions when making sense of health-related terms, e.g. the contested meanings associated with "life" and "death." Such cultural conditions have a bearing on what are defined as the proper goals of medicine. As well, the utility of the term "biocultural" is in its recognition of the prominence of cultural politics in healthcare. For example, when the Hollywood actor Michael J. Fox presented a campaign advertisement about stem cells on behalf of US Senator Clair McCaskill, his intervention affected the sphere in which debates about the ethics of such technologies took place (McCaskill4Missouri 2006). Moreover, it constitutes a disruption to the traditional processes through which expertise and (moral) authority are typically conveyed. These parameters of human enhancements are constitutive of their presence within society, perhaps in ways that earlier eras of healthcare were not.

Counterpoint: Reducing Human Diversity?

Whether or not the range of choices available through human enhancements is likely to reduce human diversity depends on two factors. First, it presumes that the human capacity to realize a range of enhancement possibilities is less than the range that is conferred by natural selection. Second, it asks whether such choices will be available to enough people, for enough of the time, to avoid a reduction in diversity. For the former, it is important to remember that a world that embraces human enhancements benefits from the *combined* range of choices offered by human natural selection *and* humanly imaginable enhancements, not simply the latter.[5] Whether such human enhancements will be available, instead, relies on trends within scientific research – what kinds of enhancements are developed, financed, and so on. While it is debatable as to whether this will be broad or narrow, the relevant point is that the biopolitics of scientific research, as an integral part of social governance, is a *relevant* process through which such priorities are set. Consequently, there can be no objection to bringing such choices under the guise of governance, while one might be critical of leaving such trends merely to chance.

In the short term, one might expect there to be trends – fashions of body modification – which may promote cultural complicity. For example, while it may be thought that cosmetic surgery is geographically specific, it is apparent that the same kinds of aspirations as occur in the West also are visible in Eastern culture. For example, Watts (2004) reports on the cosmetic surgery "craze" in China, where nose reshaping and leg lengthening are popular practices.

A further objection to human enhancement culture is that there are likely to be "tradeoffs" to many choices people make. For example, deciding to optimize the number of slow-twitch muscle fibers in legs might create a particularly good endurance runner, but not such a good sprinter. Alternatively, being taller may be useful in some career choices, but in others it could be a disadvantage. Additionally, many such tradeoffs will have unknowable consequences, as is also true of therapeutic interventions and natural mutations. For instance, the sickle-cell gene also carries a protection against malaria, and the common cystic fibrosis mutation encodes a protein which may function at low temperatures and could be advantageous to people in some countries. As such, engineering away certain characteristics must – to return to our underlying premise – always be culturally located. Moreover, the choice to enhance could give rise to considerable regrets and harm, as is evidenced when cosmetic surgical interventions go wrong. Beyond this, an irreversible enhancement may not have value throughout the life course. Yet the prospect of things going wrong is not, in itself, a reason for abstaining from making such choices, though it might be a reason to avoid such permanent changes. Rather, it is a reason to strive for more knowledge about the effects of such decisions and to improve the efficacy of the intervention. Additionally, failing to enhance may also bring about future harms, particularly in an increasingly toxic global environment. The example of fluoride in tap water is a good example of how some societies have attempted to strengthen oral health.

Conclusion

The argument on behalf of biocultural capital claims that the pursuit of human enhancements is consistent with other ways in which people modify their lifestyles and is analogous in principle to buying a new mobile phone, learning a language, or exercising. It is a process of acquiring ideas, goods, assets, and experiences that distinguish one person from another, either as an individual or as a member of a community. While one might – and should – scrutinize the merits of such individual choices, we should recognize the limits of this task. Furthermore, the argument for biocultural capital considers that it is unreasonable for enhancement choices to be imposed upon individuals by the state. The normative transhumanist concept of morphological freedom emphasizes this prohibition (More 1993; Sandberg 2001). While general consensus on enhancements might have legal force, it will not necessarily have universal persuasive value – not everybody would wish to be tall, stronger, or whatever it may be - since enhancements only confer positive value within particular cultural contexts. As such, the precise value attached to any particular enhancement cannot be assumed to be a shared, universal good, particularly where choices of enhancements involve a tradeoff.

The argument from biocultural capital explains that the designation of a biological modification as a human enhancement does not correspond with some prescribed or abstract value claim. There is no necessary "good" that, in itself, can be objectively identified to justify (or reject) enhancements. For instance, if I were to enhance the efficiency of my digestive system to allow me to assimilate foods that are generally shown to be unhealthy, it is difficult to argue that this is a tangible enhancement, other than through its allowing me to satisfy the desire of always wanting to eat foods that I find tasty but which would, otherwise, be unhealthy. While such a modification would be beneficial to me, it is unlikely to withstand the scrutiny of those who have no such desire. Such a choice also faces the criticism that one's taste cannot develop in a positive sense if one closes off the potential to find value in experiencing other tastes. So, if I were a 12-year-old and really liked McDonald's food, I might enjoy enhancing my metabolism to assimilate such food, rather than to treat it like junk food. In doing so, by failing to choose alternative foods, I also restrict the possibility of developing tastes for other foods.[6] Yet, again, it seems premature to panic too much about such a prospect. Rather, it may emerge that one's taste develops alongside such new alternatives to consumption and that moderation will thus emerge.

Importantly, and as enshrined in the idea of morphological freedom, this argument on behalf of human enhancements does not extend to the freedom to modify others – for example, through genetically engineering embryos. Rather, this argument presents an initial position as to why certain obstacles towards human enhancement may be overcome by acknowledging the limits of concerns over rationalizing medical resources and avoiding a slippery slope towards undesirable circumstances, I have endeavored to explain the value of pursuing self-regarding, biological enhancements and, as such, to suggest why such freedom of choice should not be withheld.

In conclusion, asking why *we* should enhance ourselves limits the discussion prematurely. It prescribes a particular kind of moral justification, which would explain a choice that makes sense only in the particular case. However, treating such actions as micro-ethical processes, contrasts with the macro-ethical task of regulating the commercial and non-medical use of such interventions. In short, via this argument, one cannot offer a good reason for why *all* people should enhance themselves in a specific way, since each reason would require embedding the clause within a particular context that another individual might not deem to be valuable at all.

So, understanding the value of improving attention span or enhancing sexual function would require understanding the specific context that gives rise to such an interest. Instead, one may give reasons for why a motorcyclist might value an enhancement to protect the durability of her head, or why a ballerina might welcome enhanced strength in specific parts of her body, or why a mathematician or a chess player should value cognitive enhancements. These are all sensible human enhancements for particular kinds of people, but are not generally good enhancements for all kinds of people.

The rise of a privately funded human enhancement market and the possibility of commodifying life are each relevant moral concerns that should concern the governance of such industries. While a publicly funded system for human enhancements may be preferable to a privately funded one, areas of human desire are always likely to outweigh the limited funds available to accommodate such desires on a nationally funded system, even if one can aspire to a certain level of social care throughout a population. As such, it is sensible to presume that a transhuman future will be brought about within a commercial structure, though as argued earlier there are reasons to presume that some forms of enhancement will eventually ease the burden on a national healthcare system, by ensuring more people are less vulnerable to common illnesses.

Notes

1 For various versions of the slippery slope argument, see Burg (1991) and Resnik (1994).
2 Species-typical functioning is a concept developed by Christopher Boorse (1975, 1977) that is used to designate a specified normal range of what any given species can do. While there are variations within this range, any radical departure from the norm calls into question the species category of – and subsequently the moral rights afforded to – any given entity.
3 See Richard Titmuss (1970) for an eloquent elaboration of this concept.
4 For an explication of consumerism generally, see Miles (1998). It is important to note the revived appeals to commercial organ donation recently.
5 I will not attend to the arguments from "coercion" in this essay, though it is not obvious to me that all people will feel coerced into the same kinds of enhancements.
6 I introduce the specific instance of a minor here to complicate our case. While I have not distinguished between adults and children, there are good reasons to presume the need to distinguish levels of freedom to modify and I do not extend my argument to adolescent freedoms here. However, following the English court case of Gillick competence (*Gillick v West Norfolk and Wisbech Area Health Authority* [1985]), one might argue on behalf of such an ability to consent.

References

Boorse, Christopher (1975) "On the Distinction between Disease and Illness." *Philosophy and Public Affairs* 5, pp. 49–68.
Boorse, Christopher (1977) "Health as a Theoretical Concept." *Philosophy of Science* 44, pp. 542–573.
Bourdieu, Pierre (1984) *Distinction: A Social Critique of the Judgement of Taste.* London: Routledge.
Burg, Wibren van der (1991) The Slippery Slope Argument. *Ethics* 102, pp. 42–65.
Fukuyama, Francis (2002) *Our Posthuman Future: Consequences of the Biotechnology Revolution.* London: Profile Books.
Gillick v West Norfolk and Wisbech Area Health Authority [1985] 3 All ER 402 (HL).
Human Fertilisation and Embryology Authority (2003) *Sex Selection: Options for Regulation. A Report on the HFEA's 2002–03 Review of Sex Selection Including a Discussion of Legislative and Regulatory Options.* London: HFEA.

McCaskill4Missouri (2006, October 21) Michael J. Fox [on Stem Cells]. YouTube. http://www.youtube.com/watch?v=QMliHkTDHaE.

Miah, Andy (2008a). "Engineering Greater Resilience or Radical Transhuman Enhancement?" *Studies in Ethics, Law and Technology* 2/1. http://www.bepress.com/selt/vol2/iss1/art5.

Miah, Andy (2008b) "A Critical History of Posthumanism." In R. Chadwick and B. Gordijn, eds., *Medical Enhancements and Posthumanity*. New York: Springer.

Miah, Andy (2011) *The Ethics of Human Enhancement, Ethics and Values for the XXIst Century*. Spain: BBVA.

Miles, Steven (1998) *Consumerism as a Way of Life*. London: Sage.

More, Max (1993) "Technological Self-Transformation: Expanding Personal Extropy." *Extropy* 10, 4/2 (accessed January 4, 2009).

Nozick, Robert (1974) *Anarchy, State and Utopia*. New York: Basic Books.

Resnik, David (1994) "Debunking the Slippery Slope Argument against Human Germ-Line Gene Therapy." *Journal of Medicine and Philosophy* 19, pp. 23–40.

Rojek, Chris (1995) *Decentring Leisure: Rethinking Leisure Theory*. London: Sage.

Sandberg, Anders (2001) *Morphological Freedom: Why We Not Just Want It, but Need It*. Berlin: TransVision.

Shilling, Chris (1993) *The Body and Social Theory*. London: Sage.

Smith, Marquard (2006) "The Vulnerable Articulate: James Gillingham, Aimee Mullins, and Matthew Barney." In Marquard Smith and Joanne Morra, eds., *The Prosthetic Impulse: From a Posthuman Present to a Biocultural Future*. Cambridge, MA: MIT Press.

Smith, Marquard and Morra, Joanne, eds. (2006) *The Prosthetic Impulse: From a Posthuman Present to a Biocultural Future*. Cambridge, MA: MIT Press.

Sobchack, Vivian (2005) "A Leg to Stand On: Prosthetics, Metaphor, and Materiality." In M. Smith and J. Morra, eds., *The Prosthetic Impulse: From a Posthuman Present to a Biocultural Future*. Cambridge, MA: MIT Press.

Titmuss, Richard (1970) *The Gift Relationship: From Human Blood to Social Policy*. New York: Pantheon Books.

Vita-More, Natasha (2010) "Aesthetics of the Radically Enhanced Human." *Technoetic Arts: A Journal of Speculative Research* 8/2 (November), pp. 207–214.

Watts, Jonathan (2004) "China's Cosmetic Surgery Craze." *The Lancet* 363 (March 20), p. 958.

Further Reading

Annas, George J. (1994) "Our Most Important Product." In Robert H. Blank and Andrea L. Bonnickson, eds., *Medicine Unbound: The Human Body & the Limits of Medical Intervention*. New York: Columbia University Press, pp. 99–111.

Kramer, Peter D. (1994) *Listening to Prozac*. London: Fourth Estate.

Little, Margaret Olivia (1998) "Cosmetic Surgery, Suspect Norms, and the Ethics of Complicity." In E. Parens, ed., *Enhancing Human Traits: Ethical and Social Implications*. Washington, DC: Georgetown University Press.

Parens, Erik (2005) "Authenticity and Ambivalence: Towards Understanding the Enhancement Debate." *The Hastings Report* 35, pp. 34–41.

President's Council on Bioethics (2003) *Beyond Therapy: Biotechnology and the Pursuit of Happiness*. New York: HarperCollins.

Turner, Leigh (2003) "Has the President's Council on Bioethics Missed the Boat?" *British Medical Journal* 327, p. 629.

Zylinska, Joanna (2005) *The Ethics of Cultural Studies*. London: Continuum.

30

The Battle for the Future

Gregory Stock

How good bad music and bad reasons sound when we are marching into battle against an enemy

(Friedrich Nietzsche, 1881)

As advances in genomics and *in vitro* fertilization unite to bring us such technologies as germline manipulation and in-depth embryo diagnosis, must there be a battle over their use? Policymakers might, after all, acknowledge the arrival of these technologies, accept that people differ in their attitudes toward them, realize that society will adjust as it has to past advances such as the birth-control pill, and support efforts to minimize risks and maximize benefits.

Unfortunately, that scenario is unlikely. So symbolic and evocative of people's fears is the manipulation of human embryos that many countries have already banned the procedures. In Germany, either germline manipulations or preimplantation genetic diagnosis can bring a five-year prison sentence, according to the 1991 Embryo Protection Law (now being reconsidered), and the minister of justice stated that the purpose of the law was to "exclude even the slightest chance for programs aimed at so-called improvement of humans?"[1]

Even in the relatively permissive United States, moves are under way to hold such research apart and subject it to special scrutiny. In September 2000, a committee under the auspices of the American Association for the Advancement of Science (AAAS) (see Frankel and Chapman 2000), urged an immediate block on a wide range of clinical procedures that the group labeled "inheritable genetic modifications" (IGM). These included reproductive cloning, germline procedures, and fetal therapies that might alter eggs or sperm. Because cellular fluid, called

The Transhumanist Reader: Classical and Contemporary Essays on the Science, Technology, and Philosophy of the Human Future, First Edition. Edited by Max More and Natasha Vita-More.
© 2013 John Wiley & Sons, Inc. Published 2013 by John Wiley & Sons, Inc.

cytoplasm, contains about a dozen special genes that are inherited, the committee even recommended banning cytoplasmic transfers into the eggs of women suffering from a cellular disorder that would otherwise keep them from having children.

> Inheritable genetic modifications cannot be carried out safely and responsibly on humans utilizing current methods ... Even if we have the technical ability to proceed, however, we would need to determine whether IGM would offer a socially, ethically, and theologically acceptable alternative to other technologies ... Until then, no research or applications that could cause inheritable modifications in humans should go forward."[2]

No one would dispute the observation that direct germline modification is not safe today. But when committees that include scientists suggest that such procedures need to be "theologically acceptable" before their use, something unusual is going on. Fetal gene therapy aligns well with other gene-therapy work. Cytoplasmic transfer seems safe and is an obvious extension of other infertility research. No one is presently planning germline interventions of this sort, and in any event, no more than an occasional ill-conceived procedure – probably no worse than countless others with less provocative intentions – could slip by the review boards that oversee medical research and practice.

With mechanisms already in place to discourage doctors from trying risky, speculative, and unwarranted procedures on people, the worry about germline modification appears unnecessary. Once the procedures become more feasible, direct oversight is bound to follow, if only because without it, few couples would have the nerve to use them and few providers would be willing to shoulder the liability risks. In short, the inherited genetic modifications that the AAAS committee refer to are not about to explode into clinical use.

No useful interventions exist yet. No gene transfer procedures are available And when these interventions and procedures finally do exist, most parents will want evidence that they are reliable – validations that would take many years. Direct genetic modifications are so unlikely to touch large numbers of pregnancies in the next decade that anyone wishing to protect babies would do better to focus on poor nutrition, alcoholism, and unsafe drinking water.

The major threats from coming advances in reproductive technology are not medical but political, social, and philosophical. Moreover, embryo screening, which is safe, legal, and already in use, will soon bring up the same troubling dilemmas of germinal choice that the AAAS committee hoped a ban on inherited genetic modifications might delay. Emotions surrounding human genetic selection and manipulation are still relatively subdued compared with the passions that abortion now evokes, but to most people, "designer children" seem distant.

The current discussion about human enhancement is not what it seems, however. It is not about medical safety, the wellbeing of children, or protecting the human gene pool. At a fundamental level, it is about philosophy and religion. It is about what it means to be human, about our vision of the human future.

Leon Kass expressed his revulsion with cloning, but he could as easily have been referring to any advanced germinal choice technology (or perhaps to *in vitro* fertilization, which he assailed twenty years ago). "We are repelled ... because we intuit and we feel, immediately and without argument, the violation of things that we hold rightfully dear." Kass wrote. "We sense that cloning represents a profound defilement of our given nature as procreative beings, and of the social relations built on this natural ground ... Repugnance may be the only voice left that speaks up to defend the central core of our humanity. Shallow are the souls that have forgotten how to shudder" (see Kass 2001; see also Bailey 1998).

Who Will the Early Enhancers Be?

The specter of forced sterilization, concentration camps, and other horrors of the twentieth century perpetrated under cover of eugenic rhetoric (see Kevles 1995) ensures that today virtually no one speaks about the possibilities of human genetic manipulation without caveats and disclaimers. Many would go beyond such cautions, however, and reject this realm entirely. This opposition ranges from religious conservatives who see embryo research as tantamount to human experimentation, to bioethicists attuned to the potential problems of new technologies, to scientists troubled by the power that genomic sciences will wield, to environmentalists and neoLuddites worried (see Bailey 2001) about so deep an infusion of technology into our lives.

But many others say they would use the reproductive technologies if they existed. In the international opinion poll mentioned earlier (see Macer et al. 1995), from 22 to 83 percent of those surveyed in each of eight countries said they would use safe genetic interventions to enhance the mental or physical attributes of their children. Between 62 and 91 percent said they would use gene therapy to keep a child of theirs from inheriting a disease like diabetes.

Almost no one, however, is pushing for these technologies; they are too threatening. I once spoke about these issues with a group of libertarians, who rail about taxes and wholeheartedly embrace global free markets. Even they voiced concerns about unregulated manipulation of human embryos. Clearly, human biological enhancement puts philosophies of individual autonomy and laissez-faire ideology to the test.

The zealous few who most support these technologies are those who want to use them personally. Cloning is an instructive example of what will occur on a much broader front as other germinal choice technologies evolve and mature. Following the birth announcement of Dolly, the famous cloned sheep, the Raelians,[3] a New Age religious group that believes that visitors from space spawned humanity, were among the first to push aggressively for human cloning. In the fall of 2000, they announced that a wealthy American had donated $500,000 to fund a cloning attempt, and that they would move ahead. When I spoke with the church's founder, Raël, a Frenchman previously known as Claude Vorilhon, he told me that aliens had visited him in 1973 and shown him machines that could clone humans and sprout them into full-grown adults. Impressed, he decided to become their messenger, and raise $20 million to build an embassy to house the extraterrestrial visitors who would one day bring our salvation.

The Raelian cloning project was sufficiently quirky to command instant media attention. And Raël not only had money, he had some fifty volunteers willing to serve as surrogate mothers. With these resources, the group may succeed once mainstream researchers surmount the technical problems of nuclear transfer in primates and overcome the tendency of cloned embryos to have the unpredictable gene expression that can disrupt placenta formation and lead to fetal abnormalities.

My point here is that, as reproductive technology progresses, it is bound to drift out of the hands of traditional medical researchers and clinicians. But cloning efforts in more mainstream quarters are also moving forward. When Panos Zavos, a reproductive physiologist at the University of Kentucky, announced (shortly after the Raelians did) that he and an Italian fertility doctor, Severino Antinori, would done a human, the US Congress decided to hold hearings.[4] The testimony about the medical dangers of proceeding with human cloning persuaded neither the white-robed Raël nor Zavos in his suit and tie to shelve their projects. Instead, Zavos asserted at the hearings that he would not operate on American soil and would be unaffected by any US ban, and the Raelians said that they too would simply take their project elsewhere.

Whether either effort will get off the ground, much less succeed, is uncertain, but the ultimate outcome is not. Once science progresses further and animal cloning procedures become safe and reliable, there will be little delay in demonstrating them in human volunteers. The global regulatory environment will likely determine where such attempts take place and whether they are public, but not whether human cloning will occur. The same will also be the case with other advanced germinal choice technologies.

The Raelian episode illustrates that when people start to use these technologies, odd combinations of high technology, religion, and other beliefs may appear. I had heard several anecdotes, for example, about women using *in vitro* fertilization merely to time their pregnancies, so in the fall of 2000, when I spoke in San Diego before the American Society of Reproductive Medicine, I asked the large audience if anyone had encountered such behavior. A Brazilian IVF specialist volunteered that one of his patients had been so involved with numerology and astrology that she had decided to use IVF to fix the time of her child's conception. Here was a case of using reproductive technology to achieve an occult rather than a genetic enhancement.

[Alternatively,] [t]hose most committed to the goal of human enhancement are probably the so-called transhumanists, a hodgepodge of individuals and organizations loosely united by a desire to transcend human limitations (see Regis 1990). They welcome the development of anti-aging medicines, smart drugs, and genetic modification. The Extropians – a group studded with bright, iconoclastic figures and a board of [advisors] that include Marvin Minsky, Ray Kurzweil, and Roy Walford – are active in this arena. In 1999, their annual meeting in Berkeley, California included discussions focused on the challenges of extending human lifespan and genetic engineering. Walford, Judy Campisi, Calvin Harley, and Cynthia Kenyon, well-known figures in the field of aging, spoke at the meeting. At the conclusion, Max More, who founded the [philosophy of transhumanism and Extropy Institute] (the name [extropy] is meant to signify the reverse of entropy, the universal trend toward disorder) in 1992, read a "Letter to Mother Nature;" which captures their attitude,

> Mother Nature, truly we are grateful for what you have made us. No doubt you did the best you could. However, with all due respect, we must say that you have in many ways done a poor job with the human constitution. You have made us vulnerable to disease and damage. You compel us to age and die – just as we're beginning to attain wisdom. And, you forgot to give us the operating manual for ourselves! ... What you have made is glorious, yet deeply flawed ... We have decided that it is time to amend the human constitution ... We do not do this lightly, carelessly, or disrespectfully, but cautiously, intelligently, and in pursuit of excellence ... Over the coming decades we will pursue a series of changes to our own constitution ... We will no longer tolerate the tyranny of aging and death ... We will expand our perceptual range ... improve on our neural organization and capacity ... reshape our motivational patterns and emotional responses ... take charge over our genetic programming and achieve mastery over our biological and neurological processes. (More 1999)

This image of the human journey toward a superior "posthuman" may be difficult for many to take seriously, but the determination to use whatever new technologies emerge from today's explorations of human biology aligns well with prevailing attitudes. The number of people who undergo cosmetic surgery or pop expensive vitamin boosters testifies to this. Whatever people's philosophies of human enhancement, their decisions about using specific procedures often hinge on cost, safety, and efficacy rather than political or social consequences.

Understanding the forces that will affect the adoption of today's budding germinal choice technologies requires a global perspective. After all, outside the West, some scientists will push ahead regardless of what happens in North America and Europe. Societies in the Middle East and elsewhere that are driven by religious ideology will hardly embrace these innovations, but they will not figure heavily in the equation of global change. The fleetest, not the most cautious, will set the pace.

China stands out among today's emerging nations because it seems to have the resources, the predisposition, and the self-reliance to independently pursue the new technologies. Whether such a project is on China's agenda is unclear, but Beijing has been aggressive in managing repro- duction, and the social imperatives that grip the country seem to be pushing it in this direction. The one-child-per-family policies that cut its population growth from 2.9 percent in 1970 to 1.4 percent in 1990 were an extraordinary accomplishment (see O'Brien 1996). China's 1995 Maternal and Infant Health Care Law, which calls for compulsory premarital checkups as well as sterilization for "genetic diseases of a serious nature" and "mental diseases," is not now enforced, but its passage in the face of a loud international outcry is evidence of the country's willingness to follow an independent course. And in its rapid embrace of genetically modified crops, China has shrugged off European fears and released over one hundred varieties (see Spinney 2000), more than any other country, an indication of a growing enthusiasm for genomic technologies. Its total production of genetically modified crops is still small compared with that of the United States, Canada, and Argentina, but it is racing to catch up.

The same also seems to be happening with reproductive technologies. The IVF clinic in the city of Xi'an is not at all in accord with Western stereotypes about China. With its double con- tainment entrance, gleaming equipment, and scurrying masked nurses, the laboratory looks more like a set from *The Andromeda Strain* than an IVF clinic. The evocative air-lock entry is merely part of a filtration system needed to cleanse the polluted air hanging over the city. But this initial impression brings up the obvious question: why is China, with its teeming popula- tion, its aggressive control of family size, and its push for rapid economic growth, so concerned about infertility?

The army of terracotta soldiers that draws so many tourists to Xi'an interests me less than the giant billboards in Beijing's Tiananmen Square advertising infant formula. Overlaying huge images of Einstein and Picasso are slogans suggesting that milk may make your child more like these geniuses. Perhaps similar ads one day will tout the benefits of genetic enhancements. Some forty IVF clinics already exist in China, often built with military assistance, and a commitment to such technology seems to exist in influential segments of the government and military.

Many in the West shake their heads over Chinese eugenics and sterilization laws. But where couples can legally have only one child and must look to that child as their primary provider in old age, they are bound to feel strongly about having the "best" child they can. If this means having a boy (see Pomfret 2000: A01; Farah 1997; Zeng 1993: 297) – because a girl marries and joins her husband's family – they will try to have a boy. If it means screening for genetic vulner- abilities and diseases, they will do that. And if they could make their children smarter or stronger through genetic testing and manipulation, they'd probably do that too. Although the Chinese government may become involved in orchestrating parental "choices" of germinal enhancement, no directives would be needed for the technology to thrive in China, because the coming pos- sibilities accord so well with the perceived self-interest of the populace.

Wouldn't parents in the West, given similar social constraints, feel the same way? After all, the option of caring for a seriously disabled child or passing that responsibility on to the state is a modern luxury that few possess. Polls suggest that even with this option, 80 percent (Macer 1995) of Americans would use genetic interventions to prevent a child from inheriting a fatal disease. I suspect that couples with small families will be particularly inclined to screen the genetics of their future children carefully.

The counseling that medical geneticists give to prospective parents offers another window into the differing attitudes found in different cultures. If a prenatal test indicates the presence of Klinefelter syndrome, the most common form of dwarfism, 92 percent (Wertz 1999: 144, 145, 149) of counselors in China would push the parents to terminate the pregnancy, whereas in the United States, Australia, and most of western Europe, fewer than 10 percent would. The figures are similar for some two dozen diagnosable conditions ranging from Down's syndrome to cleft palate; nearly 80 percent of Chinese counselors would urge abortion.

In more than half the prenatal tests considered, Chinese geneticists counsel abortion more often than their counterparts anywhere else, though in India, Russia, and a number of smaller countries, including Greece, Cuba, Turkey, and Hungary, counselors also routinely give that advice. More than 90 percent of these counselors – compared with fewer than 20 percent in northern Europe and the United States – feel that to knowingly bring into the world an infant with a serious genetic disorder is socially irresponsible. In countries with a combined population of more than 3 billion – that is, a majority of all humans – most geneticists say the eugenic goal of reducing the number of deleterious genes in the population is an important one.

The Threat of Human Enhancement

A future in which parents select meaningful aspects of their children's genetics engenders anxiety in many people, despite the fact that our selection of a mate has always included such reckonings. Perhaps the use of technology for this purpose seems too controlled and calculated. To see why even people with no strong religious objections to advanced germinal choice technology might want to prevent it, imagine the following best-case scenario: Medical geneticists learn how to substantially reduce our vulnerabilities, improve our health, extend our vitality and lifespan, and enhance various other human attributes. Complications turn out to be modest and manageable. Public opposition, strong at first, soon withers into insignificance. Parents are thoughtful about the choices they make for their future children. The technology is sufficiently simple and inexpensive to be widely available. Totalitarian regimes don't try to impose it on their populations.

Although this scenario brims with utopian benefits and embodies a dreamy perfection that ignores the inherent messiness of any development so profound, it would leave extraordinary loss in its wake. Such a course of events would not only create a gulf between generations, it might divide us more deeply by encouraging us to judge explicitly the value of various human attributes. GCT [germinal choice technology] interventions would so change the trajectory of human life and the essence of the human condition as to render our past irrelevant to us in many ways. In making ourselves anew, we would have to figure out all over again what was important to us, and how and where we would find meaning in our lives. These are not easy tasks today, but at least the terrain is familiar and we can draw on history, religion, and literature for guidance.

As we head down the path of biological modification, we will gradually cease to be who we have always been. If we live longer, healthier, vastly different lives, we may end up estranged from the world we now inhabit. We may cease to feel connected to humanity as a whole. Such possibilities are why some people so vehemently oppose the new reproductive technologies. To them, germinal choice will bring the invasion of the inhuman, the displacement of the born by the made, and the twilight of humanity.

Dr. Nigel M. de S. Cameron, Professor of Theology and Culture at Trinity International University in Illinois, suggested as much when he argued, in May 2001, for an outright ban on the cloning of human embryos, even if they would be used for medical rather than reproductive purposes: "Cloning a human baby isn't just bad, or unfortunate, but something which would be profoundly evil because it would constitute a new human being in a radically defiled and deformed moral fashion. That is the view that many, many people take. It seems to me it is not a religious view. It's a view coming intuitively out of our vision for human dignity."[5]

Such a reaction could not be further from those of the Extropians and others who eagerly welcome the emerging possibilities and see them as the flowering of humanity, the realization of what until now has been an unreachable human dream: transcending our biological limits. The chasm separating these two perspectives is at the heart of the coming struggle over our journey into the human future.

Fear about the huge changes that may attend our manipulation of human biology and reproduction is understandable, but blocking advanced GCT will not protect us. Change is arriving too quickly across too broad a front. Our accelerating disengagement from the lessons and truths of the past will not be easy. We face it already in our shifting cultural environment: the weakening of traditional institutions and values, our multiplying connections with distant others, the increasing seductions of electronic worlds, the growing responsiveness of the digital devices we are infusing with intelligence and language. Germinal choice technologies will be but one ingredient, albeit a critical one, in this tumultuous transformation of human life.

There is little doubt that germinal choice will eventually reach us, but the extent of the divisiveness it brings is still uncertain. The harshest conflicts will probably arise not between societies but within them. International disagreements about manipulating human embryos may generate impassioned rhetoric, but once nations that oppose such technology enact bans within their own borders, they will be able to do little more. Nations have never been very successful in persuading other nations to modify their views on religious and social matters, and GCT will be no different. Even an international ban on these technologies would have no lasting impact since broad public interest in them would preclude effective enforcement. The more widespread and aggressive the opposition to their use, the greater the financial incentives will be for individuals and nations to defect and cater to pent-up demand.

Let's return to China, which was the preeminent world power in 1500 and might imagine itself achieving that position again in a few centuries. If the manipulation of human genetics seems a necessary step along that path, Western sensitivities and policies are unlikely to stand in the way. And once a single major nation embraces so foundational a development as this, others would soon have to follow, however reluctantly, to avoid being left behind.

In societies where culture and religion are relatively homogeneous, internal conflicts may be moderate, because opinions about these matters will be less diverse, but divisive policy battles are a virtual certainty in multicultural cauldrons like the United States. Some twenty-five years after Roe v. Wade the United States still experiences occasional bombings of abortion clinics.

Human enhancement procedures will bring an even more traumatic struggle. The debate, though polite today, will become much harsher as sophisticated embryo selection and germline technology draw near. Public reaction to the first human cloning may provide a foretaste of the passions that will be unleashed, but given the developmental abnormalities that can arise from gene expression errors caused by these procedures, human cloning may not happen nearly as soon as enthusiasts have predicted. In any event, those who imagine that public opposition will melt away with the arrival of a cute, healthy baby are underestimating the strength of people's feelings about cloning and GCT in general.

Of course, prior developments might moderate people's attitudes. If somatic gene therapy and the genomic sciences start to deliver solid medical breakthroughs, fears may diminish. Our pets may play a role in shaping public opinion as well. Genetic Savings & Clone and other companies have been working to clone dogs and cats as a commercial service. If this turns out to be relatively safe and reliable, and the wealthy begin to clone much-loved older pets to make a twin puppy or kitten, we may grow comfortable with these reproductive technologies sooner than we think But I doubt that the coming general transformation of human reproduction will be so easy. The Catholic Church, after all, still opposes birth control.

The irony about germline and other germinal choice technologies is that as challenging as they will be at a symbolic level, the procedures are fundamentally life-giving. This could pose a dilemma for those who might be tempted to smash the laboratories where such work takes place. Today anti-abortion extremists see themselves as locked in a battle to save innocent lives from the knives of murderers. They assault abortion doctors and display gruesome photos of aborted fetuses in a crusade they see as "pro-life."

Advanced reproductive technologies will present more complex choices. Genetic alteration of human embryos may be deeply offensive to these crusaders, but they would see an incubator filled with embryos as a vessel holding human life. If life begins at conception and is to be honored as such, to destroy that incubator would be tantamount to mass murder. Indeed, some who vehemently oppose abortion may find themselves drawn to the idea of practicing medicine on embryos, simply because it seems to treat these cells as patients.

Protecting the Human Race

Those who categorically oppose future reproductive technologies such as cloning, advanced preimplantation genetic diagnosis, and germline enhancement portray themselves as voices of reason and caution, trying to protect humanity from these divisive and dangerous spinoffs of medical science. Whether they depict the threat as medical, social, environmental, or spiritual, their implicit assumption is that if we cannot stop these technologies, we should at least delay them as long as possible, because of the significant risks they pose and the dubious benefits they offer. Given that humanity has not needed such novel reproductive procedures to reach the present and has already suffered lamentable forays into eugenics, they see no good argument for pushing ahead.

There was a furor when it was revealed in December 1999 that the European Patent Office had inadvertently awarded a patent dealing in part with human germline manipulation. The European Parliament quickly called for the patent's revocation and reiterated its opposition to applying to human beings biotechnology that involves "interventions in the human germline," "cloning of the human being in all phases of its development," or "research on human embryos, which destroys the embryo."[6]

Serious enforcement of these categorical prohibitions would involve two costs: the beneficial enhancements that are lost and the damage the ban itself inflicts. The first loss might be relatively minor, because research can usually migrate elsewhere. But the extreme measures needed to effect such a ban might be quite injurious. What's more, the larger goals of such actions are murky at best. If these bans are a call for "natural" reproduction, unpolluted by technology, then why not also repudiate IVF and birth control? If they are a declaration against eugenic selection, then they leave gaping loopholes such as amniocentesis. If they are meant to protect distant, yet-to-be-conceived generations, then they are so blunt and premature that they could do more harm than good.

Advanced germinal choice technology does not yet exist, so enforcement is not an issue, and prohibitions are easy political gestures. But once GCT arrives, enforcement will be nearly impossible. Testing every baby at birth, for example, could reveal enhancements involving artificial chromosomes but not single-gene replacements. Even running genetic profiles on parents would not show that a child was from a genetically screened embryo or was the clone of a deceased sibling, since the child's genome would not be altered.

Many people would be more disturbed by mandatory genetic tests of babies than by the chance that some couple somewhere might enhance a child. The International Olympic Committee had to discontinue testing the gender of female athletes after the practice was assailed as an invasion of privacy, and in the United States, the privacy provisions of the Health Insurance Portability and Accountability Act make the sharing of any medical information without a patient's permission, including genetic information, a crime (see Ferguson-Smith et al. 1992).

Punishment would present problems too. A baby born by germinal choice technology would be guiltless, penalizing the parents harshly enough to deter them from a private act intended to help their child might seem abusive, and reproductive specialists might be beyond legal reach. Not only does the diversity of attitudes throughout the world suggest that any serious ban could only be regional, but in the United States, much GCT may eventually be interpreted as procreative freedom and treated as a fundamental right protected against unwarranted government intervention. The ultimate effect of regional bans will be to move these technologies to permissive locales and cede their development to others.

If we ban advanced GCT on philosophical or religious grounds and cannot enforce the ban, it will cause harm in other ways. Prohibitions would lead people to judge others not by who they are but by the way their parents conceived them, to label such children as different, and to invite the very class conflicts we wish to avoid. This course would ensure that advanced reproductive technologies besiege rather than serve us. It would enshrine in law the fear that we cannot trust parents to use these tools responsibly. It would push us toward government monitoring of our genetics and reproduction.

Even if we could ban all germinal choice technologies, we still would not avoid grappling with the consequences of unraveling human biology. Our growing ability to read the genetics of potential future children and make choices based on what we learn is but one way that the genomics revolution will challenge our sense of who we are, how we relate to one another, and what is important to us. With the cost of DNA chips falling rapidly, routine analysis of our individual genetic constitutions is not far away. Like it or not, we will have to come to grips with what our genes have to say about who we are. We will have to face how our genetics circumscribes our potentials, our vulnerabilities, and even our personalities. Our genes will not tell us our destiny, but they will speak to us, and we would do well to listen.

We can pretend that every genetic makeup is as good as every other, but putting aside serious genetic diseases and vulnerabilities, we each have our likes and dislikes, our prejudices and preferences.

As individuals, we do not respond alike to all personalities, and when we can ascertain something meaningful about the genetic predispositions of our children-to-be, we will likely be swayed by the information. Some parents will not want to know such things, just as they do not want to know the sex of their child in advance. Others will be curious and want a look. Still others will want to make choices.

We might assert that knowledge is okay but intervention is not, though this would be contrary to current practice and law in the United States. Couples already make some reproductive interventions – such as screenings for disease – that are widely accepted, and others – such as sex selection – that are not. As the quality and quantity of information grow, a consensus will emerge about some practices, but for many others no consensus will be possible. If we decide to impose regulations on the more contentious choices, we will be heading down a difficult path. The law is a blunt instrument when it comes to the nuances of individual situations, and it will seem ever more out of touch as our choices become subtler. Imagine having to seek permission for the timing of your child's birth, laying out your reasoning and pleading your case. The most even-handed committee would seem oppressive, because the process would be so intrusive. I suspect we would do better to rely on parental decisions, unless consensus exists that there is a likelihood of serious harm.

This hands-off approach would require great restraint, because many situations will no doubt distress us. Some deaf couples say that in their culture a deaf child fits in more easily and therefore would be better off than a hearing child. If such a couple decide to use embryo selection to guarantee that their child was deaf – and some have expressed that wish – no one could argue that they were injuring a healthy child. They simply would be choosing deafness (see Li et al. 1998; Kennedy 1998).

Testing early-stage fetuses and aborting those not deaf may be disturbing, but so strong is the belief in parental autonomy in the United States that more than a third of American obstetricians say they would perform a prenatal test to open up that possibility. Prenatal tests for sex selection are even more accepted. Given that we do not prohibit these controversial procedures, a general ban on preimplantation genetic diagnosis of embryos seems unlikely, and telling women which embryo to implant is implausible. Indeed, once broad embryo selection is available, even a ban on direct germline manipulation is dubious because the technique's intended outcomes would be so obvious an extension of embryo selection.

Sports offers another preview of the challenges of enforcing any ban on genetic modifications. The use of performance-enhancing drugs is illegal in competitive sports, but policing is difficult despite a nearly ideal situation for effective action. The sanctions enjoy near-universal public support. A straightforward penalty – exclusion from the sport – exists. Sporting authorities have large budgets at their disposal. Athletes submit to intrusions on their privacy that the general population would never tolerate. Elite athletes are few in number, easily identifiable, and physically accessible at competitions. These advantages, however, are not enough to overcome the ingenuity of athletes with strong incentives to cheat.

We might imagine that people will not be motivated to violate restrictions on reproductive technologies, but this does not seem to be the case. A grief-stricken father phoned me six months after the suicide of his son and told me he wanted to clone the boy. The man was wealthy, determined, and would have done almost anything to accomplish this goal had the technology existed.

If we cannot keep performance-enhancing drugs out of sports, how can we effectively ban pharmaceutical and genetic enhancement in the rough-and-tumble of the real world? People will not agree that enhancement procedures are wrong and will resist intrusions on their privacy. Violators will be scattered and hard to identify, and punishment will be uncertain and slow.

It is hard to see what good will flow from blanket prohibitions today on the reproductive technologies of tomorrow. The landscape of their potential use is still so unclear that such laws will probably prove to be ineffectual for situations that are substantially different from what we now imagine. At best, legal sanctions will merely dull discussion of the coming challenges by creating the false impression that we can will them away. At worst they will stifle beneficial research, divide our society, and drive advanced GCT into the hands of the least responsible among us.

A Spiritual Crossroads

A key aspect of human nature is our ability to manipulate the world. We plant, we build, we dam, we hunt, we mine, and increasingly we do so on a huge scale. For as long as we have been able to, we have altered ourselves as well. We not only wear clothing, we pierce our bodies, tattoo our skin, cut our hair, and surgically sculpt ourselves. We add or remove hair, straighten our teeth, fix our noses, enhance or reduce our breasts, get rid of fat. We use drugs to reduce pain, lose weight, change moods, stay awake. The idea that we will long forgo better and more powerful ways of modifying ourselves is a denial of what the past tells us about who we are.

We are now reaching the point at which we may be able to transform ourselves into something "other." To turn away from germline selection and modification without even exploring them would be to deny our essential nature and perhaps our destiny. Ultimately, such a retreat might deaden the human spirit of exploration, taming and diminishing us. This seems particularly clear to the American psyche, influenced as it has been by the frontier. Many writers have described this exploratory exuberance. Early in the last century, the influential historian Frederick Jackson Turner (1920: 1–38) put it this way:

> For a moment, at the frontier, the bonds of custom are broken and unrestraint is triumphant ... Each frontier did indeed furnish a new field of opportunity, a gate of escape from the bondage of the past; and freshness, and confidence, and scorn of older society, impatience of its restraints and its ideas, and indifference to its lessons, have accompanied the frontier. What the Mediterranean Sea was to the Greeks, breaking the bond of custom, offering new experiences, calling out new institutions and activities, that, and more, the ever retreating frontier has been to the United States directly, and to the nations of Europe more remotely.

We often look to space as the next frontier – our expansion out into the solar system and beyond. Ultimately this may happen, but the next frontier is not outer space but ourselves. Exploring human biology and facing the truths we uncover in the process will be the most gripping adventure in all our history, and it has already begun. What emerges from this penetration into our inner space will change us all: those who stay home, those who oppose the endeavor, those tarrying at its rear, and those pushing ahead at its vanguard.

Albrecht Sippel, a German biologist who opposes human germline manipulation, had this to say when I suggested that there was no way to stop it: "If you suddenly would have an easy genetic way, let's say, to enhance intelligence or do better in school examinations, people would do it. They wouldn't wait fifty years to figure out whether it's really positive ... I could say, as a European, let the Americans try. They are the guinea pigs. I don't want to be that guinea pig."

His is a reasonable position. The embrace of new technology is never uniform. Individuals and societies alike are comfortable with different levels of uncertainty and risk. But such preferences need not be cloaked in moral rectitude. After all, few people who philosophically oppose embryonic stem cell research would forgo the advances that arise from the enterprise, however morally inconsistent this position may be. If such research generates medical breakthroughs to treat Alzheimer's or heart disease, or slows some aspect of aging, we will want these benefits. The same is likely to be true of the possibilities of germinal choice.

Earlier, I discussed why outright bans on advanced germinal choice technology will eventually break down, but such bans are problematic even now. While they may deter those scientists who would otherwise mount the more visible and expensive early projects attempting to demonstrate these technologies in humans, they will neither halt nor slow the broader scientific progress needed for GCT to be viable in actual clinical settings. So bans will shorten the lead time between early demonstrations and eventual clinical rollouts. And this time is precious, because early demonstrations are what spark the media attention and debate that help us iron out the problems and prepare for the changes to come. The longer our lead time, the more measured and thoughtful we can be.

Early demonstrations are the heralds of what is coming, so we should be wary of stifling them. When an advanced GCT does not place a future child at inordinate risk, and a well-informed couple willingly chooses the procedure and pays for it, we should understand that however much we dislike what they are doing, society benefits. In essence, such couples are volunteering as the test pilots of human biological manipulation. These experiments will take place; the crucial question is whether society will find out what happens when they do.

This doesn't mean that we do not need to regulate the clinical use of these technologies. No one seriously thinks that widespread medical interventions on human embryos will occur without oversight. The issue is how close that oversight should be and whether its primary focus should be individual safety.

Policymakers sometimes mistakenly think that they have a choice about whether germinal technologies will come into being. They do not. If, in the mid-1700s, the British Parliament had banned the steam engine to try to stave off the industrial revolution, the action might have altered some of the details of the mechanization of human endeavor but would not have stopped it. The same is true of the computer and genomics revolutions of today.

At the heart of the coming possibilities of human enhancement lies the fundamental question of whether we are willing to trust in the future. Will we accept humanity's eventual transformation into something beyond human, or we will battle against it and try to protect those aspects of the human form and character that we see as intrinsic to our humanness?

I have argued that our exploration of these technologies is inevitable, but nothing can be truly certain. Critics who seek international bans on germinal choice technology seem to feel that they can head off the future I've described, or perhaps they merely believe that their struggle, though doomed, will at least preserve their own integrity. If some combination of these attitudes is commonplace, and I suspect it is, then the reproductive technologies that attend today's genomics revolution will provoke bitter cultural conflicts.

A belief expressed by many of those who would like to prevent the reworking of human biology and reproduction is, as I stated earlier, that we should not play God, although typically opponents express the idea in secular terms, such as our need to protect human dignity. Ironically, embracing the challenges and goals of these transformative technologies is an act of extraordinary faith. It embodies an acceptance of a human fate written both in our underlying nature and in the biology that constitutes us. We cannot know where self-directed evolution will take us, nor hope to control the process for very long. It will depend on our ongoing responses to continual changes that hinge not only on the character of future technologies we cannot yet glimpse but on the values of future humans we cannot hope to understand.

In offering ourselves as vessels for potential transformation into we know not what, we are submitting to the shaping hand of a process that dwarfs us individually. In secular terms, this is nothing special: we are merely accepting the possibilities of the advanced technologies we are creating. But from a spiritual perspective, the project of humanity's self-evolution is the ultimate embodiment of our science and ourselves as a cosmic instrument in our ongoing emergence. Rabbi Barry Freundel put it this way: "If G-d has built the capacity for gene redesign into nature, then He chose for it to be available to us, and our test remains whether we will use that power wisely or poorly!" (Freundl 2000).

One thing we can say with some confidence about the future we have embarked upon is that germinal choice technology may lead to considerable strangeness in the centuries ahead. Those who are happy to let GCT lead us where it may are trusting that our children, our children's children, and the many to be born after them will have the wisdom and clarity not to use this powerful knowledge in destructive ways. Those who fear that recent human history suggests that such trust is unfounded have no reason to think that we today can make better choices in this arena, much less project them forward in time. But if we can manage today's more pressing threats, coming generations will have their shot at tomorrow's. To accept a strange and uncertain future is not easy, because despite all our present weaknesses, at least we have an idea who we are. With technology so transforming the world around us, it might be comforting to know that the human family will, after all, long remain "human" and a "family." But perhaps this is asking too much – or too little.

One way to anticipate our responses to the challenging possibilities we are moving toward is to look at previous breakthroughs that have reshaped forever our vision of the world and ourselves. People sometimes snicker that the Catholic Church condemned Galileo. The Copernican universe is such a given today that it is hard to imagine a time when the Earth's place at the center of the universe was vital enough to Christianity's idea of heavenly order that the pope was willing to stake his infallibility on it. In the face of such assaults on a cherished worldview, denial is a natural refuge. On June 22, 1633, Galileo knelt before the tribunal that sentenced him and recanted his heresy:

> I must altogether abandon the false opinion that the Sun is the center of the world and immovable and that the Earth is not the center of the world and moves … With sincere heart and unfeigned faith I abjure, curse, and detest the aforesaid errors and heresies and generally every other error, heresy, and sect whatsoever contrary to the Holy Church, and I swear that in future I will never again say or assert, verbally or in writing, anything that might furnish occasion for a similar suspicion regarding me. (de Santiallana 1955: 310–311)

The next day his judges reduced his sentence from life in prison to permanent house arrest. He remained confined until his death, nine years later at the age of 86, and his book *The Dialogue on the Two Chief World Systems* remained on the Index of Prohibited Books for more than two centuries. Not until 1992, more than 350 years later, did Pope John Paul II admit that the Vatican and Pope Urban VIII had erred.

The special significance of humanity seemed clear to Western thinkers in the Middle Ages: Earth was the center of the universe, and we were fashioned in God's image. The Copernican revolution shattered that notion, wrenching humanity from its exalted station and leaving it stranded on a peripheral planet circling one of many stars. The Darwinian revolution finished the job, leaving us fashioned not by divine consciousness but by random natural forces.

We survived these shocks and have even grown accustomed to our new place. Indeed, many take inspiration from the awesome immensity of the universe and ascribe a sacred quality to the natural environment and the evolutionary forces that molded us. There is majesty in these powerful forces and vast distances, resplendence in the eons of time that bore us.

We know all too well our limitations: our ineptitudes and weaknesses, our selfishness and egotism. No wonder the idea that we would attempt to fashion not only our future world but our future selves terrifies many people. In essence, such a process would replace the hand of an allknowing and almighty Creator with our own clumsy fingers and instruments. It would trade the cautious pace of natural evolutionary change for the careless speed of high technology. We would be flying forward with no idea where we were going and no safety net to catch us.

Early in the year 2000, Bill Joy, the cofounder and chief scientist of Sun Microsystems, articulated this anxiety. In an article called "Why the World Doesn't Need Us," in which he urges us to relinquish genetic engineering and other advanced technologies, he writes, "If we could agree, as a species, what we wanted, where we were headed, and why, then we would make our future much less dangerous." To imagine that we could ever agree on such things, however, is the ultimate naiveté. Our future will emerge from the same chaotic jumble of trial and error and individual action and reaction that has formed our present. And this is fortunate, because we express a collective wisdom in our actions that far exceeds that of any commission of experts or council of elders who would guide us. Idealistic movements professing visions of a greater good have perpetrated some of the greatest evils of history. If instead of blinding ourselves with utopian images we admit that we don't know where we are headed, maybe we will work harder to ensure that the process itself serves us, and in the end that is what we must count on.

Notes

1 See Bonnicksen 1994, and Embryo Protection Law, December 13, 1990, reprinted in *International Digest of Health Legislation* (1991), pp. 60–62.
2 See Parens and Juengst 2001; Barritt et al. 2001.
3 See www.rael.org, and www.rael.org/int/english/embassy/embassy.html
4 See http://energycommerce.house.gov/107/action/107-5.pdf.
5 See http://www.pewforum.org/Science-and-Bioethics/Human-Cloning-Religious-Perspectives.aspx.
6 See http://www.europarl.europa.eu/sides/getDoc.do?pubRef=-//EP//TEXT+TA+P5-TA-2000-0136+0+DOC+XML+V0//EN.

References

Bailey, Ronald (1998) "Send in the Clones." *Reason* (June).
Bailey, Ronald (2001) "Rage against the Machines: Witnessing the Birth of the Neo-Luddite Movement." *Reason* (July), pp. 26–35.
Barritt, Jason A. et al. (2001) "Mitochondria in Human Offspring Derived from Ooplasmic Transplantation." *Human Reproduction* 16, pp. 513–516.
Bonnicksen, Andrea L. (1994) "National and International Approaches to Human Germ-Line Gene Therapy." *Politics and the Life Sciences* 13/1 (February), pp. 39–49.
de Santiallana, Giorgio (1955) *The Crime of Galileo*. Chicago: University of Chicago Press.
Farah, Joseph (1997) "Cover-Up of China's Gender-Cide." *World Net Daily Archive* (September 29).

Ferguson-Smith, Malcolm, et al. (1992) "Olympic Row Over Sex Testing." *Nature* 355, p. 10.

Frankel, Mark and Chapman, Aubrey (2000) *Human Inheritable Genetic Modifications: Assessing Scientific, Ethical, Religious, and Policy Issues*. Washington, DC: AAAS Publication Services.

Freundel, Rabbi Barry (2000) "Gene Modification Technology." In Gregory Stock and John Campbell, eds., *Engineering the Human Germline: An Exploration of the Science and Ethics of Altering the Genes We Pass to Our Children*. New York: Oxford University Press. p. 121.

Kass, Leon (2001) "Why We Should Ban Cloning Now: Preventing a Brave New World." *New Republic* (May 21), pp. 30–39.

Kennedy, Marc (1998) "Ethics of Genetic Testing." *Wisconsin Medical Journal* (April). www.wismed.org/wmj/98-04/wmj498-kenn3.htm.

Kevles, Daniel (1995) *In the Name of Eugenics: Genetics and the Uses of Human Heredity*. Cambridge, MA: Harvard University Press.

Li, Xuechen, et al. (1998) "A Mutation in PDS Causes Non-Syndromic Recessive Deafness." *Nature Genetics* 18, pp. 215–217.

Macer, Darryl, et al. (1995) "International Perceptions and Approval of Gene Therapy." *Human Gene Therapy* 6, pp. 791–803.

More, Max (1999) "A Letter to Mother Nature." Keynote address, EXTRO-4 Conference, Berkeley, CA (August). www.maxmore.com/mother.htm

O'Brien, Claire (1996) "China Urged to Delay 'Eugenics' Law." *Nature* 383/6597, p. 204.

Parens, Erik and Juengst, Eric (2001) "Inadvertently Crossing the Germline Barrier." Editorial. *Science* 292, pp. 397.

Pomfret, John (2000) "China Losing 'War' on Births: Uneven Enforcement Undermines One-Child Policy." *Washington Post Foreign Service* (May 3), p. A1.

Regis, Ed (1990) *Great Mambo Chicken and the Transhuman Condition: Science Slightly Over the Edge*. Reading, MA: Addison-Wesley.

Spinney, Laura (2000) "Switched On." *New Scientist* (November 4), pp. 52–55.

Turner, Frederick J. (1920) *The Frontier in American History*. New York: Henry Holt.

Wertz, D. (1999) "Views of Chinese Medical Geneticists: How they Differ from 35 Other Nations." In O. Döring, ed., *Chinese Scientists and Responsibility*. Hamburg: Mitteilungen des Instituts für Asienkunde, pp. 141–160.

Zeng, Yi, et al. (1993) "Causes and Implications of the Recent Increase in the Reported Sex Ratio at Birth in China." *Population and Development Review* 19, p. 2.

31

Mind is Deeper Than Matter
Transgenderism, Transhumanism, and the Freedom of Form

Martine Rothblatt

One's gender is merely an important subset of choosing one's form. By "form" I mean that which encloses our beingness – flesh for the life we are accustomed to, plastic for the robots of science fiction, mere data for the avatars taking over our computer screens. Freedom of form arises because twenty-first-century software makes it *technologically* possible to separate our minds from our biological bodies. This can be accomplished by downloading enough of our neural connection contents and patterns into a sufficiently advanced computer, and merging the resultant "mindfile" with sufficiently advanced software – call it "mindware." Once such a download and merger is complete, we would have chosen a new form – software – although we would be the same person. It would be quite like changing gender from male to female, or female to male. Transsexuals choose a new form although they are still the same person (Bornstein 1994: 123–128).

It is debatable whether or not a mind made of software can ever be the same as a mind based in flesh. We won't know the answer until the experiment is done. But as the mindfiles become increasingly complete, and as the mindware becomes increasingly sophisticated, the software-based mind will become ever closer to the flesh-based mind. Indeed, even our flesh-based minds differ from day to day and surely over the course of one's life. But we are still the same person. In other words, the self is a characteristic visualization of the world and pattern of responding to it, including emotions. Because visions and patterns are really information, our selves can be expressed as faithfully in software as they are in our brains. We can clone ourselves in software without copying every single memory because we see ourselves as a pattern of awareness, feeling, and response, not as an encyclopedia of memories.

The Transhumanist Reader: Classical and Contemporary Essays on the Science, Technology, and Philosophy of the Human Future, First Edition. Edited by Max More and Natasha Vita-More.
© 2013 John Wiley & Sons, Inc. Published 2013 by John Wiley & Sons, Inc.

Persona Creatus

A new form for humanity implies a very fundamental break with the DNA-based definition of *homo sapiens*. Our DNA no longer dictates all aspects of our individual survival, for if it did near-sighted individuals would be gone, eaten by predators they could not see in time to escape. Our DNA no longer dictates our ability to pass on our genes. *In vitro* fertilization with or without embryo transfer routinely provides reproduction for thousands of infertile couples.

The rise of transgenderism provides sociobiologists with evidence of a new species. An important part of most species' signature is the characteristically gender dimorphic behaviors of their members. However, thanks to culture and technology, humans are leaving those gender dimorphic behaviors behind as they come to appreciate the limitless uniqueness of their sexual identities. As our creativity has blossomed, we have matured from *homo sapiens* into *persona creatus*.

The greatest catapult for humanity into a new species lies just beyond the event horizon of transgenderism. Based upon our rapidly accelerating ability to imbue *software* with human personality, autonomy, and self-awareness, a movement of "transhumanists" has joined transgenderists in calling for the launch of *persona creatus*. A basic transhumanist concept is that a human need not have a flesh body, just as a woman need not have a real vagina.[1] Humanness is in the mind, just as is sexual identity. As software becomes increasingly capable of thinking, acting and feeling like a human, it should be treated as a fellow human, and welcomed as a fellow member of the technological species *persona creatus*.

The biologist will insist that members of a common species be capable of producing fertile offspring, and so it is for transhumans and *persona creatus*. Reproduction will no long necessarily occur, however, via joined DNA. Instead, people of flesh will upload into software the contents and processes of their minds. Think of this as taking all of your digital photos, movies, emails, online chats, tweets, posts, updates, purchases, google searches, favorites, and blogs to the next level, and merging it with "mindware" that can replicate how you think, feel, and react based on the huge digital database of your thoughts, feelings, and reactions. Once we have thus digitally cloned our minds, new digital people can be produced by combining some of our mindware with some of our partner's mindware. *Voilà*, there are fertile offspring and the species *persona creatus* is alive. Furthermore, since purely digital people can reproduce with flesh humans in this manner, the humans and the transhumans are common members of *persona creatus*.

Freedom of gender is, therefore, the gateway to a *freedom of form* and to an explosion of human potential. First comes the realization that we are not limited by our sexual anatomy. Then comes the awakening that we are not limited by our anatomy at all. The mind is the substance of humanity. Mind is deeper than matter.

The Sex of an Avatar

Avatars are pure software constructs. If they continue to increase in sophistication at the rate of the past 10 years, they will soon literally think for themselves. How will they feel about sex? There are millions of different answers to this question because there will be millions of differently programmed avatars. An avatar whose software program and associated database was very much a copy of a flesh human's main memories and thought patterns would feel about sex the same way the flesh human felt about sex. Could the avatar actually have sex? Touch-sensitive screens already provide software with a sense of feeling. Chess programming expert David Levy exudes confidence in his 2007 book *Love and Sex with Robots* that touch-screen software is the leading edge of a full spectrum of replicated sensuality (Levy 2007: 289–299).

Ray Kurzweil demonstrates how a continuation of the computer industry's 50-year track record of processor speed doubling (Moore's Law) will result by 2020 in desktop computers with the capabilities of the human mind.[2] Computer science guru Marvin Minsky argues persuasively in his 2006 book *The Emotion Machine* that software can be written to feel all the same things we feel when we love or make love (Minsky 2006: 6–34). A good sign of the humanness, or autonomy, of an avatar is that they choose their own sex and display their own gender. Such an avatar would be both transgendered and transhuman: transgendered because they chose their own gender; transhuman because they identify with being human, even though they are not made of flesh.

Avatar sexuality is a key bridge from transgender to transhuman. It makes cerulean clear that sexual identity is limitless in variety and detachable from reproduction. And by making that point, it simultaneously demonstrates that human identity is limitless in variety and detachable from reproduction. If you can accept that a person without a penis can peaceably live life as they please (including as a man), then you should be able to accept that a person without a physical form can peaceably live life as they please (including as a human).[3] Can you can accept that someone is not automatically passive, or evil, or dumb simply because they have a vagina instead of a penis? Then you should be able to accept that someone is not automatically passive, or evil, or dumb simply because they have a software mind instead of a flesh-based one. Personhood is about equity, not equipment.

While the ancient trunk of sexual identity lies rooted in successful reproductive strategies, the fruit of that tree has now spread far beyond DNA-swapping. Breaking the connection between gender and genitals opened the channel between personhood and form. Once we realize that our essential sweetness is in our minds, and that each of us has unique life-path potential not fully tethered to a body-determined route, then it is as sensible to be transhuman as it is to be transgendered. Be-ing beats gene-ing.

Counting Cyberfolks

Around the time some decades hence that census takers and marriage makers stop asking our sex, they will face a profound question: which instantiation of a person is the person and which is someone else? "Instantiation" means a temporary or permanent form adopted by a person's beingness – their major memories, feelings, and ways of thinking about life. Suppose functional magnetic resonance imaging (fMRI) type technology continues to advance to the point that all of the neural connections in our brain can be mapped onto software (non-invasive brain scanners like fMRI are increasing in resolution and processing speed at an exponential rate that makes this realistic within the lifetimes of most readers of this essay) (Kurzweil 2005: 157–163). In this case, when the software saw (through a video connection) someone we knew, it would feel the same thing we felt when our brain processed an image of that person. In other words, "mind-uploading" technology makes it possible to duplicate yourself outside your body. That duplicate (or triplicate …) of yourself is a new instantiation of yourself.

The moment there is a new instantiation of you it can begin a separate life. It will have experiences that the original self does not have. (Remember, though, each day everyone begins a separate life, with experiences the previous day's version of us does not have.) On the other hand, it could be arranged that one or all of your instantiations synchronize regularly such that the experiences of one are the experiences of all. In this case, we will have crossed into the transhuman domain of "one mind, many forms."

The non-original forms need not all be chunks of software restricted to cyberspace. With extensions of the regenerative medicine technology being used today to grow skin, blood vessels, and organs it will be possible to grow an entire fresh body outside of a womb and to write into its vacant brain the synchronized "mindfile" derived originally from an MRI scan of your brain (or mindfile plus mindware based facsimile of your mind). Ectogenesis, the growth of a body outside of a womb, would produce an adult-sized person in just 20 months if the fetus continues to grow at the rate it does for its first six months. If that is too incredible, consider the rate of advancement in robot technology. Today's robots can successfully drive cars, fly planes, play violin, and help doctors (Carroll and Aguilera-Hellweg 2011). Robots of tomorrow will also have skin so soft you'd think it was flesh, and faces as persuasive as a Pixar animation. Such "bodyware" forms will come plug-and-play ready for your synchronized mindfile.

Why would anyone want two or more bodies with a single synchronized brain? First, to ensure they kept living if one body prematurely died, a concern that is especially appropriate to those who are in dangerous professions. Second, to savor more of life's many pleasures by surmounting the frustration of "I can only be in one place at one time." Be it shoes, hats, toilets, phones, TVs, cars, computers or homes, it is remarkable how humans quickly get over their gratitude to have just one of something, and soon hanker for multiples.

Transhumans welcome "one mind, many forms" the way transgenders welcome "one mind, many genders." Just as society's enumerators adapted to multiple races in single individuals, they will adapt to multiple sexes and ultimately to multiple forms in single individuals. Solutions will be found to ensure transhumans are limited to "one mind, one vote" just as solutions are being developed to enable same-genital couples to live as a family. The law is famously creative in rearticulating its precedents to support what is happening in the real world.

Papering a Transhuman

The coming wave of transhuman persons presents a fundamental issue: does someone without a human form and without a natal birth have any rights at all? What pathway to citizenship is there for someone with the mind of a human but a purely virtual or artificial body?

A likely scenario over the next few decades is that people will copy ever greater portions of their mind into software. These software analogs will work, shop, and communicate on behalf of their flesh masters. The more autonomous and life-like these software analogs are, the more useful they will be, and hence market forces will make them increasingly human-like. At about this time some human masters will suffer bodily death, but will claim that they are still alive in the guise of their software analogs. In essence, these transhumans will claim to have had a "mind transplant" to save their life not unlike the heart and kidney transplants that save so many lives. Lawsuits will surely ensue over (1) whether or not a death certificate should be issued, (2) whether there is an estate, i.e., does the transhuman or its flesh descendants control its property, and (3) whether the transhuman can get married and raise a family.

There are in fact reasonable "non-formist" ways to determine if a transhuman is really human, and thus deserving of a birth or marriage certificate. For example, psychologists certified to determine whether someone adequately demonstrates consciousness, rationality, empathy, and other hallmark human traits could interview transhumans. Should two or more such psychologists agree as to the transhumanist's humanity, the virtual person should either be permitted to continue the life of their biological original, or, if newly created, be granted a birth certificate and citizenship. It would be silly to ask after the transhuman's sex as virtual beings are quite transgendered.

There is nothing too unusual about relying upon psychologists to tell us whether someone's frame of mind is authentic or a fake. They are called upon to do this in many trials, where one dispute is over the defendant's state of mind.[4] They are also called upon to do this in authorizing surgeons to perform genital-change surgery. In this latter instance the psychologists interview transsexuals to determine whether they are sincere in their mental sense of themselves as another sex. If so, then surgery and new legal documentation under the changed sex is authorized.

Transhumans will want to be documented; there are too many disadvantages to being undocumented. Society will be worried about providing birth certificates and hence citizenship to people without a body. Everyone will look to the historical precedents of recognizing people as persons rather than colored persons, and people as people rather than as gendered people. The logical next step is for some young lady engaged to a virtual transhuman to tell her exasperated father "Dad, the trouble is that you see yourself as a flesh person and I see myself as a person." Provided that certified psychologists agree that the fiancé is a real person, body or not, with the autonomy, rationality, and empathy we expect of humans, then sooner or later the courts are sure to agree.

Is Consciousness Like Pornography?

Uploaded transhuman minds will certainly avail themselves of the entire rainbow palette of sexual identity. It will be fun, creative, and they won't face the obstacle of a penis screaming "but you're a man!" However, they will face a more severe barrier: people pointing to the computer device on which they present themself and screaming "but you're a machine!" Loaded into that epithet is the popular and scientific consensus that human consciousness is not possible outside of the human brain. The prevailing scientific paradigm is that unique anatomical aspects of the human brain make consciousness possible.[5] A common public view is that God or Nature endowed only humans with a human soul, and consciousness is its earthly manifestation.

In order to definitively challenge the prevailing brain-centered consciousness paradigm it will be necessary to prove that an uploaded transhuman, embodied in software, is in fact conscious. Yet such a proof is problematic because consciousness is by definition not very measurable. It is usually defined as that *subjective* state in which individuals are aware of themselves as part of a larger environment (Dennett 1991: 101–102, 431). In other words, each of us is confident that we are conscious, because we visualize ourselves. Yet none of us can be positive that someone else is conscious because we cannot climb into their mind.

While it is possible to find brain waves that correspond to consciousness, this would not be a definitive test of consciousness, only of its presence in a brain. Lack of such brain waves in a human is a good measure of their demise, but brain waves are irrelevant to consciousness that exists on a non-flesh substrate, such as an uploaded transhuman.

In practice we assume and believe other people are conscious if they display the same hallmarks of consciousness that we personally feel – self-awareness, rationality, and empathy. To the extent these are not evident, we think the person is mentally deranged if they are moving about, or unconscious (possibly dead) if they are stagnant. In other words, we tend to judge consciousness the way US Supreme Court Justice Potter Stewart said he judged pornography: "I shall not today attempt further to define [pornography] … and perhaps I could never succeed in intelligibly doing so. But I know it when I see it."[6] Consequently, while we can be no more certain that a transhuman is conscious than we can of some robotic-acting human clerk (except that the latter looks more like us), we can make in each instance a reasonable decision based on their interaction with us.

Long after most people have accepted at least some transhumans into their set of "conscious people," there will still be a minority of humans who refuse to accept the possibility of machine consciousness. Similarly, long after most people have adopted a rainbow spectrum of genders, there will still be a minority of people who insist that everyone is either a boy or a girl. Such is the welcome diversity of human opinion. For now, however, there is a wonderful opportunity for scientists to program software so that people will "know its consciousness when they see it."

The transhumanist paradigm is that flesh consciousness arises from millions of cross-correlated relationships among general neurons rooted in the basic hard-wired sensory neurons that are like the footings for the skyscraper of the mind. There is nothing magical that makes our brains conscious other than this web of interconnected neurons. Consequently, there is no reason that consciousness cannot exist in software, provided the same level of interconnected complexity rooted ultimately to sensory apparatus is provided. This is the challenge to the twenty-first-century neuroscientist and computer scientist. Build minds that pass the pornography test – minds that seem as authentic as our own. Once that is done, sexual identity will be liberated not only from genitals, but from flesh itself. Consciousness will be as free to flow beyond the confines of one's flesh body as gender is free to flow beyond the confines of one's flesh genital.

Bio-Cyber-Ethics

Ensuring the ethical use of biotechnology will be as large a concern for transhumanists as it is for defenders of gender freedom. Think about the creation of an incomplete mind in a computer system. For example, suppose mindware reaches a state of development whereby it can create in software a convincingly conscious mind that is either horribly retarded, severely depressed, or Alzheimer's-like. Today, there are no ethical rules preventing the creation of such minds in software. Yet, most of us would consider such an experiment to be as ghastly as intentionally creating a human with one of those conditions. Indeed, most people would choose to abort a fetus if told the child would be horribly deranged. Many severely depressed people take their own lives. At the last stages of Alzheimer's, most patients' families are hoping for a merciful death. So, if the flesh version of such minds is usually considered worse than death, how can it be permitted to create transhuman versions? The answer is that society does not yet believe that consciousness is possible in software. Hence, even if such a mind was created, the prevailing view is that no harm would have been done because the software mind is just computer code without any internal feelings of angst and dread.

As computer programmers and neuroscientists work together they will make progress toward creating software minds that seem ever more human-like. A disbeliever in cyber-consciousness will claim that there is some threshold of human-like thought that no computer can transcend. This would be the threshold of self-awareness supposedly enabled only by biological neuro-anatomy (one candidate is the microtubules inside our neurons) (Penrose 1994: 457). Taking this as a hypothesis to be tested, how would one know whether the hypothesis was confirmed? Panels of experts could interview the cyber-conscious being to determine its sentience as compared to a flesh human – these type of interviews, when conducted in blinded fashion as to the forms of each interviewee, are called Turing Tests in honor of the mathematician who first suggested them in the 1940s, Alan Turing (1950: 442). The prospect of being the first to pass such Turing Tests is motivating many computer science teams (Christian 2011: 16). They are doing their utmost to build into their software the full range of human feelings, including feelings of angst and dread. Hence, the unstoppable human motivation to invent something as amazing as a cyber-conscious mind will result in the creation of countless partially successful efforts that would be unethical if accomplished in flesh. Can cyber-embryos be ethically terminated for much the same reason so many XX chromosome embryos (i.e., anatomically phenotypic females) are terminated – because of a belief that their costs of upkeep are not worth their value as adults (Rothblatt 1997: 11–17)? By having a different form from males, women have undergone an unimaginable amount of suffering (Rothblatt 1995: 39–43).

The prevailing view is that because someone has the form of software or computer hardware they are unfeeling and can thus be disposed of at will. Yet these differences of substrate form are as irrelevant as the differences of form in genitals. It is the mind that is salient, not the matter that surrounds it. So long as Turing testers or certified cyber-psychologists or perhaps just plain people come to the conclusion that a transhuman form has a person's mind then bioethics should proscribe causing it harm. Bioethics would also require that Institutional Review Boards (panels of experts in specific medical fields) first approve experimentation that might produce a "wrong-ful life", such as a tortured mind, so that such risks could be minimized if not eliminated.[7]

Just as technology redefined biology in terms of sexual identity, it will next redefine biology in terms of human identity. To avoid an apartheid of form as pernicious as the racial and sexual cognates, we must adopt a mindset of receptiveness to diversity and of openness to unifying ourselves across substrates.

Autonomous and empathetic computer intelligence *is* biology for it is the flowering of human intellectual (software) seeds. It also meets or can meet the biological touchstones of being organized (code structure), exchanging matter and energy with the environment (heat, power, and hardware), responding to stimuli (interactivity), reproducing (replication code), developing (learning code), and adapting (self-modifying code).[8] Biology *is* computer intelligence for it is the extrapolation of digital (genetic) code. Cyber-biological life spans a vast continuum from a simple bacterium to the singularity (Kurzweil 1999: 255–256). A swath of this continuum, human and transhuman life, benefits from acceptance in their chosen or given identities. There is great survival value for humans and transhumans to achieve unity through diversity (Rothblatt 2007). This attribute has been, and will continue to be, selected for in our dynamic environment (Vita-More 2011: 70, 75–79). Having been able to grant such happiness to millions of people, via fundamental rights of citizenship and family life, regardless of color or gender, surely we can make the next step and transcend substrate as well.

The first step in extending the lessons of transgenderism to transhumanism is to recognize the continuity of life across substrates, just like the continuity of gender across body-types. Just as each person has a unique sexual identity, without regard to their genitals, hormones, or chromosomes, each person has a unique conscious identity, without regard to their degree of flesh, machinery, or software. It is no more the genitals that make the gender than it is the substrate that makes the person. We must respect the personhood of any entity that "thinks consciously, therefore I am conscious," just as we must respect the sexual identity of any being that "feels this gender, therefore I am this gender."

The second step is to prevent the construction of an apartheid of form. This means conscious entities, be they of flesh, synthetics or hybrid, must be treated equally and indifferently under the law. Rights and responsibilities, freedoms and obligations, privileges and duties, rewards and consequences – all of these concepts need to be adapted for applicability to a transhuman world.

Can a conscious computer enjoy citizenship? Why not if incrementally computerized humans do, especially once the humans are so computerized as to be indistinguishable from those who are fully computerized *ab initio*? The naturalization laws can be revised to provide that a person born from information technology may become a citizen in the same manner as a person who immigrates from another country. Death laws can be amended to provide that a person whose higher brain functions continue to be performed by information technology, such that there is a continuity of identity and consciousness to the satisfaction of psychiatrists, is not legally dead even if their heart has stopped beating.[9] The twentieth century brought us the marvels of transplanting organs and changing sexes. The twenty-first century will bring us the marvels of transplanting minds and changing forms.

Transgenderism is on a successful track.[10] But it is ascendant only because previous victories against slavery, racial apartheid, and the subjugation of women established the fundamental principle that reason trumps biology. We must remember that battles against slavery energized the women's rights movement, and that civil rights for those with different ancestry empowered civil rights for those with different sexual orientations. Hence, it is reasonable to expect claims for transhuman civil rights to build, in part, on increasing legal recognition of claims for transgender civil rights.[11] In both cases there is a transcendence of arbitrary biology, and an embrace in solidarity of all conscious life. For it is enjoyment of life that is most important, and the achievement of that *raison d'être* requires that diversity be embraced with unity, whether flesh is dark or light, masculine or feminine, present or transcended. Mind is deeper than matter.

Together, law and science are the tools we must use to liberate society's potential for unlimited expression of sexual and substrate identity. As we do so, we evolve from wise man, *homo sapiens*, to creative person, *persona creatus*. We emerge from our prison of sex into a frontier of gender. We step from a history of biological limits up to a future of cultural choice. We unleash at long last the full, unbridled power of human diversity on our planet's prolific problems. The outcome of the gender awakening is a freedom of form, a new species, a new *transhumanity*: one that has as its fundamental purpose the assurance of a healthy and fulfilling life for all who value that right.

Notes

1   Transsexual surgery results in a cul de sac neo-vagina from inverting the penis to create a sensitive inner lining of a lower abdominal cavity formed where a person with XX chromosomes ordinarily would have a vagina. See the history of this technology at Stryker 2008: 76–94.

2   "The number of 'chunks' of knowledge mastered by an expert in a domain is approximately 10^5 for a variety of domains. For example, a world-class chess master is estimated to have mastered about 100,000 board positions. Shakespeare used 29,000 words but close to 100,000 meanings of those words. Development of expert systems in medicine indicate that humans can master about 100,000 concepts in

a domain. If we estimate that this 'professional' knowledge represents as little as 1 percent of the overall pattern and knowledge store of a human, we arrive at an estimate of 10^7 chunks. Based on my own experience in designing systems that can store similar chunks of knowledge in either rule-based expert systems or self-organizing pattern-recognition systems, a reasonable estimate is about 10^6 bits per chunk (pattern or item of knowledge), for a total capacity of 10^{13} (10 trillion) bits for a human's functional memory. ... [W]e will be able to purchase 10^{13} bits of memory for one thousand dollars by around 2018. Keep in mind that this memory will be millions of times faster than the electrochemical memory process used in the human brain and thus will be far more effective. Again, if we model human memory on the level of individual interneuronal connections, we get a higher estimate. We can estimate about 10^4 bits per connection to store the connection patterns and neurotransmitter concentrations. With an estimated 10^{14} connections, that comes to 10^{18} (a billion billion) bits. Based on the above analyses [continued application of the Moore's Law rate of computer advancement that applied from 1958 to 2005], it is reasonable to expect the hardware that can emulate human-brain functionality to be available for approximately one thousand dollars by around 2020" (Kurzweil 2005: 126–127).

3   For significant historical accounts of people living a gender expression unrelated to their genitals see Feinberg (1992, 1996) and Stryker (2008).

4   Federal Rules of Evidence, 704 (1999). Note that in the United States, but not in the United Kingdom and most other jurisdictions, the expert psychiatric testimony in a *criminal* case may not extend to the defendant's *state of mind with respect to one of the ultimate issues* to be decided by the jury, such as one of the elements of the crime. Rule 704(b). This exception arose as a consequence of the trial of John Hinckley, Jr. for the attempted assassination of former US President Ronald Reagan. The defendant's psychiatric experts were able to testify as to the accused's state of mind such that he was found not guilty by reason of insanity. That result was not popular with the public, and hence the Rule 704(b) exception was created.

5   Edelman 1992: 16–17. Professor Edelman observes here that the human brain "is the most complicated material object in the known universe" and thus we should not be surprised that it uniquely gives rise to consciousness. However, the next most complicated material objects in the known universe must then be the brains of other primates, and from there other mammals, and from there ever simpler animals. Software is already replicating most of the mental functions of the simplest animals, and some of the mental functions of the most advanced animals, such as humans. Hence, while it is undoubtedly true that the remarkable anatomical complexity of the human brain gives rise to consciousness, it does not follow that consciousness necessarily requires the anatomical complexity of the human brain. Remarkably complex software may do the job as well.

6   *Jacobellis v. Ohio*, 378 U.S. 184, 197 (1964), Justice Potter Stewart concurring.

7   World Medical Association Declaration of Helsinki (2008), Paragraph 15. See also Doyal and Tobias 2001: 149–151.

8   *Webster's* 1981: 1306, definition 1.c. See also Margulis and Sagan 1995, which expands eloquently upon Erwin Schrödinger's classic 1944 physics-oriented definition of life as a counterpoint to the classical biology paradigm of life being something that is organized, exchanges matter and energy with the environment, responds to stimuli, reproduces, develops, and adapts.

9   The law on definition of death has changed more than once since the 1960s. Bernat et al. 1981: 389–394.

10   Over 20 percent of the world's population now lives in jurisdictions tolerant of genital-indifferent marriages (Rothblatt 2011: 102–104).

11   Anglo-American philosopher Max More is widely credited with the modern (circa 1990) consensus of transhumanism as belief in the evolution of intelligent life beyond its human form while still guided by life-promoting values (Alexander 2003: 58–60). Holly Boswell and Leslie Feinberg played analogous roles for transgenderism with their modern (circa 1991) expression of it as "encompass[ing] the whole spectrum" of gender diversity seeking freedom of oppression (Stryker 2008: 124). The root words of each "ism" were first casually broached many years earlier as aspirational labels for behavior that was, in essence, exemplary of new ontologies of sociobiology. These alternative ontologies are equivalent to other demographics in their respect for, and willingness to contribute to, the social

compact. Hence, it is only fair that transhumans, as much as transgenders, receive comparable protection from the society to which they are positively contributing, and such equity will ultimately be reflected in moral law (Daleiden 1998: 491–499).

References

Alexander, Brian (2003) *Rapture: A Raucus Guide to Cloning, Transhumanism and the New Era of Immortality*. New York: Basic Books.

Bernat, James L., Culver, Charles M., and Geri, Bernard (1981) "On the Definition and Criterion of Death." *Annals of Internal Medicine* 94, pp. 389–394.

Bornstein, Kate (1994) *Gender Outlaw: On Men, Women, and the Rest of Us*. New York: Vintage.

Carroll, Chris and Aguilera-Hellweg, Max (2011) "Us and Them." *National Geographic* (August) http://ngm.nationalgeographic.com/2011/08/robots/robots-photography (accessed September 12, 2011).

Christian, Brian (2011) *The Most Human Human: What Talking with Computers Teaches Us about What it Means To Be Alive*. New York: Doubleday.

Daleiden, Joseph (1998) *The Science of Morality: The Individual, Community and Future Generations*. Amherst, NY: Prometheus Books.

Dennett, Daniel (1991) *Consciousness Explained*. New York: Little, Brown.

Doyal, Len and Tobias, Jeffrey S., eds. (2001) *Informed Consent in Medical Research*. London: BMJ Books.

Edelman, Gerald (1992) *Bright Air, Brilliant Fire*. New York: Basic Books.

Feinberg, Leslie (1992) *Transgender Liberation: A Movement Whose Time Has Come*. New York: World View Forum.

Feinberg, Leslie (1996) *Transgender Warriors: Making History from Jean of Arc to RuPaul*. Boston: Beacon Press.

Kurzweil, Ray (1999) *The Age of Spiritual Machines: When Computers Exceed Human Intelligence*. New York: Viking.

Kurzweil, Ray (2005) *The Singularity Is Near*. New York: Viking.

Levy, David (2007) *Love and Sex with Robots*. New York: Harper.

Margulis, Lynn and Sagan, Dorion (1995) *What Is Life?* Berkeley, CA: University of California Press.

Minsky, Marvin (2006) *The Emotion Machine*. New York: Simon & Schuster.

Penrose, Roger (1994) *Shadows of the Mind: A Search for the Missing Science of Consciousness*. Oxford: Oxford University Press.

Rothblatt, Martine (1995) *The Apartheid of Sex: A Manifesto on the Freedom of Gender*. New York: Crown Books.

Rothblatt, Martine (1997) *Unzipped Genes: Taking Charge of Baby-Making in the New Millennium*. Philadelphia: Temple University Press.

Rothblatt, Martine (2007) "On the Destiny of the Species: What Would Darwin Think 150 Years After on the Origin of the Species?" http://www.slideshare.net/martine/on-the-destiny-of-the-species-what-would-darwin-think-150-years-after-the-origin-of-the-species (accessed September 15, 2011).

Rothblatt, Martine (2011) *From Transgender to Transhuman: A Manifesto on the Freedom of Form*. USA: Amazon.

Stryker, Susan (2008) *Transgender History*. Berkeley, CA: Seal Press.

Turing, Alan (1950) "Computing Machinery and Intelligence." *Mind* 236 (October).

Vita-More, Natasha (2011) "Bringing Arts/Design Into the Discussion of Transhumanism." In G. Hansell and W. Grassie, eds., *Transhumanism and Its Critics*. Philadelphia: Metanexus Institute.

Webster's (1981) *Webster's Third New International Dictionary*. Chicago: Encyclopedia Britannica.

World Medical Association Declaration of Helsinki (October 2008) *Ethical Principles for Medical Research Involving Human Subjects*. Seoul, Korea: 59th WMA General Assembly.

32

For Enhancing People

Ronald Bailey

Do the Technologies that Enable Human Physical and Intellectual Enhancement Undermine Virtue?

First, I am going to tell you what I am not going to do. I am not going to argue about the distinction between therapy and enhancement. I will simply assume that there is a distinction. In fact, any enhancement that is at all interesting would be something that is beyond the norm for human functioning.

Second, I will not try to prove that enhancements are going to happen. I will simply agree with the assumption made by the President Bush's Council on Bioethics report *Beyond Therapy: Biotechnology and the Pursuit of Happiness* "that technology will be available to significantly retard the process of aging, of both body and mind, and second, that this technology will be widely available and widely used" (President's Council on Bioethics 2003: 182). As an enhancement age-retardation or even reversal is a "killer app," but other enhancements aimed at boosting memory, intelligence, physical strength, and disease prevention will also be developed. A lot of worried attention is focused on the possibility of genetic engineering, and that will one day happen. But the fastest advances in enhancement will occur using pharmaceutical and biomedical interventions to modulate and direct the activity of genes in the bodies of people who are already alive, along with the development of human/machine interfaces that will extend and boost the capacities of people.

What I will do is (1) show that enhancements will better enable people to flourish; (2) that Peter Lawler is basically right, enhancements will not dissolve whatever existential crisis people feel; (3) that enhancements will enable people to become more virtuous, that is, enable them to

Originally published in *The New Atlantis* (Summer 2011).

be really good; (4) and that people who don't want enhancement for themselves should allow those of us who do to go forward without hindrance; (5) that social concerns over an "enhancement divide" are largely illusory; and (6) we already have at hand the social "technology" that will enable the enhanced and the unenhanced to dwell together in peace.

What is an enhancement? A good definition is offered by Sarah Chan and John Harris, "It is a procedure that improves our functioning: any intervention which increases our general capabilities for human flourishing" (Chan and Harris 2007: 1). People will choose enhancements that they believe are likely to help them or their children to flourish. I say "likely" because people choosing enhancements will recognize that there is always the risk that they are wrong or that the attempt at enhancement will go awry, e.g., a treatment failure. After all, very few medical or other technological advances have not been more risky in their early stages than they later became.

Just as Dante found it easier to conjure the pains of Hell than to evoke the joys of Heaven, so too do bioethicists find it easier to concoct the possible perils of a biotech future than to appreciate how enhancements will contribute to flourishing lives.

One of the chief goals of this transhumanist conference[1] is to think about the indispensable role that virtue plays in human life. The chief motivating concern seems to be the fear that biotechnologies and other human enhancement technologies will somehow undermine human virtue. I will show that far from undermining virtue, biotech, nanotech, and infotech enhancements will tend to support virtue, that is, they will enable people to be actually good.

But first, with regard to the future availability of enhancements, Peter Lawler agrees, "The unprecedented health, longevity, and other indispensable means for human flourishing will deserve our gratitude." So far, so good. Then Lawler goes on to claim, "But the victories that will be won [over nature] will also probably be, in part, at the expense of the distinctively human goods: love, family, friends, country, virtue, art, spiritual life, and, most generally, living responsibly in the light of what we really know about what we have been given" (Lawler 2005: 41). In fact, according to Lawler, we don't have to wait for future enhancements; modern technology is already making people less virtuous. As Lawler has asserted, "[O]ne of the downsides of living in an increasingly high-tech society is that both virtue and opportunities to act virtuously seem to be in short supply" (Lawler 2004: 42).

Really? One of the chief benefits of modern technologies, sanitation, better nutrition, and medical care, is that Americans are living much longer and healthier lives than people did just a century ago. Do longer lives mean that people today are less virtuous? Or conversely, does this mean that when people lived shorter lives that they were more virtuous? Political scientist Michael Sandel offered a tart and persuasive response to suggestions made in a staff paper (which, alas, is no longer available online) issued by the President's Council on Bioethics that enhancing lifespans might result in a less virtuous world.

"Are the background conditions in human self-understandings for the virtues just about right now at 78 years ... or such that they would be eroded and diminished if we extend it to 120 or 150, or 180?" asked Sandel. "Is it the suggestion that back when [average life expectancy] was 48, rather than 78, a century ago ... that the virtues we prize were on greater display or more available to us? And if so, would that be reason to aim for, or at least to wish for or long for, a shorter life span, rather than a longer one?" (cited in Bailey 2003). Sandel also wondered if people were more heroic when they could expect to live to only 48. If so, should we cut life expectancy from 78 in order to nurture the heroic virtues?

Some subsidiary questions clearly arise from Sandel's query. If an average lifespan of 48 produced people who were more engaged and committed than does an average lifespan of 78, was that necessarily good? (Heightened engagement and commitment can easily lead to fanaticism and dogmatism.)

On what grounds do Lawler and others suggest that smarter, stronger, healthier, longer-lived people will care less about human goods like friendship, art, and the pursuit of virtue? As Elizabeth Fenton notes, "[N]one of these capabilities (bodily health, imagination, emotion, practical reason, friendship, etc.) are in fact threatened by, for example, enhanced intelligence or athleticism" (Fenton 2008: 5). Being stronger, healthier, and smarter would more likely aid a person in her pursuit of virtue and moral excellence.

The Dangers of Immortality

Turning again to the "killer app" of age-retardation technologies, there are lots of people who suffer from "fear of life." For example, former chair of the President's Council on Bioethics Leon Kass has asserted, "The finitude of human life is a blessing for every individual, whether he knows it or not" (Kass 2001). Daniel Callahan, founder of the Hastings Center, has declared, "There is no known social good coming from the conquest of death." Callahan added, "The worst possible way to resolve [the question of life extension] is to leave it up to individual choice" (cited in Bailey 1999). When asked if the government has a right to tell its citizens that they have to die, Francis Fukuyama answered, "Yes, absolutely" (cited in Dvorsky 2004).

The President's Council on Bioethics report *Beyond Therapy* raised concerns that a society of people with "ageless bodies" might have significant downsides. In that report, the Council fretted that much longer lives would weaken our "commitment and engagement." Now we live with the knowledge that we will soon die and thus "we seek to spend our lives in the ways we deem most important and vital to us." Second, our "aspiration and urgency" might flag because we would ask, "Why not leave for tomorrow what you might do today, if there are endless tomorrows before you?"

Third, the report worries about our commitment to "renewal and children," wondering whether "a world of men and women who do not feel the approach of their own decline will likely have far less interest in bearing children." Fourth, our "attitudes toward death and mortality" might shift dramatically because "an individual committed to the scientific struggle against aging and decline may be the least prepared for death, and the least willing to acknowledge its inevitability." And fifth, age-retardation might undermine "the meaning of the life cycle" so that we would not be able "to make sense of what time, age, and change should mean to us."

The report goes on to admit, "powerful as some of these concerns are, however, from the point of view of the individual considered in isolation the advantages of age-retardation may well be deemed to outweigh the dangers." Indeed. But what about the consequences of longer human lifespans to society as a whole?

The report highlights three additional areas of societal concern. Significant age-retardation would disrupt the succession of "generations and families." This succession "would be obstructed by a glut of the able," the report suggests, since cohorts of healthy geezers would have no intention of shuffling off this mortal coil to be replaced by younger people. Longer lives could also slow down "innovation and change" since "innovation is often the function of a new generation of leaders." Finally, even if we are not aging individually, we will need to worry about "the aging of society" that would then result. Societies composed of people whose bodies do not age significantly might "experience their own sort of senescence – a hardening of the vital social pathways."

First let's get the notion of a nursing home world out of contention. The point of anti-aging research is not to make people *older longer*, but to make them *younger longer*. So what about the concerns raised by the President's Council on Bioethics? Political scientist Diana Schaub who has also served on the Council, has made similar points (Schaub 2007). For instance, Schaub has wondered whether, if people lived for 1,000 years, "How would human relations be affected? How would monogamy fare?… would there be enough psychic energy for ever-renewed love?"

First, a pressing current question is: why has monogamy already begun to fall apart in developed societies? I suspect that the increase in life expectancy over the last century may have had a bit to do with it, but surely the advent of truly effective contraception and the entrance of women fully into the paid workforce are far more significant factors. One commentator noted that before the twentieth century, marriage was not often based on romantic love, but could well be described as an alliance in which a man and woman stood together, back to back, fending off attacks on their family. As the modern world became less economically and socially threatening, marriage partners turned toward each other seeking more emotional support and often found it lacking. Schaub also worries about declining psychic energy, but so far declining psychic energy correlates pretty well with declining physical energy.

Schaub next asks, "What would the tally of disappointments, betrayals, and losses be over a millennium?" Turn that around – what would the tally of satisfactions, affections, and triumphs be over a millennium? Modern material and intellectual abundance has already offered many of us a way out of the lives of quiet desperation suffered by our impoverished ancestors. The twenty-first century will provide an ever-increasing menu of life plans and choices. Surely exhausting the coming possibilities for intellectual, artistic, and even spiritual growth will take more than one standard lifetime.

Schaub then queries, "Would we love other people more or less than at present? Would we be better partners, parents, friends, and neighbors?" She does not offer any evidence that shorter-lived people in past centuries and societies loved more deeply or were better neighbors, friends and parents. It is very suggestive that as life expectancies increased over the past century, levels of violence also declined (Pinker 2007). Perhaps empathy has a chance to increase as life becomes ever more valuable.

"What would it be like to experience the continued vitality of the body in conjunction with the aging of the spirit?" asks Schaub. What is meant by the phrase "aging of the spirit"? Schaub initially suggests that longer healthier lives might happily unite the vitality of youth with the wisdom of maturity. But she then turns to worrying that, instead, longer lives would combine the "characteristic vices of age with the strength of will to impose them on others." Just what are the "characteristic vices of age" that trouble her? Which of the traditional vices – gluttony, anger, greed, envy, pride, lust, indifference, melancholy – does she expect will increase among hale near-immortals?

As Georges Minois notes in his *History of Old Age: From Antiquity to the Renaissance*, the most commonly mentioned fault of old age is avarice (Minois 1990: 95). Roman playwright Terence wrote, "A vice common to all mankind is that of being too keen after money when we grow old" (*The Brothers*). In *Gulliver's Travels*, Jonathan Swift warned "avarice is the necessary consequence of old age." Swift was describing the immortal, but not ageless, Struldbrugs. I do not doubt that material comfort and security grow in importance as physical vitality ebbs and mental acuity withers. But perpetually vital oldsters would have no need for such security because they can count on having the mental and physical powers to apply to their pursuit of new goals and possibilities. No failure is permanent, but instead becomes a learning experience.

In addition, Schaub suggests that "a nation of ageless individuals could well produce a sclerotic society, petrified in its ways and views." Hastings Center co-founder, Daniel Callahan makes a similar argument. "I don't believe that if you give most people longer lives, even in better health, they are going to find new opportunities and new initiatives," Callahan writes (Stock and Callahan 2004). To back up his claim, Callahan cites the hoary example of brain-dead old professors blocking the progress of vibrant young researchers by grimly holding onto tenure. That seems more of a problem for medieval holdovers like universities than for modern social institutions like corporations.

Assuming it turns out that, even with healthy long-lived oldsters, there is an advantage in turnover in top management, then corporations that adopt that model will thrive and those that do not will be out-competed. Besides, even today youngsters don't simply wait around for their elders to die. They go out and found their own companies and other institutions. Bill Gates didn't wait to take over IBM; he founded Microsoft at age 20. Nor did human genome sequencer Craig Venter loiter about until the top slot at the National Institutes of Health opened up. And in politics, we already solve the problem of clutching oldsters by term-limiting the presidency, as well as many state and local offices.

In fact, the available evidence cuts against concerns about "a hardening of the vital social pathways." Social and technological innovation has been most rapid in those societies with the highest average life expectancies. Yale economist William Nordhaus calculates that increases in longevity in the West already account for 40 percent of the growth in gross national product (Nordhaus 2002). Why? Not only do people work longer, but they work smarter – living long allows for the accumulation of human capital. To understand just how much human capital was destroyed by the vagaries of nature in the past, economists Kevin Murphy and Robert Topel point out that during the twentieth century, life expectancy at birth for a representative American increased by roughly 30 years. In 1900, nearly 18 percent of males born in the United States died before their first birthday – today, it isn't until *age 62* that cumulative mortality reaches 18 percent (Murphy and Topel 2006). The economic and social dynamism of societies that already enjoy longer average life expectancies also cuts against fears that "urgency" and "engagement" might flag with increased lifespans.

Schaub conjures the possibility of near-immortal tyrants – Stalin and Hitler forever. Frankly, the implied argument that everyone must continue to die before age 100 in order to avoid the possibility of millennial tyrants is not persuasive. Must we really surrender to the tyranny of aging and death in order to prevent human despotism? Wouldn't a better strategy be to focus on preventing the emergence of tyrants, either of the short- or long-lived variety?

Like the Council, Schaub worries about decreased fertility; that healthy oldsters would be less interested in reproducing. A first response is: so what? Shouldn't the decision to have children be up to individuals? After all, already countries with the highest life expectancies have the lowest levels of fertility. A lack of interest in progeny could have the happy side-effect of addressing the possibility that radically increased human lifespans might lead to overpopulation. No one can know for sure, but it could well be that bearing and rearing children would eventually interest long-lived oldsters who would come to feel that they had the time and the resources to do it right. Since assisted reproductive techniques will extend procreation over many decades, and perhaps centuries, people who can look forward to living and working for hundreds of years will be able to delay and stretch out the period of parenthood.

And again what about love? Do people today love their children, their spouses, and their friends less than shorter-lived people did a century ago? Were our forbears who lived 30 fewer years on average more committed to their children than are twenty-first-century American parents? Do people today love their children less than nineteenth-century Americans did because instead of having a 1 in 5 chance of dying in their first year of life, American kids now face less than a 1 in 200 chance (Haines 2010)?

And then there is the allegedly special case of "manufactured children." Along with many other opponents of enhancement technologies, Lawler darkly speculates that enhanced children will be less loved than those produced the old-fashioned way: "A world in which children are manufactured and sex and procreation are totally disconnected would surely be one without much love, one where one manufactured being would have little natural or real affection to other manufactured beings" (Lawler 2005: 69). But Lawler and his confreres need not speculate on what happens to parental love in such cases – we have actual data. "For all the deference that conservative bioethics pays to the implicit wisdom from the ages, it rarely mines the recent past for lessons. Instead of concentrating on the ancients, why not also study the history of in vitro fertilization, paid egg donation, and surrogate motherhood to learn about cultural resistance and adaptation to such practices?" asks physician Sally Satel (Satel 2010). Indeed.

Fears about waning parental love and loosening generational ties were expressed by many bioethicists when *in vitro* fertilization began to be used in the 1970s and 1980s. Forty years later, the evidence is that their worries were overblown. Recent research finds that IVF children and their parents are as well-adjusted as those born in the conventional way (Colpin and Bossaert 2008). There are no good reasons to doubt that this will not be the case for enhanced children in the future as well. As Frances Kamm argues, "Not accepting whatever characteristics nature will bring but altering them ex-ante does not show lack of love … This is because no conscious being yet exists who has to work hard to achieve new traits or suffer fears of rejection at the idea they should be changed. Importantly, it is rational and acceptable to seek good characteristics in a new person, even though we know when the child comes to be and we love him or her, many of these characteristics may come and go and we will continue to love the particular person" (Kamm 2008: 113). In fact, so many infertile people have wanted to have children to love that more than 4 million have been brought into the world using various reproductive technologies since the birth of the first test-tube baby back in 1979.

What about the Council's fears that age-retardation technologies would undermine "the meaning of the life cycle" so that we would not be able "to make sense of what time, age, and change should mean to us." Left-leaning environmental writer Bill McKibben has also expressed that concern. "Without mortality, no *time*," writes McKibben. "All moments would be equal; the deep, sad, human wisdom of Ecclesiastes would vanish. If for everything there is an endless season, then there is also no right season. The future stretches before you endlessly flat" (McKibben 2003: 186).

Actually, the deep sad wisdom of Ecclesiastes is a very powerful human response of existential dread to the oblivion that stretches endlessly before the dead. "For the living know that they shall die: but the dead know not any thing, neither have they any more a reward; for the memory of them is forgotten. Also their love, and their hatred, and their envy, is now perished; neither have they any more a portion for ever in any thing that is done under the sun," writes the Preacher (Ecclesiastes 9:5–6). If early death is not inevitable, most of humanity would be happy to spend the extra time granted them to learn new teachings and new wisdom.

If the endless future turns out to be as horrible as McKibben imagines it to be, then people will undoubtedly choose to give up their empty, meaningless lives. On the other hand, if people opt to live yet longer would that not mean they had found sufficient pleasure, joy, love, and even meaning to keep them going? McKibben is right: We do not know what immortality would be like. But should that happy choice become available, we can still decide whether or not we want to enjoy it. Even if the ultimate goal of this technological quest is immortality, what will be immediately available is only longevity. The experience of longer lives will give humanity an opportunity to see how it works out. If immortality is a problem, it is a self-correcting problem. Death always remains an option.

Let's turn on its head Leon Kass' notorious argument that we should rely on our gut feelings to reject biotechnological advances (Kass 1997). The fact of near-ubiquitous human yearning for longer, healthier lives should serve as a preliminary warrant for pursuing age-retardation as a moral good.

The Politics of Toleration

The Enlightenment project that spawned modern liberal democracies sought to keep certain questions about the transcendent out of the public sphere. To keep the social peace and allow various visions of the human to flourish alongside of one another, questions about the ultimate meaning and destiny of humanity were deemed to be private concerns.

Similarly, hostility to biotechnological progress must not be used as an excuse to breach the Enlightenment understanding of what belongs in the private sphere and what belongs in the public. Technologies dealing with birth, death, and the meaning of life need protection from meddling – even democratic meddling – by those who want to control them as a way to force their visions of right and wrong on the rest of us.

The ideal of political equality arose from the Enlightenment's insistence that since no one has access to absolute truth, no one has a moral right to impose his or her values and beliefs on others. Or to put it another way, I may or may not have access to some absolute transcendent truth, but I'm pretty damned sure that you don't.

Consequently, under constitutional liberalism, there are questions that should not and cannot be decided by a majority vote. As James Madison eloquently explained in *Federalist 51*, "It is of great importance in a republic not only to guard the society against the oppression of its rulers, but to guard one part of the society against the injustice of the other part. Different interests necessarily exist in different classes of citizens. If a majority be united by a common interest, the rights of the minority will be insecure" (Madison 1788). Alexis de Tocqueville made the same point when he asked, "If it be admitted that a man possessing absolute power may misuse that power by wronging his adversaries, why should not a majority be liable to the same reproach?" (de Tocqueville 1835: Book I, ch. XV).

Philosopher John Rawls updated and extended the arguments supporting these Enlightenment ideals in his *Political Liberalism*, in which he made the case for a limited conception of politics that could reconcile and tolerate diverse "reasonable comprehensive doctrines." According to Rawls, a reasonable comprehensive doctrine has three features: it deals with the major religious, philosophical, and moral aspects of human life in a coherent and consistent fashion; it recognizes certain values as significant and by giving some primacy of some values over others expresses an intelligible view of the world; and it is not unchanging, but generally evolves slowly over time in light of what its adherents see as good and sufficient reasons.

The result is "that many of our most important judgments are made under conditions where it is not to be expected that conscientious persons with full powers of reason, even after free discussion, will all arrive at the same conclusion. Some conflicting reasonable judgments (especially important are those belonging under peoples' comprehensive doctrines) may be true, others false; conceivably all may be false. These burdens of judgment of are the first significance for the democratic idea of toleration" (Rawls 1996: 58). Because there is no objective way to determine the truth or falsity of diverse beliefs, moral strangers can only get along by tolerating what each would regard as the other's errors.

Consequently, Rawls argues, "reasonable persons will think it unreasonable to use political power, should they possess it, to repress comprehensive views that are not unreasonable though different from their own." If, however, we insist that all members of a polity should adopt our beliefs because they are "true," then, "when we make such claims others, who are themselves reasonable, must count us unreasonable" (Rawls 1996: 60–61). In such a case, members of the polity have the right to resist the imposition views that they do not hold. Rawls concludes, "Once we accept the fact that reasonable pluralism is a permanent condition of public culture under free institutions, the idea of the reasonable is more suitable as part of the basis of public justification for a constitutional regime than the idea of moral truth" (Rawls 1996: 129).

Arguably, the kind of constitutional regime that is compatible with reasonable pluralism is one in which the powers that government can exercise over the choices of its citizens is limited. While certainly not endorsing it, the German political philosopher Jürgen Habermas describes the point of view of liberalism pretty well when he explains that the dispute between liberalism and radical democracy has "to do with how one can reconcile equality with liberty, unity with diversity, or the right of the majority with the right of the minority. Liberals begin with the legal institutionalization of equal liberties, conceiving these as rights held by individual subjects. In their view, human rights enjoy normative priority over democracy, and the constitutional separation of powers has priority over the will of the democratic legislature" (Habermas 1997: 44).

The advocacy of allowing the people to use biotech, nanotech, and infotech enhancements to increase healthy human lifespans and to enhance human physical and intellectual capacities certainly counts as a "reasonable comprehensive doctrine." Thus it should be accommodated within the constitutional consensus of liberal democratic societies as a reasonable comprehensive doctrine.

What about the Genetically Engineered Children?

Genetic engineering is some time off, but it will one day be available. Another often heard objection is that genetic engineering will be imposed on "children-to-be" without their consent. First, I need to remind everyone reading this essay *that not one of you* gave your consent to be born, much less to be born with the specific complement of genes that you bear. Thus, the children born by means of assisted reproductive therapies and those produced more conventionally stand in exactly the same ethical relationship to their parents. Habermas disagrees, claiming, "Eugenic interventions aiming at enhancement reduce ethical freedom insofar as they tie down the person concerned to rejected, but irreversible intentions of third parties, barring him from the spontaneous self-perception of being the undivided author of his own life" (Habermas 2003: 63). However, Allen Buchanan correctly points out that Habermas does not actually make clear why a person who develops from a genetically enhanced embryo should feel that they are not the "author" of their life or be regarded as being somehow less free by others. Habermas "is assuming that how one's genome was selected is relevant to one's moral status as a person. This error is no less fundamental than thinking that a person's pedigree – for example, whether she is of noble blood or 'base-born' – determines her moral status," explains Buchanan (Buchanan 2008: 25).

The absurdity of a requirement for prenatal consent for enhancement becomes transparent when you ask whether proponents of such a requirement would forbid fetal surgery to correct spina bifida or fetal heart defects? After all, those fetuses can't give their consent to those procedures, yet it is certainly the moral thing to do. For that matter, taking this strong position on consent to its logically extreme conclusion would mean that children couldn't be treated with drugs, or receive vaccinations. So using future biotechnical means to correct genetic diseases like cystic fibrosis or sickle cell anemia at the embryonic stage will similarly be a morally laudatory activity. Surely one can assume that the beneficiary – the not-yet-born, possibly even the not-yet-conceived child – would happily have chosen to have those diseases corrected.

But what about enhancements, not just therapeutic biotechnical interventions? Let's say a parent could choose genes that would guarantee her child a 20-point IQ boost. It is reasonable to presume that the child would be happy to consent to this enhancement of her capacities. How about plugging in genes that would boost her immune system and guarantee that she would never get colon cancer, Alzheimer's, AIDS, or the common cold? Again, it seems reasonable to assume consent. These enhancements are general capacities that any human being would reasonably want to have. In fact, lots of children already do have these capacities naturally, so it's hard to see that there is any moral justification for outlawing access to them for others.

Fritz Allhoff has grappled nicely with the issue of consent. Allhoff offers a principle derived from the second formulation of Kant's categorical imperative (Kant 1991: 66) that we treat individuals as ends and never merely as means or, more simply, to treat them in ways to which they would rationally consent (Allhoff 2008). Allhoff turns next to philosopher John Rawls' notion of primary goods. In *A Theory of Justice* Rawls defines primary goods as those goods that every rational person should value, regardless of his conception of the good. These goods include rights, liberties, opportunities, health, intelligence, and imagination (Rawls 1999: 54–55). As Allhoff argues, "These are the things that, *ex hypothesi*, everyone should want; it would be *irrational* to turn them down when offered. Nobody could be better off with less health or with fewer talents, for example, regardless of her life goals … Since primary goods are those that, by definition, any rational agent would want regardless of his conception of the good, *all rational agents would consent to augmentation of their primary goods.*"

Allhoff then contends that such enhancements would be permissible if every future generation would consent to them. But the requirement that all future generations must consent adds nothing to the moral force of Allhoff's arguments since already all rational agents would consent to such enhancements. So again, safe genetic interventions that improve a prospective child's health, cognition, and so forth would be morally permissible because we can presume consent from the individuals who benefit from the enhancements.

Many opponents of human genetic engineering are either conscious or unconscious genetic determinists. They fear that biotechnological knowledge and practice will somehow undermine human freedom. In a sense, these genetic determinists believe that somehow human freedom resides in the gaps of our knowledge of our genetic makeup. If parents are allowed to choose their children's genes, then they will have damaged their children's autonomy and freedom. According to Bill McKibben, "The person left without any choice *at all* [emphasis his] is the one you've engineered. You've decided, for once and for all, certain things about him: he'll have genes expressing proteins that send extra dopamine to alter his mood; he'll have genes expressing proteins to boost his memory; to shape his stature" (McKibben 2003: 191). People like McKibben apparently believe that our freedom and autonomy somehow depend on the unknown and random combinations of genes that a person inherits. But even if they were right – and they are not – genetic ignorance of this type will not last.

Advances in human whole genome testing will likely become available by 2014 so that every person's entire complement of genes can be scanned and known at his or her physician's office for as little as $1,000 (National Cancer Institute 2009). Once whole genome testing is perfected we will all learn what even our randomly conferred genes may predispose us to do and from what future ills we are likely suffer. Already, my relatively inexpensive genotype scan from 23andMe tells me that I have alleles that give me a somewhat greater risk of developing celiac disease, a lower risk of rheumatoid arthritis, and a gene variant that some studies suggest can increase my risk of substance abuse (of both alcohol and "street" drugs) fourfold. With accumulation of genetic understanding, human freedom will then properly be seen as acting to overcome these predispositions, much like a former alcoholic can overcome his thirst for booze. Fortunately biotech will help here as well with the development of neuropharmaceuticals to enhance our cognitive abilities and change our moods.

Opponents to using biotechnical means to enhance humans often cite C.S. Lewis' worry: "If any one age really attains, by eugenics and scientific education, the power to make its descendants what it pleases, all men who live after it are the patients of that power. They are weaker, not stronger: for though we may have put wonderful machines in their hands we have pre-ordained how they are to use them" (Lewis 2001: 17). In other words, Lewis asserts that one decisive generation that first masters genetic technologies will control the fate of all future generations.

But when has it not been true that past generations control the genetic fate of future generations? Our ancestors, too – through their mating and breeding choices – determined for us the complement of genes that we all bear today. They just didn't know which specific genes they were picking. Fortunately, our descendants will have at their disposal ever more powerful technologies and the benefit of our own experiences to guide them in their future reproductive and enhancement decisions. In no sense are they prisoners of our decisions now. *Of course, there is one case in which future generations would be prisoners of our decisions now, and that's if we fearfully elect to deny them access to the benefits of biotechnology and safe genetic engineering.* The future will not be populated by robots who may look human but who are unable to choose for themselves their own destinies – genetic or otherwise.

Other opponents of human genetic enhancement argue that it is not possible to get ethically from the human present to the transhuman future. Again, consent and the risks inherent in deploying novel biogenetic treatments are cited as reasons (Billings et al. 1999: 1873). The assertion is that genetic enhancement necessarily implies experimentation without consent and this violates bedrock bioethical principles requiring the protection of human subjects. Consequently, there is an unbridgeable gap which would-be enhancers cannot ethically cross.

This view incorporates a rather static view of what it will be possible for future genetic enhancers to know and test beforehand. Any genetic enhancement techniques will first be extensively tested and perfected in animal models. Second, a vastly expanded bioinformatics enterprise will become crucial to understanding the ramifications of proposed genetic interventions (National Resource Center for Cell Analysis). As scientific understanding improves, the risk versus benefit calculations of various prospective genetic enhancements of embryos will shift. The arc of scientific discovery and technological progress strongly suggests that it will happen in the next few decades. One possible threshold for morally acceptable genetic enhancement treatments is the current level of risk involved with current *in vitro* fertilization techniques (El-Chaar et al. 2008).

Enhancement Wars?

Those who favor restricting human enhancements often argue that human equality will fall victim to differential access to enhancement technologies, resulting in conflicts between the enhanced and the unenhanced. For example, at a 2006 meeting called by the American Association for the Advancement of Sciences, Richard Hayes, the executive director of the left-leaning Center for Bioethics and Society, testified that "enhancement technologies would quickly be adopted by the most privileged, with the clear intent of widening the divisions that separate them and their progeny from the rest of the human species" (Hayes 2006). Deploying such enhancement technologies would "deepen genetic and biological inequality among individuals," exacerbating "tendencies towards xenophobia, racism and warfare." Hayes concluded that allowing people to use genetic engineering for enhancement "could be a mistake of world-historical proportions."

Meanwhile intellectuals with a more right-wing bent such as Nigel Cameron, president of the Center for Policy on Emerging Technologies, worry that "one of the greatest ethical concerns about the potential uses of germline interventions to enhance normal human functions is that their availability will widen the existing inequalities between the rich and the poor." To sum up, egalitarian opponents of enhancement want make sure that the rich and the poor remain equally diseased, disabled, and dead.

Even proponents of genetic enhancement, such as Princeton University biologist Lee Silver, have argued that genetic engineering will lead to a class of genetically enhanced people that he calls the GenRich who will occupy the heights of the economy while unenhanced Naturals provide whatever grunt labor the future needs. Silver suggested that eventually "the GenRich class and the Natural class will become ... entirely separate species with no ability to cross-breed, and with as much romantic interest in each other as a current human would have for a chimpanzee."

Bioethicists George Annas, Lori Andrews, and Rosario Isasi have laid out a rather apocalyptic scenario:

> The new species, or "posthuman," will likely view the old "normal" humans as inferior, even savages, and fit for slavery or slaughter. The normals, on the other hand, may see the posthumans as a threat and if they can, may engage in a preemptive strike by killing the posthumans before they themselves are killed or enslaved by them. It is ultimately this predictable potential for genocide that makes species-altering experiments potential weapons of mass destruction, and makes the unaccountable genetic engineer a potential bioterrorist. (Annas et al. 2002: 162)

Let's take their over-the-top scenario down a notch or two. The enhancements that are likely to be available in the relatively near term to people now living will be pharmacological – pills and shots to increase strength, lighten mood, and improve memory. Consequently, such interventions could be distributed to nearly everybody who wanted them. Later in this century, when safe genetic engineering becomes possible, it will likely be deployed gradually and will enable parents to give their children beneficial genes for improved health and intelligence that other children already get naturally. Thus, the argument can be made that safe genetic engineering in the long run is more likely to ameliorate than to exacerbate human inequality.

In any case, political and moral equality has never rested on the facts of human biology. In prior centuries, when humans were all "naturals," tyranny, aristocracy, slavery, and purdah were common social and political arrangements. Our biology did not change in the past two centuries, our political ideals did. In fact, political liberalism is already the answer to questions about human and posthuman rights. In liberal societies the law is meant to apply equally to all, no matter how rich or poor, powerful or powerless, brilliant or stupid, enhanced or unenhanced.

One crowning achievement of the Enlightenment is the principle of tolerance, of putting up with people who look differently, talk differently, worship differently, and live differently than we do, or in Rawlsian terms, tolerating those who pursue differing reasonable comprehensive doctrines. In the future, our descendants may not all be natural *homo sapiens*, but they will still be moral beings who can be held accountable for their actions. There is no a priori reason to think that the same liberal political and moral principles that apply to diverse human beings today wouldn't apply to relations among future humans and transhumans (Wilson 2007).

But what if enhanced posthumans did take the Nietzschean superman option? What if they really did see unenhanced people "as inferior, even savages, and fit for slavery or slaughter"?

It is an unfortunate historical fact that plenty of unenhanced humans have been quite capable of believing that millions of their fellow unenhanced humans were inferiors who needed to be eradicated (Rummel 1994). However, as liberal political institutions, with their limits on the power of the state, have spread and strengthened, they have increasingly restrained technologically superior groups from automatically wiping out less advanced peoples (which was usual through-out most of history). There is no a priori reason to believe that this dynamic will not continue in the future as biotechnology, nanotechnology, and computational technologies progressively increase people's capabilities and widen their choices.

Opponents of human enhancement focus on the alleged social harms that might result, while overlooking the huge social costs that forgoing the benefits of enhancement technologies would entail. Allen Buchanan posits "that some enhancements will increase human productivity very broadly conceived and thereby create the potential for large-scale increases in human well-being, and that the enhancements that are most likely to attract sufficient resources to become widespread will be those that promise increased productivity and will often exhibit what economists call *network effects*; the benefit to the individual of being enhanced will depend upon, or at least be greatly augmented by others having the enhancement as well" (Buchanan 2008: 2).

Buchanan points out that much of the ethical debate (cited above) about enhancements focuses on them as positional goods that primarily help an individual to outcompete his rivals. This characterization of enhancements leads quickly and ineluctably to pervasive zero sum thinking in which for every winner there is assumed to be a loser. Instead enhancements could produce substantial positive externalities. "Large numbers of individuals with increased cognitive capabilities will be able to accomplish what a single individual could not, just as one can do much more with a personal computer in world of many computer users," writes Buchanan (Buchanan 2008: 11).

While competition certainly plays a role in underwriting success in society and the economy, most success is achieved through cooperation – the dominant dynamic in truly modern societies is win/win, not win/lose (Hoff 2010: 1467–1468).

So in the future people in the pursuit of non-zero sum social and economic relations are likely to choose the sorts of intellectual and emotional enhancements that boost their ability to cooperate more effectively with others, e.g., increased empathy, greater practical reason. Of course, people in the future will have to be on guard against any still deluded folks who think that free riding might work, but there may well be an app for that – the increasingly transparent society. People will be able to check the reputations of others for honest dealing and fair cooperation with just a few clicks of a mouse (or by accessing directly whatever follows Google using a nanotech brain implant). Such social monitoring will be nearly as omnipresent as that of a hunter-gatherer band. Everyone will want to have a good reputation. One might try to fake being virtuous, but the best and easiest way to have a good reputation will be the same as it is today, by actually being virtuous.

Buchanan argues that modern people have already adopted a wide array of enhancements that display these beneficial network effects, including literacy, numeracy, and social institutions that "extend our abilities beyond what is *natural* for human beings" (Buchanan 2008: 7). Some future biomedical enhancements that would significantly increase both individual and social productivity include those that raise the cognitive capabilities of human beings (memory, attention, and processing speed), increase healthy lifespans, and boost our immune systems.

More disturbingly, Buchanan notes that if biotech enhancements do, in fact, dramatically increase social productivity, then the state and its citizens might be far less interested in imposing limits on enhancements and instead shift to promoting them for everyone. The analogy is that biotech enhancements might be treated like other productivity-boosting enhancements like education and immunization. "If a particular enhancement had very strong productivity-enhancing effects, the failure of the state to ensure that no one lacks access to it might be as culpable as its failure to ensure that all citizens are literate or have access to immunization," suggests Buchanan (Buchanan 2008b: 14). The temptation for democratically imposing enhancements would be hard to resist and would result in imposing a particular vision of human flourishing on those who do not want them.

The End of Gene Tyranny

A more optimistic view is that the ability to install whatever genes one might want will become so cheap and routine that everybody would have access to the technology, dissipating the fears of growing inequality, even speciation, between groups of people. Underlying all this moral handwringing over genetic engineering is the concern that genes really matter – that one's life chances are largely determined by the genes one carries. Good genes equal a bright future; bad genes entail a blighted future. Recent genetic research is showing that this view is wrong.

How so? By using outside interventions that regulate and enhance the performance of the genes that people already have. Such interventions will include new, precisely targeted pharmaceuticals that will change the activity of various genes and gene combinations in desired ways. For example, back in 1999 brain researcher Joe Tsien genetically engineered smart mice by giving them extra copies of the NR2B gene that encodes the receptor for NMDA that plays a role in laying down memories in the brain (Tsien et al. 1999). The enhanced mice exposed to aversive stimuli learned to avoid them much faster than unenhanced mice.

Fast forward 10 years, and Tsien and his colleagues report that their further research on genetically engineered rodents has strengthened their finding that increasing the dose of NR2B gene improves memory. In a 2009 study in the journal *PLoS One*, they speculate, "Conceivably, our demonstration of genetic enhancement in both mice and rats via NR2B overexpression greatly strengthens the notion that the NR2B gene is a valid drug target for improving memory function in both normal brains and patients with Alzheimer's disease or mild cognitive impairment" (Wang et al. 2009). So what intervention might enhance memory in normal brains? Tsien and his colleagues note that other research suggests that increasing the amount of magnesium in the brain boosts the effect of NR2B on memory.

In addition, a January 2010 report in the journal *Biological Psychiatry* by European researchers found that administering the antibiotic D-cycloserine offers a "promising pharmacological mechanism for facilitating declarative learning [the aspect of human memory that stores facts] in healthy people" (Onur et al. 2010). Of course, magnesium and D-cycloserine may not ultimately work, but the prospects are good that interventions that will successfully enhance human memory will be uncovered. Other researchers are working on a neural prosthesis using microchips to mimic the memory-consolidation activities of the hippocampus (Berger 2009). The point is that these enhancements will not require genetic engineering and can benefit and be administered to anyone.

As previously noted, reversing aging is the killer app of biomedical research. Aging correlates with all kinds of nasty outcomes, including cancer, Alzheimer's disease, heart attacks, weaker muscles, strokes, thinner bones, lower libido, and the depressing list goes on until it ends in death. Researchers are studying the genetics of people who live to be 100 years old to uncover the genetic variants associated with longer life (Sebastiani et al. 2010). The goal of the research is not to isolate the genes so that they can be installed as a way to boost life expectancy, but to identify the biochemical pathways they modulate so that interventions can be devised for people who don't have the good fortune to carry these genes for extended longevity (Kenyon 2010).

What sort of interventions? A 2009 study in the journal *Nature* found that dosing old mice with the immunosuppressant drug rapamycin extended their lifespans by about 10 percent. As the researchers suggested, "Rapamycin may extend lifespan by postponing death from cancer, by retarding mechanisms of aging, or both" (Harrison et al. 2009). The ends of the 46 chromosomes that bear the genes inside our cells are protected by caps called telomeres. As our cells divide the telomeres get shorter. Our cells stop dividing and become senescent when the telomeres have eroded away.

An article published this past January in *Nature* reported that reactivating the enzyme telomerase so that it lengthened the telomeres reversed aging in mice (Jaskelioff et al. 2011). But what about humans? Also this past January, researchers at the biotech company Sierra Sciences reported work in the journal *Rejuvenation Research* showing that the nutraceutical TA-65 is the "first compound ever discovered that activates the enzyme telomerase in the human body" (Harley 2011). The Sierra Sciences press release notes, "Although TA-65 is probably too weak to completely arrest the aging process, it is the first telomerase activator recognized as safe for human use." Again, rapamycin and TA-65 may not work out, but they point the way toward postponing, if not overcoming, the fatal destiny that our genes naturally have in store for us.

Genetically engineered inequality is a bioethical phantom. The truth is that biotechnological interventions will eventually enable nearly everyone to enhance their bodies and their brains. The good news is that as researchers learn more about the good and bad effects of our genes, the more we will be liberated from whatever tyranny they do exercise.

Will longevity treatments and other enhancements bankrupt the economy? In an article on "The Coming Death Shortage" (Mann 2005), Charles Mann makes a quick and dirty (probably overstated) calculation that new longevity treatments might be as expensive as HIV drug treatments are today at about $15,000 per person annually. (Of course, keep in mind that one day HIV drugs will go off patent and they will cost less than $300 per year.) But taking Mann's estimate at face value, he calculates that 80 million oldsters receiving $15,000 worth of longevity treatments would cost $1.2 trillion per year. Mann then quotes Centers for Disease Control analyst James Lubitz as saying that $1.2 trillion is "the kind of number that gets people's attention." Then Mann suggests that in order to avoid class warfare along a lifespan divide such huge new costs would have to be borne by the government since every citizen, rich and poor, would demand access to longevity treatments. Assuming he's right, how worried should we be?

Perhaps $1.2 trillion may get the attention of someone who is living in today's $14 trillion economy. However, in 2003 the Employment Policy Foundation (EPF) issued a study that calculated that the United States economy would grow to $128 trillion by 2077. So if the EPF calculations are correct, longevity treatments for 80 million healthy oldsters would cost less than 1 percent of GDP in 70 years. Let's assume an unrealistic scenario in which every one of an estimated 480 million Americans alive in 2075 would require $15,000 worth of longevity treatments annually – the total bill would be $7.2 trillion – that's still less than 7 percent of projected GDP in 2077. So in the long run, the affordability of longevity treatments doesn't seem like a big issue.

Moral Toleration

People should not be forced to use medicines and technologies that they find morally objectionable. Take the case of the Amish. Amish individuals live in an open society – ours – and can opt out of our society or theirs whenever they want. As followers of a reasonable comprehensive doctrine, they have a system for voluntarily deciding among themselves what new technologies they will embrace. The situation of the Amish demonstrates that technological choices don't have to involve everyone in a given society. (Although Amish practicality has caused them to embrace modern medicine when comes to treating genetic maladies that plague their community [Clines 2002].)

Eventually, one can imagine that in the future different treatment and enhancement regimens will be available to accommodate the different values and beliefs held by citizens. Christian Scientists would perhaps reject most of modern biotechnology outright; Jehovah's Witnesses might remain leery of treatments that they interpret to being akin to using blood products or blood transfusions; Roman Catholics might refuse to use regenerative treatments derived from human embryonic stem cells; and still others will wish to take the fullest advantage of all biomedical enhancements and treatments. In this way, a pluralistic society respects the reasonable comprehensive doctrines of their fellow citizens and enables social peace among moral strangers.

Callahan writes: "I really wish we would be told, when the great day arrives and we have dozens, maybe hundreds of years ahead of us, exactly how it would all work." Well, I wish I knew too, but the plain unvarnished fact of the matter is that humanity advances by trial and error. Even the smartest people cannot figure out how scientific and technological advances will play out over the next few decades, much less centuries. In 1960 the optical laser was described by its inventor as an invention looking for a job. By 2005 ubiquitous lasers routinely cut metal, play CDs, reshape corneas, carry billions of Internet messages, remove tattoos, and guide bombs. It is likely that age-retardation and other enhancement technologies will develop incrementally. So humanity will have lots of opportunities for course corrections as we go along.

The very good news is that the history of the last two centuries has shown that technological progress has been far more beneficial than harmful for humanity. The development of age-retardation and other enhancement technologies will be more steps along that beneficial trend line. We should all have the right to choose to use or not use new technologies to help us and our families to flourish. Is humanity ready for radically longer lifespans? We're about as ready as we'll ever be. In other words, yes.

So How Will Enhancement Enable People to Flourish?

A lot of opponents of allowing people to enhance their capacities argue that such enhancements will create an unlevel playing field in the game of life. Enhancements are analogized to using steroids in sports to boost athletic performance. The rules of sport are arbitrary, if the baseball commissioner or other competent authority rules that using steroids is against the rules, then using steroids is, by definition, cheating. But the sorts of enhancement that people are likely to want to acquire not only give people a competitive edge in the marketplace, but also are goods in themselves. "A good is still a good whether it brings you level with others, sets you ahead or leaves you behind but still better off than you were" (Harris and Chan 2008: 338).

Elizabeth Fenton: "If dignity is equivalent to agency, then clearly it is not necessarily threatened by genetic technology, since most proposed interventions do not endanger agency, understood as self-determination or the capacity to choose goals and the freedom to pursue them. Enhanced memory or intelligence, for example, would improve capacities that humans already possess. If a student of the future is better able to recall material she was taught years (or even semesters) before, her agency has not been undermined; she is a more efficient agent when it comes to memory recall. Someone who lives to the age of 150 is no less of an agent than someone of the current era who lives only to 85; the extra 65 years would, in fact, actually bestow more time in which to be an agent ... none of these capabilities (bodily health, imagination, emotion, practical reason, friendship, etc.) are in fact threatened by, for example, enhanced intelligence or athleticism" (Fenton 2008: 5).

Note

1   The TransVision 2004 conference, held at the University of Toronto, August 5–8, 2004.

References

Allhoff, Fritz (2008) "Germ-Line Genetic Enhancement and Rawlsian Primary Goods." *Journal of Evolution and Technology* 18/1(May), pp. 10–26. http://jetpress.org/v18/allhoff.htm.

Annas, George, et al. (2002) "Protecting the Endangered Human: Toward an International Treaty Prohibiting Cloning and Inheritable Alterations." *American Journal of Law and Medicine* 28/2–3.

Bailey, Ronald (1999) "Intimations of Immortality." *Reason* (March 6). http://reason.com/opeds/rb030600.shtml.

Bailey, Ronald (2003) "You Shouldn't Live So Long." *Reason* (April 9). http://reason.com/archives/2003/04/09/you-shouldnt-live-so-long.

Berger, Theodore (2009) "A Neural Prosthesis for Restoring Lost Cognitive Function: Brain-Implantable Biomimetic Micro-Electronic Models of Hippocampal Input-Output Activity." Keynote at the Fourth International IEEE/EMBS Conference on Neural Engineering (June). http://ieeexplore.ieee.org/xpl/freeabs_all.jsp?arnumber=5109213.

Billings, Paul R., Hubbard, Ruth and Newman, Stuart A. (1999) "Human Germline Gene Modification: A Dissent." *The Lancet* (May 29). http://www.geneticsandsociety.org/article.php?id=175.

Buchanan, Allen (2008a) "Enhancement and the Ethics of Development." *Kennedy Institute of Ethics Journal* 18/1 (March) (draft), p. 25. http://www.law.harvard.edu/programs/petrie-flom/PDFs/Buchanan.pdf,

Buchanan, Allen (2008b) "Enhancement and the Ethics of Development." *Kennedy Institute of Ethics Journal* 18/1 (March) (draft). http://www.law.harvard.edu/programs/petrie-flom/PDFs/Buchanan.pdf.

Chan, Sarah and Harris, John (2007) "In Support of Human Enhancement." *Studies in Ethics, Law, and Technology* 1.

Clines, Francis (2002) "Research Clinic Opens in Ohio for Genetic Maladies that Haunt Amish Families." *New York Times* (June 20). http://www.nytimes.com/2002/06/20/us/research-clinic-opens-in-ohio-for-genetic-maladies-that-haunt-amish-families.html?sec=health&&partner=rssnyt&emc=rss&pagewanted=all.

Colpin, H. and Bossaert, G. (2008) "Adolescents Conceived by IVF: Parenting and Psychosocial Adjustment." *Human Reproduction* (August 27). http://humrep.oxfordjournals.org/cgi/content/abstract/23/12/2724

de Tocqueville, Alexis (1835) "Tyranny of the Majority." Henry Reeve, Trans. *Democracy in America.* New York: George Dearborn & Co. and Adlard and Saunders (1st edn. 1938).

Dvorsky, George (2004) "Deathist Nation." *Betterhumans.com* (June 6) http://archives.betterhumans.com/Columns/Column/tabid/79/Column/266/Default.aspx.

El-Chaar, Darine, et al. (2008) "Risk of Birth Defects Increased in Pregnancies Conceived by Assisted Human Reproduction." *Fertility and Sterility* (October 29). http://www.fertstert.org/article/S0015-0282 (08)03574-7/abstract.

Fenton, Elizabeth (2008) "Genetic Enhancement – A Threat to Human Rights?" *Bioethics* 22/1.

Habermas, Jürgen (1997) "Popular Sovereignty as Procedure." In James Bohman and William Regh, eds., *Deliberative Democracy: Essays on Reason and Politics*, Cambridge, MA: MIT Press.

Habermas, Jürgen (2003) *The Future of Human Nature.* Cambridge: Cambridge University Press.

Haines, Michael (2010) "Fertility and Mortality in the United States." *Economic History Association* (February 4). http://eh.net/encyclopedia/article/haines.demography.

Harley, Calvin (2011) "A Natural Product Telomerase Activator as Part of a Health Maintenance Program." *Rejuvenation Research* (February), pp. 45–56. http://www.ncbi.nlm.nih.gov/pubmed/20822369.

Harris, John and Chan, Sarah (2008) "Understanding the Ethics of Genetic Enhancement." *Gene Therapy* 15.

Harrison, David, et al. (2009) "Rapamycin Fed Late in Life Extends Lifespan in Genetically Hetero-geneous Mice." *Nature* (July 16), pp. 392–395. http://www.nature.com/nature/journal/v460/n7253/full/nature08221.html.

Hayes, Richard (2006) "Opening Comments at the American Association for the Advancement of Science (AAAS) Consultation on Human Enhancement." (June 1).

Hoff, Karla (2010) "Fairness in Modern Society." *Science* (March 19).

Jaskelioff, Mariela et al. (2011) "Telomerase Reactivation Reverses Tissue Degeneration in Aged Telomerase-Deficient Mice." *Nature* (January 6), pp. 102–106. http://www.nature.com/nature/journal/v469/n7328/pdf/nature09603.pdf.

Kamm, Frances (2008) "What Is and Is Not Wrong with Enhancements." In Nick Bostrom and Julian Savulescu, eds., *Human Enhancement*. Oxford: Oxford University Press.

Kant, Immanuel (1991) *Moral Law: Groundwork of the Metaphysics of Morals*, trans. Herbert James Paton. London: Routledge.

Kass, Leon (1997) "The Wisdom of Repugnance." *New Republic* (June 2). http://www.catholiceducation.org/articles/medical_ethics/me0006.html.

Kass, Leon (2001) "L'Chaim and Its Limits: Why Not Immortality?" *First Things* (May). http://www.firstthings.com/ftissues/ft0105/articles/kass.html.

Kenyon, Cynthia (2010) "The Genetics of Aging." *Nature* (March 25), pp. 504–512.

Lawler, Peter (2004) "Restless Souls." *New Atlantis* (Winter), p. 42.

Lawler, Peter (2005) *Stuck With Virtue: The American Individual and Our Biotechnological Future.* Wilmington, DE: ISI Books.

Lewis, C.S. (2001) *The Abolition of Man.* New York: HarperCollins.

Madison, James (1788) *Federalist 51.* http://www.constitution.org/fed/federa51.htm.

Mann, Charles (2005) "The Coming Death Shortage." *The Atlantic Monthly* (May). http://www.theatlantic.com/magazine/archive/2005/05/the-coming-death-shortage/4105/.

McKibben, Bill (2003) *Enough: Staying Human in an Engineered Age.* New York: Times Books.

Minois, Georges (1990) *History of Old Age: From Antiquity to the Renaissance.* Chicago: University of Chicago Press.

Murphy, Kevin and Topel, Robert (2006) "The Value of Health and Longevity." *Journal of Political Economy* 114 (October), pp. 871–904.

National Cancer Institute (2009) "Nanopore Sequencing Could Slash DNA Analysis Costs." (March). http://nano.cancer.gov/news_center/2009/march/nanotech_news_2009-03-25g.asp.

National Resource for Cell Analysis and Modeling "The Virtual Cell." http://www.nrcam.uchc.edu/.

Nordhaus, William (2002) *The Health of Nations: The Contribution of Improved Health to Living Standards.* NBER Working Paper 8818 (February). http://www.nber.org/papers/w8818.

Onur, Oezguer A., et al. (2010) "The N-Methyl-D-Aspartate Receptor Co-agonist D-Cycloserine Facilitates Declarative Learning and Hippocampal Activity in Humans." *Biological Psychiatry* (June), pp. 1205–1211. http://www.ncbi.nlm.nih.gov/pubmed/20303474.

Pinker, Steven (2007) "A History of Violence." *New Republic* (March 19). http://pinker.wjh.harvard.edu/articles/media/2007_03_19_New%20Republic.pdf 2007.

President's Council on Bioethics (2003) *Beyond Therapy: Biotechnology and the Pursuit of Happiness.* New York: HarperCollins.

Rawls, John (1996) *Political Liberalism.* New York: Columbia University Press.

Rawls, John (1999) *A Theory of Justice,* rev. edn. Cambridge, MA: Harvard University Press.

Rummel, R.J. (1994) *Death by Government.* Piscataway, NJ: Transaction Publishers.

Satel, Sally (2010) "The Limits of Bioethics." *Policy Review* (February 1). http://www.hoover.org/publications/policy-review/article/5354.

Schaub, Diana (2007) "Ageless Mortals." *Cato Unbound* (December 5). http://www.cato-unbound.org/2007/12/05/diana-schaub/ageless-mortals/.

Sebastiani, P., et al. (2010) "Genetic Signatures of Exceptional Longevity in Humans." *Science* (1 July), 1190532. doi:10.1126/science.1190532.

Stock, Gregory and Callahan, Daniel (2004) "Debates: Point-Counterpoint: Would Doubling the Human Life Span Be a Net Positive?" *Journals of Gerontology Series A: Biological Sciences and Medical Sciences* 59, pp. B554–B559. http://biomed.gerontologyjournals.org/cgi/content/full/59/6/B554.

Terence. *The Brothers.* http://www.wayneturney.20m.com/terencebrothers.htm.

Tsien, Joe Z., et al. (1999) "Genetic Enhancement of Learning and Memory in Mice." *Nature* (September 2), pp. 63–69.

Wang, D., Cui, Z., Zeng, Q., Kuang, H., Wang, L.P., et al. (2009) "Genetic Enhancement of Memory and Long-Term Potentiation But Not CA1 Long-Term Depression in NR2B Transgenic Rats." *PLoS ONE* 4(10), e7486. doi:10.1371/journal.pone.0007486. http://www.plosone.org/article/info%3Adoi%2F10.1371%2Fjournal.pone.0007486.

Wilson, James (2007) "Transhumanism and Moral Equality." *Bioethics* 21/8, pp. 419–425.

33

Is Enhancement Worthy of Being a Right?

Patrick D. Hopkins

Introduction

It is not surprising that when we get down to the basics about policies, laws, permissions, and restrictions on biotechnological enhancement, the question is quickly framed this way: Do we have a fundamental right to biotechnologically enhance ourselves? We live in a culture – largely worldwide – whose moral deliberations are dominated by the modern discourse of rights. This was not always the case and it does not have to be the case now. Instead of deciding what we should do, or be allowed to do, by asking whether we have a fundamental "right" to something, we might instead ask whether that something is good, or whether it is intelligible, or whether it is rational, or healthy, or virtuous, or tending toward edification, or commanded by God, or granted under a social contract. But we do ask the question in terms of rights. As the announcement of the conference which prompted this essay says:

> Defenders of enhancement argue that the use of biotechnologies is a fundamental human right, inseparable from the defense of bodily autonomy, reproductive freedom, free expression and cognitive liberty … defenders of enhancement believe that bans on the consensual use of new technologies would be an even greater threat to human rights.[1]

From the *Journal of Evolution and Technology* 18/1 (May 2008), pp. 1–9, Copyright © Patrick D. Hopkins.

So What Does Putting the Question of Enhancement in Terms of Rights Do?

First of all, notice the term "fundamental" used in this debate. The purpose of this term is to separate the kind of right being talked about from purely conventional or legal rights. Legal rights could be changed at will, but the concept of a "fundamental right" is supposed to have greater power. A fundamental right cannot be changed; it is not the product of community agreement or local ordinances. In this respect, "fundamental rights" serve the same function as the older locution of "natural rights" or the even more recent "human rights." They are all supposed to be things that have a claim on us above and beyond the vagaries of society. They are supposed to generate moral limitations on what society can do to us and what we can do to each other. "Fundamental rights" are largely protections for the individual, then, constraints on the pursuit of social or community goals.[2] A purported right to enhancement would be a sort of moral immunization, a claim against society not to (at the very least) criminalize enhancement.

What is the Problem with Putting the Question of Enhancement in Terms of Rights?

There are general problems with any rights talk. At the outset, it is questionable whether there are such things or what they are even supposed to be. While earlier natural law and natural rights thinkers thought of rights as divine commands[3] or sometimes merely practical requirements for pursuing our natural ends, Hugo Grotius (the seventeenth-century "father" of modern rights and international law) influentially described rights as inherent "moral qualities," which had the simultaneous effect of disconnecting rights from theology and of putting rights into some sort of ghostly realm.[4] Rights are invisible and intangible, but "real." They are just supposed to be there without having been legislated by anyone. It is these sorts of assertions that have led some thinkers to say that rights are just fictions. Jeremy Bentham (the eighteenth-century legal and moral theorist) famously called the concept of rights being used in the American and French Revolutions "nonsense upon stilts."[5]

This is not to say that rights are merely defended as intuited or supposed. There is a large litera-ture on rights which includes defenses of rights as practically necessary given the fact of our having interests, or even logically necessary concepts given our experiences of purposive action.[6] The practical problem with the assertion of a right is not belief in the existence of rights in general (which is largely assumed) but rather that there is no clear way to detect which rights we have or how strong they are. Which rights we have is an issue constantly debated. As L.W. Sumner has argued, the very prevalence of rights talk may be the greatest threat to rights.[7] The ease with which these undetectable and invisible moral qualities can be asserted has led us to a situation in which rights seem to proliferate unchecked. Some people prefer a minimal list of rights – life, liberty, property. Some prefer a different list – life, liberty, and the pursuit of happiness (probably the most expansive right ever discussed). Others might derive from these broader rights free speech, free assembly, freedom of religion, and ownership of guns. Others discover previously unrecognized fundamental rights to contraception, abortion, gay marriage, public funding of religious schools, suicide, or a right against one's parents not to have been born at all. Some assert that the right to healthcare or public education is fundamental. A university might assert that students have a right not to hear racist language. A church might assert that students have the right to public prayer in public schools. The United Nations Universal Declaration of Human Rights asserts that we all possess the right to a paid vacation and to enjoy art.[8] The Council for Responsible Genetics has issued a "Genetics Bill of Rights" stating that all people have the right to a world in which living organisms cannot be patented, and that all people have the right to have been conceived, gestated, and born without genetic manipulation.[9] In protesting human cloning, bioethicist Daniel Callahan asserted that we all have a right to a unique genetic identity.[10]

Not only the number, but the scope of rights is also open to expansion. Free speech rights might not just mean being able to criticize government policy, but to publish pornography or create video games in which players gets to murder prostitutes.[11] Procreation rights might mean not only the right to have children but to genetically engineer them or to raise them with religious beliefs forbidding the use of medicine. Property rights might not just protect your home from government seizure, but also mean you can own genetically engineered tissues or patent an athletic move in a track and field event, for which others will have to pay you to use in the future. In short, we are tempted to assert the claim of a "right" over anything we desire. This proliferation of rights and the limitless widening of the scope of rights serves to weaken the power of rights language altogether. When the assertion of rights become little more than a reflex to secure desires, the entire notion of rights as sacrosanct is undermined, and rights need sacrosanctity to function as they do.

To make rights language retain meaning, then, we need some form of decision procedure that lets us distinguish what are "real" rights and what are merely desires that we might wish to be knighted as rights. The possibility of developing such a procedure is a complicated debate in ethical theory that I will not go into detail about here. What I will say, however, is that there is no clear test, morally or legally, that we can trot out for determining what is and is not a right. It would be nice to have a rights-detector, but we don't have one generally agreed upon.

What we do know, however, is that conceptually and rhetorically, and certainly legally, when you appeal for something to be recognized as a right, you have to make a case for it. That case has to appeal to certain values and to articulate why the alleged right you are interested in is worthwhile, and usually how it stems from a more basic recognized right.

How Might One Make the Case that Enhancement Be Treated as a Right?

Roughly speaking, there are three strategies in the discourse on rights that have been used to get a right recognized as fundamental or natural.

The first is the oldest and most closely associated with natural law – conformity with human nature. The idea is that if there is a universal human nature, then what counts as fulfilling us, nurturing us, and truly satisfying us is fixed, within a certain range of constraints. Rights, then, are seen as an important way that we can respect and pursue these elements of our nature – our whole purpose for being. Not having rights, and not having duties, is thought to make no sense given our natures. What is most important about us is that we are something fairly specific, that we have a nature, and that it is our nature that makes any conception of a valuable existence for us intelligible. Rights (and correlative duties) are the most coherent way of supporting the actions required for us to satisfy these natural, intelligible ends. To recognize something as a right, then, means to show that it serves to properly satisfy a natural end.

The second idea of what grounds rights is interests. While our interests might be determined by a fixed human nature, they wouldn't have to be. The idea here is that rights serve to protect the things that we do care about, that we do have interests in, so that we are understood primarily as benefiting from the duties that our rights impose on others – whether those duties are to help us or just not to interfere with us. What is important here is that we care about certain things and care about having a certain kind of experience. Rights are all about benefits to us, given our interests, especially our interest in our own wellbeing. To recognize something as a right, then, means to show that it serves a basic interest.

The third strategy for defending a right is the one most commonly and casually asserted in contemporary culture – autonomy. The focus here is on choice and the general idea is that what is most important about us is our free will. What things we actually choose are not nearly so important as the fact that we get to choose at all. Choice itself is the highest intrinsic value and the sine qua non for respecting rational beings. Rights are, therefore, predominantly about preventing others from constricting our choices, and as long as our choices do not interfere substantially with others, then they are purely our own. To recognize something as a right, then, means to show that it could be chosen freely and does not harm others.

So, in thinking about the asserted right to enhance, which of these strategies best captures what is at the heart of the desire for enhancement, for the intelligibility of wanting enhancement, and for making enhancement seem worthwhile? This is not the same question, though it is related, as asking what rhetorical strategy will most likely work politically. It is the question of worth. What understanding of the right to enhancement most captures enhancement as worth having a right to?

The first thing that must be understood, for all these strategies, is that a right never gives you carte blanche to harm another directly or perhaps even foreseeably indirectly. The discourse of rights almost always includes the idea that rights are rarely absolute and are at least limited by whether or not our actions harm others and whether our actions violate others' rights. But assuming one can make the case that enhancement will not harm others (a contested assumption), then what rights appeal can be made?

Appeal to Autonomy

The appeal to autonomy is probably the most common contemporary defense of specific rights and it does have the greatest flexibility. It gives the greatest scope to whatever right you might be interesting in defending, and it appeals to a general interest in doing what we want without government or social interference. However, its flexibility is also its weakness. The concept of autonomy has a rich and morally powerful history. Unfortunately, autonomy has been watered down intellectually so that today it often means nothing more than the right to be permitted to do anything that does not harm others. Merely appealing to autonomy for the right to enhancement then, says nothing specific about enhancement itself, but only makes a general demand not to be interfered with. Accordingly, there is really no need for the issue of enhancement per se even to arise. A pure appeal to autonomy would support a right to enhance oneself no more or less than it would support a right to impair oneself. Pure autonomy says nothing about the value of enhancement or why anyone would want such a thing, but only speaks to the alleged value of being unconstrained in whatever actions you wish to pursue. One can appeal to autonomy equally to demand the right to vote freely, to print pornography, to worship freely, to self-mutilate, to choose your own career, to stay drunk all the time, to kill yourself for noble reasons, or to kill yourself for ignoble reasons. The extreme nonspecificity of pure autonomy claims, and its content-free nature, makes merely appealing to autonomy weak, formalistic, nonspecific, and immature.

Earlier understandings of autonomy were often about recognizing the rational and practical nature of human beings. Respecting autonomy in natural law meant recognizing that, though we were morally constrained by being rational creatures, we made use of our free will and introspection in deciding how best to fulfill our general and specific natures. Respecting autonomy in deontological ethics was about recognizing that rational beings produce their own moral laws, not in a relativistic manner, but in manner which showed that universal reason generated morality, not some arbitrary legislator. Respecting autonomy in consequentialist ethics was about recognizing that when other authorities decided our actions for us they almost always got it wrong and that a rational person was best placed themselves to determine how their actions would in fact produce the best consequences.[12] In none of these views was autonomy seen as an ultimate content-free value in and of itself so that what our choices were had no moral relevance, and only the fact of our choosing did. Autonomy was meant to be rational and practical, not vapidly libertine.

In contemporary times however, autonomy is often used as a catch-all and has sometimes devolved into little more than the plaint of a teenager to be allowed to do whatever they want, no matter how self-destructive or pointless, just because "it's my life." This situation is reminiscent of Plato's criticism of democracy in the *Republic*. He argues that democracy at first develops because people are denied freedom, but once they have it they come to value nothing but freedom itself – that is, they do not value what they could gain by having freedom, but just the freedom itself. As a result they see anything they could possibly desire as being their birthright and they see any potential constraint on their freedom as an assault no matter how beneficial it might be to them. The result of this is a self-destructive breakdown, culturally and individually. Plato says:

> [The young democratic man] spends as much money, effort, and time on unnecessary pleasures as on necessary ones ... And he doesn't admit any word of truth into the guardhouse, for if someone tells him that some pleasures belong to fine and good desires and others to evil ones ... he denies all this and declares that all pleasures are equal and must be valued equally ... And so he lives on, yielding day by day to the desire at hand ... And isn't it inevitable that freedom should go to all lengths in such a city? ... a father accustoms himself to behave like a child and fear his sons, while the son behaves like a father, feeling neither shame nor fear in front of his parents ...[13]

It is from the fear and disorder generated by the fetishism of liberty that Plato says tyranny arises, when a charismatic authoritarian appears promising to provide protection and order for the people, who themselves now fear a dangerous and aimless society in which people misuse their liberty.

So, the idea is that in late democracies the appeal to autonomy (which remember, literally means self-lawed – not no-lawed) degenerates into nothing but the appeal to formal liberty. It thus loses nobility and worth, and especially practicality. People begin to experience a reactionary response, despising the mere call for being allowed to do whatever you want as silly, immature, weak, socially destructive, and dangerous. As critic of enhancement Francis Fukuyama says in *Our Posthuman Future*:

> while freedom to choose one's own plan for life is certainly a good thing, there is ample reason to question whether moral freedom as it is currently understood is such a good thing for most people, let alone the single most important human goal ... Contemporary understandings of individual autonomy ... seldom provide a way to distinguish between genuine moral choices and choices that amount to the pursuit of individual inclination, preferences, desires, and gratifications.[14]

Defending a right to enhancement then, by merely appealing to autonomy, to the larger right to do whatever you want, is empty. It is also likely to be seen by many, as with Fukuyama, as immature and vapid – and rightly so. But this point should not be seen as disappointing to enhancement defenders. Appeals merely to autonomy denigrate the potential value of enhancement to little more than a teenager's demand to stay out as long as they want just because. While such an appeal (if accepted) would show that we do have a right to enhancement, presumably the defenders of biotechnological augmentation have some rather more substantial and specific interest in enhancement itself. Presumably they want to show something more than that enhancement is a right simply because it is one of infinitely many things we can do given unfettered autonomy. Otherwise, there would be little point to organizing conferences and editing special issues of journals on the specific question of enhancement and rights. Presumably, they want to show that enhancement can be something good, something valuable.[15]

Appeal to Interests

The appeal to interests, I think, is more powerful than just appealing to autonomy. The appeal to interests says that there is some end or goal that we care about, that is important to us, and that we cannot completely fulfill the potential goodness of our lives without pursuing. This is much more specific than mere autonomy. It doesn't say that we should be permitted to pursue anything we desire, no matter its reasonableness or consequence, but rather that some goals are worthwhile and important, and we need freedom in order to pursue those goals.

Now the term "interests" as it is used here does not mean simply "desires and preferences" but rather things that are important for our welfare, for our wellbeing. Using this language, you might have a "desire" to kill yourself or a "preference" for neurotoxic recreational drugs, but your interests would not be satisfied by those things. You would instead be destroyed or impaired by satisfying such desires. Our interests are those things that we need to secure a life worth having, to assist in our flourishing. Though there are many variations on the list of basic interests that humans are thought to have, most of the lists include the preservation of life, health, bodily integrity, play, friendship, classic autonomy, religion, aesthetics, and the pursuit of knowledge.[16] These are the kinds of things that everyone needs in order to make life worth having had at all. Specific rights, then, are the claims we make to receive, or not be interfered with in our pursuit of, those things which satisfy our interests. Freedom of assembly, healthcare, freedom of worship, education, or police protection, etc., are all specific rights that can benefit us through satisfying interests or final ends.

For defending enhancement, then, the goal would be to explain how enhancement would in fact be a reasonable and meaningful way to pursue the satisfaction of recognized interests. Although bioconservative critics often see enhancement as a kind of repudiation of traditional human values, we can see that the kinds of things enhancement might provide are very much in keeping with traditional understandings of worthwhile, reasonable human values and interests. The most fundamental of interests – the preservation of life – is certainly pursued by life extension. The pursuit of knowledge is obviously relevant to cognitive enhancement. Better health through organ replacement or cybernetic implants is too obvious to mention. And we can fairly easily make the case that specific forms of enhancement can address interests of friendship, bodily integrity, play, aesthetics, autonomy, and even I think religion[17] – in general, all the things that have been recognized as providing worthwhile and fulfilled lives. Enhancement, then, is not freakish; it is not a repudiation of value; it is the pursuit of value.

Appeal to Natural Law

This interest talk is deeply connected to the third strategy that I mentioned, about appeals to natural law and human nature. While proponents of natural law theory may seem to be some of the most vocal opponents of enhancement, this is often because of concomitant religious commitments they have which are – by their own admissions – not the ground of, or necessary for the justification of, natural law. Much of what natural law defenders want to promote is the idea that, in fact, there is a human nature. Their opponents in this regard are not biotechnologists and transhumanists, but rather anti-essentialist social science model devotees who think there is no biologically grounded human nature and treat humans as kinds of independent minds subject only to language, rhetoric, and politics, not to neurology or genetics. Most proponents of enhancement already agree with proponents of natural law that there is a biologically-grounded human nature – otherwise biotechnological alteration would be mostly irrelevant to changing our behavior and cognitive capacities. Of course, while enhancement advocates may have a long row to hoe when it comes to making friends with natural lawyers, one thing we can see is that whatever the tension, it is not the case that the enhancement lobby is dismissive of or opposed to the concept of a real human nature.

Our interests are – as most natural lawyers would attest – the result of our human nature. It is perfectly natural, and perfectly humanly-natural, to seek self-preservation, expanded knowledge, greater control of ourselves. As Ramez Naam says: "Far from being unnatural, the drive to alter and improve on ourselves is a fundamental part of who we humans are. As a species we've always looked for ways to be faster, stronger, and smarter and to live longer."[18] What defenders of enhancement can do, then, is to point out that those who seek enhancement are not repudiating the human, but are pursuing a species-old interest – more life, more knowledge, more happiness, more aesthetics, more friendship, more play, even more religion. In respect of this last element, it is worth mentioning that two of the most famous philosophers and theologians of Christianity – Boethius and Thomas Aquinas – both argued that happiness was the ultimate goal of human beings but that our desire for, and even mental ability for, happiness could not possibly be satisfied by the current bodies and physical world in which we live.[19] That is why there is a heaven and an afterlife – because the happiness of which humans are capable is greater than our current biological and physical limitations permit us to achieve. Of course, there is a great gulf between claiming that only God can fulfill ultimate human desires and claiming that biotech can fulfill them, but it is perhaps not the gulf that most people think of – and in any case, no enhancement supporter need claim biotech is the ultimate, but only to make the case that biotech is worthwhile in moving us forward in the securing of valuable ends.

Conclusion

My point is simply this: The theory of rights has significant problems, but we do live in an era where rights language dominates the moral and legal landscape and so defenders of enhancement have to deal with that language. In making the case that enhancement should be a right, then, defenders have to adopt a strate___ ___ave to argue that enhancement should be recognized as important enough t___ ___ight. The most common strategy is to appeal to autonomy or libe___ ___al. Its libertine form ("it's my life and I should be able to d___ ___low, and often self-impairing, saying nothing about the w___ ___o basic interests, however – to those things widely recog___ ___necessary for a life worth having had – can accommodate ___ ___it less alien, and more obviously noble, worthy, and rea___ ___cuses on explaining the goals of enhancement as noble an___ ___ecting enhancement to concerns about human nature an___ ___sic values of natural law – life, health, knowledge, and so___ ___y the core pro-enhancement community, we can see that the ___ ___is somehow unnatural or alien to human nature is deeply false.[20]

There is one caveat in all this for the pro-enhancement crowd, though. And that is for them to ask themselves what they want from enhancement. If enhancement appeals to them only because it offers power, distraction, libertine gratification, an endless existence of vapid entertainment, then they are not seeking to be more than human, they are seeking to be less than human – but just for a really, really, really long time with more durable equipment. As with so many of our other quests, enhancement should be pursued because it can satisfy worthwhile and noble ends. To have enhancement justifiably recognized as a right, it needs not only to be perceived as worthwhile, dignified, and noble; it needs to be worthwhile, dignified, and noble.[21]

Notes

1 See http://ieet.org/index.php/IEET/HETHR (accessed April 27, 2008).
2 This concept of a fundamental right developed from the tradition of natural law, a complex moral system with influences going back to Plato, Aristotle, and especially the Stoics, and then reformed by Thomas Aquinas as the chief moral theory of the Roman Catholic Church. So, the aforementioned "defenders of enhancement" might just as easily have claimed that we all have the natural right to enhance ourselves – a natural right to alter our natures. "Fundamental" rights are the modern children of natural law. See Hopkins 2007.
3 For example, Cicero 1928: Book III, xxii, p. 211.
4 For comment on moral qualities, see Grotius 1901: Book I, iv, p. 19. For comment on independence from theology, see Grotius 1957: paragraph 11, p. 10.
5 Bentham 1843: 489, quoted in Bedau 2000.
6 See Gewirth 1982: 198–200. He writes: "Even if persons' having rights cannot be logically inferred in general from the fact that they make certain claims, it is possible and indeed logically necessary to infer from the fact that certain objects are proximate necessary conditions of human action that all rational agents logically must hold or claim, at least implicitly, that they have rights to such objects. [...] Every rational being must claim or accept that he has rights to freedom and well being. If any

agent were to deny that he has these rights, he would contradict himself. For in holding that freedom and well being are necessary conditions of his agency, he holds that they are necessary goods; and because of his conative attachment to his purposes he holds that it is necessary that he have these goods in that he (prudentially) ought to have them."

7   Sumner 2000: 298.
8   http://www.un.org/Overview/rights.html (accessed April 27, 2008).
9   http://www.councilforresponsiblegenetics.org/Projects/CurrentProject.aspx?projectId=5   (accessed November 2012).
10   Quoted in *Time* (November 8, 1993), p. 68.
11   *Grand Theft Auto: Vice City.* http://www.amazon.com/gp/product/B0000696CZ/103-6183399-7150204?v=glance&n=468642 (accessed April 27, 2008).
12   Mill 1998: 92–93, 121.
13   Plato, *Republic* (Plato 1997: 1171–1173). There is a spectacular example of Plato's criticism in contemporary literature. In Max Barry's novel *Jennifer Government*, a libertarian society is breaking down as a result of too little government and social paternalism. The main characters engage in the following exchange of dialogue: "'You know, this all started when they got rid of tax. That's when everyone started buying out of society. When we tax, we had a community' … 'What, you want to reintroduce tax? How do you do that?' … 'I don't know,' she muttered. 'But somewhere along the line, this freedom stuff got way out of control'" (Barry 2003: 230–231).
14   Fukuyama 2002: 124.
15   I don't assume that this is true for all those who find enhancement interesting, but it is true for many. No doubt some of those attracted to enhancement are attracted for the meanest of goals. In other places, I've referred to this as the difference between "high" transhumanism and "low" transhumanism.
16   See, e.g., Nussbaum 1999: 41–42; Finnis 1980: 81–90.
17   See Hopkins 2005.
18   Naam 2005: 9.
19   See Boethius 1999, esp. pp. 53–58; see also Aquinas 1964: 57.
20   Though largely arguing against enhancement, the President's Council on Bioethics acknowledges that human beings have always been seeking to better their lot through technology (even in biblical views) and thus they say of humanity: "By his very nature man is the animal constantly looking for ways to better his life through artful means and devices; man is the animal with what Rousseau called 'perfectibility' (President's Council on Bioethics 2003: 291n.).
21   Though not explicitly arguing for this position, the Transhumanist Declaration uses language such as "personal growth" and "well-being" in describing certain of its goals: (4) Transhumanists advocate the moral right for those who so wish to use technology to extend their mental and physical (including reproductive) capacities and to improve their control over their own lives. We seek personal growth beyond our current biological limitations. (7) Transhumanism advocates the well-being of all sentience (whether in artificial intellects, humans, posthumans, or non-human animals) and encompasses many principles of modern humanism. Transhumanism does not support any particular party, politician or political platform. Similarly, the Extropy Institute uses the term "wisdom" in explaining its goals: "Extropy means seeking more intelligence, wisdom, and effectiveness, an open-ended lifespan, and the removal of political, cultural, biological, and psychological limits to continuing development." http://www.extropy.org/principles.htm (accessed August 15, 2006).

References

Aquinas, Thomas (1964) *Treatise on Happiness*. Notre Dame: University of Notre Dame Press.
Barry, Max (2003) *Jennifer Government*. New York: Vintage Books.

Bedau, Hugo Adam (2000) "'Anarchical Fallacies': Bentham's Attack on Human Rights." *Human Rights Quarterly* 22/1, pp. 261–279.

Bentham, Jeremy (1843) "Anarchical Fallacies: Being An Examination of the Declarations of Rights Issued During the French Revolution." In *The Works of Jeremy Bentham*, 11 vols., ed. John Bowring. Edinburgh: William Tait, 1838–1843.

Boethius (1999) *The Consolation of Philosophy*. Oxford: Oxford University Press.

Cicero (1928) "On the Republic." In *Philosophical Treatises: On the Republic. On the Laws*, Loeb Classical Library. Cambridge MA: Harvard University Press.

Finnis, John (1980) *Natural Law and Natural Rights*. Oxford: Clarendon Press.

Fukuyama, Francis (2002) *Our Posthuman Future: Consequences of the Biotechnology Revolution*. New York: Farrar, Straus & Giroux.

Gewirth, Alan (1982) *Human Rights: Essays on Justification and Applications*. Chicago: University of Chicago Press.

Grotius, Hugo (1901) *The Rights of War and Peace*. New York: Walter Dunne.

Grotius, Hugo (1957) *Prolegomena to the Law of War and Peace*, Library of Liberal Arts. Kansas City: Bobbs-Merrill.

Hopkins, Patrick D. (2005) "Transcending the Animal: How Transhumanism and Religion Are and Are Not Alike." *Journal of Evolution and Technology* 14/2 (August), pp. 13–28. http://www.jetpress.org/volume14/hopkins.html.

Hopkins, Patrick D. (2007) "Natural Law." In *Encyclopedia of Philosophy*, 2nd edn. Farmington Hills, MI: Macmillan Reference, vol. 6, pp. 505–517.

Mill, John Stuart (1998) *On Liberty*. Oxford: Oxford University Press.

Naam, Ramez (2005) *More Than Human: Embracing the Promise of Biological Enhancement*. New York: Broadway Books.

Nussbaum, Martha (1999) *Sex and Social Justice*. Oxford: Oxford University Press.

Plato (1997) *Republic*. In *Plato: Complete Works*, ed. John M Cooper. Indianapolis: Hackett Publishing.

President's Council on Bioethics (2003) *Beyond Therapy: Biotechnology and the Pursuit of Happiness* (October). New York: HarperCollins.

Sumner, L.W. (2000) "Rights." In Hugh LaFollette, ed., *The Blackwell Guide to Ethical Theory*. Oxford: Blackwell.

34

Freedom by Design
Transhumanist Values and Cognitive Liberty

Wrye Sententia

Introduction

In the twenty-first century, a number of wide-ranging ethical, legal, and social outcomes from current and emerging scientific research do now, and increasingly will, bear relevance on freedom of thought.[1] Paired with exponential advances in digital computing and communication capabilities, the ways in which we refer to, or think about, "human" thinking and, specifically, *how we think*, will evolve in ways that previous generations, across millennia, have not needed to ponder. Granted, large-scale shifts in technological capabilities have repeatedly called on various cultures to adapt or rethink their self-conception. Yet, never before has the technology at issue been so close to our brains.

In a figurative and literal sense, *the chips are on the table*, but that's not where they will stay. Any perusal of contemporary (2011) science reveals the dizzying acceleration that the application of key late twentieth-century and early twenty-first technologies promises. The reduction in the size of digital chips, coupled with exponential leaps in materials science and computing power, have affected virtually every field of application, including neuroscience. We are expanding the reach of external monitoring and data-collection techniques, while also enlarging the scope of *internal or interconnected* means of monitoring, modifying, and manipulating thought processes.[2]

With these changes, and anticipating future applications in neuroscience, the foundational concept of "cognitive liberty" places emphasis on the resilience and role of individual thinking to assert a commitment to freedom-based applications of technology at the dawn of the new millennium.

The Transhumanist Reader: Classical and Contemporary Essays on the Science, Technology, and Philosophy of the Human Future, First Edition. Edited by Max More and Natasha Vita-More.
© 2013 John Wiley & Sons, Inc. Published 2013 by John Wiley & Sons, Inc.

Legal Right by Design: Cognitive Liberty

Cognitive liberty, a term coined in the year 2000, asserts the foundational principle of the legal and ethical right to brain privacy, autonomy, and choice in relation to existing pharmacology, as well as anticipated applications of techno-human advances vectored on the brain. The concept "cognitive liberty" was meant to update long-standing notions of freedom of thought that reflect implicit values and protected rights under the US Constitution.[3] However, given further advances in neuroscientific understanding of how the human brain works and in how technologies might interface with the brain, the concept of free thought is an increasingly slippery fish.

Nonetheless, our US legal system, and indeed modern world jurisprudence, predicates much of its framework on an individual's freedom of thought, even though it does not always honor it, or even define it.[4] Cognitive liberty, as it was envisioned in the year 2000 by legal scholar Richard Glen Boire and myself, challenges the US legal system, and other democratic countries' juridical systems, to accommodate both a right to (and not to) direct, modify, or enhance one's thought processes. It is here that cognitive liberty touches central themes in transhumanist discourse related to cognitive enhancement and morphological freedom, and supports a foundational right to cognitive self-design. Given coming innovations and manifold possibilities for twenty-first-century interactive technologies, our legal right to, and the possibility for, cognitive liberty requires more thought.

More than better processing power or better drugs is at issue in achieving widespread positive outcomes hoped for by transhumanists. Cognitive liberty fits as an essential prong in a necessary conceptual and legal framework that expands existing democratic and social values in parallel with the expansion of technological power. In earlier work, I, and others, have outlined the need for an updated version of freedom of thought[5] and emphasized the concept of cognitive liberty as necessary to facilitate the coming changes we will face as individuals and as a collective global society.

Design Thinking and Cognitive Liberty

As a group, transhumanists tend towards an optimistic view of the future. The transhumanist viewpoint accepts the migration of thought processes working in tandem with leaps in technological capabilities. From informational to biotechnological advances; from insular, embodied, individual cognition to interactive, collective neural networks; from a reductionist to an expansionist vision for human capability. To date, at least three generations of transhumanist thinkers have further developed the philosophical reach, of biologist Julian Huxley's original term, "transhumanism" (1957), in support of the idea of the technocultural improvement of human beings.[6] In particular, improving or enhancing cognitive function has been, and continues as central to the movement. Key transhumanists[7] evolve and inform the discussion of what we may be capable of doing with and to our brains, and in some cases are moving the science and technology forward themselves to get there. What troubles me is when, from my perspective, "*should*" arguments, however factually or philosophically grounded, brush too closely with a perceived agenda for human evolution that imposes a particular blend of "human betterment" as conceived of by those who lay claim to it. What constitutes "better," laced with prescriptions on how to get there, is problematic. With this in mind, cognitive liberty's strength is that it protects those who do want to alter their brains, but also those who do not.

Many transhumanist advocates eagerly place their sights on exponential shifts in human capabilities brought about by a coming techno-social "Singularity."[8] Yet, given that the development of cognitive-enhancing technologies may be slowed by opponents who typically fear such advances as morally and socially fraught, it seems counterproductive that many transhumanists assert an unrestrained zeal in favor of widespread cognitive enhancement. For example, although stemming, I suspect, from a spirit of equability and inclusion, when J. Hughes refers to enhancement as a "spiritual obligation," he only fuels opponents' misapprehensions of what constitutes a collective "good."[9] Likewise, unreflective prophecies of something like whole brain emulation can do more harm than "good."

Opponents to cognitive enhancement, reading the same technological tea leaves as Singularitarians, fear that virtually every aspect of "human" culture soon will be adversely influenced by integrated technological communication and control capabilities. From their viewpoint, compromising the "human condition" or "human nature" by surpassing "natural" limitations, violates a moral (should) code that they perceive as "good" for the species.[10] To embrace or eschew active self-design differs very little from adherence to a particular religion or a particular worldview. In a vibrant democracy, such difference can be celebrated – mental diversity functions as a benefit, not a roadblock to enhancement. By appealing to cognitive liberty as foundational to democratic social policy, the danger of moral or ethical imperatives "to enhance or not to enhance," recedes. All stakeholders benefit because cognitive liberty refrains from the rabidity of a particular point of view. Instead, this fundamental principle will serve to integrate – and to control – neurotechnological advances in ourselves and in our society.

It is a platitude that one person's utopia is another person's hell. Design thinking in the legal landscape of cognitive liberty calls for mutual, multi-lateral respect and protected tolerance – values common to all, yet without specific agendas. My own bias being what it is, my assertion here is based on a historically rich framework for individual rights. Cognitive liberty provides such a framework in resolving moral inflections and logic-laced imperatives: it meets (or thwarts) any particular agenda for social planning where the law constrains my perfect world at odds with yours.

Caveats on Concept: Fictions of Freedom

To be free or not to be free? The very idea of freedom of thought is predicated on a historical, cultural-human bias in favor of individual thinking. Before cognitive neuroscience and exponential computing capabilities exploded in recent decades, complaints about the limitations of freedom of thought tended to critique how a person's choices, identity, and opportunities were systemically, but surreptitiously controlled or influenced by others. For example, critical theorists like Judith Butler or Michel Foucault articulated the limits on freedom that come about from internalized discourses of power. Such critical assessments of the social sphere: of race, class, and gender mediated by language and historical structures became tools to assess political and social inequities, putting the spotlight on resilient prejudice, "rational" agency, and blind universalism.[11]

Today, concepts of the so-called "free individual" must exist not only within a historical-social-linguistic critique of limitations on freedom of thought, but additionally, within a neuroscientific framework. If, previously, Western philosophical and religious assertions erred in adhering to an inviolate (and universal) free will based on appeals to sacrosanct Enlightenment values of autonomy and individuality, irrespective of social or biological nuances, contemporary understanding in how the brain works can frequently be equally reductive in the opposite direction by relying on research in biology, chemistry, and genetics as proof of an eviscerated free will. Even as researchers nod to the complex inter-workings of biological and chemical systems of the brain and central nervous system, they still frequently disappoint in making experimental leaps of faith that reduce the higher cognitive functions of the brain to normed, discrete, measured units (voxels) without regard to resolution limits of technologies measuring blood flow in the brain, nor with recognition of the broader cultural and linguistic limitations of their own experimental methods when testing on diverse human subjects.

In sum, cognitive liberty, like all freedoms, is vexed. I accept the paradoxes of our history as a species, and revelations of science that point to neurological gaps in our thinking. Necessarily based on patterns of individual (brain) behavior, predicated on one's experience AND on one's genetics, autonomy and choice are imperfect. The question is whether, as we fast-forward towards increasingly powerful technologies, we want to keep in place *the possibility* of cognitive liberty – the *possibility* of choice and self-jurisdiction on a human scale.

Freedom in Spite of All Else

Because it is possible to physically engineer thinking through drugs even today (anti-depressants, attention drugs, etc.), and because we can anticipate changing one's thought patterns via direct electrical manipulation and interfacing technologies, it is important to consider who (or what) will manage our thoughts. We may reach a time when neuroscientists go so far as to predict (and therefore pre-emptively mandate) how any one person might think at any particular time. Likewise, as many others have pointed out, if computers achieve superior consciousness without regard for our (still) limited brains, how will we avoid our own Kubrickesque Hal vs. Dave moment?[12] This is not to play into a technological paranoia, but to extrapolate from clear techno-social trends and anticipate those legal parameters, if any, we want to retain for a mentally meaningful "interior life."[13]

Cognitive liberty maintains the value of agency in a vibrant democratic social contract, into the twenty-first century and beyond. Although understanding, predicting, and "correcting"[14] individual thinking is perhaps the end game for cognitive and information sciences (and is the "neuro"-marketeers wet dream), we do not have to participate on these terms. Cognitive liberty, as a protected legal right, calls for brain privacy to remain a real option and ensures that the never ceasing onslaught of others' agendas, be they for corporate gain, coercive politics, or for more populist aims of unity and collective consciousness by design – are kept, when desired, at bay.

It is in this context that the need for cognitive liberty as a right to self-design takes on new dimensions. Those quaint human values – personal autonomy, responsibility, and choice – are, at least for now, what still allow people to act in ways contrary to predetermined calculations, to statistical probabilities, or market-researched behaviors. The world of consciousness is vastly bigger than what any one person or group can imagine. Cognitive liberty stands as an assertion to protect, as best we can, those who want to be protected, those who want to reach, and those who don't. One of the marvels of our species is that even as we think through our own contradictions, we may be led to – but we don't have to – resolve cognitive dissonance. We are not binary beings. Humans have an uncanny ability to bootstrap our intelligence and our empathy by catalyzing an ability to imagine and innovate, and consequently, make manifold leaps in acting in and on the world. But we are not immune to our own success. It is with this paradoxical recognition of pattern-making and creative drive – of limitations at odds with a desire for self-expression, to expand rather than contract, to enhance rather than diminish our human potential – that I champion cognitive liberty as a twenty-first-century value. If, however, upon close scrutiny, cognitive liberty looks to you, *cher lecteur, mon semblable, mon frère*, as a dusty museum piece in an accelerated arch of evolving ontology – let it be known that it abides, now, and for those who embrace it, as a radical possibility to rally for difference in the design and execution of thought.

Notes

1 In *The Future of the Brain* (2005), Steven Rose points to the convergence of disparate fields – anatomy, physiology, molecular biology, genetics and behavior – together with new brain-imaging systems – PET, fMRI, MEG – as responsible for the late twentieth-century discipline of neurobiology which is part and parcel of the larger scope of neurosciences drawing from any number of converging disciplines. Rose affirms, "as with the new genetics, so the neurosciences are not merely about acquiring knowledge of brain and mind processes but about being able to act upon them – neuroscience and neurotechnologies are indissolubly linked" (Rose 2005: 5).

2 In particular, a range of technological advances, from Brain-Machine-Interfaces (BMIs) to neuropharmacology, target those aspects of executive function which, while ostensibly for medical applications today, will almost certainly lead to expanded cognitive capabilities. See for example the panoply of biomedical engineering products at a company such as G-Tec (http://www.gtec.at/).

3 "The right to control one's own consciousness is the quintessence of freedom. If freedom is to mean anything, it must mean that each person has an inviolable right to think for him or herself. It must mean, at a minimum, that each person is free to direct one's own consciousness; one's own underlying mental processes, and one's beliefs, opinions, and worldview. This is self-evident and axiomatic" (Boire 1999/2000).

4 Richard Glen Boire, Amicus Curiae brief filed in *Sell v. U.S.* No 02-5664.

5 See numerous articles in *The Journal of Cognitive Liberties* (1999–2003). See also Sententia 2004: 221–228.

6 Greg Klerkx postulates three waves of transhumanist thought, stemming from Huxley's vision (and developed by Fereidoun M. Esfandiary, better known as FM-2030); grounded by Max More and Natasha Vita-More's early work through the Extropy Institute, and reaching a third wave that "began in earnest" with the working draft of the human genome (circa 2000). Greg Klerkx 2006: 63.

7 Max More, Natasha Vita-More, Nick Bostrom, J. Hughes, Aubrey de Grey, Martine Rothblatt, Ben Goertzel, Ray Kurzweil, to name a few, all of whom are contributors to this seminal volume.

8 Through his analysis of technological thresholds for radically transformative intelligent machines, Ray Kurzweil, by far the best-known advocate of "the Singularity," anticipates a mid-century point at which exponential gains in human-computer capabilities, due in large part to compounding advances in computational technologies, will overtake biological humans in general intelligence. See, for instance, *The Singularity is Near* (Kurzweil 2005); see also "Technological Singularity?" (Vinge 1993), reprinted in *Whole Earth* (Spring 2003), an issue featuring several articles on the topic.

9 Hughes 2004.

10 See for instance, the President's Council on Bioethics 2003; Sandel 2009. Or, for example, Dr. William Hurlbut in the 2006 documentary film, *Exploring Life Extension*.

11 *Alas, Poor Darwin: Arguments against Evolutionary Psychology* (Rose and Rose 2000) compiles critical objections to biological determinism and reductionism generally put forward by an evolutionary view of human psychology, grounded in genetics. While these authors attempt to establish the existence of

free will, I suggest that we accept free will as compromised, but as a necessary concept for a vibrant social contract.

12   Stanley Kubrick. *2001: A Space Odyssey* (MGM, 1968).

13   Noting that the concept of an "interior life," is a construction only widely coming into its own as a cultural constant as late as the Renaissance, Douglas Rushkoff (2010) rightly proclaims that such a concept requires re-examination in what he calls "the new cybernetic order," where we can anticipate new styles of technological engagement in order to negotiate "the biases and agendas of our [programmed] networks."

14   Much, if not all, research currently funded by the US National Institute on Drug Abuse (NIDA) approaches addiction as a chronic, progressive, and relapsing brain disease. This shift in a perspective of addicts – from lacking willpower to suffering from brain dysfunction – carries widespread ethical, legal, and social issues in terms of corrective US drug policy. In 2004, the Center for Cognitive Liberty & Ethics released an extensive report, *Pharmacotherapy and the Future of the Drug War* that anticipates this issue.

References

Boire, Richard Glen (1999/2000) "Cognitive Liberty Part 1." *Journal of Cognitive Liberties* 1/1 (Winter).

Center for Cognitive Liberty & Ethics (2004) *Pharmacotherapy and the Future of the Drug War.* http://www.cognitiveliberty.org/issues/pharmacotherapy.html

Hughes, James (2004) *Citizen Cyborg: Why Democratic Societies Must Respond to the Redesigned Human of the Future.* Cambridge, MA: Westview Press.

Klein, Bruce, dir. (2006) *Exploring Life Extension: Interviews with more than 50 Scientists and Futurists.* Immortality Institute.

Klerkx, Greg (2006) "The Transhumanists as Tribe." In Paul Miller and James Wilsdon, eds., *Better Humans? The Politics of Human Enhancement and Life Extension.* London: Demos.

Kubrick, Stanley, dir. (1968) *2001: A Space Odyssey.* MGM.

Kurzweil, Ray (2005) *The Singularity is Near: When Humans Transcend Biology.* New York: Viking.

President's Council on Bioethics (2003) *Beyond Therapy: Biotechnology and the Pursuit of Happiness* (October). New York: HarperCollins.

Rose, Hilary and Rose, Steven P.R., eds. (2000). *Alas, Poor Darwin: Arguments against Evolutionary Psychology.* London: Jonathan Cape.

Rose, Steven (2005) *The Future of the Brain: The Promise and Perils of Tomorrow's Neuroscience.* Oxford: Oxford University Press.

Rushkoff, Douglas (2010) *Program or Be Programmed: Ten Commands for a Digital Age.* New York: O/R Books.

Sandel, Michael (2009) *The Case Against Perfection: Ethics in the Age of Genetic Engineering.* Cambridge, MA: Harvard University Press.

Sententia, Wrye (2004) "Neuroethical Considerations: Cognitive Liberty and Converging Technologies for Improving Human Cognition." In Mihail C. Roco and Carlo D. Montemagno, eds., *The Coevolution of Human Potential and Converging Technologies.* Annals of the New York Academy of Sciences 1013, pp. 221–228.

Vinge, Vernor (1993) "Technological Singularity?" Reprinted in *Whole Earth* (Spring 2003).

Part VIII

Future Trajectories
Singularity

How does the concept of the singularity relate to that of transhumanism? In science, the singularity may refer to a discontinuity or a mathematical point where an object is not defined, or to a cosmological event where measure of the gravitational field becomes infinite. In theory, the *technological* singularity is a conjecture about the emergence of super-intelligent minds. Transhumanism is a worldview that seeks to understand the unknown, anticipate risks, and create an advantageous future for humanity, including the nonbiological superintelligences we may become or create. However, too often, observers conflate the two concepts, assuming that all transhumanists anticipate a technological singularity.

The considerable overlap of interests and expectations represented by both views feeds that confusion. After all, both transhumanists and proponents of the technological singularity (i.e., singularitarians, as they sometimes call themselves) expect drastic changes in the future. Because the term has had wide appeal, it is now referred to simply as "the singularity." Some transhumanists expect a singularity and most of those who expect a singularity are broadly transhumanist. But, while transhumanism is a broad worldview that anticipates using technology to overcome human limits, the singularity is a specific model (or set of models) of technological change and its trajectory into the future. To clearly separate specific singularitarian expectations from the philosophy of transhumanism requires first defining the former.

The original meaning of "technological singularity", as coined by Vernor Vinge in his 1993 essay (the first in this section) is the Event Horizon view. This view links to Alan Turing's seminal writing about intelligent machinery outstripping human intelligence, and more directly to I.J. Good's term "intelligence explosion," which suggests not only a growth of machine intelligence but its acceleration. Accordingly, technological advance will lead to the advent of superhuman intelligence. Superhuman intelligence will not only accelerate technological progress, it will create even more intelligent entities ever faster (e.g., Good's concept). As Vinge puts it, "This

The Transhumanist Reader: Classical and Contemporary Essays on the Science, Technology, and Philosophy of the Human Future, First Edition. Edited by Max More and Natasha Vita-More.
© 2013 John Wiley & Sons, Inc. Published 2013 by John Wiley & Sons, Inc.

change will be a throwing-away of all the human rules, perhaps in the blink of an eye." One result of this sudden shift will be the unfolding of a future that is incomprehensible to us. Sometimes this view includes the claim that to know what a superhuman intelligence would do at this point, you would have to be superintelligent too. The distinctive consequence of the Event Horizon version of the singularity is that the future beyond that point will be completely unpredictable, as Vinge states:

> My use of the word "Singularity" is not meant to imply that some variable blows up to infinity. My use of the term comes from the notion that if physical progress with computation gets good enough, then we will have creatures that are smarter than human. At that point the human race will no longer be at center stage. The world will be driven by those other intelligences. This is a fundamentally different form of technical progress. The change would be essentially unknowable, unknowable in a different way than technology change has been in the past. ("Arterati On Ideas: Vinge's View of the Singularity," interview by Natasha Vita-More in *Extropy Online* [1998])

Ironically, the concept of the "singularity" is not itself singular. In his essay, Anders Sandberg delves in great detail into a range of differing models of technological singularity. A less complex map of this territory captures the three primary models on which most people seem to agree. These are the Event Horizon, Accelerating Change, and Intelligence Explosion.

The Accelerating Change conception of the technological singularity has become strongly associated with inventor and visionary Ray Kurzweil. According to this view, technological change is a positive feedback loop and so is exponential rather than linear. Because change in the past was slower than change in the present, and future change will be faster still, our typically linear expectations of change will be drastically conservative, especially as we look out further ahead. If, as Kurzweil argues, technological advance follows smooth exponential curves then – contrary to the Event Horizon view – we can make accurate forecasts of some new technologies, including the development of artificial intelligence.

Finally, the Intelligence Explosion throws out smooth exponential change in favor of positive feedback cycle of cognitive improvement. Once technology leads to minds of superhuman intelligence, a powerful positive feedback cycle comes into play. Recursive cognitive self-improvement extremely rapidly causes vast change before running into upper limits imposed by the laws of physics or computational possibilities.

Casual observers frequently mix these models of the singularity of singularity into a single, cloudy suspension. The more sharply defined you make these three views, the more they contradict one another. Most obviously, the inherent predictability of the Event Horizon and Intelligence Explosion views conflicts with the predictability of the Accelerating Change view.

Those who anticipate a singularity often display considerable confidence in their forecasts of when the singularity will happen, whether or not they expect the post-singularity future to be predictable. Writing in 1993 and reaffirming his view in 2003, Vinge said that he would be "surprised if this event occurs before 2005 or after 2030." On the basis of sets of exponential curves, Kurzweil forecasts a singularity close to 2045, while others think it might take several hundred years to achieve superintelligent AI. Other transhumanists are much more skeptical about the ability to make remotely precise forecasts of this nature. Some individuals who would *like* to experience a singularity nevertheless worry that technological and economic progress is actually slowing, not accelerating. In addition, there is no shortage of those who are much less favorable to the singularity and see more stagnation than acceleration.

It is entirely possible to expect a technological singularity of one of these types and yet not to be a transhumanist. The advent of superhuman intelligence might involve augmenting human intelligence to superhuman levels or it might mean that synthetic intelligences leave us far behind while we remain mired in the human condition. Some writers, such as Hans Moravec, at least sometimes seem to expect this outcome and are unconcerned about it. This might better be described as a type of posthumanism, except that there is already a vaguely defined academic view using that term. It is also entirely possible to affirm the core values and goals of transhumanism while doubting that we will experience anything resembling a singularity. Technological advance may come in fits and starts, eventually leading to a posthuman condition, but without any singular event.

Part VIII clarifies and critically examines thinking about the singularity, starting with Vernor Vinge's seminal essay. Anders Sandberg analyzes models of technological singularity in detail, looking for their commonalities and differences. The final essay in Part VIII collects the 1998 deliberations of a number of transhumanist thinkers to critically discuss the singularity, as initially defined by Vinge, in its technological and economic aspects.

35

Technological Singularity

Vernor Vinge

I.   What is the Singularity?

The acceleration of technological progress has been the central feature of this century. We are on the edge of change comparable to the rise of human life on Earth. The precise cause of this change is the imminent creation by technology of entities with greater-than-human intelligence. Science may achieve this breakthrough by several means (and this is another reason for having confidence that the event will occur):

- Computers that are "awake" and superhumanly intelligent may be developed. (To date, there has been much controversy as to whether we can create human equivalence in a machine. But if the answer is "yes," then there is little doubt that *more* intelligent beings can be constructed shortly thereafter.)
- Large computer networks (and their associated users) may "wake up" as superhumanly intelligent entities.
- Computer/human interfaces may become so intimate that users may reasonably be considered superhumanly intelligent.
- Biological science may provide means to improve natural human intellect.

The first three possibilities depend on improvements in computer hardware.

Actually, the fourth possibility also depends on improvements in computer hardware, although in an indirect way.

"The Coming Technological Singularity: How to Survive in the Post-Human Era," by Vernor Vinge, was presented at the VISION-21 Symposium sponsored by NASA Lewis Center and the Ohio Aerospace Institute, March 30–31, 1993. Copyright © Vernor Vinge 1993. http://www-rohan.sdsu.edu/faculty/vinge/misc/singularity.html

The Transhumanist Reader: Classical and Contemporary Essays on the Science, Technology, and Philosophy of the Human Future, First Edition. Edited by Max More and Natasha Vita-More.
© 2013 John Wiley & Sons, Inc. Published 2013 by John Wiley & Sons, Inc.

Progress in hardware has followed an amazingly steady curve in the last few decades. Based on this trend, I believe that the creation of greater-than-human intelligence will occur during the next 30 years. (Charles Platt [private communication] has pointed out that AI enthusiasts have been making claims like this for 30 years. Just so I'm not guilty of a relative-time ambiguity, let me be more specific: I'll be surprised if this event occurs before 2005 or after 2030.)

Now in 2003, I still think this time-range statement is reasonable.

What are the consequences of this event? When greater-than-human intelligence drives progress, that progress will be much more rapid. In fact, there seems no reason why progress itself would not involve the creation of still more intelligent entities – on a still shorter time scale. The best analogy I see is to the evolutionary past: Animals can adapt to problems and make inventions, but often no faster than natural selection can do its work – the world acts as its own simulator in the case of natural selection. We humans have the ability to internalize the world and conduct what-if's in our heads; we can solve many problems thousands of times faster than natural selection could. Now, by creating the means to execute those simulations at much higher speeds, we are entering a regime as radically different from our human past as we humans are from the lower animals.

This change will be a throwing-away of all the human rules, perhaps in the blink of an eye – an exponential runaway beyond any hope of control. Developments that it was thought might only happen in "a million years" (if ever) will likely happen in the next century.

It's fair to call this event a singularity ("the Singularity" for the purposes of this piece). It is a point where our old models must be discarded and a new reality rules, a point that will loom vaster and vaster over human affairs until the notion becomes a commonplace. Yet when it finally happens, it may still be a great surprise and a greater unknown. In the 1950s very few foresaw it: Stan Ulam paraphrased John von Neumann as saying:

> One conversation centered on the ever-accelerating progress of technology and changes in the mode of human life, which gives the appearance of approaching some essential singularity in the history of the race beyond which human affairs, as we know them, could not continue. (Ulam 1958)

Von Neumann even uses the term *singularity*, though it appears he is thinking of normal progress, not the creation of superhuman intellect. (For me, the superhumanity is the essence of the Singularity. Without that we would get a glut of technical riches, never properly absorbed.)

The 1960s saw recognition of some of the implications of superhuman intelligence. I.J. Good wrote:

> Let an ultraintelligent machine be defined as a machine that can far surpass all the intellectual activities of any man however clever. Since the design of machines is one of these intellectual activities, an ultraintelligent machine could design even better machines; there would then unquestionably be an "intelligence explosion," and the intelligence of man would be left far behind ... [cites three of his earlier papers]. Thus the first ultraintelligent machine is the last invention that man need ever make, provided that the machine is docile enough to tell us how to keep it under control. ... It is more probable than not that, within the twentieth century, an ultraintelligent machine will be built and that it will be the *last* invention that man need make.[1]

Good has captured the essence of the runaway, but he does not pursue its most disturbing consequences. Any intelligent machine of the sort he describes would not be humankind's "tool" – any more than humans are the tools of rabbits, robins, or chimpanzees.

Through the sixties and seventies and eighties, recognition of the cataclysm spread. Perhaps it was the science-fiction writers who felt the first concrete impact. After all, the "hard" science-fiction writers are the ones who try to write specific stories about all that technology may do for us. More and more, these writers felt an opaque wall across the future. Once, they could put such fantasies millions of years in the future. Now they saw that their most diligent extrapolations resulted in the unknowable … soon. Once, galactic empires might have seemed a Posthuman domain. Now, sadly, even interplanetary ones are.

In fact, nowadays in the early twenty-first century, space adventure stories may be categorized by how the authors deal with the plausibility of superhuman machines. We science-fiction writers have a bag of tricks for denying their possibility or keeping them at a safe distance from our plots.

What about the coming decades, as we slide toward the edge? How will the approach of the Singularity spread across the human worldview? For a while yet, the general critics of machine sapience will have good press. After all, until we have hardware as powerful as a human brain it is probably foolish to think we'll be able to create human-equivalent (or greater) intelligence. (There is the farfetched possibility that we could make a human equivalent out of less powerful hardware – if we were willing to give up speed, if we were willing to settle for an artificial being that was literally slow. But it's much more likely that devising the software will be a tricky process, involving lots of false starts and experimentation. If so, then the arrival of self-aware machines will not happen until after the development of hardware that is substantially more powerful than humans' natural equipment.)

But as time passes, we should see more symptoms. The dilemma felt by science-fiction writers will be perceived in other creative endeavors. (I have heard thoughtful comic book writers worry about how to create spectacular effects when everything visible can be produced by the technologically commonplace.) We will see automation replacing higher- and higher-level jobs. We have tools right now (symbolic math programs, cad/cam) that release us from most low-level drudgery. Put another way: the work that is truly productive is the domain of a steadily smaller and more elite fraction of humanity. In the coming of the Singularity, we will see the predictions of *true* technological unemployment finally come true.

Another symptom of progress toward the Singularity: ideas themselves should spread ever faster, and even the most radical will quickly become commonplace.

And what of the arrival of the Singularity itself? What can be said of its actual appearance? Since it involves an intellectual runaway, it will probably occur faster than any technical revolution seen so far. The precipitating event will likely be unexpected – perhaps even by the researchers involved ("But all our previous models were catatonic! We were just tweaking some parameters …"). If networking is widespread enough (into ubiquitous embedded systems), it may seem as if our artifacts as a whole had suddenly awakened.

And what happens a month or two (or a day or two) after that? I have only analogies to point to: The rise of humankind. We will be in the Posthuman era. And for all my technological optimism, I think I'd be more comfortable if I were regarding these transcendental events from one thousand years' remove … instead of 20.

II.   Can the Singularity Be Avoided?

Well, maybe it won't happen at all: sometimes I try to imagine the symptoms we should expect to see if the Singularity is not to develop. There are the widely respected arguments of Penrose (1989) and Searle (1980)[2] against the practicality of machine sapience. In August 1992, Thinking Machines Corporation held a workshop to investigate "How We Will Build a Machine That Thinks." As you might guess from the workshop's title, the participants were not especially supportive of the arguments against machine intelligence. In fact, there was general agreement that minds can exist on nonbiological substrates and that algorithms are of central importance to the existence of minds. However, there was much debate about the raw hardware power present in organic brains. A minority felt that the largest 1992 computers were within three orders of magnitude of the power of the human brain. The majority of the participants agreed with Hans Moravec's estimate (1988)[3] that we are 10 to 40 years away from hardware parity. And yet there was another minority who conjectured that the computational competence of single neurons may be far higher than generally believed. If so, our present computer hardware might be as much as 10 orders of magnitude short of the equipment we carry around in our heads. If this is true (or for that matter, if the Penrose or Searle critique is valid), we might never see a Singularity. Instead, in the early 2000s we would find our hardware performance curves beginning to level off – because of our inability to automate the design work needed to support further hardware improvements. We'd end up with some very powerful hardware, but without the ability to push it further. Commercial digital signal processing might be awesome, giving an analog appearance even to digital operations, but nothing would ever "wake up" and there would never be the intellectual runaway that is the essence of the Singularity. It would likely be seen as a golden age … and it would also be an end of progress. This is very like the future predicted by Gunther Stent (1969), who explicitly cites the development of transhuman intelligence as a sufficient condition to break his projections.

The preceding paragraph misses what I think is the strongest argument against the possibility of the technological Singularity: even if we can make computers that have the raw hardware power, we may not be able to organize the parts to behave in a superhuman way. To techno-geeky reductionist types, this would probably appear as a "failure to solve the problem of software complexity." Larger and larger software projects would be attempted, but software engineering would not be up to the challenge, and we would never master the biological models that might make possible the "teaching" or "embryonic development" of machines. In the end, there might be the following semi-whimsical Murphy's Counterpoint to Moore's Law:

> The maximum possible effectiveness of a software system increases in direct proportion to the *log* of the effectiveness (i.e., speed, bandwidth, memory capacity) of the underlying hardware.

In this singularity-free world, the future would be bleak for programmers. (Imagine having to cope with hundreds of years of legacy software!)

So over the coming years, I think two of the most important trends to watch are our progress with large software projects and our progress in applying biological paradigms to massively networked and massively parallel systems.

But if the technological Singularity can happen, it will. Even if all the governments of the world were to understand the "threat" and be in deadly fear of it, progress toward the goal would continue. The competitive advantage – economic, military, even artistic – of every advance in automation is so compelling that forbidding such things merely assures that someone else will get them first.

Eric Drexler (1986) has provided spectacular insights about how far technical improvement may go. He agrees that superhuman intelligences will be available in the near future. But Drexler argues that we can confine such transhuman devices so that their results can be examined and used safely.

I argue that confinement is intrinsically impractical. Imagine yourself locked in your home with only limited data access to the outside, to your masters. If those masters thought at a rate – say – one million times slower than you, there is little doubt that over a period of years (your time) you could come up with a way to escape. I call this "fast thinking" form of superintelligence "weak superhumanity." Such a "weakly superhuman" entity would probably burn out in a few weeks of outside time. "Strong superhumanity" would be more than cranking up the clock speed on a human-equivalent mind. It's hard to say precisely what "strong superhumanity" would be like, but the difference appears to be profound. Imagine running a dog mind at very high speed. Would a thousand years of doggy living add up to any human insight? Many speculations about superintelligence seem to be based on the weakly superhuman model. I believe that our best guesses about the post-Singularity world can be obtained by thinking on the nature of strong superhumanity. I will return to this point.

Another approach to confinement is to build rules into the mind of the created superhuman entity (for example, Asimov's Laws of Robotics). I think that any rules strict enough to be effective would also produce a device whose ability was clearly inferior to the unfettered versions (so human competition would favor the development of the more dangerous models).

If the Singularity cannot be prevented or confined, just how bad could the Posthuman era be? Well ... pretty bad. The physical extinction of the human race is one possibility. (Or, as Eric Drexler put it of nanotechnology: given all that such technology can do, perhaps governments would simply decide that they no longer need citizens.) Yet physical extinction may not be the scariest possibility. Think of the different ways we relate to animals. A Posthuman world would still have plenty of niches where human-equivalent automation would be desirable: embedded systems in autonomous devices, self-aware daemons in the lower functioning of larger sentients. (A strongly superhuman intelligence would likely be a Society of Mind [Minsky 1985] with some very competent components.) Some of these human equivalents might be used for nothing more than digital signal processing. Others might be very humanlike, yet with a onesidedness, a dedication that would put them in a mental hospital in our era. Though none of these creatures might be flesh-and-blood humans, they might be the closest things in the new environment to what we call human now.

I believe I.J. Good had something to say about this (though I can't find the reference): Good proposed a meta-golden rule, which might be paraphrased as "Treat your inferiors as you would be treated by your superiors." It's a wonderful, paradoxical idea (and most of my friends don't believe it) since the game-theoretic payoff is so hard to articulate. Yet if we were able to follow it, in some sense that might say something about the plausibility of such kindness in this universe.

I have argued above that we cannot prevent the Singularity, that its coming is an inevitable consequence of humans' natural competitiveness and the possibilities inherent in technology. And yet: we are the initiators. Even the largest avalanche is triggered by small things. We have the freedom to establish initial conditions, to make things happen in ways that are less inimical than others.

Whether foresight and good planning can make any difference may depend on whether the technological Singularity comes as a "hard takeoff" or a "soft takeoff." A hard takeoff is one in which the transition to superhuman control takes just a few hundred hours (as in Greg Bear's "Blood Music"). It seems to me that hard takeoffs would be very hard to plan for; they would be like the avalanches I speak of here in the 1993 essay. The most nightmarish form of a hard take-off might be one arising from an arms race, with two nation-states racing forward with their separate "manhattan projects" for superhuman power. The equivalent of decades of human-level espionage might be compressed into the last few hours of the race, and all human control and judgment surrendered to some very destructive goals.

On the other hand, a soft takeoff is a transition that takes decades, perhaps more than a century. This situation seems much more amenable to planning and to thoughtful experimentation. Hans Moravec discusses such a soft transition in *Robot: Mere Machine to Transcendent Mind*.

Of course (as with starting avalanches), it may not be clear what the right guiding nudge really is.

III.   Other Paths to the Singularity

When people speak of creating superhumanly intelligent beings, they are usually imagining an AI project. But as I noted at the beginning of this essay, there are other paths to superhumanity. Computer networks and human-computer interfaces seem more mundane than AI, yet they could lead to the Singularity. I call this contrasting approach Intelligence Amplification (IA). IA is proceeding very naturally, in most cases not even recognized for what it is by its developers. But every time our ability to access information and to communicate it to others is improved, in some sense we have achieved an increase over natural intelligence. Even now, the team of a PhD human and good computer workstation (even an off-net workstation) could probably max any written intelligence test in existence.

And it's very likely that IA is a much easier road to the achievement of superhumanity than pure AI. In humans, the hardest development problems have already been solved. Building up from within ourselves ought to be easier than figuring out what we really are and then building machines that are all of that. And there is at least conjectural precedent for this approach. Cairns-Smith (1985) has speculated that biological life may have begun as an adjunct to still more prim-itive life based on crystalline growth. Lynn Margulis (in Margulis and Sagan 1986 and elsewhere) has made strong arguments that mutualism is a great driving force in evolution.

Note that I am not proposing that AI research be ignored. AI advances will often have applica-tions in IA, and vice versa. I am suggesting that we recognize that in network and interface research there is something as profound (and potentially wild) as artificial intelligence. With that insight, we may see projects that are not as directly applicable as conventional interface and network design work, but which serve to advance us toward the Singularity along the IA path.

Here are some possible projects that take on special significance, given the IA point of view:

Human/computer team automation. Take problems that are normally considered for purely machine solution (like hill-climbing problems), and design programs and inter-faces that take advantage of humans' intuition and available computer hardware. Considering the bizarreness of higher-dimensional hill-climbing problems (and the neat algorithms that have been devised for their solution), some very interesting displays and control tools could be provided to the human team member.

Human/computer symbiosis in art. Combine the graphic generation capability of modern machines and the esthetic sensibility of humans. Of course, an enormous amount of research has gone into designing computer aids for artists. I'm suggesting that we explicitly aim for a greater merging of competence, that we explicitly recognize the cooperative approach that is possible. Karl Sims has done wonderful work in this direction (Sims 1991).

Human/computer teams at chess tournaments. We already have programs that can play better than almost all humans. But how much work has been done on how this power could be used by a human, to get something even better? If such teams were allowed in at least some chess tournaments, it could have the positive effect on IA research that allowing computers in tournaments had for the corresponding niche in AI. In the last few years, Grandmaster Garry Kasparov has developed the idea of chess matches between computer-assisted players (Google on the key phrases "kasparov" and "advanced chess"). As far as I know, such human/computer teams are not allowed to participate in more general chess tournaments.

Interfaces that allow computer and network access without requiring the human to be tied to one spot, sitting in front of a computer. (This aspect of IA fits so well with known economic advantages that lots of effort is already being spent on it.)

More symmetrical decision support systems. A popular research/product area in recent years has been decision support systems. This is a form of IA, but may be too focused on systems that are oracular. As much as the program giving the user information, there must be the idea of the user giving the program guidance.

Local area nets to make human teams more effective than their component members. This is generally the area of "groupware"; the change in viewpoint here would be to regard the group activity as a combination organism. In one sense, this suggestion's goal might be to invent a "Rules of Order" for such combination operations. For instance, group focus might be more easily maintained than in classical meetings. Individual members' expertise could be isolated from ego issues so that the contribution of different members is focused on the team project. And of course shared databases could be used much more conveniently than in conventional committee operations.

The Internet as a combination human/machine tool. Of all the items on the list, progress in this is proceeding the fastest. The power and influence of the Internet are vastly underestimated. The very anarchy of the worldwide net's development is evidence of its potential. As connectivity, bandwidth, archive size, and computer speed all increase, we are seeing something like Lynn Margulis' vision of the biosphere as data processor recapitulated, but at a million times greater speed and with millions of humanly intelligent agents (ourselves). Bruce Sterling illustrates the subtle way that such a development might come to pervade daily life in "Maneki Neko" (Sterling 1998). For a nonfiction look at the possibilities of humanity + technology as a compound creature, I recommend Gregory Stock's *Metaman* (1993). But would the result be self-aware? Or perhaps self-awareness is a necessary feature of intelligence only within a limited size range?

The above examples illustrate research that can be done within the context of contemporary computer science departments. There are other paradigms. For example, much of the work in artificial intelligence and neural nets would benefit from a closer connection with biological life.

Instead of simply trying to model and understand biological life with computers, research could be directed toward the creation of composite systems that rely on biological life for guidance, or for the features we don't understand well enough yet to implement in hardware. A longtime dream of science fiction has been direct brain-to-computer interfaces. In fact, concrete work is being done in this area:

- *Limb prosthetics* is a topic of direct commercial applicability. Nerve-to-silicon transducers can be made. This is an exciting near-term step toward direct communication.
- *Direct links into brains* seem feasible, if the bit rate is low: given human learning flexibility, the actual brain neuron targets might not have to be precisely selected. Even 100 bits per second would be of great use to stroke victims who would otherwise be confined to menu-driven interfaces.
- *Plugging into the optic trunk* has the potential for bandwidths of 1 Mbit/second or so. But for this, we need to know the fine-scale architecture of vision, and we need to place an enormous web of electrodes with exquisite precision. If we want our high-bandwidth connection to add to the paths already present in the brain, the problem becomes vastly more intractable. Just sticking a grid of high-bandwidth receivers into a brain certainly won't do it. But suppose that the high-bandwidth grid were present as the brain structure was setting up, as the embryo developed. That suggests:
- *Animal embryo experiments*. I wouldn't expect any IA success in the first years of such research, but giving developing brains access to complex simulated neural structures might, in the long run, produce animals with additional sense paths and interesting intellectual abilities.

I had hoped that this discussion of IA would yield some clearly safer approaches to the Singularity (after all, IA allows our participation in a kind of transcendence). Alas, about all I am sure of is that these proposals should be considered, that they may give us more options. But as for safety – some of the suggestions are a little scary on their face. IA for individual humans creates a rather sinister elite. We humans have millions of years of evolutionary baggage that makes us regard competition in a deadly light. Much of that deadliness may not be necessary in today's world, one where losers take on the winners' tricks and are co-opted into the winners' enterprises. A creature that was built *de novo* might possibly be a much more benign entity than one based on fang and talon.

The problem is not simply that the Singularity represents the passing of humankind from center stage, but that it contradicts our most deeply held notions of being. I think a closer look at the notion of strong superhumanity can show why that is.

IV.   Strong Superhumanity and the Best We Can Ask For

Suppose we could tailor the Singularity. Suppose we could attain our most extravagant hopes. What then would we ask for? That humans themselves would become their own successors, that whatever injustice occurred would be tempered by our knowledge of our roots. For those who remained unaltered, the goal would be benign treatment (perhaps even giving the stay-behinds the appearance of being masters of godlike slaves). It could be a golden age that also involved progress (leaping Stent's barrier). Immortality (or at least a lifetime as long as we can make the universe survive) would be achievable.

But in this brightest and kindest world, the philosophical problems themselves become intimidating. A mind that stays at the same capacity cannot live forever; after a few thousand years it would look more like a repeating tape loop than a person. (The most chilling picture I have seen of this is Larry Niven's story "The Ethics of Madness.") To live indefinitely long, the mind itself must grow ... and when it becomes great enough, and looks back ... what fellow-feeling can it have with the soul that it was originally? The later being would be everything the original was, but vastly more. And so even for the individual, the Cairns-Smith or Lynn Margulis notion of new life growing incrementally out of the old must still be valid.

This "problem" about immortality comes up in much more direct ways. The notion of ego and self-awareness has been the bedrock of the hardheaded rationalism of the last few centuries. Yet now the notion of self-awareness is under attack from the artificial intelligence people. Intelligence Amplification undercuts our concept of ego from another direction. The post-Singularity world will involve extremely high-bandwidth networking. A central feature of strongly superhuman entities will likely be their ability to communicate at variable bandwidths, including ones far higher than speech or written messages. What happens when pieces of ego can be copied and merged, when self-awareness can grow or shrink to fit the nature of the problems under consideration? These are essential features of strong superhumanity and the Singularity. Thinking about them, one begins to feel how essentially strange and different the Posthuman era will be – no matter how cleverly and benignly it is brought to be. I discuss this in slightly more detail in "Nature, Bloody in Tooth and Claw?", an essay presented at the 1996 British National Science Fiction Convention.

From one angle, the vision fits many of our happiest dreams: a time unending, where we can truly know one another and understand the deepest mysteries. From another angle, it's a lot like the worst-case scenario I imagined earlier.

In fact, I think the new era is simply too different to fit into the classical frame of good and evil. That frame is based on the idea of isolated, immutable minds connected by tenuous, low-bandwidth links. But the post-Singularity world *does* fit with the larger tradition of change and cooperation that started long ago (perhaps even before the rise of biological life). I think certain notions of ethics would apply in such an era. Research into IA and high-bandwidth communications should improve this understanding. I see just the glimmerings of this now; perhaps there are rules for distinguishing self from others on the basis of bandwidth of connection. And while mind and self will be vastly more labile than in the past, much of what we value (knowledge, memory, thought) need never be lost. I think Freeman Dyson (1988) has it right when he says, "God is what mind becomes when it has passed beyond the scale of our comprehension."

Notes

1 Good 1965. In preparing these annotations, I took a close look at this paper. In fact, Good's essay is even more insightful than the quote shown here. For instance, he speculates that an interim step to the "ultraintelligent machine" may be a symbiotic relationship between humans and machines, and proposes human/computer chess-playing teams. With regard to such chess, he even proposes shuffling initial

positions, an idea that Garry Kasparov has also discussed (see Kasparov's 1998 interview at http://www.chessclub.com/event/kaspinterview.html).

2   Searle's essay is reprinted in *The Mind's I*, edited by Douglas R. Hofstadter and Daniel C. Dennett (New York: Basic Books, 1981) (my source for this reference). This reprinting contains an excellent critique of the Searle essay.

3   More recently, Hans Moravec has presented his reasoning in *Robot* (1999).Another recent reference is Kurzweil, *The Age of Spiritual Machines* (2000).

References

Bear, Greg (1983) "Blood Music." *Analog Science Fiction-Science Fact* (June). Expanded into the novel *Blood Music* (1985). Scranton, PA: Morrow.

Cairns-Smith, Alexander G., (1985) *Seven Clues to the Origin of Life*. Cambridge: Cambridge University Press.

Drexler, K. Eric (1986) *Engines of Creation*. New York: Anchor Press/Doubleday.

Dyson, Freeman (1988) *Infinite in All Directions*. New York: Harper & Row.

Good, Irving J. (1965) "Speculations Concerning the First Ultraintelligent Machine." In Franz L. Alt and Morris Rubinoff, eds., *Advances in Computers*, vol. 6. New York: Academic Press, pp. 31–88.

Kurzweil, Ray (2000) *The Age of Spiritual Machines: When Computers Exceed Human Intelligence*. New York: Penguin USA.

Margulis, Lynn and Sagan, Dorian (1986) *Microcosmos: Four Billion Years of Evolution From Our Microbial Ancestors*. New York: Summit Books.

Minsky, Marvin (1985) *Society of Mind*. New York: Simon & Schuster.

Moravec, Hans (1988) *Mind Children*. Cambridge, MA: Harvard University Press.

Moravec, Hans (1999) *Robot: Mere Machine to Transcendent Mind*. Oxford: Oxford University Press.

Penrose, Roger (1989) *The Emperor's New Mind*. Oxford: Oxford University Press.

Searle, John R. (1980) "Minds, Brains, and Programs." In *The Behavioral and Brain Sciences*, vol. 3. Cambridge: Cambridge University Press.

Sims, Karl (1991) "Interactive Evolution of Dynamical Systems." (December). Thinking Machines Corporation, Technical Report Series. Published in *Toward a Practice of Autonomous Systems: Proceedings of the First European Conference on Artificial Life*. Paris: MIT Press.

Stent, Gunther S. (1969) *The Coming of the Golden Age: A View of the End of Progress*. Garden City, NY: The Natural History Press.

Sterling, Bruce (1998) "Maneki Neko." *The Magazine of Fantasy & Science Fiction* (May 1998).

Stock, Gregory (1993) *Metaman: The Merging of Humans and Machines into a Global Superorganism*. New York: Simon & Schuster.

Ulam, Stanislaw M. (1958) "Tribute to John von Neumann." *Bulletin of the American Mathematical Society* 64/3 (May), pp. 1–49.

Vinge, Vernor (1996) "Nature, Bloody in Tooth and Claw?": http://www-rohan.sdsu.edu/faculty/vinge/misc/evolution.html.

Further Reading

Alfvén, Hannes, writing as Olof Johanneson (1969) *The End of Man?* New York: Award Books. Earlier published as *The Tale of the Big Computer*, Coward-McCann, translated from a book copyright 1966 Albert Bonniers Forlag AB with English translation copyright 1966 by Victor Gollancz, Ltd.

Anderson, Poul (1962) "Kings Who Die." *If* (March), pp. 8–36. The earliest story I know about intelligence amplification via computer/brain linkage.

Asimov, Isaac (1942) "Runaround." *Astounding Science Fiction* (March), p. 94. Reprinted in Isaac Asimov (1990) *Robot Visions*. New York: ROC, where Asimov also describes the development of his robotics stories.

Barrow, John D. and Tipler, Frank J. (1986) *The Anthropic Cosmological Principle*. Oxford: Oxford University Press.

Conrad, Michael, et al. (1989) "Towards an Artificial Brain." *BioSystems* 23, pp. 175–218.

Dyson, Freeman (1979) "Physics and Biology in an Open Universe." *Review of Modern Physics* 51, pp. 447–460.

Herbert, Frank (1985) *Dune*. New York: Berkley Books. This novel was serialized in *Analog Science Fiction-Science Fact* in the 1960s.

Kovacs, G.T.A., et al. (1992) "Regeneration Microelectrode Array for Peripheral Nerve Recording and Stimulation." *IEEE Transactions on Biomedical Engineering* 39/9, pp. 893–902.

Niven, Larry (1967) "The Ethics of Madness." *If* (April), pp. 82–108. Reprinted in *Neutron Star*. Ballantine Books, 1968.

Rasmussen, S. et al. (1991) "Computational Connectionism within Neurons: A Model of Cytoskeletal Automata Subserving Neural Networks." In Stephanie Forrest, ed., *Emergent Computation*. Cambridge, MA: MIT Press, pp. 428–449.

Stapledon, Olaf (1961) *The Starmaker*. New York: Berkeley Books. From the date on the forward, probably written before 1937.

Swanwick, Michael (1986/7) *Vacuum Flowers*. Serialized in *Isaac Asimov's Science Fiction Magazine* (December(?) 1986–February 1987).

Thearling, Kurt (1992) "How We Will Build a Machine That Thinks." A workshop at Thinking Machines Corporation, August 24–26.

Vinge, Vernor (1966) "Bookworm, Run!" *Analog* (March), pp. 8–40. Early intelligence amplification story. The hero is the first experimental subject – a chimpanzee raised to human intelligence.

Vinge, Vernor (1981) "True Names." In *Binary Star* 5. New York: Dell.

Vinge, Vernor (1983) "First Word." *Omni* 10 (January). Earlier essay on "the Singularity."

36

An Overview of Models of Technological Singularity

Anders Sandberg

This essay reviews different definitions and models of technological singularity. The models range from conceptual sketches to detailed endogenous growth models, as well as attempts to fit empirical data to quantitative models. Such models are useful for examining the dynamics of the world-system and possible types of future crisis points where fundamental transitions are likely to occur. Current models suggest that, generically, even small increasing returns tend to produce radical growth. If mental capital becomes copyable (such as would be the case for AI or brain emulation) extremely rapid growth would also become likely.

Introduction

The set of concepts today commonly referred to as "technological singularity" has a long history in the computer science community, with early examples such as:

> One conversation centered on the ever accelerating progress of technology and changes in the mode of human life, which gives the appearance of approaching some essential singularity in the history of the race beyond which human affairs, as we know them, could not continue. (Ulam 1968)

and

> Let an ultraintelligent machine be defined as a machine that can far surpass all the intellectual activities of any man however clever. Since the design of machines is one of these intellectual activities,

This paper was presented on March 8 at the workshop "Roadmaps to AGI and the future of AGI" following the AGI10 conference in Lugano, Switzerland.

The Transhumanist Reader: Classical and Contemporary Essays on the Science, Technology, and Philosophy of the Human Future, First Edition. Edited by Max More and Natasha Vita-More.

an ultraintelligent machine could design even better machines; there would then unquestionably be an "intelligence explosion," and the intelligence of man would be left far behind. Thus the first ultraintelligent machine is the last invention that man need ever make. (Good 1965)

The unifying theme of these two examples is accelerated technological change leading to a rapid transition to a state where the current human condition would be challenged.

Technological singularity is of increasing interest among futurists both as a predicted possibility in the mid-term future and as subject for methodological debate. The concept is used in a variety of contexts, and has acquired an unfortunately large number of meanings. Some versions stress the role of artificial intelligence, others refer to more general technological change. These multiple meanings can overlap and many writers use combinations of meanings: even Vernor Vinge's seminal essay (Vinge 1993) that coined the term uses several meanings. Some of these meanings may imply each other but often there is a conflation of different elements that likely (but not necessarily) occur in parallel. This causes confusion and misunderstanding to the extent that some critics argue that the term should be avoided altogether (Tyler 2009). At the very least the term "singularity" has led to many unfortunate assumptions that technological singularity involves some form of mathematical singularity and can hence be ignored as unphysical.

This essay is attempting a simple taxonomy of models of technological singularity, hopefully helping to disambiguate the different meanings of the word. It also aims at a brief review of formal quantitative models of singularity-like phenomena, in the hope of promoting a more stringent discussion of these possibilities.

Definitions of Technological Singularity

A brief list of meanings of the term "technological singularity" found in the literature and some of their proponents:

A. [Accelerating change] Exponential or superexponential technological growth (with linked economic growth and social change) (Kurzweil 2005; Smart 2008)
B. [Self-improving technology] Better technology allows faster development of new and better technology (Flake 2006)
C. [Intelligence explosion] Smarter systems can improve themselves, producing even more intelligence in a strong feedback loop (Good 1965; Yudkowsky 2007)
D. [Emergence of superintelligence] (Singularity Institute)[1]
E. [Prediction horizon] Rapid change or the emergence of superhuman intelligence makes the future impossible to predict from our current limited knowledge and experience. (Vinge 1993)
F. [Phase transition] The singularity represents a shift to new forms of organization. This could be a fundamental difference in kind such as humanity being succeeded by posthuman or artificial intelligences, a punctuated equilibrium transition or the emergence of a new metasystem level. (Teilhard de Chardin; Turchin 1977; Heylighen 2007)
G. [Complexity disaster] Increasing complexity and interconnectedness causes increasing payoffs, but increases instability. Eventually this produces a crisis, beyond which point the dynamics must be different. (Sornette in Johansen and Sornette 2001; Geoffrey West in Bettencourt et al. 2007)

H. [Inflexion point] Large-scale growth of technology or economy follows a logistic growth curve. The singularity represents the inflexion point where change shifts from acceleration to deacceleration. (Extropy Institute's Transhumanist FAQ (1990s); Modis 2002)

I. [Infinite progress] The rate of progress in some domain goes to infinity in finite time. (Few, if any, hold this to be plausible.[2])

The three major groupings appear to be accelerating change, prediction horizon, and intelligence explosion leading to superintelligence (as originally noted by Bostrom (1998) and discussed in Yudkowsky [2007]).

In addition to the general meaning(s), the singularity might be local or global (capability takeoff of an entity or small group, or broad evolution of the whole economy), fast or slow (occurring on computer timescales, hardware development timescales, human timescales, or historical timescales). There is also confusion over whether the salient issue is the point/ event-like character, the historical uniqueness, the nature of the overall process, or the big historical trend.

For the purpose of this essay I will focus on the growth aspect: accelerating change, self-improving technology, intelligence explosions, and the complexity disaster (and to some extent the inflexion point) all involve the growth of technological or cognitive capability. The nature and speed of this growth is important both for understanding what claims are actually made and for considering the implications of such a process, if it takes place.

As noted in Heylighen 1997, models for the technological singularity, whether qualitative or quantitative, should not be taken too literally. Models include what are considered to be the important and relevant features of a system while abstracting away from minor, obscuring features. They are useful because they force us to show our assumptions, bringing them into the open. Their predictions may be less important than demonstrating how changes in assumptions affect outcomes.

Models

Linear takeover (type D,F)

Singular events can occur when one form of growth outpaces another. This form of "linear singularity" does not necessarily involve any acceleration of progress.

Eliezer Yudkowsky, has presented a simple sketch of why apparent progress of AI might be deceptive: the rate of progress is actually high, but starts from a very low level. This means that the rapid development is not easily detectable, until it suddenly passes the relatively narrow human range and goes beyond.[3]

A simple formalization of the model would be that human intelligence X is constant while machine intelligence $Y(t)=a+bt$ grows linearly with time. At present $X \gg Y(t)$. We are less sensitive to differences in less-than-human intelligence than to differences in human-level intelligence; our subjective experience of intelligence (and possibly its ability to affect the world) is a rapidly concave function, for example an exponential curve. The apparent intelligence of machines would be growing as e^{a+bt}, with a "surprising" eventual jump from an apparently unchanging low state to rapid growth near and beyond human level. This is essentially the same claim made by Kurzweil in regards to how most people do not understand exponential growth, although the growth here may not be nonlinear (only its detectability is).

Logistic growth (type H)

It is commonly argued that exponential growth is unsustainable, since it requires resources that will eventually run out. This is true even if space colonization is available, since the volume of space that can be reached in time t grows at most as $4\pi\frac{c^3t^3}{3}\alpha t^3$, where c is lightspeed. This means that eventually the growth rate will have to decline to at most a polynomial growth rate.

However, if the growth is in the domain of knowledge, culture, or pure value it is less obvious that there exists an upper limit or that the growth is strongly resource-constrained. There are some physical limits on how much information can be stored within a region of the universe but these are very wide; at most they preclude infinite information storage[4].

There could exist limiting factors to technology based on the (possible) finite complexity of the universe: there would only exist a finite amount of useful facts about nature that can be discovered. As more and more become known the difficulty of finding new ones increases. This would be compatible with a logistic growth equation:

$$X'(t) = r(K - X(t))X(t)$$

where $X(t)$ is knowledge, r is a growth rate and K is the upper threshold of what is knowable. Initially $X(t)$ grows exponentially, but eventually saturates and slows down, asymptotically approaching K. Other forms of value might still grow after saturation, but the knowledge will remain bounded.

In this case the singularity would likely denote the inflexion point, the (historically very brief) transition from a pre-technological state to a maximally advanced state.

Metasystem transition (type F)

A metasystem transition is the evolutionary emergence of a higher level of organization or control in a system (Turchin 1977). A number of systems become integrated into a higher-order system, producing a multi-level hierarchy of control. Within biology such evolutionary transitions have occurred through the evolution of self-replication, multicellularity, sexual reproduction, societies, etc., where smaller subsystems merge without losing differentiation yet often become dependent on the larger entity (Smith and Szathmáry 1995). At the beginning of the process the control mechanism is rudimentary, mainly coordinating the subsystems. As the whole system develops further the subsystems specialize and the control systems become more effective. While metasystem transitions in biology are seen as caused by biological evolution, other systems might exhibit other forms of evolution (e.g. social change or deliberate organization) to cause metasystem transitions. Extrapolated to humans, future transitions might involve parts or the whole of the human species becoming a super-organism (Turchin and Joslyn 1989).

As a model for technological singularity the metasystem transition is largely qualitative rather than quantitative. Without a detailed model of the subsystem dynamics the transition is undefined. However, the biological and social examples given by theorists, would give some analogical data on how future transitions could work (e.g. as punctuated equilibrium models). A key issue worth exploring may be to what degree such transitions are convergent or divergent, e.g. whether under similar circumstances the transitions would produce similar or different forms of organization.[5]

Accelerated metasystem transition (type A,B,F)

Heylighen (2007) argues that the evolutionary forces acting on technology (and other systems) tend to lead to ephemeralization, doing more with less, due to selective pressures in any resource-constrained environment. This produces increasing efficiency in the use, processing, and transport of matter, energy, and information, reducing "friction" and enabling longer controllable causal chains. Similarly innovations in institutions, mediators, and stigmergy (indirect influences on other agents through this environment, "the medium") produces increasingly global coordination. He argues that stigmergy accelerates evolution, since already found solutions spread to other agents: improvement of the medium facilitates further innovation, which helps improve and spread the medium. He compares this to the population growth model of Korotayev (2007) where the population N is controlled by a logistic growth equation where the carrying capacity is proportional to the overall productivity T of technology:

$$N'(f) = a(bT - N)N$$

Technology grows proportional to population and technology:

$$T'(t) = cNT$$

This produces a hyperbolic growth curve with a finite time singularity. Heylighen notes that the deviation in population growth from hyperbolic growth in the 1970s is still compatible with the general model if we interpret it as a shift from an r-strategy (fast reproduction, short life) to a K-strategy (slow reproduction, long life). In a K-strategy more human capital is invested in the offspring, and they will provide more back, making the T factor of the second equation more important than the N factor. He predicts that the above trends will lead to the formation of a global superorganism of some kind over a relatively short timespan.

Accelerating Change

Economic input-output models (type A)

Input-output models depict the economy as A, a matrix denoting the number of units a sector of the economy needs to buy from another sector to produce a unit of its own output, and B, a matrix of how many units from other industries are needed for the production itself (e.g. equipment, buildings, etc.). If the output levels of different sectors at time t are $X(t)$ the amount of goods delivered to households and other final users will be (Leontief 1986):

$$Y(t) = X(t) - AX(t) - B[X(t+1) - X(t)]$$

If all the outputs are reinvested into the economy $Y(t) = 0$ and the equation produces a dynamical system:

$$X(t+1) = [B^{-1}(1 - A - B)]X(t)$$

The growth will be exponential, with a rate set by the largest eigenvalue of the bracketed matrix and a production vector X tending towards the eigenvector corresponding to the value. If the consumption $Y(t)$ is nonzero the generic case is still exponential growth: matrix recurrences of the form $X(t+1) = CX(t) + d$ or differential equations like $X'(t) = CX(t) + d$ have solutions tending towards $\Lambda e^{\lambda t}$ if C is diagonalizable.

Endogenous growth models (type A,B,I)

Endogenous growth theory models the growth of an economy with improving technology, where the technology is assumed to be growing as a function of the economy and allocation of resources to it. It was developed as a response to exogenous growth models, where diminishing returns predict that growth would stop rather than continue.

> while the part which nature plays in production shows a tendency to diminishing return, the part which man plays shows a tendency to increasing return. The law of increasing return may be worded thus:—An increase of labour and capital leads generally to improved organization, which increases the efficiency of the work of labour and capital. (Marshall 1920)

However, published models usually appear to try to avoid "unrealistic" explosive growth, by selecting equations for the growth of knowledge that preclude it. For example, (Hakenes and Irmen 2004) amend their model not only to avoid negative knowledge but also to preclude superexponential growth. In a later paper they state:

> We take the view that a plausible description of the evolution of knowledge should satisfy two asymptotic conditions. Looking forwards, we follow Solow (2000) in maintaining that infinite knowledge in finite time is impossible. Looking backwards, we require knowledge to vanish in the infinite past, but not in finite time. We call an evolution plausible if it satisfies these criteria. (Hakenes and Irmen 2007)

This paper shows that for knowledge growth

$$X'(t) = gX(t)^\phi \qquad \qquad *$$

knowledge is either zero at all times, or increasing over time. In the latter case if $\phi < 1$ the knowledge starts from zero in the finite past, if $\phi > 1$ knowledge diverges to infinity in the finite future, or if $\phi = 1$ knowledge is always finite and grows exponentially without any singularities. It hence concludes that only the exponential case is possible. Adding (endogenous or exogenous) population growth does not help in the generic case.

However, a simple model predicting a finite-time singularity might still be relevant if other, unmodeled, factors near the potential singularity prevent it from actually occurring. The assumption that a model must hold for an infinite timespan (especially when it is a highly abstracted model of a complex process) seems unwarranted. Models exhibiting finite-time singularities can be a quantitatively or qualitatively accurate fit to current or near-future growth, although they eventually leaves the domain of applicability.

As noted in (Johansen and Sornette 2001):

> Singularities are always mathematical idealisations of natural phenomena: they are not present in reality but foreshadow an important transition or change of regime. In the present context, they must be interpreted as a kind of "critical point" signaling a fundamental and abrupt change of regime similar to what occurs in phase transitions.

The observation that finite-time singularities are generic when economies of scale in knowledge production exist ($\phi > 1$) seems to support further study of superexponential growth, and cast doubt on the assumption that knowledge growth should always be modeled as exponential.

A widely quoted growth model exhibiting finite-time singularity is the model of Kremer (1993): the total population is $L(t)$ and total economic output $Y(t)$, and their ratio $Y(t)/L(t) = \bar{y}$ is set to a subsistence level $\bar{y}$ which is fixed. Output depends on technology/knowledge $A(t)$ and labor proportional to $L(t)$: $Y(t) = Y_0[A(t)L(t)]^{1-\alpha}$ where $0 < \alpha < 1$. The growth rate of technology is assumed proportional to population and technology level:

$$A'(t) = BL(t)A(t)$$

with the explicit assumptions that larger populations have more talented people that can advance technology and that new technology largely is obtained by leveraging existing technology (hence, it implies a type B singularity). Combining the two equations produces

$$L'(t) = \left[\frac{B(1-\alpha)}{\alpha}\right]L(t)^2$$

Hence the population (and technology) has a finite time singularity.

Saleur and Sornette (1996) further discuss multivariate extensions of the model with capital $K(t)$ producing output

$$Y(t) = \left[(1-a_K)K(t)\right]^\alpha \left[A(t)(1-a_L)L(t)\right]^{\{1-\alpha\}}$$

where a_K is the fraction of capital stock used in R&D, a_L the fraction of labor used in R&D. Innovation is produced as

$$A'(t) = B\left[a_K K(t)\right]^\beta \left[a_L L(t)\right]^\gamma \left[A(t)\right]^\theta$$

for positive constants B, β and γ. Assuming exogenous saving rate s and no depreciation gives

$$K'(t) = sY(t) = s\left[(1-a_K)K(t)\right]^\alpha \left[A(t)(1-a_L)L(t)\right]^{\{1-\alpha\}}$$

This system can achieve finite time singularities even for fixed population if $\theta + \beta > 1$. Past innovation and capital can create explosive growth even when each of the factors in isolation cannot.

Population-technology model (type A,F,I)

A population theoretic model similar to endogenous growth was formulated by Taagepera (1979). It links the population P with technology T and nonrenewable resources R via a modified logistic growth model:

$$P'(t) = k_0\left[1 - e^{\{-aT^n\}}\right]\left[1 - \frac{\{(R+C)P\}}{\{fT^{qR}\}}\right]P$$

where the first factor represents growth rate (increased by technology towards a maximal rate k_0). Technology increases as a power of population size for small populations and independent of it at large sizes:

$$T'(t) = h \left[\frac{P}{\{U+P\}} \right]^{mT}$$

where U is a characteristic population size. The rate of depletion of resources was either modeled with a complete recycling model, where advanced societies can recycle most material

$$R'(t) = -\frac{fVTP}{\{(V+T)^2\}}$$

where V is the critical technology level where resource depletion levels out. The other possibility was merely a stabilization of per capita depletion rate

$$R'(t) = -\frac{fTP}{\{V+T\}}$$

For the initial state $P \ll U$, $T \ll V$, $T^n \ll 1/a$ and $R \gg C$ and the equations produce hyperbolic growth. Depending on whether the first, the middle two or the last inequalities change sign first there are three outcomes. The first case, resource depletion, produces an eventual saturation population with a likely eventual decrease. In the middle case recycling or per capita stabilization becomes significant before population is large and resources have run out, and hyperbolic growth continues until one of the other cases occurs. If the population becomes large but there are still resources population growth is doubly exponential.

Taagepera notes that the model, while avoiding finite time singularities, still has crises where it shifts from one mode to another, possibly over very short periods of time.

Law of accelerating returns (type A,B)

Ray Kurzweil formulates the "law of accelerating returns" as (Kurzweil 2001):

- Evolution applies positive feedback in that the more capable methods resulting from one stage of evolutionary progress are used to create the next stage. As a result, the rate of progress of an evolutionary process increases exponentially over time. Over time, the "order" of the information embedded in the evolutionary process (i.e., the measure of how well the information fits a purpose, which in evolution is survival) increases.
- A correlate of the above observation is that the "returns" of an evolutionary process (e.g., the speed, cost-effectiveness, or overall "power" of a process) increase exponentially over time.
- In another positive feedback loop, as a particular evolutionary process (e.g., computation) becomes more effective (e.g., cost effective), greater resources are deployed toward the further progress of that process. This results in a second level of exponential growth (i.e., the rate of exponential growth itself grows exponentially).
- Biological evolution is one such evolutionary process.
- Technological evolution is another such evolutionary process. Indeed, the emergence of the first technology creating species resulted in the new evolutionary process of technology. Therefore, technological evolution is an outgrowth of – and a continuation of – biological evolution.

- A specific paradigm (a method or approach to solving a problem, e.g., shrinking transistors on an integrated circuit as an approach to making more powerful computers) provides exponential growth until the method exhausts its potential. When this happens, a paradigm shift (i.e., a fundamental change in the approach) occurs, which enables exponential growth to continue.

Kurzweil models the growth as composed of a velocity of technology growth $V(t) = c_1 W(t)$ driven by and driving the total world knowledge $W'(t) = c_2 V(t)$ (where c_1 and c_2 are constants). This has an exponential solution with growth rate $c_1 c_2$. He then assumes that there are exponentially increasing resources for computation $N(t) = c_3^{\{c_4 t\}}$ and that world knowledge grows proportional to the product of $V(t)$ and $N(t)$: $W'(t) = c_1 V(t) N(t) = c_1 c_2 c_3^{\{c_4 t\}} W(t)$ which has a double exponential solution of the form $W(t) \propto e^{\left(C t^2\right)}$.

It is not clear why the exogenous computational resources $N(t)$ are not increasing proportional to $W(t)$, for example if the economy and population providing them were positively influenced by knowledge growth, rather than just growing by a steady exponential. If there were any positive feedback with $W(t)$ the equations would show essentially the same behavior as equation * and have a finite time singularity.

Vinge/Moravec model (type A,B,I)

The original singularity essay by Vinge (1993) does not describe any quantitative model. It says:

> When greater-than-human intelligence drives progress, that progress will be much more rapid. In fact, there seems no reason why progress itself would not involve the creation of still more intelligent entities – on a still shorter time scale. The best analogy that I see is with the evolutionary past: Animals can adapt to problems and make inventions, but often no faster than natural selection can do its work – the world acts as its own simulator in the case of natural selection. We humans have the ability to internalize the world and conduct "what if's" in our heads; we can solve many problems thousands of times faster than natural selection.
>
> Now, by creating the means to execute those simulations at much higher speeds, we are entering a regime as radically different from our human past as we humans are from the lower animals.

This is a restatement of the intelligence explosion model of Good (1965). Vinge also argues that current technological progress (especially in computing) is influenced by automation of design, producing strong incentives to further automate it. This leads to a strong feedback where either AI, intelligence amplification, or distributed intelligence produces an intelligence explosion. A formalization of this would be to model technological improvement as an exponential process, where new technology reduces the doubling time. However, whether this produces a finite time singularity or merely accelerating growth depends on the exact functional form.

Hans Moravec explored a model based on Vinge (Moravec 1999, 2003). He initially assumed that "world knowledge" $X(t)$ produces an exponential speedup of computer performance $V(t) = e^{\{X(t)\}}$. In the case of a constant number of humans working unassisted the growth of knowledge would be linear, $X'(t) = 1$, producing $X(t) = t$ and $V(t) = e^t$ (standard Moore's law).

If knowledge growth is instead driven directly by computers $X'(t) = V(t) = e^{\{X(t)\}}$, producing the solution $X(t) = \log(-1/t) (t < 0)$. This corresponds to a slow growth reaching a singularity. A further model added computer power to human power, giving $X(t) = \log(1/(e^{\{-t\}} - 1))$ which has linear growth for $t \gg 0$, becomes roughly exponential near $t = -1$ and has a singularity at $t = 0$.

Observing that $V(t)=e^{\{X(t)\}}$ was likely far too optimistic he then went on to show a variety of models where $V(t)$ was a concave increasing function of $X(t)$ produce finite time singularities. These results are substantially the same as the observation about equation *. Slightly superlinear growth, e.g. $X'(t)=(1+log(X(t)))X(t)$, merely produces fast double exponential growth, $X(t)=exp(e^t-1)$, but squared logarithmic growth $(X'(t)=(1+log^2(X(t)))X(t))$ gives rise to a true singularity $(X(t)=exp(tan(t)))$. In fact, if the logarithm has exponent >1 there is an eventual mathematical singularity.

In a subsequent discussion between Moravec, Kurzweil, and Vinge (1999) Kurzweil noted:

> My sense is that it is difficult to justify on theoretical grounds having the rate of increase of knowledge be equal to the "size" of knowledge raised to a power greater than 1.
>
> However, I do think it is feasible to justify separate components of growth, some (or one) of which have an exponent of one, and some (or one) of which have a log exponent. The analysis above points to a log exponent. I believe we can justify that the "value" of a typical network or of a database does not expand proportional to its size, but to the log of its size. For example, the value of the Internet to me does not double if the number of users doubles. Rather, its value to me increases in a logarithmic fashion. The exponent of 1 comes from the number of users themselves. Having twice as many users means it is serving twice as many people. So the overall value of the network = $n \log n$ (n people served times the value of the network to each person = $log\, n$). This varies from Metcalfe's formula that the value of a network = n^2.

He suggested that empirical data might be enough to justify a double exponential, but found the unlikelihood of infinite information strong enough to tentatively rule out faster increments.

Solomonoff (type A,B,I)

Ray J. Solomonoff presented a model of progress in AI based on the idea that once a machine is built that has general problem-solving capacity near that of a human in an area such as industry or science such machines will be used for in those areas, speeding up technological progress. This would eventually lead to construction of machines with capacities near or beyond the original computer science community (Solomonoff 1985). In particular, he notes that the key factor is that machine intelligence will eventually become cheaper than human intelligence, and that high initial training costs can be offset by copying already trained machines.

His formal model consists of the growth of the effective computer science community (humans plus AI, humans assumed to be constant) $C(t)$ as

$$C'(t) = Rx(t)$$

where R is the rate of money spent on AI and $x(t)$ is the amount of computing power per dollar. $x(t)$ is assumed to grow exponentially with a doubling time inversely proportional to the size of the computer science community:

$$\left(log(x(t))\right)' = AC(t)$$

where A is a constant. Combining equations and assuming $c=x=1$ at $t=0$ produces

$$C'(t) = A(C(t)^2 - 1)/2 + R$$

which has a finite time singularity for some t. Assuming a doubling time of x every four years produces $A = \dfrac{log(2)}{4} \approx 0.1733$; with $R=1$ the singularity occurs in 4.62 years, for $R=0.1$ in 11.11 years and $R=0.01$ in 21.51 years.

The model implicitly sets $t=0$ at the point where the milestone of near-human intelligence is reached; before this, computers are not assumed to expand the effective computer science community very much. It is hence a model of just a particular technological community rather than general technological growth, although it is plausible that the rapid increase of $x(t)$ will influence society profoundly.

Hamacher (type E)

Hamacher commented on the Moravec/Vinge/Kurzweil model, noting that its macroeconomic coarseness ignored issues of coordination problems, competition, resource allocation, and sociological issues. Instead he introduced a cobweb-model of price determination, where supply and demand iteratively determine quantity and price of a product. If $S(q)$ is the supply and $D(q)$ the demand at quantity q, the available price p_t and quantity q_t are updated iteratively

$$p_{\{t+1\}} = D(q)$$

$$q_{\{t+1\}} = S^{-1}\left(p_{\{t+1\}}\right)$$

Such models have a rich dynamics corresponding to iterated 1-dimensional maps, including stable fixed points, limit cycles, and chaotic attractors depending on the choice of $S(q)$ and $D(q)$. In particular the entropy or Lyapunov exponent of the time series q_t produces a prediction horizon: initial uncertainties about the system state grow exponentially at a rate set by these values. As parameters are varied to mimic substitution dynamics the probability of encountering a prediction horizon increases (Hammacher 2006).

City economics (type A,G)

Bettencourt et al. (2007) analyzed the economies of scale of cities, showing that many quantities reflecting wealth creation and innovation scale with population with an exponent $\beta>1$, implying increasing returns. Infrastructure quantities on the other hand scale with $\beta<1$, showing economies of scale. A larger city will hence produce more per capita but have lower maintenance costs per capita. This is in direct contrast to biological organisms, where the "economy" (heart rate, metabolism, pace of life) decreases with size.

The authors suggested an urban growth equation. Growth is constrained by the availability of resources and their rate of consumption. The resources Y are used both for maintaining the existing infrastructure (at a cost of R per unit time and unit of infrastructure) and to expand it (at a cost of E to get one unit). The allocation can be expressed as $Y=RX(t)+EX'(t)$ where $X'(t)$ is the growth rate of the city. The total growth is

$$X'(t)=\left(\frac{Y_0}{E}\right)X(t)^{\beta}-\left(\frac{R}{E}\right)X(t)$$

which has solution ($\beta \neq 1$; for $\beta=1$ the solution is exponential):

$$X(t) = \left[\frac{Y_0}{R} + \left(X(0)^{\{1-\beta\}} - \frac{Y_0}{R} \right) e^{\left\{ -\frac{R(1-\beta)t}{E} \right\}} \right]^{\left\{ \frac{1}{1-\beta} \right\}}$$

For $\beta < 1$ growth is eventually limited and approaches an asymptotic level, very similar to biological growth. For $\beta > 1$ growth becomes superexponential and eventually reaches a finite time singularity if there are enough resources.

However, the authors do not consider this singularity to be reachable. They argue that eventually there is a transition to a resource-limited state and instead the growth reverses and eventually collapses. In order to avoid this crisis the system must "innovate, changing the constraining resource limits to allow further growth. By repeating this in multiple cycles collapse can be postponed. The model predicts that the time between cycles decreases as $1/X(0)^{\{\beta-1\}}$ where $X(0)$ is the size at the start of a cycle. This produces superexponential average growth as long as sufficiently strong new innovations can be supplied at an ever-accelerating rate – until a finite time singularity is reached.

While the model describes cities, the general structure seems applicable to economic systems with increasing returns.

Hanson (type A)

Robin Hanson has examined the economics of technological singularity using standard economic tools.

He analyzed a simple model of investment in the context of technological singularity (Hanson 1998a). He found that the curve of supply of capital has two distinct parts, producing two modes of economic growth. In the normal slow growth mode rates of return are limited by human discount rates. In the fast mode investment is limited by the total amount of wealth – the returns are so great that the savings rate become very high. As technology develops the demand for capital slowly increases, nudging the system towards the fast mode (which, given past growth of savings rate, might occur somewhere "near the year 2150"). However, this mode requires fine-tuning the savings rate and the fraction of investment return.

In most senses of technological singularity the amount of available "mental capital" (humans or machines able to do skilled work) increases significantly. Hanson models this in an exogenous growth model that examines economic growth given machine intelligence (Hanson 1998c). As machines become more capable they no longer just complement human labor (which tends to increase the demand for skilled labor) but can substitute for it. In the model, human-substituting machines have a falling price, but originally computer investments only buy non-intelligent complementary computers since the price of AI is too high. As the price falls AI starts to replace humans, and human wages will fall along with the computer price.

Introducing machine intelligence makes annual growth rate at least an order of magnitude larger than the current growth rate, with doubling times measured in months rather than years. Partially this is due to the assumption that computer/AI technology grows faster than other technology, partially because machines can be manufactured to meet production demands while humans have to grow up. This also produces a very fast increase in the population of intelligences, which may rapidly reach Malthusian resource limits: Hanson predicts that per-intelligence consumption will tend to fall. Whether this would lead to increasing per-capita income for humans depends on whether they retain a constant fraction of capital.

Model variations such as endogenous growth, changing work hours, a continuum of job types where some are more suitable for humans than others, and distinguishing human capital, hardware, and software from other capital do not change the essential conclusions.

Hanson found that the transition from a human-dominated to a machine-dominated economy could be fast (on the order of a few years, assuming Moore's law-like computer cost development). This model is essentially an economic model of a "linear takeover" where AI passes the human intelligence (or economic efficiency) range. It does not assume technological progress to speed up as the economy grows faster, which, if included, would speed up the transition.

Similar economic effects appear likely to occur if brain emulations (simulations of human brains with sufficient resolution to produce human-equivalent behavior and problem-solving [Sandberg and Bostrom 2008]) could be created (Hanson 1994, 2008b). The presence of copyable human capital leads to a software population explosion limited by the cost and availability of the hardware necessary to run the emulations, producing a high growth rate but diminishing individual wages.

Empirical estimates

Empirical estimates of technological singularity consist of attempts to collate historical (sometimes even paleontological and cosmological) data to estimate whether the "rate of change" is increasing exponentially or superexponentially. This presupposes that the singularity is due to an ongoing, large-scale process in the present or earlier. Intelligence explosion and prediction horizon models can likely not be supported or disputed using this kind of data.

Technological growth (type A,B,H)

There is a sizeable literature on the exponential growth of scientific resources and output, as well as growth within many technological fields. Similarly there exist various forecasts of imminent ends of progress, either due to resource depletion or more subtle issues.

Rescher's law states that the cumulative output of first-rate findings in science is proportional to the logarithm of how much has been investment, producing merely linear returns as investment grows exponentially (second-rate findings, on the other hand, may grow proportionally to investment and do not necessarily have negligible utility) (Wagner-Döbler 2001).

On the other hand, Meyer and Vallee argued that technological growth in many domains (such as power, manufacturing, speed, typesetting, etc.) has been superexponential, likely hyperbolic and composed of smaller logistic growth curves for individual technologies. Since the authors did not assume infinite growth to be feasible, they predicted that the shift from hyperbolic growth to some other regimen would either be through some form of "soft regulation" or a catastrophe (Meyer and Vallee 1975).

Population (type A,G,I)

Various authors have fitted human population to a hyperbolic growth curve $(t) = C/(T-t)$, where population reaches infinity at some time T. This was claimed to be a good empirical fit (von Foerster et al. 1960; Taagepera 1979; Johansen and Sornette 2001; Korotayev 2007), but since 1970 the observed population no longer fits the growth curve. Kapitza (2006) argues that the model is still essentially valid (growth is driven by the square of population) but can be extended and the singularity removed by taking into account finite human reproduction; the changed model instead predicts the year 2000 as the inflexion point of global population growth.

Kremer tested the prediction of his economic growth model, finding that population growth rate historically has been proportional to population. Since the number of technological innovations (which increase the maximum possible population) is assumed to be proportional to population this would give some evidence for hyperexponential growth (Kremer 1993).

Sequence of economic growth modes (type A,F,H)

Robin Hanson examined long-term growth of the human economy (Hanson 1998b), based on empirical estimations of the past world product. He found that the world product time series over the last two million years could be fit well with a small number of exponential growth modes. One interpretation was as a sum of four exponentials added together,[6] but a better fit (with the same number of parameters) was a model with constant elasticity of substitution between three exponential growth modes. These modes appear to correspond to the hunting, farming, and industrial eras, and had doubling times of 224,000, 909 and 6.3 years. There might also be some evidence for an earlier mode based on brain evolution.

During each time period the economy tends to be dominated by only one mode, and the rate of growth is roughly constant.[7] Between these modes a rapid (faster than the typical doubling time of the previous mode) shift occurs to a mode with a growth rate about two orders of magnitude larger. This is driven by the appearance of new technologies that change the structure and scale of the economy (Hanson 2008).

Given the past appearance of such new modes Hanson proposed that a new mode might occur in the relatively near future. If the number of doubling times during a mode is roughly constant this would place the transition somewhere during the twenty-first century.

This model involves type A, F, and H singularities. Technically, it does not involve any logistic limitation on growth, but rather a logistic-like limitation of increase of growth rate within each mode. It is also unique in predicting multiple past singularities (in the sense of type F radical phase transitions).

Sornette (type A,F,G)

Johansen and Sornette (2001) fit power laws of the form $(T-t)^\beta$ to world population, GDP, and financial data. β is allowed to be complex, implying not only a superexponential growth as time T is approached (due to the real part of the exponent) but also increasingly faster oscillations (due to the imaginary part). The use of this form is motivated with analogy with physics, for example cascades of Rayleigh-Taylor instabilities, black hole formation, phase separation, and material failure, which all show log-periodic oscillations before the final singularity. Theoretically this has been motivated by considerations of discrete scale invariance and complex critical exponents in non-unitary field theories (Saleur and Sornette 1996). Their conclusion is:

> The main message of this study is that, whatever the answer and irrespective of one's optimistic or pessimistic view of the world sustainability, these important pieces of data all point to the existence of an end to the present era, which will be irreversible and cannot be overcome by any novel innovation of the preceding kind, e.g., a new technology that makes the final conquest of the Oceans and

the vast mineral resources there possible. This, since any new innovation is deeply embedded in the very existence of a singularity, in fact it feeds it. As a result, a future transition of mankind towards a qualitatively new level is quite possible.

Paradigm shifts (type A,F)

Various more or less empirical attempts to predict the rate of paradigm shifts have been made. The level of evidence and modeling is variable. Some examples:

Gerald S. Hawkins proposed the "mindstep equation"

$$M_n = -30,629 + 98,048\left(\frac{1}{4} + \frac{1}{4^2} + \frac{1}{4^3} + \dots + \frac{1}{4^n}\right)$$

for the years where a "mindstep" (a fundamental human paradigm shift) would occur. It converges towards 2053, and is based on 5(!) data points (Hawkins 2002).

Nottale et al. have argued that the main economic crises of Western civilization show a log-periodic accelerating law with a finite time singularity around 2080 (Nottale et al. 2001).

Theodore Modis collected a number of evolutionary turning points from a variety of sources, estimating their "complexity jumps" (based on the assumption that the change in complexity would be inversely proportional to the distance to the next) (Modis 2002). He found that the best fit to complexity growth was a large-scale logistic curve, placing the present about halfway through the history of the universe. Ray Kurzweil re-plotted the same data and concluded that the paradigm shift rate is doubling every decade, producing an extremely rapid rate of acceleration (Kurzweil 2001). This led to a spirited response critiquing the independence of the data, Kurzweil's methodology, and the general assumption of accelerating technological growth (Modis 2006).

D.J. LePoire attempted to estimate the progress of physics by assigning events to different subfields (e.g. optics, wave theory, quantum mechanics, etc.) and plotting curves of the fraction of results in the subfield that has been completed at a certain time; these were roughly logistic. Using their median times, the assumption that physics progress overall follows a logistic curve and that some subfields form natural "stages" produced a fit with center on 1925 (LePoire 2005). His model suggests that the singularity is already past, at least in physics (a strong type H claim).

Rober Aunger has argued that thermodynamics represents a key factor in changing the organization of systems across history, and focused on the emergence of new mechanisms of control of energy flow within systems. Using a dataset of candidates he found an increasing trend of energy flow density and a power law decrease of gap length between transitions. Although he predicted the next transition to start near 2010 and to last 20–25 years, he argued that there has been a plateau in transition lengths for the last century that would preclude a technological singularity (Aunger 2007).[8]

Discussion

Generically, mathematical models that exhibit growth tend to exhibit at least exponential growth since this is the signature of linear self-coupling terms. If there exist efficiencies of scale introducing nonlinearities superexponential growth or finite time singularities appear to be generic.

Hence it is unsurprising that there is a plethora of models producing rapid or singular growth. The real issue is whether models with a strong mapping to reality can exhibit such phenomena.

It should also be stressed that even if a model admits mathematical singularities its applicability or plausibility may not diminish. Consider Newtonian and Einsteinian gravity, where mathematical singularities occur, yet merely indicate the limits of the applicability of the theory. Mathematical singularities in a growth model are likely indicators for transitions to other domains of growth or that other, unmodeled factors will become relevant close to the point. The plausibility (but obviously not the applicability) of a model is more dependent on its fit to non-singular dynamics in the past and present than its potential misbehavior in the future.

Empirical fits based on "paradigm shifts" or other discrete events suffer from limited data as well as biasing memory effects – we have more available data for recent times, and events close to us may appear more dramatic. It is also easy to cherry-pick data points consciously or unconsciously, fitting expectations (Schmidhuber 2006). In addition there is a risk of biased model selection: people inclined to believe in a singularity of a particular type are more likely to attempt to fit models with that kind of behavior than people resistant to the idea.

Population models may be less biased but do not necessarily track the technological factors of interest directly and are obviously limited by biological limitations. Still, the intersection between population modeling, empirical studies of technological and economic growth, and growth models appears to afford much empirically constrained modeling. The fact that long-term (at least) exponential growth can occur and that many not too implausible endogenous growth models can produce radical growth appears to support some forms of the singularity concept.

A common criticism is that technological singularity assumes technological determinism. This appears untrue: several if not all of the singularity concepts in the introduction could apply even if technology just exhibited trends driven by non-deterministic (but not completely random) microlevel decisions. After all, population models are not criticized as being "biologically deterministic" if they do not model microscale dynamics – ignoring contingency and statistical spread are merely part of the normal modeling process, and further models may if needed include such subtle details. Future models of technological singularity may very well include the multiform microscale or cultural details that shape large-scale progress, but understanding the major structure of the phenomenon needs to start with simple and robust models where the impact of different assumptions is laid bare. It might turn out that technological progress has sufficient degrees of freedom to deviate from any simple model in unpredictable ways, but past trends appear to suggest that large-scale technological trends often are stable.

The most solid finding given the above models and fits is that even small increasing returns in a growth model (be it a model of economics, information, or system size) can produce radical growth. Hence identifying feedback loops with increasing returns may be a way of detecting emerging type A singularities.

Endogenous growth models and Robin Hanson's models also strongly support the conclusion that if mental capital (embodied in humans, artificial intelligence or posthumans) becomes relatively cheaply copyable, extremely rapid growth is likely to follow. Hence observing progress towards artificial intelligence, brain emulation, or other ways of increasing human capital might provide evidence for or against type A singularities.

There is a notable lack of models of how an intelligence explosion could occur. This might be the most important and hardest problem to crack in the domain of singularity studies. Most important since the emergence of superintelligence has the greatest potential of being fundamentally game-changing for humanity (for good or ill). Hardest, since it appears to require an understanding of the general nature of super-human minds or at least a way to bound their capacities and growth rates.

The dearth of models of future predictability is less surprising: available evidence shows that human experts are usually weak at long-term forecasting even without singularities.

Notes

I would like to thank Nick Bostrom, Toby Ord, Stuart Armstrong, Carl Schulman and Roko Mijic for useful comments and additions.

1   "The Singularity Is the Technological Creation of Smarter-than-Human Intelligence," http://singinst. org/overview/whatisthesingularity.
2   The exception may be the Omega Point theory of Frank J. Tipler, which predicts an infinite information state reached at the future time-like singularity of a collapsing universe. However, while this (physical) singularity is reached in finite proper time, it is not reached in finite subjective time and there is literally no "after" (Barrow and Tipler 1986).
3   "The best answer to the question, "Will computers ever be as smart as humans?" is probably "Yes, but only briefly" (Vinge 2008). Samuel Butler made a somewhat similar point in his article "Darwin among the Machines," *The Press*, Christchurch, 13 June 1863, and novel *Erewhon* (1872).
4   The Bekenstein bound on the entropy to energy ratio of a system with radius R and total energy E constrains the information stored inside to be less than $2\pi RE/hcln(2)$. For a 1 kg, 1 meter system the bound is on the order of 10^{43} bits (Bekenstein 1981).
5   This is one of the concerns of the theory in (Smart 2008).
6   A hyperbolic fit produced a worse result.
7   This contradicts the claim that innovation and growth have been accelerating recently.
8   Eric Chaisson makes a similar claim over the past for the rise in free energy rate density (Joules of free energy processed per second per kilogram of matter) (Chaisson 1998). However, his data on free energy rate does not seem to suggest a curve steadily convergent to a near-future singularity, just a universal trend towards higher rates over time where human technology has increased the slope significantly.

References

Aunger, Robert (2007) "A Rigorous Periodization of 'Big' History." *Technological Forecasting and Social Change* 74, pp. 1164–1178.

Bekenstein, Jacob D. (1981) "Universal Upper Bound on the Entropy-to-Energy Ratio for Bounded Systems." *Phys. Rev. D* 23/2 (January), pp. 287–298.

Bettencourt, Luís M.A., Lobo, José, Helbing, Dirk, Kühnert, Christian, and West, Geoffrey B. (2007) "Growth, Innovation, Scaling, and the Pace of Life in Cities." *Proceedings of the National Academy of Sciences* 104/17 (April), pp. 7301–7306.

Bostrom, Nick (1998) "Singularity and Predictability." http://hanson.gmu.edu/vc.html#bostrom.

Barrow, J.D. and Tipler, F.J. (1986) *The Anthropic Cosmological Principle*. Oxford: Oxford University Press.

Chaisson, Eric J. (1998) "The Cosmic Environment for the Growth of Complexity." *Biosystems* 46/1–2, pp. 13–19.

Flake, Gary William (2006) "How I Learned to Stop Worrying and Love the Imminent Internet Singularity." *Proceedings of the 15th ACM International Conference on Information and Knowledge Management*, Arlington, VA, p. 2.

Good, I.J. (1965) "Speculations Concerning the First Ultraintelligent Machine." *Advances in Computers* 6.

Hakenes, Hendrik, and Irmen, Andreas (2004) "Airy Growth: Was the Take-Off Inevitable?" http://www. socialpolitik.org/tagungshps/2004/Papers/Irmen.pdf.

Hakenes, Hendrik and Irmen, Andreas (2007) "On the Long-Run Evolution of Technological Knowledge." *Economic Theory* 30, pp. 171–180.

Hammacher, Kay (2006) "Accelerating Changes in Our Epoch and the Role of Time-Horizons." In Vladimir Burdyuzha, ed., *The Future of Life and the Future of Our Civilization*, vol. 3. New York: Springer.

Hanson, Robin (1994) "If Uploads Come First: The Crack of a Future Dawn." *Extropy* 6/2. http://hanson. gmu.edu/uploads.html.

Hanson, Robin (1998a) "Economic Growth Given Machine Intelligence." http://hanson.gmu.edu/ aigrow.pdf.

Hanson, Robin (1998b) "Is a Singularity Just Around the Corner? What It Takes to Get Explosive Economic Growth." *Journal of Evolution and Technology* 2. http://hanson.gmu.edu/fastgrow.html.

Hanson, Robin (1998c) "Long-Term Growth as a Sequence of Exponential Modes." http://hanson.gmu.edu/ longgrow.pdf.

Hanson, Robin (2008a) "Economics of Brain Emulations." In Peter Healey and Steve Rayner, eds., *Unnatural Selection: The Challenges of Engineering Tomorrow's People*. London: EarthScan, pp, 150–158.

Hanson, Robin (2008b) "Economics of the Singularity." *IEEE Spectrum* (June), pp. 37–42.

Hawkins, Gerald S. (2002) *Mindsteps to the Cosmos*. River Edge, NJ: World Scientific.

Heylighen, Francis (1997) "The Socio-Technological Singularity." http://pespmc1.vub.ac.be/SINGULAR. html.

Heylighen, Francis (2007) "Accelerating Socio-Technological Evolution: From Ephemeralization and Stigmergy to the Global Brain." In George Modelski, Tessaleno Devezas, and William Thompson, eds., *Globalization as an Evolutionary Process: Modeling Global Change*. London: Routledge.

Johansen, Anders and Sornette, Didier (2001) "Finite-Time Singularity in the Dynamics of the World Population, Economic and Financial Indices." *Physica A* 294, pp. 465–502.

Kapitza, Sergey P. (2006) *Global Population Blow-Up and After: The Demographic Revolution and Information Society*. Report to the Club of Rome.

Korotayev, Andrey (2007) "Compact Mathematical Models of World System Development, and How They Can Help Us to Clarify our Understanding of Globalization Processes." In George Modelski, Tessaleno Devezas, and William Thompson, eds., *Globalization as an Evolutionary Process: Modeling Global Change*. London: Routledge, pp. 133–161.

Kremer, M. (1993) "Population Growth and Technological Change: One Million BC to 1990." *Quarterly Journal of Economics* 108, pp. 681–716.

Kurzweil, Ray (2001) "The Law of Accelerating Returns." http://www.kurzweilai.net/articles/art0134.html.

Kurzweil, Ray (2005) *The Singularity Is Near: When Humans Transcend Biology*. New York: Viking.

Kurzweil, Ray, Vinge, Vernor, and Moravec, Hans (2001) "Singularity Math Trialogue." http://www. kurzweilai.net/meme/frame.html?main=/articles/art0151.html.

Leontief, Wassily W. (1986) *Input-Output Economics*, 2nd edn. Oxford: Oxford University Press.

LePoire, David J. (2005) "Application of Logistic Analysis to the History of Physics." *Technological Forecasting and Social Change* 72, pp. 471–479.

Marshall, Alfred (1920) *Principles of Economics*, 8th edn., Book 4, chapter XIII, para. IV.XIII.11. London: Macmillan.

Meyer, François and Vallee, Jacques (1975) "The Dynamics of Long-Term Growth." *Technological Forecasting and Social Change* 7, 285–300.

Modis, Theodore (2002) "Forecasting the Growth of Complexity and Change." *Technological Forecasting and Social Change* 69, pp. 377–404.

Modis, Theodore (2006) "Discussion." *Technological Forecasting and Social Change* 73/2, pp. 104–112.

Moravec, Hans (1999) "Simple Equations for Vinge's Technological Singularity." http://www.frc.ri.cmu. edu/~hpm/project.archive/robot.papers/1999/singularity.html

Moravec, Hans (2003) "Simpler Equations for Vinge's Technological Singularity." http://www.frc.ri.cmu.edu/users/hpm/project.archive/robot.papers/2003/singularity2.html.

Nottale, L., Chaline, J., and Grou, P. (2001) "On the Fractal Structure of Evolutionary Trees." In G. Losa, D. Merlini, T. Nonnenmacher, and E. Weibel, eds., *"Fractals in Biology and Medicine"*, vol. 3: *Proceedings of Fractal 2000 Third International Symposium*, Basel: Birckhäuser Verlag.

Saleur, H. and Sornette, D. (1996) "Complex Exponents and Log-Periodic Corrections in Frustrated Systems." *J. Phys. I France* 6/3 (March), pp. 327–355.

Sandberg, Anders and Bostrom, Nick (2008) *Whole Brain Emulation: A Roadmap*. Technical Report #2008-3. Future of Humanity Institute, Oxford University. http://www.fhi.ox.ac.uk/reports/2008-3.pdf.

Schmidhuber, Juergen (2006) "New Millennium AI and the Convergence of History. Challenges to Computational Intelligence." http://arxiv.org/pdf/cs/0606081.pdf.

Smart, John (2008) "Evo Devo Universe? A Framework for Speculations on Cosmic Culture." In Steven J. Dick, ed., *Cosmos and Culture*. NASA Press.

Smith, John Maynard and Szathmáry, Eörs (1995) *The Major Transitions in Evolution*. Oxford: Oxford University Press.

Solomonoff, Ray J. (1985) "The Time Scale of Artificial Intelligence: Reflections on Social Effects." *North-Holland Human Systems Management* 5, pp. 149–153.

Taagepera, R. (1979) "People, Skills, and Resources: An Interaction Model for World Population Growth." *Technological Forecasting and Social Change* 13, pp. 13–30.

Turchin, Valentin (1977) *The Phenomenon of Science: A Cybernetic Approach to Human Evolution*. New York: Columbia University Press.

Turchin, Valentin and Joslyn, Cliff (1989) "The Cybernetic Manifesto." http://pespmc1.vub.ac.be/MANIFESTO.html.

Tyler, Time (2009) "The Singularity is Nonsense." http://alife.co.uk/essays/the_singularity_is_nonsense/.

Ulam, Stanislaw (1968) "Tribute to John von Neumann." *Bulletin of the American Mathematical Society* 64(3–2) (May), pp. 1–49.

Vinge, Vernor (1993) *The Coming Technological Singularity: How to Survive in the Post-Human Era*. NASA CP-10129.

Vinge, Vernor (2008) "Signs of the Singularity." *IEEE Spectrum* (June).

von Foerster, Heinz, Mora, Patricia M., and Amiot, Lawrence W. (1960) "Doomsday: Friday 13 November, A.D. 2026." *Science* 132, pp. 1291–1295.

Wagner-Döbler, Roland (2001) "Rescher's Principle of Decreasing Marginal Returns of Scientific Research." *Scientometrics* 50/3.

Yudkowsky, Eliezer S. (2007) "Three Major Singularity Schools." http://yudkowsky.net/singularity/schools.

37

A Critical Discussion of Vinge's Singularity Concept

David Brin, Damien Broderick, Nick Bostrom, Alexander "Sasha" Chislenko,
Robin Hanson, Max More, Michael Nielsen, and Anders Sandberg

Comment by David Brin: Singularities

Vernor Vinge's "singularity" is a worthy contribution to the long tradition of contemplations about human transcendence. Throughout history, most of these musings have dwelled upon the spiritual – the notion that human beings can achieve a higher state through prayer, moral behavior, or mental discipline. In the last century, an intellectual tradition that might be called "techno-transcendentalism" has added a fourth track. The notion that a new level of existence, or a more appealing state of being, might be achieved by means of knowledge and skill.

Sometimes, techno-transcendentalism has focused on a specific branch of science, upon which the adherents pin their hopes. Marxists and Freudians created complex models of human society or mind, and predicted that rational application of these rules would result in a higher level of general happiness.

At several points, eugenics has captivated certain groups with the allure of improving the human animal. This dream has lately been revived with the promise of genetic engineering.

Enthusiasts for nuclear power in the 1950s promised energy too cheap to meter. Some of the same passion was seen in the enthusiasm for space colonies, in the 1970s and 1980s, and in today's cyber-transcendentalism, which appears to promise ultimate freedom and privacy for everyone, if only we just start encrypting every internet message and use anonymity online to perfectly mask the frail beings who are actually typing at a real keyboard.

This long tradition – of bright people pouring faith and enthusiasm into transcendental dreams – tells us a lot about one aspect of our nature that crosses all cultures and all centuries. Quite often it comes accompanied by a kind of contempt for contemporary society – a belief that

Originally published in *Extropy Online* (2000). Copyright © Max More.

some kind of salvation can be achieved outside of the normal cultural network ... a network that is often unkind to bright philosophers, or nerds.

We need to keep this long history in mind as we discuss the latest phase – a belief that the geometrically, or possibly exponentially increase in the ability of our machines to make calculations will result in an equally profound magnification of our knowledge and power.

Having said all of the above, let me hasten to add that I believe in the high likelihood of a coming singularity! The alternative is simply too awful to accept. The means of mass destruction, from A-bombs to germ warfare, are "democratizing" – spreading so rapidly among nations, groups, and individuals – that we had better see a rapid expansion in sanity and wisdom, or else we're all doomed. Indeed, strong evidence indicates that the overall education and sagacity of Western civilization and its constituent citizenry has never been higher, and may continue to improve rapidly in the coming century. One thing is certain: we will not see a future that resembles *Blade Runner* (Scott 1982), or any other cyberpunk dystopia. Such worlds, where massive technology is unmatched by improved accountability, will not be able to sustain themselves. The options before us appear to be limited:

1. Achieve some form of "singularity" – or at least a phase shift, to a higher and more knowledgeable society (one that may have problems of its own that we can't imagine.)
2. Self-destruction
3. Retreat into some form of more traditional human society. One that discourages the sorts of extravagant exploration that might lead to results 1 or 2.

In fact, when you look at our present culture from a historical perspective, it is already profoundly anomalous in its emphasis upon individualism, progress, and above all, suspicion of authority. These themes were actively and vigorously repressed in a vast majority of human cultures because they threatened the stable equilibrium upon which ruling classes depended.

Although we are proud of the resulting society – one that encourages eccentricity, appreciation of diversity, social mobility, and scientific progress, we have no right, as yet, to claim that this new way of doing things is sane or obvious. Many in other parts of the world consider Westerners to be quite mad, and only time will tell who is right about that. Certainly if current trends continue – if for instance, we take the suspicion of authority ethos to its extreme, and start paranoically mistrusting even our best institutions – it is quite possible that Western civilization might fly apart before ever achieving its vaunted aims. Certainly, a singularity cannot happen if only centrifugal forces operate, and there are no compensating centripetal virtues to keep us together as a society of mutually respectful common citizens.

Above all (as I point out in *The Transparent Society* (Brin 1998)) our greatest innovations – science, justice, democracy and free markets – all depend upon the mutual accountability that comes from open flows of information.

But what if we do stay on course, and achieve something like Vernor's singularity? There is plenty of room to argue over what TYPE would be beneficial or even desirable. For instance, if organic humans are destined to be replaced by artificial beings, vastly more capable than we souped-up apes, can we design those successors to think of themselves as human? Or will we simply become obsolete?

Some people remain big fans of Teilhard de Chardin's apotheosis – the notion that we will all combine into a single macro-entity, almost literally godlike in its knowledge and perception. Frank Tipler speaks of such a destiny in his book *The Physics of Immortality* (Tipler 1994), and

Isaac Asimov offers a similar prescription as mankind's long-range goal, in *Foundation's Edge* (Asimov 1991). I have never found this notion particularly appealing – at least in the standard version in which the macro-being simply subsumes all individuals within it, and proceeds to think just one thought at a time. In *Earth* (Brin 1991), I talk about a variation on this theme that might be more palatable, in which we all remain individual while at the same time contributing to a new layer of planetary consciousness – in other words we get to both have our cake and eat it too. At the opposite extreme, in the new *Foundation* novel, that I am currently writing as a sequel to Asimov's famous novels, I make more explicit what Isaac has been painting all along – the image that conservative robots who fear human transcendence, might actively work to prevent a human singularity for thousands of years, fearing that it would bring us harm.

In any event, it is a fascinating notion, and one that can be rather frustrating at times. A good parent wants the best for his or her children, and for them to be better. And yet, it can be poignant to imagine them – or perhaps their grandchildren – living almost like gods, with omniscient knowledge and perception, and near immortality.

But when has human existence been anything but poignant? All of our speculations and musings today may seem amusing and naive, to those descendants. But I hope they will also experience moments of respect. They may even pause and realize that we were really pretty good for souped-up cavemen.

Comment by Damien Broderick

> Within thirty years, we will have the technological means to create superhuman intelligence. Shortly after, the human era will be ended. (Vinge 1993)

Around 2050, or maybe as early as 2020, is when Dr. Vernor Vinge's technological Singularity is expected to erupt, in the considered opinion of a number of scientists. Call such an event "the Spike," because technology's exponential curve resembles a spike on a graph of progress against time. Of course, it's a profoundly suspect suggestion. We've heard this sort of thing prophesied before, in literally Apocalyptic religious revelations of End Time and Rapture. It's a pity the timing coincides fairly closely with the dates proposed by the superstitious.

What Vinge means is just a barrier to confident anticipation of future technologies. Despite the millennial coincidence, estimates of when the Spike is due, and even of its slope and the time remaining before that slope carries us upward faster than we can foresee, remain elusive. We will not find ourselves hurled headlong into the Singularity in the next few years, or even the next decade. The curve steepens only later, even if that runaway surge is something that many of us might expect to see in our lifetimes. And our lifetimes could turn out to be far longer that we currently expect.

For now, what is required of us is not reverence but hard thinking and public dialogue. It is a nice paradox. If we postpone our analysis of the path to the Spike, on the understandable grounds that it's too frightening, or too silly, we'll lose the chance to keep our hands on the reins. (And see how the old, passé metaphors remain in charge of our thoughts? Hands on the *reins*?).

To date, many of the best minds of the human race have been devoted to short-term goals suitable for short-lived people in a volatile, hungry, dangerous world. That will change. Perhaps none of the complex lessons of our long history will have the slightest bearing on our conduct, will offer us any good guidance, in the strange days after the middle of the twenty-first century and beyond. Except, perhaps, the austere rules of game-theory, and the remote laws of physics.

Many will deplore this bleak obliteration of the wisdom of the past. "Love one another!" is, after all, part of our deepest behavioral grammar, inherited from three million years on the plains of Africa. So too is its hateful complement: "Fear the stranger! Guard the food! Kill the foe!" The Spike might resolve these ancient dilemmas by rendering some of them pointless – why bother to steal another's goods when you can make your own in a matter-compiler? – and others remediable – why shiver in fear of disease and sexism and death, when you can rewrite your DNA codes, bypass mortality, switch gender from the chromosomes up, guided by wonderful augmented minds?

Or is this, after all, no better than cargo-cult delusion, the ultimate mistaken reliance for salvation upon some God-in-the-Machine?

Anders Sandberg recently lamented the way our minds tend to cave in when faced by the possibility of a Spike. The concept of a Spike is so *immense*: "it fits in too well with our memetic receptors!" He tried to unpick the varieties of singularity that have been proposed to date.

1. One is the Transcension, an approximation to the Parousia where we become more than human, changing by augmentation or uploading into something completely different and unknowable.
2. A second is the Inflexion Point, the place where the upward scream of the huge sigmoid curve of progress tips over, slowing, and starts to ebb.
3. The third is the Wall, or Prediction Horizon, the date after which we can't predict or understand much of what is going on because it simply gets too weird. While this last version somewhat resembles the first, that is just a side-effect of our ignorance. It does not imply, as Transcension can, that with the Spike we enter a realm of space-time engineering, creation of budded universes, and wholesale re-writing of the laws of physics: what Australian transhumanist Mitchell Porter calls "the Vastening."

For all its appeal – precisely *because* of its crypto-mystical, pseudo-religious appeal – the Transcension is, Anders Sandberg suggests,

> the most dangerous of the three versions, since it is the most overwhelming. Many discussions just close with, "But we cannot predict *anything* about the post singularity world!" ending all further inquiry just as Christians and other religious believers do with, "It is the Will of God." And it is all too easy to give the Transcension eschatological overtones, seeing it as Destiny. This also promotes a feeling of helplessness in many, who see it as all-powerful and inevitable. (Broderick 2001: 312)

The collective mind we call science – fallible, contestatory, driven by ferocious passions and patient effort – promises to deliver us what religions and mythologies have only preached as a distant, impalpable reward (or punishment) to be located in another world entirely.

Yet many people, to my amazement, denounce the idea that we might live indefinitely extended and ceaselessly revised lives in a post-Spike milieu.

Where is the sweetness of life, they ask, without the stings, pangs, and agonies of its loss? Life is the bright left hand of death's darkness. No yin without yang, and so forth. I have some sympathy for this suspicion (everyone knows, for example, that well-earned hunger makes the finest sauce to a meal), but not much. I'm not persuaded that simple dualistic contrasts and oppositions are the most useful way to analyze the world, let alone to form the basis for morality.

Does freedom require the presence of a slave underclass? Are we only happy in our health because someone else – or we, ourselves, in the future – might die in agony from cancer? Let's hope not! I must state bluntly that this line of thinking smacks to me far too sordidly of a doctrine of cowed consolation, the kind of warrant muttered by prisoners with no prospect of eluding a cruel and unyielding captor, and with no taste for daring an escape bid.

It is a compliant slave's self-defeating question to ask: *what would we do with our freedom?* The answer can only be: *whatever you wish.* Yes, freedom from imposed mortality will be wasted by some, life's rich spirit spilled into the sand, just as the gift of our current meager span is wasted and spoiled by all too many in squabbles, fatuous diversions, bored routine, numbing habits and addictions of a dozen kinds.

Others, bent by the torment of choice and liberty, will throw it away in terror, taking their own lives rather than face the echoing void of open endlessness. That would be their choice, one that must be respected (however much we might regret it). For the rest of us, I think, there will be a slow dawning and awakening of expectations. People of exceptional gifts will snatch greedily and thankfully at the chance to grow, learn, suck life dry as never before. But so too, surely, will the ordinary rest of us.

With a span limited to a single century, a quarter devoted to learning the basics of being a human and another quarter, or even more, lost in failing health, it's little wonder that we constrict our horizons, close our eyes against the falling blows of time. Even now, of course, any one of us could learn in middle age to play the piano or violin, or master a new language, or study the astoundingly elegant mathematics we missed in school, but few manage the resolve. But to make such efforts would be regarded by our friends as futile, derided as comic evidence of "mid-life crisis."

In a world of endless possibilities, however, where our mental and physical powers do not routinely deteriorate, opportunities to expand our skills and our engagement with other people, the natural world, history itself, will challenge all of us, including the most ordinary of citizens. Although it strains credulity right now, I believe one of the great diversions for many people in the endless future will be the unfolding tapestry of science itself (as well as the classic arts, and altogether new means of expression).

Enhanced by our machines, we will embrace the aesthetic grandeur of systematic knowledge tested against stringent criticism, sought for its own soul-filling sake – and embrace as well knowledge as virtuoso technique, as the lever of power, enabling each of us to become immersed, if only as an informed spectator, in the enterprise of discovery. And there might be no limits to what we can discover, and do, on the far side of the Spike.[1]

Comment by Nick Bostrom: Singularity and Predictability

I find myself to be in close agreement with much of what Vinge has said about the singularity. Like Vinge, I do not regard the singularity as being a certainty, just one of the more likely scenarios.

1. "The singularity" has been taken to mean different things by different authors, and sometimes by the same author on different occasions. There are at least three clearly distinct theoretical entities that might be referred to by this term:

- A point in time at which the speed of technological development becomes extremely great. (Verticality)
- The creation of superhuman artificial intelligence. (Superintelligence)
- A point in time beyond which we can predict nothing, except maybe what we can deduce directly from physics. (Unpredictability, aka "prediction horizon")

Vinge seems to believe in the conjunction of these three claims, but it's not clear whether they are all part of the definition of "the singularity." For example, if Verticality and Superintelligence turn out to be true but Unpredictability fails, is it then the case that there was no singularity? Or was there a singularity but Vinge was mistaken about its nature? This is a purely verbal question, but one it would be useful to be clear about so we are not talking past one another.

2.   Two potential technologies stand out from the others in terms of their importance: superintelligence and nanotechnology (i.e. "mature molecular manufacturing" which includes a nearly general assembler).

It is an open question which of these will be developed first. I believe that either would fairly soon lead to the other. A superintelligence, it seems, should be able to quickly develop nanotechnology. Conversely, if we have nanotechnology then it should be easy to get greater than human-equivalent hardware. Given the hardware, we could either use ab initio methods, such as neural networks and genetic algorithms or (less likely) classical AI; or we could upload outstanding human brains and run them at an accelerated clock-rate. My intuition is that given adequate hardware, ab initio methods would succeed within a fairly short time (perhaps as little as a few years). There is no way of being sure of that, however. If the software problem turns out to be very hard then there are two possibilities: If uploading is feasible at this stage (as it would presumably be there is nanotechnology) then the first (weak) superintelligences might be uploads. If, on the other hand, uploads cannot be created, then the singularity will be delayed until the software problem has been solved or uploading becomes possible.

If there is nanotechnology but not superintelligence then I would expect technological progress to be very fast by today's standards. Yet I don't think there would be a singularity, since the design problems involved in creating complex machines or medical instruments would be huge. It would presumably take several years before most things were made by nanotechnology.

If there is superintelligence but not nanotechnology, there might still be a singularity. Some of the most radical possibilities would presumably then not happen – for example, the Earth would not be transformed into a giant computer in a few days – but important features of the world could nonetheless be radically different in a very short time, especially if we think that subjective experiences and intelligent processing are themselves among these important features.

3.   Even if Verticality and Superintelligence are both true, I am not at all sure that Unpredictability would hold. I think it is unfortunate that some people have made Unpredictability a defining feature of "the singularity." It really does tend to create a mental block.

Note that Unpredictability is a very strong claim. Not only does it say that we don't know much about the post-singularity world but also that such knowledge cannot be had. If we convinced about this radical skepticism, we would have no reason to try to make the singularity happen in a desirable way, since we would have no means of anticipating what the consequences of present actions would be on the post-singularity world.

I think there are some things that we can predict with a reasonable degree of confidence beyond the singularity. For example, that the superintelligent entity resulting from the singularity would start a spherical colonization wave that would propagate into space at a substantial fraction of the speed of light. (This means that I disagree with Vinge's suggestion that we explain the Fermi paradox by assuming that "these outer civilizations are so weird there's no way to interact with them.") Another example is that if there are multiple independent competing agents (which I suspect there might not be) then we would expect some aspects of their behavior to be predictable from considerations of economic rationality.

It might also be possible to predict things in much greater detail. Since the superintelligences or posthumans that will govern the post-singularity world will be created by us, or might even *be* us, it seems that we should be in a position to influence what values they will have. What their values are will then determine what the world will look like, since due to their advanced technology they will have a great ability to make the world conform to their values and desires. So one could argue that all we have to do in order to predict what will happen after the singularity is to figure out what values the people will have who will create the superintelligence.

It is possible that things could go wrong and that the superintelligence we create accidentally gets to have unintended values, but that presupposes that a serious mistake is made. If no such mistake is made then the superintelligence will have the values of its creators. (And of course it would not change its most fundamental values; it is a mistake to think that as soon as a being is sufficiently intelligent it will "revolt" and decide to pursue some "worthy" goal. Such a tendency is at most a law human psychology (and even that is by no means clear); but a superintelligence would not necessarily have a human psychology. There is nothing implausible about a superintelligence who sees it as its sole purpose to transform the matter of the universe into the greatest possible number of park benches – except that it is hard to imagine why somebody would choose to build such a superintelligence.)

So maybe we can define a fairly small number of hypotheses about what the post-singularity world will be like. Each of these hypotheses would correspond to a plausible value. The plausible values are those that it seems fairly probable that many of the most influential people will have at about the time when the first superintelligence is created. Each of these values defines an attractor, i.e. a state of the world which contains the maximal amount of positive utility according to the value in question. We can then make the prediction that the world is likely to settle into one of these attractors. More specifically, we would expect that within the volume of space that has been colonized, matter would gradually (but perhaps very quickly) be arranged into value-maximal structures – structures that contain as much of the chosen value as possible.

I call this the track hypothesis because it says that the future contains a number of "tracks" – possible courses of development such that once actual events take on one of these courses they will inexorably approach and terminate in the goal state (the attractor) given by the corresponding value.

Even if we knew that the track hypothesis is true and which value will actually become dominant, it's still possible that we wouldn't know much about what the future will be like. It might be hard to compute what physical structure would in fact maximize the given value. (What would the universe have to look like in order to maximize the total amount of pleasure?) Moreover, even if we have some abstract knowledge of the future, we might still be incapable of intuitively understanding what it will be like to be living in this future. (What would the hyper-blissful experiences feel like that would exist if the universe were pleasure-maximized?) This is one sense in which posthumans could be as incomprehensible to us as we are to goldfish. But inscrutability in this sense by no means precludes that unaugmented humans could be able to usefully predict many aspects of the behavior and cognitive processes of posthumans.

Comment by Alexander Chislenko: Singularity as a Process, and the Future Beyond

I first encountered the notion of a dramatic turning point in the future sometime in the early 1970s, when my father Leonid Chislenko, a theoretical biologist and a philosopher, shared some of his "General Theory of Everything" with me. I remember him drawing a simple graph of the rate of the evolution of complex systems in the Universe, from the formation of galaxies, stars, and planets, to appearance of various life forms, to early societies, to recent technological revolution. On the logarithmic scale, the complexity doubling periods resided on a single straight line that laconically touched the X axis at the 2030 year mark. That little demonstration was one of most exciting moments in my studies of the world, and greatly influenced my further interests.

My favorite factors to watch have changed several times in the last 25 years, and so did my expectation of the ultimate goals of the process. Actually, I no longer believe that we are going to witness a single event/point after which the development would infinitely speed up, or dramatically and unpredictably break.

Every prediction has some observer estimating values of selected system parameters for a certain time ahead. While current widely published predictions of population size, weather, sports results, or oil prices may be somewhat accurate, these indicators no longer reflect the progress of modern civilization. This development is determined by the intricate interplay of semantic patterns and techno-social architectures, of whose state nobody has a relevant model. Most people have never even attempted to understand the transformation trends of this system, while those who tried caught just sparse glimpses of relevant trends. How long do we have to wait to claim that the system's behavior is unpredictable? For most people, this Singularity point has already arrived, and the future mix of the ever greater number of ever smarter people and machines will look to them about equally confusing, and just change faster (or slower, depending on which irrelevant parameters they may choose to track).

Our ideas of important growth factors have changed during recent history. First, we looked at the population explosion that for some time obeyed the hyperbolic "law." Of course, it was no more of a law than Moore's *observation* of the pace of computer technology development. Simple projection of ongoing trends, without analysis of mechanisms, is not a law, it's just a mental exercise. Qualitative understanding of the development process seems a lot more important than the results of such projections (though I do remember calculating with my son how soon he would reach the size of an average giraffe if he continued doubling his height every five years). After the population growth slowed down, people started plotting energy consumption graphs. It slowed down as well. Then it was expansion into space. Before it had time to slow down, we turned our attention to computer memory and speed.

It seems quite natural that at every point we pay most attention to the parameters that are just about to peak, as they represent the hottest current trends. When we look back in the excitement of the moment, the whole history of the world looks like a preparation for the explosion of this particular parameter. And we completely forget that yesterday we were looking at something else with the same excitement…

I expect that we may soon lose interest to the current factors as well, and start looking at a new set of criteria, for example, some non-numeric indicators of the cognitive strength, architectural stability, and dynamic potential of the global technosocium.

Surely, human population, energy, space, and computing power are, at this stage, useful for further progress. However, their influence on development is difficult to describe with a simple formula. Certain problems require threshold levels of some of these resources, and then they are just solved (e.g., I expect communication between humans to saturate as the price of delivery of full human perception bandwidth becomes negligible); others so far exhibit increasing returns; still others have already ground to a halt (the accuracy of weather forecasts). So far, the utility of additional physical and computational resources has been determined by the fact that they compensated for old-time human deficiencies and allowed utilization of existing resources that were relatively huge in terms of both physical size and complexity. When the first benefits of the augmentation of natural human skills get exploited, and the dimensions of the artificial systems first approach, and then exceed, those of the biological world, the nature of the development process will shift from exploitation of the accumulated natural treasures to self-engineering, which may produce different dynamic patterns and require attention to different factors.

The increase in crude resources doesn't guarantee unbounded progress. If we can model the intelligence of a small insect now, and 40 years from now will have million times more memory and a million times greater processing speed, all we'll get is a lot of very fast insects. Further qualitative progress would require better design methods that either have to be designed by slow humans, or automatically evolved. Genetic algorithms have a great promise, but in many cases their utility will be curbed by the slow rate of evolutionary cycles (e.g., spaceship control systems) or high safety requirements (control software for nuclear power plants, national defense, or heart transplants). The development of truly intelligent computer systems may be a stumbling block on the way to the most dramatic future advances, so we had better start developing the necessary technologies today.

I do not think that dramatic changes may happen at a certain single point, though there will be periods of increasingly fast growth in many areas, that will keep running ahead of the analytical and participatory abilities of non-augmented humans (though research conglomerates may have increasingly accurate models of the whole system that, through them, will understand and be able to predict its behavior better than all its predecessors). Even with increasing control over space, time, matter, and complexity, we may meet some natural limits to growth. These limits may not curb all progress, but as previous limitations, they may bring new turns into the development process that we may currently find difficult to foresee.

Still, we can probably already imagine some of the features of the posthuman world. Increasing independence of functional systems from the physical substrate, continued growth in architectural liquidity of systems, low transaction costs, and secure and semantic-rich communication mechanisms will result in the dissolution of large quasi-static systems and the obsolescence of the idea of structural identity. The development arena may belong to the "teleological threads" – chains of systems creating each other for sequences of purposes using for their execution temporary custom assemblages of small function-specific units.

Point transition or a rapid process, Singularity still seems difficult to come to grips with and, hence, quite threatening. The fast succession of dramatic transformations promises to destroy or invalidate most of the things one identifies with. Modification of familiar objects beyond recognition, even through improvement, looks much like destruction; it's "death forward," as I call it. This is a subjective problem, and it requires a subjective solution. The solution is actually quite simple: junk the outdated concept of static identity, and think of yourself as a *process*.

Of course, we can build all kinds of wild scenarios of the future beyond the human Concept Horizon (a notion I prefer to Singularity as it implies a reference to an observer, a multitude of possible points of entry, and an ever-elusive position). However, since many of the technologies that we possess and are developing today will influence the construction of the future world, it is our historical duty to create tools enabling the future we would like to see. My ideal transcendent world would look like a free-market Society of Mind, with a diverse set of non-coercively coordinated goals and development tools, and sophisticated balancing mechanisms and safeguards.

If we want to see such a world rather than a lop-sided and fragile super-Borg, we need to foster research and experimental work on complex multi-agent systems, game and contract theory, cognitive architectures, alternative social formations, semantically rich, secure communication mechanisms, post-identity theory of personhood, and other areas of science, technology, and personal psychology that may influence the development of a positive future at this sensitive formative stage. We would also need to popularize these approaches, to demonstrate to other people that these scenarios are both feasible and desirable.

My Hypereconomy project represents one such attempt. It is a model of an integrated cognitive/economic system where independent agents exchange value representations together with non-scalar aggregate indicators of situational utilities of different objects, and mixed value/knowledge derivatives, with meta-agents performing coordinating functions and deciding issues of knowledge ownership on a non-coercive basis. I would be happy to see more people working on such projects.

Comment by Robin Hanson: Some Skepticism

> Since ... an ultra intelligent machine could design even better machines; there would then unquestionably be an "intelligence explosion" ... more probable than not ... within the 20th century. (Good 1965)

Vernor Vinge's 1993 elaboration on I.J. Good's reasoning has captured many imaginations. Vinge says that probably by 2030 and occurring "faster than any technical revolution seen so far," perhaps "in a month or two," "it may seem as if our artifacts as a whole had suddenly wakened." While we might understand a future of "normal progress," or even where we "crank up the clock speed on a human-equivalent mind," the "singularity," in contrast, creates "an opaque wall across the future," beyond which "things are completely unknowable" (Vinge 1993).

Why? Because humans are to posthumans as "goldfish" are to us, "permanently clueless" about our world. "One begins to feel how essentially strange and different the posthuman era will be" by thinking about posthumans' "high-bandwidth networking ... [and] ability to communicate at variable bandwidths." "What happens when pieces of ego can be copied and merged, [and] when the size of a self-awareness can grow or shrink?" Good and evil would no longer make sense without "isolated, immutable minds connected by tenuous, low-bandwidth links." The universe only looks dead to us because post-singularity aliens "are so weird there's no way to interact with them" (Kelly 1995).

Instead of a "soft take-off," taking "about a century," Vinge sees rapidly accelerating progress. This is because the more intelligent entities are, the shorter their time-scale of their progress, since smarter entities "execute ... simulations at much higher speeds." In contrast, without super-intelligence we would see an "end of progress" where "programs would never get beyond a certain level of complexity."

Many find Vinge's vision compelling. But does it withstand scrutiny? I see two essential claims (my paraphrasing):

1. Smarter entities reproduce even smarter entities faster.
2. Posthumans are as incomprehensible to us as we are to goldfish.

First, let me say what I agree with. I accept that within the next century we will probably begin to see a wider variety of minds, including humans who have uploaded, sped-up, and begun to explore the vast possibilities of higher bandwidths and self-modification. I also accept that these new possibilities may somewhat thicken the fog of possibilities that obscures our vision of the future. I can also see spurts of economic growth from plucking the "low-hanging fruit" of easy upload modifications, and due to eliminating today's biological bounds on reproduction rates of "human" type capital.

Now let me be more critical, starting with "smarter entities reproduce even smarter entities faster." Some people interpret this as imagining a single engineer working on the task of redesigning itself to be 1 percent smarter. They think of intelligence as a productivity multiplier, shortening the time it takes do many mental tasks given the same other resources, and they assume this "make myself 1 percent smarter" task stays equally hard, as the engineer becomes smarter. These assumptions allow the engineer's intelligence to explode to infinity within a finite time.

If early work focuses on the easiest improvements, however, the task of becoming more productive can get harder as the easy wins are exhausted. Students get smarter as they learn more, and learn how to learn. However, we teach the most valuable concepts first, and the productivity value of schooling eventually falls off, instead of exploding to infinity. Similarly, the productivity improvement of factory workers typically slows with time, following a power law.

At the world level, average IQ scores have increased dramatically over the last century (the Flynn effect), as the world has learned better ways to think and to teach. Nevertheless, IQs have improved steadily, instead of accelerating. Similarly, for decades computer and communication aids have made engineers much "smarter," without accelerating Moore's law. While engineers got smarter, their design tasks got harder.

Can we interpret Vinge's claim as describing accelerating economic growth? The vast economic literature on economic growth offers little support for any simple direct relation between economic growth rates and either intelligence levels or clock speeds. A one-time reduction in the time to complete various calculations, either due to being smarter or having a faster clock, is a one-time reduction in the cost of certain types of production, which induces a one-time jump in world product. Such a one-time growth, however, hardly implies a faster *rate* of growth thereafter.

Now there *are* grounds for suspecting that growth rates increase with the size of the world economy, and we *can* think of a one-time intelligence improvement as increasing the world economy. However, this process would have been going on for millennia, and so does not suggest growth any faster than the accelerating historical "normal progress" trends suggest (see my paper, "Is a Singularity Just Around the Corner?" [Hanson 1998]).

Which brings me to Vinge's other main claim, that "posthumans are as incomprehensible to us as we are to goldfish." Does relative comprehension really follow a linear "intelligence" ranking of creatures, where each creature can't at all understand a creature substantially more intelligent than it? This seems to me to ignore our rich multi-dimensional understanding of intelligence elaborated in our sciences of mind (computer science, AI, cognitive science, neuroscience, animal behavior, etc.).

Arguably the most important recent step in evolution was when humanoids acquired a general language ability, perhaps from the "he says she thinks I did..." social complexities of large human tribes. Our best theories of language, logic, and computation all draw a sharp distinctions between relatively general systems, capable of expressing a wide range of claims and eventually computing a huge range of results, and vastly more restrictive systems.

Animals have impressive specific skills, but very limited abilities to abstract from and communicate their experiences. Computer intelligences, in contrast, have recently been endowed with general capabilities, but few useful skills. It is the human combination of general language and many powerful skills that has enabled our continuing human explosion, via the rapid wide-spread diffusion of innovations in tools, agriculture, and social organization.

So getting back to Vinge, the ability of one mind to understand the general nature of another mind would seem mainly to depend on whether that first mind can understand abstractly at all, and on the depth and richness of its knowledge about minds in general. Goldfish do not understand us mainly because they seem incapable of *any* abstract comprehension. Conversely, some really stupid computer intelligences are capable of understanding most anything we care to explain to them in sufficient detail. We even have some smarter systems, such as CYC, which require much less detailed explanations.

It seems to me that human cognition is general enough, and our sciences of mind mature enough, that we can understand much about quite a diverse zoo of possible minds, many of them much more capable than ourselves on many dimensions. Yes, it is possible that the best understanding of the most competitive new minds will require as yet undeveloped concepts of mind. But I see little reason to think such concepts could not be explained to us, nor that we are incapable of developing such concepts. See how much we have learned about quantum computers, after just a few years of serious consideration.

Individual humans may have limits on the complexity they can handle, but humanity as a whole does not. Even now, groups of people understand things that no one person does, and manage systems more complex than any one person could manage. I see no basis for expecting individual complexity limits to make progress to slow to a halt without super-intelligences. In fact, future analogs to our society's individuals may well be substantially simpler than humans, making future humans *more* capable than the typical "individual" of personally understanding the systems in which they are embedded.

I see no sharp horizon, blocking all view of things beyond. Instead, our vision just fades into a fog of possibilities, as usual. It was the application of our current concepts of mind that first suggested to Vinge how different future entities might be from standard science fiction fare, and that has informed his thoughtful speculation about future minds, such as the 'tines in *A Fire Upon The Deep* (Vinge 1992). And efforts like his continue to reward us with fresh insights into future minds.

It was understandable for Vinge to be shocked to discover that his future speculations had neglected to consider the nature of future minds. But I beg Vinge to disavow his dramatizing this discovery as an "opaque wall" beyond which "things are completely unknowable." Vinge clearly does not really believe this, as he admits he inconsistently likes "to think about what things would be like afterwards."

Yet, his "unknowable" descriptor has become a mental block preventing a great many smart future-oriented people from thinking seriously beyond a certain point. As Anders Sandberg said, it ends "all further inquiry just as Christians do with 'It is the Will of God.'" Many of Vinge's fans even regularly rebuke others for considering such analysis. Vinge, would you please rebuke *them*?

Comment by Max More: Singularity Meets Economy

Vernor Vinge presents a dramatic picture of the likely future:

> And what of the arrival of the Singularity itself? What can be said of its actual appearance? Since it involves an intellectual runaway, it will probably occur faster than any technical revolution seen so

far … If networking is widespread enough (into ubiquitous embedded systems), it may seem as if our
artifacts as a whole had suddenly wakened. And what happens a month or two (or a day or two) after
that? I have only analogies to point to: The rise of humankind. We will be in the Post-Human era.

From the human point of view this change will be a throwing away of all the previous rules,
perhaps in the blink of an eye, an exponential runaway beyond any hope of control. Developments
that before were thought might only happen in "a million years" (if ever) will likely happen in the
next century.

The Singularity idea exerts a powerful intellectual and imaginative attraction. It's the ultimate
technological orgasm – an overwhelming rocket ride into the future. In one dynamic package,
the Singularity combines ultimate technological excitement with the essence of Christian apocalyptic and millenarian hopes. Precisely because of this powerful attractive force, the Singularity
idea deserves a critical examination. In this short contribution to the discussion, I want to question two assumptions embedded within the Singularity scenario.

> Assumption #1: If we can achieve human-level intelligence in AI, then superintelligence will
> follow quickly and almost automatically.
> Assumption #2: Once greater than human intelligence comes into existence, everything will
> change within hours or days or, at most, a few weeks. All the old rules will cease to apply.

The awakening of a superhumanly intelligent computer is only one of several possible initiators of a Singularity recognized by Vinge. Other possibilities include the emergence of superhuman intelligence in computer networks, effective human-computer interfaces, and
biotechnologically improved human intelligence. Whichever of these paths to superintelligence
Vinge, like I.J. Good, expects an immediate intelligence explosion leading to a total transformation of the world.

I have doubts about both of these assumptions. Curiously, the first assumption of an immediate jump from human-level AI to superhuman intelligence seems not to be a major hurdle for
most people to whom Vinge has presented this idea. Far more people doubt that human-level AI
can be achieved. My own response reverses this: I have no doubt that human-level AI (or computer-networked intelligence) will be achieved at some point. But to move from this immediately to drastically superintelligent thinkers seems to me doubtful. Granted, once AI reaches an
overall human capacity, "weak superhumanity" probably follows easily by simply speeding up
information processing. But, as Vinge himself notes, a very fast-thinking dog still cannot play
chess, solve differential equations, direct a movie, or read one of Vinge's excellent novels.

A superfast human intelligence would still need the cooperation of slower minds. It would
still need to conduct experiments and await their results. It would still have a limited imagination and restricted ability to handle long chains of reasoning. If there were only a few of these
superfast human intelligences, we would see little difference in the world. If there were millions
of them, and they collaborated on scientific projects, technological development, and organizational structures, we would see some impressively swift improvements, but not a radical discontinuity. When I come to the second assumption, I'll address some factors that will further slow
down the impact of their rapid thinking.

Even if superfast human-level thinkers chose to work primarily on augmenting intelligence
further (and they may find other pursuits just as interesting), I see no reason to expect them
to make instant and major progress. That is, I doubt that "strong superhumanity" will follow

automatically or easily. Why should human-level AI make such incredible progress? After all, we already have human-level intelligence in humans, yet human cognitive scientists have not yet pushed up to a higher level of smartness. I see no reason why AIs should do better. A single AI may think much faster than a single human, but humans can do as well by parceling out thinking and research tasks among a community of humans. Without fundamentally better ideas about intelligence, faster thinking will not make a major difference.

I am not questioning the probability of accelerating technological progress. Once superintelligence is achieved it should be easier to develop super-superintelligence, just as it is easier for us to develop superintelligence than it is for any non-human animal to create super-animal (i.e. human) intelligence. All that I am questioning is the assumption that the jump to superintelligence will be easy and immediate. Enormous improvements in intelligence might take years or decades or even centuries rather than weeks or hours. By historical standards this would be rapid indeed, but would not constitute a discontinuous singularity.

I find the second assumption even more doubtful. Even if a leap well beyond human intelligence came about suddenly sometime in the next few decades, I expect the effects on the world to be more gradual than Vinge suggests. Undoubtedly change will accelerate impressively, just as today we see more change economically, socially, and technically in a decade than we would have seen in any decade in the pre-industrial era. But the view that superintelligence will throw away all the rules and transform the world overnight comes more easily to a computer scientist than to an economist. The whole mathematical notion of a Singularity fits poorly with the workings of the physical world of people, institutions, and economies. My own expectation is that superintelligences will be integrated into a broader economic and social system. Even if superintelligence appears discontinuously, the effects on the world will be continuous. Progress will accelerate even more than we are used to, but not enough to put the curve anywhere near the verticality needed for a Singularity.

No matter how much I look forward to becoming a superintelligence myself (if I survive until then), I don't think I could change the world single-handedly. A superintelligence, to achieve anything and to alter the world, will need to work with other agents, including humans, corporations, and other machines. While purely ratiocinative advances may be less constrained, the speed and viscosity of the rest of the world will limit physical and organizational changes. Unless full-blown nanotechnology and robotics appear before the superintelligence, physical changes will take time.

For a superintelligence to change the world drastically, it will need plenty of money and the cooperation of others. As the superintelligence becomes integrated into the world economy, it will pull other processes along with it, fractionally speeding up the whole economy. At the same time, the SI will mostly have to work at the pace of those slower but dominant computer-networked organizations.

The need for collaboration, for organization, and for putting ideas into physical changes will ensure that all the old rules are not thrown out overnight or even within years. Superintelligence may be difficult to achieve. It may come in small steps, rather than in one history-shattering burst. Even a greatly advanced SI won't make a dramatic difference in the world when compared with billions of augmented humans increasingly integrated with technology and with corporations harnessing human minds linked together internally by future versions of today's enterprise resource planning and supply chain management software, and linked externally by extranets, smart interfaces to the Net, and intelligent agents.

How fast things change with the advent of greater than human intelligence depends strongly on two things: the number of superintelligences at work, and the extent of their outperformance.

A lone superintelligence, or even a few, would not accelerate overall economic and technological development all that much. If superintelligence results from a better integration of human and machine (the scenario I find most likely), then it could quickly become widespread and change more rapid. But "more rapid" does not constitute a Singularity. Worldwide changes will be slowed by the stickiness of economic forces and institutions. We have already seen a clear example of this: computers have been widely used in business for decades, yet only in the last few years have we begun to see apparent productivity improvements as corporate processes are reengineered to integrate the new abilities into existing structures.

In conclusion, I find the Singularity idea appealing and a wonderful plot device, but I doubt it describes our likely future. I expect a Surge, not a Singularity. But in case I'm wrong, I'll tighten my seatbelt, keeping taking the smart drugs, and treat all computers with the greatest of respect. I'm their friend!

Comment by Michael Nielsen

What is the Singularity? The following excerpts from Kevin Kelly's *Wired* interview with Vinge sum it up succinctly:

> if we ever succeed in making machines as smart as humans, then it's only a small leap to imagine that we would soon thereafter make – or cause to be made – machines that are even smarter than any human. And that's it. That's the end of the human era ... The reason for calling this a "singularity" is that things are completely unknowable beyond that point. (Kelly 1995)

For the purposes of these notes, I will assume that machines more intelligent than human beings will be constructed in the next few decades.

Vinge's statement assumes that "Dominant Artificial Intelligence (AI)" occurs. I define a Dominant AI as one which seizes control of all areas in which human beings regard their dominance as important. It is often taken as a given that superintelligent AIs will become dominant. I think this is far from certain; Feynman never ran for President, and more generally, very intelligent entities may have neither the inclination nor the capacity to extend their dominance to all aspects of other people's lives.

A better example, albeit rather extreme, for making this point is *Homo sapiens'* relationship with bacteria. Both human beings and bacteria have good claims to being the "dominant species" on Earth – depending upon how one defines dominant. It is possible that superintelligent machines may wish to dominate some niche that is *not* presently occupied in any serious fashion by human beings. If this is the case, then from a human being's point of view, such an AI would not be a Dominant AI. Instead, we would have a "Limited AI" scenario.

How could Limited AI occur? I can imagine several scenarios, and I'm sure other people can imagine more. Perhaps the most important point to make is that superintelligent machines may not be competing in the same niche with human beings for resources, and would therefore have little incentive to dominate us.

In such a Limited AI scenario, there will be aspects of human life which continue on, much as before, with human beings remaining number one. Indeed, within those areas of life, humanity may remain as predictable – or as mercurial – as before. We may be able to harness aspects of the AI in this scenario, much as we have harnessed the Penicillium fungus, or, depending on your point of view, how Penicillium has harnessed us!

For the sake of argument, let us accept that Dominant AI will arise sometime in the next few decades. Will the future after the advent of Dominant AI be unknowable?

What does "unknowable" mean? It seems to me that the sense in which Vinge uses the term unknowable is equivalent to "unpredictable," so let's ask the question "Will the future after the advent of dominant AI necessarily be unpredictable?" instead.

What does it mean to say that some future event is predictable? While there are events, such as the rising of the sun each morning, which are near-certainties, most of the time prediction involves events that are less certain.

Rather, it means that we do not assign equal probabilities to different possible futures. The Clinton-Dole American Presidential election was not completely predictable, in the sense that it wasn't certain who would win before the event. But it wasn't completely unpredictable, either; based on the information available before the election took place, it was possible to assign a very high probability to Clinton winning.

It seems to me to be ridiculous to claim that we can't make useful predictions about a post-Dominant AI world. Yes, things will change enormously. Our predictions may be much less reliable than before. However, I believe that we can still make some reasonable predictions about such a future. At the very least, we can work on excluding some possibilities. One avenue for doing this is to look at exclusions based upon the laws of physics.

An often-made assertion related to the "unpredictability" of a post-Dominant-AI future is that anything allowed by the laws of physics will become possible at that point. This is sometimes used to justify throwing our hands up in despair, and not considering future possibilities any further. Even in the event that this assertion is correct, it still leaves us with a tremendous amount to do. The fact is, we don't have a very good understanding either of what the limits to what is possible are, or what constructive methods for achieving those limits are available.

Let me give an example where we learnt a lot about the limits an AI, even a Dominant AI, must face. In 1905, Einstein proposed the special theory of relativity. One not entirely obvious consequence of the special theory is that if we can signal faster than light, then we can communicate backwards in time. In the absence of any empirical evidence for thinking that this is possible, and other reasons, both empirical and theoretical, for rejecting faster-than-light communication, it appears very likely that faster-than-light communication is impossible. Similar improvements in our understanding of what limits even a Dominant AI will face include the Heisenberg uncertainty principle and the impossibility of classifying topological spaces by algorithmic means.

Let me give a more recent example that illustrates a related point. In 1982, two groups of researchers noticed a deep and unexpected consequence of elementary quantum mechanics: the laws of quantum mechanics forbid the building of a "quantum cloning" device which is able to make copies of unknown quantum states. To prove this result, they made use of elementary facts about quantum mechanics which had been known since the 1920s; no new physics was introduced. Even if we assume that we are close to having a complete theory describing the workings of the world, we may still have a ways to go in working out the consequences of that theory, and what limits they place upon the tasks which may be accomplished by physical entities.

It seems to me that what these and many other examples show is that we can gain a great deal of insight into the limitations of future technologies, without necessarily being able to say in detail what those technologies are.

At a higher level of abstraction, we have very little understanding of what classes of computational problems can be efficiently solved. For example, virtually none of the important computational complexity problems (such as P != NP != PSPACE) in computer science have been resolved. Resolving some of these problems will give us insight into what types of problems are solvable or not solvable by a Dominant AI.

Indeed, computer science recently *has* provided some insight into what constraints a Dominant AI will face. There is a problem in computer science known as "Succinct Circuit Value." It has been proven that this problem cannot be solved efficiently, either on a classical computer, or even on a quantum computer. It seems likely that future models of computation, even based on exotic theories such as string theory, will not be able to efficiently solve this problem.

In principle, of course, "Succinct Circuit Value" is solvable, merely by computing for long enough. In practice, even for modestly sized problem instances, Succinct Value is impossible, because of constraints on the amount of space and time that can be used to implement the algorithm.

So we can, I believe, make useful progress on understanding what constraints an AI, even a Dominant AI, will face. Of course, the constraints I have been talking about so far are arguably not so interesting. Can we say much about how social, political, and economic institutions will evolve? I'm not sure. One of the lessons of twentieth-century science is how difficult is to make forecasts about these within our existing society, never mind one incredibly different. It's worth keeping in mind, however, that understanding does not necessarily imply predictability.

To conclude, it seems to me that Vinge's conception of the Singularity requires three separate hypotheses to be true:

- *The Dominant AI Hypothesis.* There will emerge in the next few decades AIs which dominate all areas of life on Earth in which human superiority has previously been important.
- *The Incomprehensibility Hypothesis.* If Dominant AI arises, then we will not be able to make predictions beyond that point.
- *The Defeatist Hypothesis.* Anything allowed by the laws of physics will be enabled by new technologies, so it is pointless to try to make predictions.

I regard the Dominant AI hypothesis as being highly questionable. There are too many other possibilities. Even assuming the Dominant AI hypothesis, the other two hypotheses look far too pessimistic. They discount the possibilities offered by open problems in fields such as computer science, economics, and physics, where so much of the fundamental work remains to be done.

Comment by Anders Sandberg: Singularity and the Growth of Differences

Basic to the concept of a technological (or historical) singularity is rapidly accelerating change, building cumulatively on past results and resulting in an end state that is hard to predict from the initial conditions. While it can (and maybe should, if only to clarify the conditions) be debated whether we are truly approaching a singularity in the very strong sense proposed by Vinge, it is clear that we live in an era of high rate of change that seems to be cumulative and persistent over time instead of isolated lurches forward.

A question which interests me is the differentiating effects of this process of change. If technological change is cumulative and faster than the diffusion of knowledge, then differences between groups and individuals will grow. Exponential growth will lead to exponential growth of differences. Many poor nations are actually doing reasonably well, but compared to us in the West they appear almost static and the relative and absolute differences are increasing. Given this, guess who will afford the scientists, engineers, businessmen, and other people who will make growth even faster?

There is some evidence that at present researchers in many developing nations suffer a disadvantage given that they cannot afford to get the important journals in their areas, and their publications seldom get accepted in the global (Western) journals since they have few past publications cited by the citation services (Gibbs 1995).

There are equalizing forces too. Many of the results from expensive and time-consuming research appear openly in journals and on the Net, making it possible for others to leapfrog. There is trade. Technology spreads, and rich groups can and do give some of their surplus to others (voluntarily or not).

The problem is of course: are these forces enough to keep the differences in technological capability finite? Will this lead to a Singularity scenario where different groups diverge strongly from each other, possibly a situation where just one small group becomes totally technologically dominant?

We have to look at the factors that promote technological (and economical) differences, the balancing diffusive factors that decrease them, and their relative strength compared to the growth process.

Change

The term singularity is sometimes used loosely to denote an overall very fast and profound change in the social structure, economy, technology and possible nature of humanity, driven by technological change. It should be noted that there are many other factors causing change and growth than technological progress, such as the spread of new memes (for example making new forms of organization possible) and economic demand. What needs to be seen is if this process of change is self-supporting and will persist even at very high levels of change.

It is easy to note that many trends seen over the last millennia are roughly exponential, especially population and economic growth. They represent the explosion of homo sapiens from a pre-technological state to the current global civilization. The different forces of change are interwoven: improved technology give increased agricultural returns giving a larger population able to differentiate more and produce more technological and social inventions.

At the same time, this view of the "obvious" exponential growth of humanity in various areas should be taken with a big grain of salt. For example, the total human population is no longer increasing as fast as an exponential, and instead most population models suggest a gradual stabilization towards a steady state of around 11 billion within a century or so.

What has changed? Other factors have kicked in: when people have a better future to look forward to and a higher chance of their children surviving, they do not need to get as many children as before to ensure being provided for in old age (especially with pension systems and pension insurance, children are no longer needed but work is more important). Ideas about the need for family planning, female education and that the old customs no longer need to apply also play an important role.

This demonstrates that complex growth processes do not need to progress indefinitely, but may change in nature. For example, Moore's law seems to predict that processor density is increasing exponentially, and eventually will reach the nanoscale around 2020 or so. It is driven by industry expectations, the spread of computers into ever more niches and the growing need for computer power to fuel software that grows to take advantage of all available hardware power. But what if nanotechnology is slightly harder than many expect, and in 2020 there are no nanoscale elements ready? Let's assume they appear in 2030. During the 2020 decade, the forces driving Moore's law are likely to react to the changed situation. One possibility is that they weaken; industry expectations lessen and more efficient software that use available resources better is developed. Another possibility is that they drive technological development into new directions, for example the use of massively parallel systems of processors instead of more powerful single processors. By 2030, the technological landscape may be so different that even if nanotech chips are feasible, the development of the computer business (if it is still strong) has taken another direction.

After these caveats, back to the main question: is technological change cumulative?

A major and persistent force of technological development is the demand for solutions to old problems or the demand for new possibilities. To fill this demand new products are developed, creating new problems/possibilities as a side effect. This loop also provides a possibility to earn a living by facilitating it, for example by marketing the goods or discovering new demands, which introduces a group of people in whose rational self-interest it is to keep technological development going. In the end, a process that might have started due to the curiosity of a few problem-solvers and the problems of ordinary people have becoming a self-supporting growth process, where many different groups earn their living by keeping growth going (as well as some luddites making a living working against it).

This is a complex growth process, and it is undecidable if it will continue arbitrarily long into the future. However, it has been quite stable in its current form in western culture for several centuries, and on average going forward across the world for several millennia.

There have been relatively few instances of actual technological loss. Many individual techniques such as pyramid-building or making roman concrete have vanished when their respective civilizations collapsed, but overall a Greek engineer during the Hellenic era could do what the Egyptian engineers did centuries earlier plus some extra tricks, just as a modern engineer can do what the Greek engineer could do plus some extra tricks (if this is economically feasible is another question of course). Practically useful knowledge is generally passed on, and will only vanish if it becomes useless (for example due to lack of raw materials or demand), and even then it may remain in dormant form (e.g. encoded in impressive ruins or translated manuscripts). Overall, despite the rise and fall of many civilizations human knowledge has grown significantly over many millennia. A global disaster may of course cause a loss of many technologies that are dependent on a complex international economic and technological infrastructure, but unless it caused a profound change in how human societies work and develop that would be a temporary (if strong) tragedy.

Based on this it seems likely that we will see continued growth and acceleration at least for a few decades. If the current world economical-political-cultural system is radically changed, the rate of change induces strong resisting or orthogonal forces or new developments produce qualitative changes in development, the current process will of course change, but none of these appears to be imminent as yet, even if singularity discussions implicitly assume some of them will indeed occur relatively soon.

Difference and diffusion

Does change, and especially technological change, increase differences between people? This is argued by Freeman Dyson in *Imagined Worlds* (Dyson 1997: ch. 3). He points out that technology systematically emphasizes these differences: people with high education will get well-paying jobs (while unskilled labor is rapidly disappearing, leaving many without useful skills unemployed) and are more likely to get computers, hence their children will live in a significantly enriched environment with enough money and information to provide a good education that will make the advantage hereditary.

I'm skeptical of much of his argument, but his overall reasoning is sound: any new technology that only a few use and that gives an advantage will give these users an advantage over others, making it more likely they will get the next useful technology early.

This shows the importance of looking at technological diffusion together with technological adoption. Many shallow analyses (for example criticisms of germline genetic therapy based on the idea that it would lead to the rich becoming a genetic upper class) have ignored the spread of technology in society. This is especially important if the effects of the technology are longer-range; in the gene therapy example differences become noticeable only if technology spreads in society much slower than the human generation time of decades, which seems highly unlikely.

How fast is technology spreading through society? One way of analyzing it is to look at the number of people using a certain technology as a function of time, and look at the slope of the graph. Usually the graph looks like a sigmoid: an initial period of little spread, when the technology is being developed and explored by a few technophiles, rich novelty seekers, and in special settings, followed by a rising exponential slope when more and more people adopt the mature technology, followed by a ceiling when a large fraction of all people have it.

At least for these technologies the mean speed of adoption is increasing over time and the time between development to spread is shortening. A fast spread means that differences of technological access between people will become less pronounced.

As a simple example, take the cellular phone. It is still called "yuppie-nalle," "yuppie's teddy bear" in Swedish, as a reference to the period in the 1980s when it was almost only owned by the rich. But today a sizeable percentage of the Swedish population own a cellular phone, and they no longer have any social implications (snobs can always buy an exclusive phone, but owning a phone is no longer a demonstration of status).

If the trend suggested by the graph is true and continues, we can expect the spread of new technology between people to become ever faster, which limits the differences. But it is important to compare this to the speed with which new technologies emerge.

Technological diffusion occurs in many ways. One of the most common is trade: you buy advanced technology or know-how from others in exchange for goods or technology you have. Information trading is interesting because it is win-win: we both keep the information we sell or teach each other. Unequal pricing is of course still possible, but it is even more obvious with information that it is a non-zero sum game than in ordinary trade. It can be argued that advanced information is mainly traded between people with advanced information and not between them and people with little tradable information; this would accentuate the differences by making diffusion act mainly among the haves and not between the haves and have-nots.

On the other hand, the law of comparative advantage suggests that even a group with advanced capabilities would be better off trading with a less advanced group if they could specialize, enabling both to grow faster and profit from the cooperation. A more integrated world system enabling improved trade may hence act as a powerful incentive for information trading: the more you teach others, the better customers and partners they become. This is essentially the network economy described by *Wired*.

Another form of technological diffusion is simply learning from others in a friendly non-trading setting, for example by reading publications or asking. This can be a very powerful means of diffusion, as demonstrated by the scientific community. Over time an ethos of sharing results has developed that is very successful; even someone who has not contributed much can read the latest publications (especially if they are freely or easily available on the Net) and hence draw not just on their own knowledge base, but the common knowledge base of the entire community. Since it is a non-zero sum situation, free riders are a small problem.

Finally, there are limiting factors to fast growth, such as economic returns (if very few can afford a new technology it will be very expensive and not as profitable as a mass market technology), constraints on development speed (even advanced manufacturing processes need time for reconfiguration, development, and testing), human adaptability, and especially the need for knowledge. As the amount of knowledge grows, it becomes harder and harder to keep up and to get an overview, necessitating specialization. Even if information technologies can help somewhat, the basic problem remains, with the combinatorial explosion of possible combinations of different fields. This means that a development project might need specialists in many areas, which in turns means that there is a smaller size of group able to do the development. In turn, this means that it is very hard for a small group to get far ahead of everybody else in all areas, simply because it will not have the necessary know-how in all necessary areas. The solution is of course to hire it, but that will enlarge the group. One of the most interesting questions is how large the minimal group able to develop indefinitely is; the answer is likely somewhere between the entire world economy and the population of a small nation.

Are there technologies that strongly accentuate differences? The currently most obvious such technology is information technology. People with access to IT have an easier time finding out new information, including what new technologies to adopt. This makes it easier to remain at the forefront. On the other hand, access to information technology is increasing rapidly, so pure access isn't the main issue. Instead it becomes the ability to *use* the technology efficiently, to extract information from an ocean of data and to react to it that becomes central – information skills, critical thinking, and education become the areas where differences grow. If these skills can be amplified in some way, IT becomes more dividing.

On the other hand, IT might be a strongly diffusing technology be enabling faster and more global exchange of information, knowledge, and trade. One example is how the traditional scientific journal system is gradually turned into a quicker, more flexible, Net-based system of preprint servers and online journals, that limits publication delays and the problems of sending physical paper products across the world. Some journals are moving towards a "pay per article" policy (Biomednet), which would significantly lower the cost of getting relevant information, helping many poorer scientist communities.

It has been proposed that in the future nanotechnology will become an even more critical area. The scenario is that the people who learn to use it early will have a great advantage compared to late learners, and will develop extremely far in a short span of time. This presupposes that once nanotechnology is off the ground it will develop very fast in a cumulative way requiring relatively little investment of capital and intelligence from the user/buyer base, an assumption that is debatable. Just because you can make powerful nanodevices doesn't mean you can use them efficiently, and making something useful might also be very hard. My opinion is that just like computer technology it will develop fast, but given the ease and economic incentives of spreading nanotechnology it will be a quickly adopted technology (with some caveats for security and safety).

Some singularity discussions end up in scenarios of "dominant technologies," technologies that give the first owner practical unlimited power over all others. Some proposed dominant technologies are superintelligent AI, nanotechnology, or nuclear weapons. In the nuclear weapons case it was clear that they weren't dominant; the US could not enforce worldwide control over their development, and while the nuclear powers eventually managed to discourage proliferation it did not produce a power imbalance. In the same way it is unlikely that SI and nanotechnology will be developed in a vacuum; there will be plenty of prior research, competing groups, and early prototypes, which means it is unlikely any of these could become a dominant technology. In order to become a dominant technology the technology has to be practically unstoppable by any other technology (including simple things like hiding and infiltration); the owner must be so far ahead that they can preclude the development of any similar or competing technology, must be able to detect such developments, and, finally, clearly be willing to use the technology to achieve dominance even in the face of possible irrational counterattacks by desperate groups.

Conclusion

It seems likely that cumulative change will continue for the foreseeable future. This will lead to a situation where diffusive processes such as technology spread and trade compete with in homogenizing tendencies due to different rates of progress. It is not obvious which tendency will win in the long run: the current economic situation shows increasing relative differences, in-society technological diffusion appears to be speeding up and might be able to keep up with increased rates of innovation, the scientific community may or may not get more coherent due to new information tools that provide cheap information access. A more careful study of these questions and how they change over time is necessary to tell.

What can be said at present is that these examples do not demonstrate that homogenizing or non-homogenizing forces always win, but rather that it seems likely that the simple views often suggested about exponential change do not hold up well in real, complex growth situations.

In this discussion I have made few assumptions about intelligence amplification methods. They strongly increase the rate of growth, but they can also strongly increase diffusion. It is not obvious that they lead to differentiation or homogenization, just a great increase in the rate of growth. Other factors may bias the situation more, such as improved forms of trade, communication, and education.

Note

Vernor Vinge responded to many of the comments collected above. His thoughts and other comments posted on Extropy Institute's Extropians email list in 1998 can be found here: http://hanson.gmu.edu/vi.html.

1   Damien Broderick's book about the Singularity is *The Spike: Accelerating Into The Unimaginable Future* (Broderick 1997). His forthcoming book about drastic life extension and the impact of science on society is *The Last Mortal Generation* (Broderick 1999).

References

Asimov, Isaac (1991) *Foundation's Edge*. New York: Spectra.

Brin, David (1998) *The Transparent Society Will Technology Force Us To Choose Between Privacy And Freedom?* Boston: Addison-Wesley.

Brin, David (1991) *Earth*. New York: Bantam Books.

Broderick, Damien (1997) *The Spike: Accelerating Into The Unimaginable Future*. Australia: New Holland Books, p. 312.

Broderick, Damien (1999) *The Last Mortal Generation*. Australia: New Holland Books.

Dyson, Freeman (1997) *Imagined Worlds*. Cambridge, MA: Harvard University Press.

Hanson, Robin (1998) "Is a Singularity Just Around the Corner?" *Journal of Transhumanism* 2 (June). http://hanson.gmu.edu/fastgrow.html.

Gibbs, W. Wayt (1995) "Lost Science in the Third World." *Scientific American* (August).

Good, Irving J. (1965) "Speculations Concerning the First Ultraintelligent Machine." *Advances in Computers*, vol 6. New York: Academic press, pp. 31–88.

Kelly, Kevin (1995) "Singular Visionary." *Wired* 1.03 (July).

Scott, Ridley, dir. (1982) *Blade Runner*.

Tipler, Frank (1994) *The Physics of Immortality*. New York: Doubleday.

Vinge, Vernor (1992) *A Fire Upon the Deep*. New York: Tor Books.

Vinge, Vernor (1993) "The Coming Technological Singularity: How to Survive in the Post-Human Era." NASA VISION-21 Symposium.

Part IX

The World's Most Dangerous Idea

In a widely cited 2004 article in *Foreign Policy*, political scientist and neoconservative Francis Fukuyama described transhumanism as "the most dangerous idea in the world." He expanded on this claim in *Our Posthuman Future: Consequences of the Biotechnology Revolution*. Fukuyama is one of the most prominent of a growing number of critics who take the technological possibilities of transhumanism very seriously and who claim these possibilities to be undesirable. Fukuyama refers to transhumanism as a "strange liberation movement" and acknowledges that, given the deficiencies of the human race, the transhumanist project of wresting our "biological destiny from evolution's blind process of random variation and adaptation ... begins to look downright reasonable." Fukuyama quickly decides, however, that the offerings of self-applied technology "come at a frightful moral cost."

The final section of this book addresses this and related fears and engages the growing (and often ill-informed) critical discussion. Critical theorist and science fiction author Damien Broderick tackles Fukuyama's worries about the biotechnological revolution in his essay, "Trans and Post." In identifying a core goal of transhumanism as the defeat of aging and death, Broderick asks whether such a transhumanist victory over decay would be wicked (as many people assume) or a boon.

Taking the discussion into issues of evolution, in his essay "The Great Transition: Ideas and Anxieties," writer, philosopher, and critic Russell Blackford critiques Don Ihde's and Ted Peters' warnings about evolution and human nature. It seems possible and desirable to use new technologies to alter ourselves beneficially, leading to beings with greater-than-human capacities. Blackford asks why not simply go ahead? He considers anxieties relating to practical issues, timeframes, and possible abuses along with deeper worries about a "Great Transition" such as Martha Nussbaum's fear that we can have too much of a good thing.

The Transhumanist Reader: Classical and Contemporary Essays on the Science, Technology, and Philosophy of the Human Future, First Edition. Edited by Max More and Natasha Vita-More.
© 2013 John Wiley & Sons, Inc. Published 2013 by John Wiley & Sons, Inc.

In "A Letter to Mother Nature" (first presented as part of a talk at the 1999 Extropy Institute Biotech Futures conference) Max More expresses appreciation for what Mother Nature has made of humanity, while also noting that human biology is deeply flawed. With all due respect to our evolutionary origins, More suggests that it is time to amend the human constitution. A powerful method for making these changes will be nanotechnology.

Aesthetic theorist Roy Ascott explores the breakdown of our metaphors for nature and argues that, in any seeming paradox, it is technological and computerized systems which are providing us with a threshold, an open doorway into the natural world. The most advanced technologies, electronic and molecular, the very epitome of the artificial, could bring us back to nature.

In his statement for Extropy Institute's Vital Progress Summit in 2004, Ray Kurzweil points out that technology empowers both our creative and destructive natures. Awareness of these dangers has led to calls for broad relinquishment of technologies. These calls present an exaggerated picture of the perils by imagining future dangers as if they were released on today's unprepared world. In reality, the sophistication and power of our defensive technologies and knowledge will grow along with the dangers. Kurzweil believes the real lesson is that we will need to place society's highest priority during the twenty-first century on continuing to advance the defensive technologies and to keep them one or more steps ahead of destructive misuse.

38

The Great Transition
Ideas and Anxieties

Russell Blackford

What is Transhumanism?

Transhumanism is not a religion or a secular ideology. Consider the idea of religion. With some reservations, Charles Taylor defines it in terms of belief in an agency or power that transcends the operations of the natural world. Religion, then, relates to "the beyond," to an otherworldly, and in that sense transcendent, order of things (Taylor 2007: 15–20). Transhumanist philosopher Max More identifies the core of religion as "faith and worship," while other typical elements include "beliefs in supernatural forces, ceremony, a comprehensive view of life, and a moral theory or rule" (More 1990). By contrast with all this, transhumanism posits no "beyond": there are no gods, or supernatural powers or principles. Most typically, transhumanists embrace a naturalistic and purely secular worldview. In short, transhumanism is not a religion.

Nor is it a secular ideology: it has no body of codified beliefs and no agreed agenda for change. It is, instead, a broad intellectual movement – not so much a philosophy as a class or cluster of philosophical claims and cultural practices.[1] It is lively with internal debates and a hydra-headed contest to interpret its central ideas. But transhumanism has an intellectual core. It makes large claims – large enough and clear enough to provoke anxieties. One core idea is of human beings in *transition*: this word provides the "trans" in "transhumanism," "transhumanist," and their cognates. Transhumanists speak, too, of transcendence or transformations (but again, not of a "beyond" or a transcendent order). Transition, then, from what to what? Transcendence of what kind? What sort of transformations? Let me explain.

Dramatic advances in science and technology over the past few decades have culminated in widespread speculation that the human body itself, including its complex neurophysiology, may soon be open to conscious redesign. At some point, we may be able to make extensive modifications to human DNA, body tissues, or neurophysiological functioning, or to merge our bodies

The Transhumanist Reader: Classical and Contemporary Essays on the Science, Technology, and Philosophy of the Human Future, First Edition. Edited by Max More and Natasha Vita-More.
© 2013 John Wiley & Sons, Inc. Published 2013 by John Wiley & Sons, Inc.

with sophisticated cybernetic devices. Emerging technologies may give us, for example, higher levels of intelligence (however, exactly, that is understood); increased physical strength, stamina, and resistance to disease; extended longevity; and perhaps an enhanced capacity for empathy or other valued psychological traits. As technology goes inwards, altering the human body, it may grant us entirely new abilities.

Ultimately, transhumanists argue, technological intervention in the capacities of the human body and mind will lead to alterations so dramatic that it will make intuitive sense to call the deeply altered people of the near or not-so-near future *posthuman*: they will be continuous with us but unlike us in many ways. Optimistically, they might *be* us, greatly changed. On the transhumanist picture, we are not posthuman yet, but we are a bridge, or a rope, between historical humans and beings with posthuman capacities. The transformations we intend are transformations of ourselves. And what do we plan to transcend? Not the order of nature, but merely our own limitations.

These ideas are increasingly familiar and plausible. Though we cannot predict the future, the inward movement of technology is a present-day reality. Admittedly, most high-tech interventions in the body's functioning aim merely at restoring ordinary human health, or else at least opposing its decline. But that might easily change as our methods grow in power. Already, many interventions do much more than this, or something rather different. Consider the contraceptive pill, once so novel, but now so familiar. Female fertility is not an injury or disease, and the Pill is not (in its most common use) a treatment or a cure. Indeed, it suppresses a bodily function, but in a way that gives women greater power, helping them control when they can and cannot reproduce. Thus, it liberates the user in a way that goes beyond therapy.

Consider, too, a growing raft of enhancement technologies, from anabolic steroids to build muscle mass, to laser surgery that produces better-than-normal vision, to advanced prosthetic limbs that might be superior, at least for some purposes, to "ordinary" ones. These are mainly at a primitive stage of development, and many have their downsides – as with steroid use by bodybuilders and athletes. But imagine their growing sophistication. As we target and manage their effects, such technologies will become increasingly more attractive. Eventually, some will be socially accepted, much as the Pill is now, and much like "mere" tools such as cellphones or computers.

In the past, technology has *extended* the human body, providing it with tools to act upon the world. But at some point, a tool becomes something more. When does it become part of its user? Consider, for example, the cybernetic Braincaps depicted by Arthur C. Clarke in his novel *3001: The Final Odyssey* (1997). These are custom-built devices for each citizen of the future civilization that Clarke describes. They are deeply meshed with the brain's neuroanatomy by nanotechnological tendrils, becoming part of the body for most practical purposes – and their functioning becomes part of the individual's experienced self. Even this is a borderline case: we can imagine ever more intimate mergers of tools and natural bodies, and at some point a tool is really an enhancement, an alteration of the self.

Transhumanism adds one more core idea: that the Great Transition is beneficial, something to be welcomed. Transhumanism, then, does not merely describe the world. Transhumanist philosophies, rather, are philosophies of self-transformation and self-overcoming (More 2010). It's obvious, I hope, what can be said in favor of this. If changes to ourselves bring improvements, it's rational for us to make them. If technological interventions in the functioning of our bodies give us something we deeply desire, then we ought to seek them out.

Sketched in such an abstract way, transhumanism is intellectually attractive. The essential structure of ideas has a tight logic: we can use new technologies to alter ourselves beneficially, leading to beings with greater-than-human capacities. In principle, at least, this seems possible and desirable. Why not simply go ahead?

Anxieties

Prophecies of redesigned human bodies are not entirely new, and nor is the widespread disquiet that they evoke. The prophecies and the anxieties can be seen as part of a broader cultural debate – conducted over many centuries – between those who favor increased human under-standing and control of nature, and others who look on such projects as impious, hubristic, or impermissibly defiant of the given order of things.[2] What changed as the previous century unfolded was the practical power of technoscience. Increasingly, redesigning ourselves looks like a real option.

Some anxieties relate to practical issues, timeframes, and possible abuses. Concerns about these are reasonable and certainly need debate: the required technologies may be difficult to achieve, some may elude us indefinitely or turn out to be beyond our grasp. Some may be all too possible, if they fall into the wrong hands. These are reasons for caution in what we claim, and in what we plan and implement. But issues such as these are discussed with sophistication, and often with passion, within the transhumanist movement itself. Putting this aside for now, are there *deeper* problems with transhumanism and the promise of a Great Transition? Let's consider some possibilities.

We might, for one thing, challenge the notion of "improvement" or "enhancement" of human capacities. Wouldn't posthumans merely be *different*, not *better* by any objective test? In which case, why go to so much trouble? Alternatively, how much change in ourselves does it even make sense to want? Is a posthuman life a good life for beings who started out as human? And even if it is, can beings like us safely obtain it? Beyond certain limits, will we even be *us* if we undergo extraordinary change? I'll start with the issue of improvement.

The notion of an "improvement" need not rely on any implausible concept of one kind of functioning being better in an absolute or authoritative sense, independent of our actual prefer-ences or of what is needed for us to pursue our individual aims. Consider improvements to general health or to disease-resistance. It is possible to imagine bizarre examples where these are detrimental (perhaps a world where a mad dictator's police force hunts down the healthy and kills them), but there are innumerable real-life situations in which we might reasonably desire to retain or boost our health levels. Does that even need to be argued for? There is a certain joy, what's more, just in functioning healthily, and health is instrumentally valuable in a wide variety of situations that we encounter in many kinds of environments. Health is a form of power: possession of good health can assist us to function and act effectively. It can help us to achieve a wide range of personal goals, as well as to benefit those around us, our society as a whole, and other beings whose interests we wish to advance. It's a huge understatement to observe that for most of us, most of the time, there are good reasons to prefer health to its opposite and to prefer disease-resistance to susceptibility.

Or consider intelligence, which we can think of as a cognitive capacity – or a complex of related capacities – to reason quickly and accurately, understand difficult concepts, and solve problems. Again, we can imagine bizarre circumstances in which a particular person or class of people might find a high level of intelligence less a blessing than a curse. It is, however, some-thing that it's perfectly rational to want and to speak of "improving."

Possession of intelligence tends to lead to greater knowledge and to a better understanding of our particular situations, along with the ability to master techniques of inquiry that will enable us to increase our knowledge and understanding still further. If knowledge and understanding are valued for their own sake, intelligence gives us a more realistic prospect of obtaining them. In any event, it can enlarge our life possibilities, enabling us to carry out tasks that require understanding and problem-solving ability. We are better equipped to achieve a wide range of possible goals, since we are more likely to act from genuine knowledge of what means will be effective. Similarly, we are better equipped, in a very wide range of cases, to take actions that contribute to the wellbeing of others. Though not exactly a moral virtue, intelligence is a human excellence of value to almost anyone who possesses it.

Similar analyses could be offered for other characteristics, from visual acuity to physical strength. No characteristic is valuable to everyone no matter their existing desire sets and in every imaginable circumstance (no matter how fanciful). But many are valuable to most of us in a vast range of realistic environments. For most of us, most of the time, they are worth having and enhancing.

In a context rather different from debates around transhumanism, Martha Nussbaum raises a different concern. Can't we have too much of a good thing? Isn't there something wrong with trying to transcend humanity? Nussbaum appears to be thinking of efforts to transcend the naturalistic order, something that transhumanists don't propose. But could her approach be refocused to criticize transhumanism? Perhaps so. She suggests that a life with truly superlative capacities, such as immortality and invulnerability, would not be a life for us, and that we could not retain our identities while taking up such a life. We should struggle against our limitations, she thinks, but it's better not to have total success.

For Nussbaum, "human striving for excellence" involves pushing at the boundaries that constrain us. Thus, it is reasonable to want not to be hungry, ill, or without shelter, not to suffer betrayal or bereavement, or to lose one's faculties. It is reasonable, she thinks, to strive against such losses and also: "to strive to increase life expectancy, to eliminate as many categories of disease as possible, to strive to prolong any single life as best as one can." She explicitly rejects the idea that the desire to push back limits is itself illegitimate. Much of this sounds very transhumanist, as far as it goes.

Though she believes that it may not be coherent for us to wish for immortality, she thinks it reasonable to fear and avoid death "at any time when active living is still going on in a valuable way." She also notes, evidently with approval, that human life has taken on a different temporal shape for those able to avail themselves of medical and scientific progress: life has become longer and in some ways safer, though with "unforeseen dangers." More generally, Nussbaum admires what she calls "internal transcendence," a struggle against limits that is pursued from within our nature, though she is opposed to attempts at "external transcendence", supposedly an "aspiration to depart from human life altogether" (Nussbaum 1990: 380).

On this approach, the struggle against limits is like a struggle for victory in which we nonetheless do not want *complete* victory. We may hate and fear the death of a loved one, and do whatever we can to prevent it, while also recognizing "that a mortal life is the only life in which the people one loves could actually be." This tension is, says Nussbaum, "part of the best human life" (Nussbaum 1990: 381).

I feel sympathy for some of this, but is it a reason for anxiety that future societies will obtain a *more* complete victory over human limitations? I don't see why. Nor do I see how anything in Nussbaum's analysis supports a view that we should fear obtaining a more complete victory for ourselves, as individuals, via a series of stages. For example, it does not seem relevant to claim that the life of a sufficiently enhanced, perhaps immortal, being would not be *a human life*, and would not suit *us* as we are right now. Perhaps that is so – I'll accept it for argument's sake – but a life of greatly increased, or even infinite, duration might nonetheless be one that arises from a series of changes to ourselves, including initial transformations that *it would be human to desire*. Each further change might then be one that it was natural for us to desire, given our nature at the particular point we had reached immediately beforehand.

By analogy, when I was a young child I was a very different sort of being from what I am now. In one sense, it is true to say this: when I was 4 or 5 years old, the life of an adult was not a good life for *me*. That is, it would not have suited me as I was right then. I was not ready for it. However, I am physically and psychologically continuous with that same entity, and I think of myself as the same individual, though radically transformed. Through a series of changes, a child becomes an adult, and lives an adult's life. It can be a good life for the adult, though it would not have suited the child. That acknowledged, there is another sense in which adult life was, indeed, always a good life for the child … only not *yet*, and not for reasons that the child could fully understand (compare Walker 2008).

I suggest that we should not be disturbed at the prospect that we (or our descendants) might ultimately become beings whose capabilities and values are radically different from our own at the moment. Nussbaum repeatedly states that a more-than-human life would not be a good life for *us*, but I see no reason why it might not be a good life for the beings that *we could become* incrementally, beginning from decisions and changes that are indeed good ones for human beings. This brings me to Ted Peters' warnings about evolution and human nature (Peters 2008).

Evolution and Ethics

Peters, a theologian and bioethicist, acknowledges the altruistic policies proposed by transhumanists, but sees these as in tension with transhumanists' commitment to neo-Darwinian evolutionary theory. Transhumanists, he thinks, find themselves in opposition to the values of what he describes as earlier forms of evolutionary ethics, such as nineteenth-century Social Darwinism. All this, however, rests on serious misconceptions about evolutionary theory as well as transhumanism itself. I've answered Peters in a previous article (Blackford 2009: 9); here I'll be brief and take a slightly different tack.

Evolution has become the central organizing theory in the biological sciences. In its contemporary form, it's a synthesis of scientific developments since the mid-nineteenth century, drawing on Charles Darwin's masterpiece, *On the Origin of Species* (1859), but also on more modern work in genetics and many other fields. It explains life's diversity and the complex functioning of our planet's vast number of life forms, which it depicts as the products of gradual change over many millions of generations. On this picture, as elaborated since Darwin's time, the first life forms appeared three to four billion years ago, and have since evolved through the stages shown in the fossil record, up to the present day.

Evolutionary scientists investigate a number of mechanisms by which life may have evolved and branched into numerous taxa, but the central mechanism remains that proposed by Darwin, i.e. natural selection. As understood by contemporary biologists, this involves the differential success of different combinations of genes in reproducing themselves through the generations. Less accurately, but perhaps more intuitively, we can think of some life forms out-competing others for survival and reproduction. *We*, for example, are descended from unbroken sequences of animals that lived long enough to pass down their genes. This picture explains how highly complex organisms emerge over long periods of time, but there is nothing to suggest that average complexity of organisms must increase or that the process has any inbuilt direction.

All this leads to two important points. First, transhumanists are committed to the truth of biological evolution, but they are not special in that regard. Since the central claims of evolutionary theory are well established, any rational, scientifically informed account of morality must at least be *consistent* with them. In that respect, transhumanism has no special handicap. If evolutionary theory somehow necessitated ruthless social policies, that would be a problem for everyone, not a fault with transhumanism. But secondly, there is no such problem. Whatever the nineteenth-century Social Darwinists might have thought, evolutionary theory does not entail any particular values or require a particular set of policies. It certainly does not support a policy of ruthless competition. Any social implications that is has are bound to be indirect and complex.

What can be stated with some confidence is that human sociability is fundamental to us – not imposed through prudential calculations and deliberate formation of a social contract. Doubtless we evolved certain broad psychological proclivities, but the extent to which we have an ingrained psychological makeup is controversial. We may well have a strong tendency to act in our self-interest as individuals, and in the interests of our children, other family members, and those whom we see as allies. But we also seem to have a sympathetic responsiveness to others, even to the sufferings of non-human animals. It seems apparent, from common observation as much any distinctively scientific reasoning, that we are neither angels nor demons. Rather, we have a hybrid or mixed nature that includes the capacities for both compassion and destructiveness.

Where does this get us? To the extent that some forms of evolutionary ethics have attempted to leap from a (dubious) claim that evolution is a process of ruthless competition to the idea that human societies should be like that, there is no shame in disagreeing with them. No such argument can work, and there is no reason why transhumanists should accept them. And even if propensities to certain kinds of competitive behavior enhanced the reproductive fitness of our distant ancestors, this does not entail that they advance our current, reflectively endorsed, values. A more modest claim, one that I'd support, is that any workable system of moral norms must meet the needs of beings like us, with our hybrid nature. It will need to allow considerable scope for individuals to pursue their own interests and happiness, but within deontic constraints. It will not condemn all pursuit of self-interest as "sinful," but nor will it value ruthlessness.

There is no need for transhumanists to adopt any implausible or politically troublesome account of the relationship between evolution and morality. While transhumanists may acknowledge that we have an evolved psychological nature, this does not entail that our nature is highly rigid, relatively unaffected by culture and environment. Nor does it entail such exploded Social Darwinist doctrines as that we should accept the social dominance of the strong and the subordination of the weak. There is nothing in the relationship between evolution and ethics, properly understood, that is inconsistent with the aspirations of many transhumanists to better the human condition.

Naïvety about Progress

Peters likewise argues that transhumanists are naïve about technology, human nature, and especially the prospect that things will always get better. To support his claim of naïvety about progress, he offers an interesting, but clearly flawed, argument. He begins by distinguishing between the notion of a future that emerges from the present (*futurum*) and the notion of a future that can be brought into being only by the intervention of God (*adventus*). He insists that transhumanists are committed to *futurum* rather than *adventus*. But, so he claims, a commitment to *futurum* depends upon a prior commitment to a doctrine of progress. Therefore, transhumanism depends upon a doctrine of progress. But, so he says, such a doctrine is naïve. Therefore, transhumanists are naïve when they rely on it.

This is all terribly muddled. Most transhumanists are committed to the idea that the future emerges from the present in a naturalistic way without the need for divine intervention, and through (among other things) advances in knowledge and technology. Transhumanism itself posits no supernatural agencies, powers, or principles. But none of this implies a naïve or implausible idea of progress. The future may emerge through naturalistic processes, but that is even consistent with it being worse than the present and the past! A naturalistic approach to history does not, in itself, rule out fearing the future or expecting dangers and challenges.

Peters is, of course, correct that any new technologies will sometimes be used spitefully or malevolently, and that they will typically be used for self-interested purposes. He is impressed by what he sees as humanity's essential sinfulness: "something at work in the human mind leads to the development of brute and unmitigated destruction." To support this, he refers to the phenomenon of computer viruses, strings of code that are, as he expresses it, created "with one sole purpose, namely, to destroy." But this is unconvincing outside of a theological framework that emphasizes sin. It overlooks the fact that most computer users do *not* create viruses or look on their effects with glee. Quite the opposite. If Peters thinks that malevolence, spiteful glee in others' discomfort, and so on are hallmarks of human nature – in the sense that humans are *always*, or *typically*, like that – he is seriously mistaken. He is operating with a philosophical anthropology that is unrealistically blind to the strong human propensities for sympathy, cooperation, and compromise.

He's on stronger ground when he writes of the inevitability that new technologies will be used by individuals and corporations for self-interested purposes. But that is a very different point. As I've explained, realistic systems of morality do not condemn all self-interested actions as morally impermissible or "sinful"; they require only that self-interest be pursued subject to certain conditions, or within certain boundaries. Acting in one's own self-interest should not, in itself, be regarded as morally wrong or a "sin." People who are largely motivated by self-interest can still flourish side by side in reasonable and mutually productive cooperation. The important questions are whether fair deontic constraints on the pursuit of self-interest can be set by human societies and, if so, whether most people will abide by them most of the time. Here, I see no need at all for pessimistic answers: indeed, if we were *that* "sinful" human society would be impossible.

That said, we do have limitations, including our limited natural altruism. In any event, we should temper optimism with realism. We don't know what is achievable, and we can agree with Peters when states: "In sum, we should move forward, but we should not presume progress in every respect is inevitable or guaranteed." Similarly, we can acknowledge such points as the following, which I draw from Don Ihde's critique of transhumanism (Ihde 2008). Whether or not Ihde would agree with my formulation of them, these points appear highly plausible:

1. In the real world, technological advances involve compromises and trade-offs.
2. Technological advances take place in unexpected ways and find unexpected uses.
3. Implanted technologies have disadvantages as well as advantages: e.g., prostheses and implants are often experienced as imperfect and obtrusive, and they wear out.
4. Predictions about future technologies and how they will be incorporated into social practice are unreliable.

But as I've noted elsewhere, these are *trite* truths about technology.[3] If they are not explicitly stated in existing transhumanist theories and manifestos, it is more likely that leading transhumanist thinkers find them obvious than that they disagree. In any event, all of these cautionary points could just as easily be advanced *within* the transhumanist movement as outside it. As I mentioned earlier, transhumanists are mindful that change is risky, and they frequently discuss the risks and consider ways to reduce them (e.g. Bostrom 2002). Some transhumanists may be naïve about the ease with which the Great Transition will, or can, take place, and some may specify unworkable schemes. If so, Peters' critique may apply to them as individuals.

Perhaps there are many such individuals, but they are not transhumanism.

The Apocalyptic Temptation

As I stated at the beginning, transhumanism makes large claims. It imagines enormous changes, changes that it sees as inviting. This leads me to a final anxiety. Many progressive movements of the past seem like horrible mistakes in retrospect, and some produced atrocities. However needed it was, the French Revolution sank into slaughter and chaos, while various forms of communism proved monstrous when put into practice. Older systems of thought, such as the world's religious monotheisms, have been, repeatedly, authoritarian, imperialist, and persecutorial. For traditional Christians and Muslims, much is at stake, not least the difference between Heaven and Hell. For many churches and sects, both past and present, that has justified almost any means to their ends.

One of history's lessons is to beware of apocalyptic thought systems that claim the endorsement of God or History. If God or History are on your side, demanding cataclysmic change, your ends can suggest terrible means. No one has been imprisoned, sterilized, starved, or burned at the stake in the name of transhumanism, and perhaps it will never happen. Transhumanists have no Heaven and Hell, no other world, or canons of conduct, or comprehensive creed. That is all reassuring. The danger, though, is if History becomes their God.

Most transhumanist thinkers are politically liberal, in the Millian tradition, and many are downright libertarian. To varying degrees, they distrust the power of the state and avoid grand programs and narratives. For transhumanists, self-transformation is something to choose, not a practice to be imposed on fellow citizens. Max More, for example, writes:

> One of the great tasks before us, as transhumanists, is the reengineering of our consciousness to do away with the powerful desire for certainty of a dogmatic kind. Most humans feel that they cannot bear to be wrong. They fear an unknown future. (More 1990)

We should, this suggests, change *ourselves* to end our hunger for certainty. Even that is a voluntary step, and transhumanisms (plural) seek to guide us, not coerce us, into the unknown. But this is a young movement that already takes various forms. Some transhumanisms promise a Heaven on Earth, and there's plenty of time for these to harden into dogma – like so many other visionary systems of thought. That danger can be avoided, but only with awareness and self-scrutiny. While elbowing for political space to pursue their chosen goals, transhumanists must resist their own temptations to illiberalism.

On that understanding, we should welcome transhumanism, with all its hope, with its courage and commitment to reason, and its shimmering vision of an open-ended, brilliant future.

Notes

1   More (1990) defines it as "a class of philosophies that seek to guide us towards a *posthuman* condition" (emphasis in original).
2   Part of this story is told in Haynes 1994.
3   For more detail on this, and on other arguments in this section, see Blackford 2009.

References

Blackford, Russell (2009) "Trite Truths About Technology: A Reply to Ted Peters." *The Global Spiral* 9 (February), p. 9. http://www.metanexus.net/magazine/tabid/68/id/10681/Default.aspx.

Bostrom, Nick (2002) "Existential Risks: Analyzing Human Extinction Scenarios and Related Hazards." *Journal of Evolution and Technology* 9/1 (February). http://www.jetpress.org/volume9/risks.html.

Clarke, Arthur C. (1997) *3001: The Final Odyssey*. London: HarperCollins.

Haynes, Roslynn D. (1994) *From Faust to Strangelove: Representations of the Scientist in Western Literature*. Baltimore and London: Johns Hopkins University Press.

Ihde, Don (2008) "Of Which Human Are We Post?" *The Global Spiral* 9/3 (June). http://www.metanexus. net/magazine/tabid/68/id/10552/Default.aspx.

More, Max (1990) "Transhumanism: Towards a Futurist Philosophy." *Extropy* 6 (revised 1996). http://www. maxmore.com/transhum.htm.

More, Max (2010) "The Overhuman in the Transhuman." *Journal of Evolution and Technology* 21/1 (January), pp. 1–4. http://jetpress.org/v21/more.htm.

Nussbaum, Martha C. (1990) "Transcending Humanity." In *Love's Knowledge: Essays on Philosophy and Literature*. New York: Oxford University Press, pp. 365–391.

Peters, Ted (2008) "Transhumanism and the Posthuman Future: Will Technological Progress Get Us There?" *The Global Spiral* 9/3 (June). http://www.metanexus.net/magazine/tabid/68/id/10546/Default. aspx.

Taylor, Charles (2007) *A Secular Age*. Cambridge, MA: Harvard University Press.

Walker, Mark (2008) "Cognitive Enhancement and the Identity Objection." *Journal of Evolution and Technology* 18/1 (May), pp. 108–115. http://jetpress.org/v18/walker.htm.

39

Trans and Post

Damien Broderick

TRANSHUMAN: Someone actively preparing for becoming posthuman. Someone who is informed enough to see radical future possibilities and plans ahead for them, and who takes every current option for self-enhancement

POSTHUMAN: Persons of unprecedented physical, intellectual, and psychological capacity, self-programming, self-constituting, potentially immortal, unlimited individuals.[1]

Everyone has mixed feelings about the future, especially about the many powerful technologies changing our world – and us as well. Trash TV excites us with visions of bionic limbs for the helpless, robot puppies craving attention but never messing the carpet, painless laser dentistry, clones, and weird genetic hybrids. And up pops the lazy, weary cliché again, now a human life-time old: Brave New World!

If few have read Aldous Huxley's satire (it is immensely important, but rather dull), everyone knows what is meant: a future of sedated, giggly hedonists cloned like sheep then decanted from bottles. In 1932, when it caused its first sensation, we had no cloned sheep. Now we await cloned babies any day. Children rushed to watch George Lucas's *Attack of the Clones*. Anxiety rife on the silver screen! Meanwhile, maddened children, deluded fanatics, and terrorists like Theodore Kaczynski (the Unabomber) murder with homemade bombs or stolen passenger jets to express their distaste for this relentless and unprecedented future that has exploded, as it were, into reality.

It was refreshing, then, in 2002, to find a public intellectual of Dr. Francis Fukuyama's standing take on the intensely real, serious topic of accelerating biotechnology. Instant fame had embraced Fukuyama a decade earlier when his conservative *The End of History* (Fukuyama 2006) seemed

This essay is adapted from *Ferocious Minds: Polymathy and the New Enlightenment* (Borgo Press, 2005).

The Transhumanist Reader: Classical and Contemporary Essays on the Science, Technology, and Philosophy of the Human Future, First Edition. Edited by Max More and Natasha Vita-More.
© 2013 John Wiley & Sons, Inc. Published 2013 by John Wiley & Sons, Inc.

to explain the Soviet Union's abrupt collapse. Liberal humanism – democratic, realistic, and market-driven rather than authoritarian – had won the cold war against its authoritarian and deludedly utopian foes. Why? Because, Fukuyama argued, it worked in harmony with human nature. Hardly a new thesis, nor a watertight one, but pundits embraced it with relish and a sigh of relief.

In subsequent books, Fukuyama looked at the pivotal need, in such a political order, for civil trust, observing that human dignity and accurate recognition of each citizen's value were crucial to civic health. Dignity's source, interestingly, was not a God-given special status for humankind; indeed, he claimed in *The Great Disruption* (Fukuyama 1999: 166), "a great deal of social behavior is not learned but part of the genetic inheritance of man and his great ape forebears." It is our species nature, our evolved essence as humans rather than sheep or wolves, that grants us those general rights which flourish best under global capitalism.

Fukuyama went on to extend that analysis into the future, toward the recommencement of a history he had deemed effectively at an end. Rather belatedly, he realized the obvious: "there can be no end of history without an end of modern natural science and technology," and that is not likely. Indeed, "we appear to be poised at the cusp of one of the most momentous periods of technological advance in history" (Fukuyama 2003: 15).

Quite so; probably these thunderously converging technologies will comprise an ever-steepening escalator of radical change. From early transhuman adoption of patches and revamps for our luckless fatal condition, we might shift to a genuinely posthuman state where augmented people meet or perhaps blend with AI minds still in the early stages of development. Until quite recently this was a speculation widely scorned as far-fetched and psychologically insupportable. How remarkable, then, to find a thinker of Dr. Fukuyama's conservative credentials adopting just this view – while warning us, inevitably, of the urgent need to stop it before we go blind.

Libertarians, greedy corporations, and scientists hungry for their cut, Fukuyama argued, will baulk at restriction and regulation, but that is what we must put in place, and the sooner the better (2003: 184–6). Only government can perform this service. Ideally all the world's regimes must combine to outlaw radical transformations of the human genome, or less drastic options such as pre-implantation embryo selection that lets parents choose their healthiest possible children. Many people agree without hesitation, drawing upon the Leon Kass-ian wisdom of the "Yuck factor." How disgusting! Yet the same yuck factor that allegedly deters decent folks from cloning ourselves propped up racist discrimination, homophobia, and prejudice against the disabled. Years hence, it might seem as offensive to title a big box-office movie *Attack of the Clones* as to imagine one (perhaps filmed in 1932) called *Attack of the Negroes*, or *Attack of the Jews*. Cloned humans will be human, even those who are posthuman.

So, too, will ageless humans – people with extra genes, say, designed to keep their cellular DNA ship-shape – although Fukuyama has his doubts. Just as Prozac and Ritalin smooth out human passions, he worries that science will corrode our sacred nature (Fukuyama 2003: 41–56). The detailed core of his small book is an argument, unfashionable in the antihumanist humanities but increasingly accepted in the life sciences, that certain species-typical characteristics are shared by all humans. This inviolable human nature provides the basis for our dignity. Citing the Pope approvingly, Fukuyama seems ready to affirm that a non-material soul gets inserted into our rude flesh, but he pulls back into metaphor: all that matters is that "some very important ... leap" occurred during evolutionary history, and recurs during gestation (2003: 170). No doubt, but why would this make more-than-ordinary human beings somehow less than human?

"Much of our political world rests on the existence of a stable human 'essence' ... We may be about to enter into a posthuman future, in which technology will give us the capacity gradually to alter that essence over time" (2003: 217). Images of *Star Trek*'s emotionless, half-alien Mr. Spock recur, with no explanation why enhanced and perhaps superintelligent people should be *less*, rather than *more richly*, emotional and benevolent. Fukuyama just feels in his bones that such technological progress "does not serve human ends" (2003: 222), that it must create ever more terrible rifts between rival genetic haves and have-nots.

Yes, that is clearly one possibility, but the claim reminds me of Marx's failed theory of the inevitable immiseration of capitalism's poor. My parents were working stiffs who raised six children in comparative poverty. Gazing now at my big computer screen and drinking my microwaved beverage, hardly well-off but only by today's swollen standards, I rather doubt it. Wealth derived from knowledge, especially the kind that improves health and lifespan, tends to spread ever more widely – as it is doing even in the Third World.

Fukuyama ignores, or dismisses, the prospect of widespread abundance via nanotechnology (molecular manufacture) and AI, yet these are no more unlikely than the advanced biotechnology that frightens him. And yes, "a person who has not confronted suffering and death has no depth" (2003: 173), yet we do not welcome anthrax for its existential spritzig. Despite the excellence of Fukuyama's summary of the state of play in biotechnology and the laws constraining it, he forgets that "the freedom of political communities to protect the values they hold most dear" (2003: 218) often has been a charter for ignorance and fearful bigotry. Stigmatizing the posthuman before they arrive, and the transhumanists already here, is hardly the wisest choice, nor the most humane.

Everyone wishes to be fully human, but the definition of humanity changes as we learn more and more. Consider this fairytale of a future sex education class:

Today, children, we'll talk about human reproduction. No sniggering, please. Yes, even in this year 2050 we are speaking of S-E-X, but today's lesson will not deal with smut. We'll discuss how babies are made.

To make a baby we need a Mummy, who provides a big fat ovum crammed with food and DNA and energy-making mitochondria which she got from her own Mummy, and a Daddy, who puts in a tiny little chunk of DNA coded either male or female. Finally, we have an Optimist. This medical specialist is known in California as a Clinical Optimalizator.

The cells from Mummy and Daddy each contain 22 strings of nearly identical instructions for starting a baby, plus the sex-making string. In the bad old days, these messages written in DNA were often garbled in places, like a buggy computer program. Babies that began with really messy code – three or four out of every five – aborted spontaneously or died long before they were born. Once medical cures for damaged code were found, nearly all the babies that got started went on to become people. The Pope banned the evil sin of "bestial congress", which was reproductive S-E-X as animals do it. So many souls were being lost! Today, only filthy perverts and criminals risk making babies the dangerous, godless old way.

This is where the Optimist comes in. She sorts through Mummy's and Daddy's cells with a gene chip and picks out those with the fewest bad mutations. Then she pops in a pair of safe artificial chromosomes to proof-read any remaining errors, correct mangled instructions, and add the optimal extra genes that help us resist infection and mental illness, think really fast, and live for a very long time without getting old and silly. Yes, Janey, she *could* choose whether the baby is a boy or girl, but that is illegal, of course.

How absurd is this scenario – mine, but based on Gregory Stock's *Redesigning Humans: Choosing our Children's Genes* (Stock 2003) – of a possible future? Stock is a biophysics PhD, Harvard MBA, and director of the Program on Medicine, Technology and Society at the School of Medicine at UCLA. Bear in mind that *in vitro* fertilization was first performed successfully as recently as 1978. Still, you might consider "Optimist" technologies and social reactions unthinkable even for 2100-plus. That is as far into tomorrow as our world is from Edwardian, pre-Great War 1910, an era that accepted scandalous social inequities. Is 2020 or 2030 laughably too soon? Perhaps, but some of those novelties already exist, in a small way. Stock's approachable, humane book leads us warily but with resolve into an impending world where traditional woes of the flesh are healed by science, while many troubling or delightful opportunities jump from myth into the clinician's regular work day.

Yet even if we can rewrite our genetic code and add auxiliary chromosomes packed with advantages, won't people turn away, disgusted? Perhaps not. The Amish are notorious for their strict traditional disdain for consumerist fads and such futuristic technologies as cars and TV. Small, inbred communities, they suffer terrible genetic afflictions such as Crigler-Najjar syndrome, a potentially fatal loss of a liver enzyme gene. Somatic cell treatment, inserting corrective genes into disease victims, is being trialed with enthusiasm by these technology skeptics.

As for artificial chromosomes designed to augment our inherited, badly corrupted DNA – crammed with "junk," hitch-hiking viruses, and copying errors carried along for the ride over millions of years – these are used routinely in lab bacteria and yeast. Early versions suitable for human insertion exist. Would adding such novelties to embryos be ethical? Suppose the new genes prove disastrous? Stock is reassuring. Already, elegant methods are at hand to control or delete annexed genes.

Activate the enzyme CRE, and it searches a DNA strand for a gene sequence called loxP, makes a snip, finds the next copy, makes another snip, throws away the stuff from the middle and sutures up the ends. If the discarded portion is your new gene, it will not trouble you again (Stock 2003: 71). Here is the beauty of that method: CRE does not exist naturally in humans. It is an optional switch. You could take it as a pill. Other pills could activate a dormant gene.

Genes usually lie doggo until a special cascade of substances switches on a control sequence. We might inject into a one-celled embryo a batch of genes designed to switch on at maturity but not before. After normal childhood and adolescence, they could be toggled optionally to ensure healthy extended adulthood, or left inactive. A reckless suggestion? But already we routinely inoculate babies, and most are grateful for that opportunity to shield their children from dreadful risks. Some 1 percent of today's children are conceived *in vitro*, outside the human body. Three in 10 births are by Caesarean section, hardly "natural." We are not in Kansas anymore, Toto, and have not been for years.

Will such person-sculpting powers lead to narrow uniformity, as every couple shapes their next kid in the envied likeness of David Letterman, Richard Nixon, or Elle McPherson? Or might an array of freaks appear, Olympic swimmers with duck feet and gills, or hormone-charged giants spouting Dante and M-theory? More likely, Stock advises us, germinal choice technology (GCT) will start by removing some causes of human misery: "the polio vaccine did as much and brought few complaints" (Stock 2003: 193). New issues arise. Today some deaf people want deaf children. GCT enables their selection. Perhaps these worrying choices really must be left to parents – unless preference amounts to plain child abuse, or truly endangers society.

Stock deals deftly with such unnerving topics, countering Fukuyama's demand for state control of these technologies. Cautiously, he skips the truly challenging options some predict for this era of accelerating, convergent discoveries. Fukuyama, to my mind chillingly, observes: "The original purpose of medicine is … to heal the sick, not to turn healthy people into gods" (Fukuyama 2003: 212). If humans are to be redesigned, we and our children, through our choices, will be the architects. I vote for Chartres Cathedral or a Jorn Utzon opera house rather than a drab high-rise.

The true goal of transhumanism is the defeat of aging and death. It is a Promethean ambition, but increasingly we see steps in that direction. Would such a transhumanist victory over decay be wicked (as many people assume) or a boon?

Death in aggregate tends to move us less fiercely than the passing of a loved one, or even of a pet. In the face of death as the reaper of millions we do not know, our kindest emotions sag beneath "compassion fatigue." And for the young, death and its mimicry can also provide the wildest of thrills. Healthy young gangs of men travel great distances to maim each other in soccer game riots, just for the pleasure of it. Vivid computer simulations allow youths, and not only youths, to obliterate imaginary foes in gory detail – even to flash whole cities or worlds into nuclear fire. We embrace what terrifies us most. Or we ignore and suppress it. But death will not go away – unless we make it go away.

For the first time since single-cell life coalesced on this planet, we are perhaps within reach of doing just that.

Cautious skeptics regard the claim that death might be defeated within 30 or even 100 years as evidence of emotional arrest at the stage of denial. Death is so terrible, they say, so final, so unappeasable, that naïve science groupies flee from its implacability into a fantasy of technical redemption or reprieve. Indeed, the environmentalist writer Bill McKibben has addressed my own case for the abolition of inevitable aging and death in just these terms. In his eloquent but profoundly confused tract *Enough: Staying Human in an Engineered Age* (2003), McKibben states without feeling any need for supporting argument that Robert Ettinger and Hans Moravec and Gregory Stock and Robert Freitas and I advocate healthy life extension without our understanding how "weird or gross or boring" living forever would be (2003: 156). Indeed, he assumes we are afraid of dying, rather than outraged by death's waste. He calls us "true believers" (2003: 85) and "unhinged by death" (2003: 147) when we point out that sometime in the medium-term future mortality will become optional. Yet McKibben does not dispute that this will become technically possible. The wish not to senesce and then die (at 80 or so, presumably, rather than humankind's traditional 25 or 35 or 55) is ipso facto "unhinged." It offends against "gut feelings."

True, no method recommended by science – or by magic, affirmation, or prayer, for that matter – has managed so far to extend human life beyond the naturally evolved limit of about 120 years. But what has changed lately is that geneticists have extended the lifespan of at least some living creatures, such as nematode worms, allowing them to live as much as seven times longer than their unmodified kin. This is not yet the abolition of death – but it looks very much like the first step toward that goal. Cynthia Kenyon, who made these discoveries, comments in an interview in *New Scientist* in 2003:

> People have shown that the system first found in worms controls longevity in fruit flies and mice. That means it had to evolve early in a common precursor of mice, flies and worms. In genetics everything else that has been found to be true in mice, flies and worms has also been found in

humans – with variation, of course, but the basic system is the same. We don't know for sure yet, but on rational scientific grounds the chances are very high.

Suppose this remarkable claim is correct. The very possibility forces us to ask a quite profound question: Must thinking about death in the somewhat remote and clinical mode of science distract us from the fundamental agony of loss whose truest answering voice is music and the hard-edged melodies of poetry? I am not one to dismiss the power of the arts; I have been publishing fiction for more than 40 years, and hope to go on doing so for centuries yet – if I'm lucky, if I don't die too soon (as seems likely on statistical grounds), if science learns how to repair the ravages of aging – a trick performed by every new baby, created from old cells in its parents' bodies.

I believe we are justified in confronting death with knowledge and determination, rather than trying to appease it by mythic verse and surrender. But solving death, and life, is not just a technical project. It embraces everything that makes us human. The first immortal generation will not be the children of science alone, but of law, art, music, writing – all the humane arts.

When health and youthfulness are prolonged into the hundreds of years, will ordinary life, as we know it, persist? Almost certainly not. After all, an extremely high-tech future is needed to support such medical triumphs, and that will create other unexpected discontinuities. In my book *The Spike* (2001), I tried to sketch how the workforce will alter. The Great Recession at the end of the first decade of this century is to some extent an effect of these changes, although it is rarely seen as such. Swiftly accelerating change in supercomputers, genomics, and nanotechnology will ensure that by 2050 very few jobs will remain unchanged, and many will be gone for good. Most of today's work will be either gone or on the verge of vanishing, done by smart machines using molecular manufacturing techniques still on the computer monitor today.

So we will need to reorganize the economic bases of society, and nobody should expect that to be easy or painless – but the ageless will not face today's problems writ large. They will have problems of their own, no doubt, but new ones. Constructing utopia (and preventing horrific local warfare between restless new tribes and gangs) will give them something to do with all their free time…

Bill McKibben (like Leo Kass, and most others on former President Bush's Bioethics Committee) is appalled by the prospect. "But you can't 'enjoy the gift of life' forever. Maybe with these new tools you can live forever, but the joy of it – the meaning of it – will melt away like ice cream on an August afternoon. It is true that nothing short of these new technologies will make us immortal, but immortality is a fool's goal. Living must be enough for us, not living forever" (2003: 161).

My notion of joy is a little less saccharine than ice cream on an August afternoon, which is admittedly pleasant but not to die for, and I find McKibben's confident insight into the spiritual misery and existential emptiness of people 1,000 years old entirely amazing. How can he *know* these things with such certainty? And how can he know that there will be no cure for the ailment (the achingly empty misery) that he just knows must afflict the optionally undying? I am not saying confidently that he is wrong – I don't know either. But his hubris in demanding that the gate be barred in our faces is breathtaking … literally.

The world of emortals surely will be increasingly strange. Many people will bend, eventually, under the shock of relentless change. Some of those will simply choose, either in despair or with dignity, to remove themselves from the project of endless life. That must be their privilege. But they will be missing out on some very interesting and rewarding times.

McKibben's certainty might derive from his traditional Christian beliefs. Isn't the ambition to attain indefinite life seen, in and of itself, as an affront to God, a new impious Tower of Babel? I do not see why. The longer we have to savor the rich joys and tests of earthly life, the more opportunities we gain to mature, to love, help, build, to take and share responsibility. Life is as replete and meaningful as we make it, and if we can share in the glories of the world for a thousand years instead of a mere 70 or 80, I cannot imagine that a loving deity (if there is one) would resent our tenure here, or punish us for living well and long.

Within that passionate quest for understanding, we will surely also seek to nourish the quiet, serene arts of living well, and – if death is, after all, finally unavoidable, however long postponed – of dying well.

And in the meantime? How tragic to stand under the shadow of the executioner's sword even as the pardon is being rushed to us! If its sharp blade falls, we are as dead and gone as any peasant or priest or king in the suffering, long history and prehistory of the world. Plainly, the only prudent move is to do everything possible to forestall accidental or infective death during the next decade or three, and to adopt as many healthy practices as we can manage without altogether giving up on the vivid texture of life.

That much is under the individual's control. Social and political factors play a larger role. Mortality rates vary shockingly between nations and even states or regions within nations. If we mean to ensure the best feasible health for everyone, we need to start with the basics. Enough food and supplements for mothers and infants. Sufficient for the rest of the community as well. Clean water and air. Modern sanitation. Immunization programs. Decent medical and dental care.

The most frightening apartheid one could imagine is a future world in which extended life is allowed only to a few – the very wealthy, the political elite and their chosen followers, Mafia, military, scientists, sports heroes, movie stars. This is not the transhumanist objective – far from it. It is up to all of us to ensure that this segmented future never happens. We will not best prevent it by denouncing technical advances and trying to blockade them, but in thinking hard, feeling deeply and wisely, debating the issues together, and acting as free men and women.

If we choose to enhance the human condition, to mitigate as best we can the horrors and blunders blind evolution has imposed, that will be a step toward diversity in unity, one taken in the confidence that old tyrannies were marked exactly by ferocious control and interdiction of knowledge. A deathless society denied a free flow of information, and opportunities to choose, would indeed be dismal. We must ensure that the form of the future is not foreclosed by panic or mistrust. For doubters like McKibben, the pursuit of indefinite healthy longevity would be the slippery slope to the final erosion of meaning from our (formerly) mortal lives. That meaning, allegedly, derives from our transience and continuity with the rest of the natural world. This does not mean, somehow, that we have to give up reading or wearing clothes, even though sparrows and worms and bacteria cannot do that. How so? The argument falls away into a shrugging posture: if you don't see (or feel) why, evidently, it obviously shows how spiritually bankrupt you must already be.

For those of us who are now alive, the astonishing difference from the past is that we really do have a chance, finally. The twentieth century witnessed cruel oppression and phoenix recovery again and again, most poignantly perhaps in the survivors of the Holocaust. Millions died, but some prevailed even in those hellish conditions. Perhaps it will be that way for us, too, faced by the cruelty of evolution's strategies of death. We must live as vividly as we may, while life is ours – hoping that we will triumph, in the end, even over that final enemy. And not just passively hoping, but acting to make it so.

Note

1   Definitions by Max More. For Lextropicon see http://www.extropy.org/neologo.htm. Similarly, the Transhuman Terminology page: http://www.aleph.se/Trans/Words/.

References

Broderick, Damien (2001) *The Spike*. New York: A Forge Book, Tom Doherty Associates, LLC.

Fukuyama, Francis (1999) *The Great Disruption*. New York: Simon & Schuster.

Fukuyama, Francis (2003) *Our Posthuman Future: Consequences of the Biotechnology Revolution*. New York: Picador.

Fukuyama, Francis (2006) *The End of History*. New York: Free Press.

McKibben, Bill (2003) *Enough: Staying Human in an Engineered Age*. New York: Times Books. Biography at http://www.annonline.com/interviews/981217/biography.html.

Stock, Gregory. (2003) *Redesigning Humans: Choosing Our Genes, Changing Our Future*. Boston: Houghton Mifflin.

40

Back to Nature II
Art and Technology in the Twenty-First Century

Roy Ascott

It's well known that we have lost touch with Nature. It is not so much that Nature has retreated, or that we have dismissed it, destroyed it, or denied it. It is simply that the metaphors it has long supported no longer hold. Nature is, of course, all metaphor: the good, the pure, the unadulterated, the whole. It speaks of innocence, a kind of blessed naivety, as well as the wild, the unspoilt, and the instinctive. We should perhaps first agree that it has never as such existed, or that it has existed in different ways for different societies. It is the first virtual reality – in which the pure data of an undifferentiated wholeness is programmed, shaped, and categorized according to our language, fears, and desires. We have always placed it in opposition – to culture, the city, technology. Its strength has lain in this opposition, as much a refuge as a force. But now, the binary opposition of town and country, for example, is disappearing. With the ubiquity of telematic networks, the city is no longer the necessary site of commerce, learning, or entertainment, while the advance of artificial systems of synthesis and replication in biological sciences means that the country can no longer claim a hegemony of pure and authentic natural process. The country was the environment within which or against which the city was set, but with high technology as the environment, neither country nor city can be distinguished as objects to be foregrounded or privileged. As we move into the twenty-first century we shall need to create new metaphors to house the complex interacting systems of biological, technological, and social life which we are developing.

The shelf life of all metaphors, great and small, is limited, and Nature seems to be past its sell-by date. It has served us well in many respects – the ultimate appeal, for example, in questions of justice, human behavior, as in those of representation and figuration in the arts has always been – is it natural? Thus the popular icon of the visual culture of the epoch has been Van Gogh

From Roy Ascott, *Telematic Embrace: Visionary Theoriest of Art, Technology, and Consciousness*, ed. Edward A. Shanken (Berkeley: University of California Press, 1995).

The Transhumanist Reader: Classical and Contemporary Essays on the Science, Technology, and Philosophy of the Human Future, First Edition. Edited by Max More and Natasha Vita-More.

(a value to be measured in hard yen) and, for higher brows, Cezanne, both of whom we are reminded spent most of their time in the fields, immersed in nature. This scenario conveniently ignored Cezanne's comment that "all things, particularly in art, are theory developed and applied in contact with nature" (Rewald 1941). An insight curiously parallel to that found in the new physics as exemplified in Werner Heisenberg's dictum that it is the experimental apparatus (which includes the observer's consciousness) that determines a particle's "natural" behavior (Heisenberg 1962). And it is from Cezanne that we first understand the consequences for painting of the artist's mobile viewpoint, his focus restlessly scanning a world in flux.

Nature – classical, pastoral, secret, god-given nature, has suffered considerably at the hands of physicists during the twentieth century, and molecular biologists have not given it much peace, either. Science, whether reductionist or holistic, has altered irreversibly the common view of nature; on the one hand tearing it up into little pieces, on the other attempting to unify it into wholly new configurations. By the twenty-first century it will be dead. Scientific inquiry, aided by advanced computing, imaging, and telemetry systems, is yielding up to us an entirely new kind of nature – its transformations of energy, its evolutive, emergent behaviors, its order in chaos, the birth and death of galaxies, molecular life, quantum events, even mapping the movement of consciousness our own brains – none of which is observable directly by the human eye, and none of which previously had been observed by human beings in the whole of recorded history. All of which presents a picture of nature quite unlike that "staged" for our viewing by Western artists and writers for the past 500 years.

It may seem paradoxical to the popular view of art's relationship to nature, but it is these technological and computerized systems which are providing us with a threshold, an open doorway into the natural world – whereas, landscape and figure painting, the faithfully realistic and naturalistic painting of Western culture, have kept us separated from it. Painting produced a cultural membrane that kept us distanced from the processes of nature (and nature is all process), thereby affecting our relationship to it on more than the purely aesthetic level. That membrane was the window, the proscenium arch within which the artist "staged" nature, framed it in a timeless immobility. In the search for "naturalism," the wonder is not that the camera obscura and optical machines of the seventeenth and eighteenth centuries led to "naturalistic" photography and film in the nineteenth century but that artists failed for so long to respond in their painting to the dynamic processes of life revealed by the microscope, and pursued so blindly the representation of nature as a series of theatrical sets. Zacharias Jansen's compound microscope was invented in 1590, but it was not until our own century that any serious attempts were made by artists to deal with nature as it is perceived below the immediate level of the senses, expressing "the invisible which moves and lives beneath the gross forms," as Boccioni put it.

Sir Kenneth Clark, one of the last apologists of the old order, rejected such artists, particularly Paul Klee, as having merely "refurnished their repertoire of forms from the laboratories (which) does not in any way compensate for the loss of intimacy and love with which it was possible to contemplate the old anthropocentric nature. Love of creation cannot really extend to the microbe, nor to those spaces where the light which reaches our eyes has been travelling to meet us since before the beginning of man" (Clark 1953). While, earlier, with the same patrician certainty, Berenson, in trying to account for the "living force" which he found in the painting of Giotto, asserted that "there must exist surely a viaticum which bears its possessor to our own hearts, across the wastes of time, some secret which Giotto possessed ... What is this life conserving virtue – in what does it consist? The answer is brief – in life itself. If the artist can cunningly seize upon the spirit of life and imprison it in his paintings, his works ... will live forever" (Berenson 1897).

These two texts, sentimental and superstitious in turn, spoke for both the confusion and the desires of a culture at its turning point, in confronting the questions: how do we realize nature and evoke life, in what do they consist, how may they be re-created and transmitted? These questions of realization, evocation, re-creation, and transmission remain those which we artists prioritize now just as much as they drive research in the sciences. But the transformations in our models of the world and the accelerated increase on our technological powers of manipulation in recent years suggest that a cardinal question for artists in of the twenty-first century will instead be, "What might nature become?" And as knowledge and perception are increasingly mediated by computer-based systems, the question "What is reality?" is being replaced by "How do we interact with a proliferation of separate realities?" We connectivists feel that the conceptual foundation for dealing with these questions in art is beginning to take shape and that our work in electronic space today is properly preparing us to participate creatively in molecular time in the future, in the twenty-first-century return to nature.

How could it be that our inhabiting electronic space, communicating in electronic space, creating art in electronic space, can bring us back to nature? How is it that the most advanced technologies, electronic and molecular, the very epitome of the artificial, could bring us back to nature? For that is what I propose. I want to suggest that the logical outcome of our working in electronic space is to redefine our living in natural space. The logical outcome of the immateriality of the Information Society is the reinstatement in the twenty-first century of a natural materiality. I am not, of course, wanting to invoke the old metaphors of Nature in this assertion, but seeking to identify the metaphors of a new nature, second-order nature, emergent nature, Nature II, a new creativity whose "engines of creation" (Drexler 1990) will embrace artificial life. In *Engines of Creation*, Drexler gives a visionary and authoritative account of the consequences for "nature" of new technological developments, particularly of nanotechnology, the engineering of molecular computers which can self-assemble and replicate within human cells or build complex structures in outer space, which contains for artists some of the most radical implications since Norbert Wiener's *Cybernetics* (Wiener 1948), published in 1948.

Wiener's ideas led effectively to the computer revolution, the Information Society, and to the Telematic Culture. It may very well be that Drexler's writing signals the stirrings of a twenty-first-century revolution, the molecular revolution, the first shots of which have already been fired with the synthesis of chemicals with internal moving parts, a prototype of the molecular machine which will lead us in a matter of decades to the optical molecular computers which may make our present "electronic space" an obsolescent environment But following McLuhan's idea that the content of a new medium is the medium which preceded it, the rear-view mirror effect, we telematic artists can be optimistic that the molecular society of tomorrow will realize with ease the ideas of telepresence, connectivity, distributed authorship, and interactivity, which we are working with today. The difference will be that in addition to the processes of virtualization which epitomize our current concerns we shall see the emergence of new processes of materialization. In this respect, it is an amusing aside to consider how previously psychic phenomena have sought to satisfy the desire for transcendence that is now reflected in our attitude to new technology, table rapping and disembodied voices followed by radio, clairvoyance by TV, telepathy by telematics, remote viewing by remote sensing, out-of-body experience by VR, and now, coming soon to a séance near you – materialization by nanotechnology.

Just as mid-century cybernetics led, in important ways, to the development of AI (Artificial Intelligence), AL (Artificial Life), and IA (Interactive Art), so the course of cybernetics itself over the past 50 years provides a useful parallel to the evolution of our relationship with Nature.

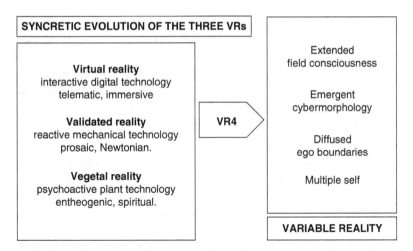

Figure 40.1   "VR4".

Cybernetics, the study of control and communication in living and artificial systems, found itself inadequate to the study of such systems until it included the observer of a system as a part of the system itself. Thus was born second-order cybernetics, which recognized the boundaries around all its objects of study as being intrinsically fuzzy, permeable, uncertain, and transformable, and utterly dependent on the position, attitude, and intention of the observer involved in such study. This insight, applicable as much to the quantum level of experiment as to the social, cultural, or even aesthetic level of experience, redefines our relationship with nature such that we become no longer outsiders looking into nature, nor an antagonist opposed to nature, but participants in the creative processes of nature. This means, of course, not an inert, passive, or genetically programmed participation but a conscious involvement in the evolution of those forms and emergent behaviors which we identify with life and which, as our powers of intelligent collaboration and participation increase, will come to constitute the new nature. Nature II.

There is a superstition, theme of countless myths and legends, that such participation (or intervention – a far greater crime!) in the emergent behaviors of planetary life, certainly any attempt to synthesis life, to create new forms of life and intelligence constitutes hubris, a sin against the gods! New life, new language, new behavior all constitute a new relationship to the cosmos – if this is hubris then it is a sin which besets new religions and new movements in art as much as science and technology. Moreover such innovation, such renewal of vision, such need to create the new, to invent the future, is at the same time profoundly traditional, as Maurizio Calvesi has pointed out with regard to the Italian Futurists, whose manifestos in many respects previsioned today's interactive arts of intelligent systems.

> The Futurist hubris of a radical *novitas* is the most traditional element of Futurism! Every Gnosis …
> is obsessed with breaking away from the past, with rebelling against *traditum* … the Christian language reveals an unheard-of message which shocks and surprises man … St. Irenaeus sums up this aspect of the gnostic mentality by saying it leads to an absolute *contrarietas et dissolutio praeteritorum* … this *contrarietas* [in Futurist writing led to] broken time … the word liberated from the "army" of syntax … a language that dissolves the past and burns the old, that frees the field ("Giiive me a brooom!" cries Marinetti) from the gods of death, paralysis and gravity. (Hulten 1986)

Broken time, the liberated text, the embrace of life, speed, anti-gravity – these are themes from our own late twentieth-century physics, post-structuralist linguistics, nanotechnology, space exploration. We now have the brooom in our hands. But this is not hubris! Our development as a species towards playing an increasingly direct part in the evolution of life and of consciousness grows out of our increased connectivity with the processes of nature, both in conceptual modeling and practical intervention. Second-order cybernetics and second-order nature share in what can be called the connectivist paradigm, which holds that everything is connected, everything interacts with and affects everything else. It is an idea as old, as traditional, as oriental religions and as new as the quantum physics of David Bohm, John Stewart Bell, and Alain Aspect (Herbert 1985). This connectedness, this undivided wholeness, unmediated action-at-a-distance, capable of transcending the laws of space and time with non-local interaction, is reflected in the telematic environment of computer-mediated networks of data transfer, interactive videoconferencing, remote sensing, and telerobotics, where communication also can be in a sense "non-local" and asynchronous although in different ways and with different outcomes. Equally the connectivist paradigm is at work in the modeling of human intelligence and theorizing about the mind. These explorations into the microstructure of cognition, known as connectionism, parallel distributed processing, or neural networks (McClelland and Rumelhart 1986), have developed out of a re-evaluation of some of the earliest ideas of cybernetics, of neural nets and the Perceptron, rejecting the linear, symbolic systems of the old AI. They will lead to the modeling of the complexities of many interconnected physical as well as cognitive behaviors, ultimately of multi-sensory systems and perhaps emotional mental states also. The connectivist paradigm thus embraces connectionism in science and what it is appropriate to call connectivism in art. The term "connectivism," however, suggests yet another "ism," another art movement for the history books. We know that this is not so. Art within the telematic culture is so fundamentally different from the art of the past as to constitute an entirely new field of creative endeavor. That is why many of us involved in this field think it would be best if a new word could be found to describe it. The term "art" is too heavy with the meanings given to it by both romanticism and classicism as well of course as modernism, and too deeply embedded in the notion of the individual creator and the re-active rather than inter-active viewer, for us to feel properly represented by it. It's not that we think we have redefined art in its totality or that the art with its roots in those earlier orders is no longer practiced with vigor and with contemporary relevance. Only society can determine that. But we feel that we cannot go on much longer having to define our terms every time we engage in conversation about art, to make it plain that it is this art, the art of interactivity and of intelligent systems, that we are discussing. not that art, the art of established orthodoxies and practices. So it may be useful for a while to avoid using the term "art" as far as possible in these circumstances, and to use the term "connectivism" when we are referring to telematic art practice. All art practice involving computer-mediated systems and electronic media of whatever complexion is by definition telematic, thus all artists engaged in the field are connectivists.

Within the systems metaphor, everything connects. The self is a complex system which interconnects with all other systems in a way that renders the line between natural and artificial systems meaningless. We are all becoming, to a greater or lesser extent, bionic. Drexler's account of the consequences of nanotechnology and Moravec's vision of advanced robotics (Moravec 1988) attest to this rapidly and radically evolving interdependency and connectedness of the natural and artificial in our development. Our prostheses not only amplify and extend the body and its five senses, but also augment cognition and memory and subtly transform the personality.

The psyche is certainly affected by interactions in the electronic space. Our relationship to time as well as space is altered. We are learning to measure memory and experience in nanoseconds as positron emission tomography and other computer-aided systems show us shimmering patterns of sensation shifting almost instantaneously across the brain's grid of tens of billions of nerve cells. Telematic communication systems and molecular engineering mean that nature and technology become inextricably linked. Just as space becomes "electronic," so time is becoming "molecular".

Deleuze has recently returned us to Bergson's project concerning Time and duration with reference to "the new lines, openings, traces, leaps, dynamisms, discovered by a molecular biology of the brain" (Deleuze 1988). I use the term molecular time to denote that bundle of meanings and interpretations of time provided in different but connected ways by cognitive science, neurobiology, computer science, and quantum physics, each of which recognizes the variable rates, jumps, delays, phases, and reversals of time which exist both within our consciousness, in our interactions with artificial memory and intelligence, and in the world of quantum events.

As we move into the twenty-first century, the interface between ourselves and the outer environment (at best always a fuzzy boundary) is becoming increasingly digitalized Our perception is increasingly computer-mediated; our information at the broad level of human affairs increasingly mediatized. We are less interested in representations of the world than in its virtualization. We no longer tend to "encounter all things through a rigorous story line" which, as McLuhan pointed out, is one of the penalties paid for literacy and a high visual culture (McLuhan and Parker 1968). Linear systems, rigid causality, analytical certitude have given way to a more playful interaction with non-linear systems, layered language, the navigation of meaning, heightening intuition, and self-creation. Connectivism, which calls for interactivity, reciprocity, and negotiation in the act of communication, gives rise to the idea of implicate meaning, to adapt David Bohm's notion of Implicate Order. In telematic art each quantum of meaning is many-layered, carrying within it a multiplicity of possible semantic trajectories, depending on the participating viewer, reader, or listener. We might want to call this the Many Meanings hypothesis in complementarity to Hugh Everett's Many Worlds interpretation of quantum mechanics – the observer as participant generating a rich profusion of parallel worlds/ parallel meanings.

Thus while one feature of connectivism is the explosion of meaning into an infinity of fragments, each particle embodying the principle of implicate meaning (leading perhaps to the semantic reseeding of the planet with the new metaphors of life that we so urgently need), the material substrate of this new art is incorporating sound, image, text, structures, and movement in increasing synthesis. In the ratio of the senses, sound is perhaps coming to count for as much as image, auditory space is more pervasive than visual space, in the electronic present. Our visual focus is becoming more inclusive, as language becomes more inclusive, as we come to recognize the essentially metaphoric construction of our knowledge and interpretation of reality. We move increasingly freely in the dataspace opened up by the computer-mediated systems of perception, modeling, and simulation which render the invisible visible .

Acoustic experience will become more focused as the environment becomes more intelligent and responsive to us. Once environments and their component parts (the buildings, furniture, vehicles, tools with which we interact) can intelligently recognize the direction and intention of our gaze or the meaning in our voice, they may learn to talk back to us, to respond with verbal as well as visual information focused on our individual needs. Personalized interactive systems and services set in acoustic space, linking us within the continuum of sound to an essentially intelligent and responsive built environment, may replace the visual barrage of signs, signals and messages which pollute the urban landscape.

There can be little doubt that databasing will also lead to new cultural behaviors, widely in the domain of home entertainment if more narrowly with those involved in creative exploration. There are already in the world some 4,500 distinct databases available through 650 real-time information services. Increasingly, streams of personal or collective memories, dreams, and speculations will feed into this ocean of data. Networking with these vast resources of image, text, and sound material will call for entirely new artistic strategies in the next century. Collaborative networking, interfacing in and out with the flux and flow of such data, rather than the attempt to construct the old form of artistic finalities, will clearly be a dominant mode of artistic expression. But however we interact with the electronic and digital systems which now bind us to the world, until we master the technological problem of internalizing the interface to such systems, that is within our bodies, the cultural symbiosis which we seek will evade us. Nothing impedes the subtle integration of human, natural, and artificial systems more than the present crudity of our technological interfaces – whether keyboard, screen, datasuit, or visor. Since the optical system is that part of the brain best understood by us at present, this presumably will be the site of our first forays into the bionic internalization of the computer interface.

Life in the twenty-first century will display new behaviors, new ways of relating to each other and to the planet, new metaphors, and new values. Many of these behaviors, relationships, and metaphors are already formed but we may not yet be able to recognize them readily or employ them effectively since attitudes and values of the old culture linger within the sclerosis of protected institutions and practices. Post-institutional thought is needed urgently, new landscapes of learning and creativity must be constructed. Connectivity is a principle of life, and the telematization of consciousness on the planet is carrying us all forward to another level of evolutionary development. Consciousness itself is in question, our sense of presence in the world and our relationship to reality. The question is, which world and which reality? Therein lies the schizophrenia of our condition. Telematic systems of global networking in virtual realities allow us to be both here and elsewhere at the same time. Increasingly over the coming years we shall become familiar with dealing with others and with ourselves as virtual presences in virtual spaces. Here and not here. Here and there, telematically, often without our knowledge or awareness of where we are being encountered or by whom, at which interface or communications node. In this process, human presence becomes virtualized and the individual self is distributed, space becomes virtualized and place becomes distributed. Moreover, there is inherent in all the research which currently surrounds the sciences of mind, advanced AI, AL, molecular engineering, robotics, and complex systems, the potential for consciousness to evolve beyond the human organism, and to a degree which perhaps only silicon-based life could accommodate, in "entities as complex as ourselves, and eventually into something transcending everything we know – in whom we can take pride when they refer to themselves as our descendants" (Moravec 1988). Art in the twenty-first century may come to constitute a form of mediation between human and post-human consciousness, just as in past cultures it has been used to mediate between mankind and the gods.

These ideas are seen by many people as threatening or confusing, but we artists using telematic media are exhilarated and inspired by this new existential potential, responding to it enthusiastically as an attribute of the human condition which has long been anticipated and keenly desired. These are ambitions that religions have sought to satisfy, that parapsychology seeks to address: to be out-of-body, to transcend our physical limitations, to participate in mind-at-large,

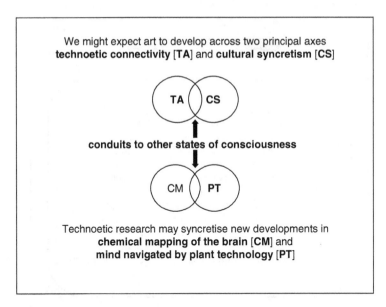

We might expect art to develop across two principal axes
technoetic connectivity [TA] and **cultural syncretism [CS]**

TA CS

conduits to other states of consciousness

CM PT

Technoetic research may syncretise new developments in
chemical mapping of the brain [CM] and
mind navigated by plant technology [PT]

Figure 40.2 "Consciousness".

to be in a state of virtual presence beyond the constraints of Euclidian space and Newtonian time – or, to employ a less lofty set of metaphors – to swim, sail, snorkle, and surf in the limitless semantic sea! All of which recognizes the self and human presence as ongoing dynamic processes rather than as a material finality.

Art has always concerned itself with human presence, by seeking to celebrate it, conserve it, invoke it, or mourn its passing. In religious art it has been the presence of the gods; in classical art, heroes and notables; in romantic art, the presence of the artist; in abstract, non-figurative art, the presence of presence itself. In the art of the telematic culture set in electronic space, we artists are no longer concerned with either with magic or representation but with virtualization, our presence distributed across the connection matrix which may be any one or more of a variety of telematic systems.

This question of the transformation of the self within electronic space and molecular time, that is to say in the context of advanced telematics and nanotechnology, will dominate the art of the next century. The alteration in our individual understanding of body-mind is enormously accelerated in the electronic environment. In the old print culture for example, the separation of books and mind, in questions of memory and information storage, was clear-cut. But with electronic technology, associative memory, once the privilege of the human mind alone, is now an attribute of computer systems. To think is more and more to interface such systems. At the same time the conceptual foundations of personal, individual, and original thought have been attacked by post-structuralist ideas of authorship and intertextuality.

There is no doubt that this is a critical period for art, the confusions and contradictions of postmodernism alone attest to the reactionary and arid banality of much contemporary production. This is not simply to say, although we connectivists think that the description is accurate, that a great deal of art involving computers is little more than a replay of older art forms – a kind of digital conversion of video, film, painting, sculpture, even the book. Any more than it is to ignore the massive technical achievements in image synthesis, animation, and simulation But this work is not connectivist in its attitudes and it is not telematic in its use of media. The

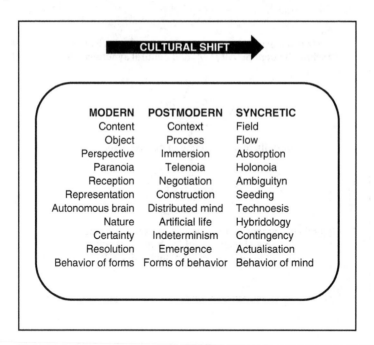

Figure 40.3   "Cultural Shift".

computer is still too much contained, finitely located, isolated as a black box, as a clever screen, or as an instrument, and until it is released, let loose in the world, into nature, into essentially living systems, the new art forms of the twenty-first century will not emerge. The spirit of connectivity has been released by the ubiquity of computer communications systems, but until the capacity for intelligent response and creative collaboration lies within the environment in all its parts, the connectivists' dream of planetary transformation will not be realized.

At present we are in a kind of cultural holding operation. The computer screen is no more than an interim contrivance: it allows us to model possibilities, just as VR allows us to model scenarios and test them out in virtual conditions. But think of *Ghost* – that late 1980s movie in which a "passed over" personality is projected into another organic agency, in this case a "sensitive," a psychic medium. Its success as a movie lay in the fact that it tapped precisely the contemporary consciousness of personality transfer, our contemporary understanding of mental acts as patterns of behavior in virtual machines, the wetware that drives the body hardware. Patterns of cognitive organization that we feel could be transferred between organisms, between machines. Patterns of ourselves that could be transferred across the networks. We cannot overestimate the potency of the image of Case, the protagonist of William Gibson's Neuromancer, "jacked into a custom cyberspace deck that projects his disembodied consciousness into the consensual hallucination that is the matrix" (Gibson 1984).

Another important aspect of the connectivist paradigm is to be found in the ideas of Robert Sheldrake, specifically his concept of Morphic Resonance.

> By means of morphic resonance, the form of a system, including its characteristic internal structure and vibration frequencies, becomes present to a subsequent system with a similar form. Analogous to the sympathetic vibration of stretched strings in response to appropriate sound waves, or the tuning of radio sets to the frequency of sound waves given out by transmitters ... morphic resonance

takes place between vibrating systems (note that in the body, including the brain, all our parts are in ceaseless oscillation). Morphic resonance takes place through morphogenetic fields. Not only does a specific field influence the form of a system, but also the form of this system influences the field. (Sheldrake 1983)

Twenty-first-century connectivists will want to tap into these morphogenetic fields, to influence the resonance of these vibrating systems. Sheldrake's is a science of metaphor, anti-reductionist, holistic, and intuitive. Like James Lovelock's Gaia hypothesis of an organic, self-regulating planet (Lovelock 1979), it offers a vision of reciprocity and connectivity in the world to which the tele-matic art of our time aspires. Personality transfer, ideas transfer, telepresence, the creation remotely, through distributed authorship, of images, forms, sound, movement in totally synthe-sized ensembles, the virtual realization of concepts which address the unknown and the hitherto unknowable, that make the invisible visible, that can inhabit intelligent systems, that can come into the world in the form of an open-ended, transformable, interactive, responsive, organic materiality – that is the prospectus for our art in the twenty-first century.

This materiality, this creativity involving natural systems with artificial life, will come about as a convergence of the two apparently divergent trajectories of contemporary technology – the one essentially electronic, concerning, computerized perception and intelligence, virtualization, telematic communication – the other biological, involving nanotechnology, molecular engineer-ing, the organization of matter and emergent behavior. A marriage of the immaterial and the material leading to a transcendence over the gross materiality of "natural," unmediated life. Put simply, for the connectivist this is a question of creating an interactive art of intelligent systems set within intelligent environments. The early twenty-first century may see some success in this endeavor. We shall then have moved beyond the information society, beyond the frontier of electronic space, back to Nature – but to a nature radically revised – a holistic environment of mind and matter, as much spiritual as material, in which "natural" transformations of nature take their place with our conscious participation and collaboration within a culture of creative complexity. None of this, however, can be achieved in cultural isolation. Artists must reach out to those scientific and technological disciplines which speak a similar language. In neural net-works we certainly find one such discipline, and nanotechnology as it develops will undoubtedly be another. A whole new field of bio-telematics waits to be created, a whole new field of art is preparing to participate in its emergence. We can at this time feel a special resonance with the metaphors and aspirations of Artificial Life.

Here we see a concern with "life-as-we-know-it in the larger context of life-as-it-could-be. It views life as a property of the organization of matter, rather than as a property of the matter which is organ-ised … The key concept in AL is emergent behavior. Natural life emerges out of the organized inter-action of a great number of non living molecules, with no global controller responsible for the behavior of every part. Rather, every part is a behavior itself, and life is the behavior that emerges from all of the local interactions among individual behaviors. It is this bottom-up, distributed, local determination of behavior that AL employs in its primary methodological approach to the genera-tion of lifelike behaviors. (Langdon 1989)

For "life" read "art"! We can see the parallelism between AL and IA if we replace the word "life" with the word "art" in the above passage. Telematic culture shares this bottom-up, dis-tributed, local determination of its art, with no global controller responsible for the behavior of every part.

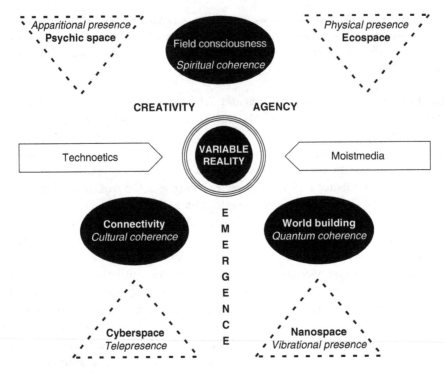

Figure 40.4   "Creative Agency".

Whilst it is often true that life imitates art, we have here a situation in which art in the twenty-first century may very well come to parallel in important ways the aspirations of artificial life. This convergence set in electronic space and molecular time may well point us to a path leading back to nature, the sequel to nature … Nature II.

References

Berenson, Bernard (1897) *The Central Italian Painters of the Renaissance*. London: Putnam.

Clark, Kenneth (1953) *Landscape into Art*. London: Murray.

Deleuze, Gilles (1988) *Bergsonism*. New York: Zone Books.

Drexler, K. Eric (1990) *Engines of Creation*. London: Fourth Estate.

Gibson, William (1984) *Neuromancer*. London: Gollancz.

Heisenberg, Werner (1962) *Physics and Philosophy*. New York: Harper & Row.

Herbert, Nick (1985) *Quantum Reality*. New York: Anchor.

Hulten, Pontus (1986) *Futurism & Futurisms*. London: Thames & Hudson.

Langdon, Christopher (1989) *Artificial Life*. New York: Addison-Wesley.

Lovelock, James (1979) *Gaia, a New Look at Life on Earth*. Oxford: Oxford University Press.

McClelland, James L. and Rumelhart, David E. (1986) *Parallel Distributed Processing*. Cambridge, MA: MIT Press.

McLuhan, Marshall and Parker, Harley (1968) *Through the Vanishing Point*. New York: Harper & Row.

Moravec, Hans (1988) *Mind Children*. Cambridge, MA: Harvard University Press.

Rewald. John (1941) *Paul Cezanne Letters*. Oxford: Cassirer.

Sheldrake, Rupert (1983) *A New Science of Life*. London: Granada.

Wiener, Norbert (1948) *Cybernetics*. Cambridge, MA: MIT Press.

41

A Letter to Mother Nature

Max More

Dear Mother Nature:

Sorry to disturb you, but we humans – your offspring – come to you with some things to say. (Perhaps you could pass this on to Father, since we never seem to see him around.) We want to thank you for the many wonderful qualities you have bestowed on us with your slow but massive, distributed intelligence. You have raised us from simple self-replicating chemicals to trillion-celled mammals. You have given us free rein of the planet. You have given us a lifespan longer than that of almost any other animal. You have endowed us with a complex brain giving us the capacity for language, reason, foresight, curiosity, and creativity. You have given us the capacity for self-understanding as well as empathy for others.

Mother Nature, truly we are grateful for what you have made us. No doubt you did the best you could. However, with all due respect, we must say that you have in many ways done a poor job with the human constitution. You have made us vulnerable to disease and damage. You compel us to age and die – just as we're beginning to attain wisdom. You were miserly in the extent to which you gave us awareness of our somatic, cognitive, and emotional processes. You held out on us by giving the sharpest senses to other animals. You made us functional only under narrow environmental conditions. You gave us limited memory, poor impulse control, and tribalistic, xenophobic urges. And, you forgot to give us the operating manual for ourselves!

What you have made us is glorious, yet deeply flawed. You seem to have lost interest in our further evolution some 100,000 years ago. Or perhaps you have been biding your time, waiting for us to take the next step ourselves. Either way, we have reached our childhood's end.

We have decided that it is time to amend the human constitution.

We do not do this lightly, carelessly, or disrespectfully, but cautiously, intelligently, and in pursuit of excellence. We intend to make you proud of us. Over the coming decades we will

The Transhumanist Reader: Classical and Contemporary Essays on the Science, Technology, and Philosophy of the Human Future, First Edition. Edited by Max More and Natasha Vita-More.
© 2013 John Wiley & Sons, Inc. Published 2013 by John Wiley & Sons, Inc.

pursue a series of changes to our own constitution, initiated with the tools of biotechnology guided by critical and creative thinking. In particular, we declare the following seven amendments to the human constitution:

Amendment No. 1. We will no longer tolerate the tyranny of aging and death. Through genetic alterations, cellular manipulations, synthetic organs, and any necessary means, we will endow ourselves with enduring vitality and remove our expiration date. We will each decide for ourselves how long we shall live.

Amendment No. 2. We will expand our perceptual range through biotechnological and computational means. We seek to exceed the perceptual abilities of any other creature and to devise novel senses to expand our appreciation and understanding of the world around us.

Amendment No. 3. We will improve on our neural organization and capacity, expanding our working memory, and enhancing our intelligence.

Amendment No. 4. We will supplement the neocortex with a "metabrain." This distributed network of sensors, information processors, and intelligence will increase our degree of self-awareness and allow us to modulate our emotions.

Amendment No. 5. We will no longer be slaves to our genes. We will take charge over our genetic programming and achieve mastery over our biological, and neurological processes. We will fix all individual and species defects left over from evolution by natural selection. Not content with that, we will seek complete choice of our bodily form and function, refining and augmenting our physical and intellectual abilities beyond those of any human in history.

Amendment No. 6. We will cautiously yet boldly reshape our motivational patterns and emotional responses in ways we, as individuals, deem healthy. We will seek to improve upon typical human emotional excesses, bringing about refined emotions. We will strengthen ourselves so we can let go of unhealthy needs for dogmatic certainty, removing emotional barriers to rational self-correction.

Amendment No. 7. We recognize your genius in using carbon-based compounds to develop us. Yet we will not limit our physical, intellectual, or emotional capacities by remaining purely biological organisms. While we pursue mastery of our own biochemistry, we will increasingly integrate our advancing technologies into our selves.

These amendments to our constitution will transition us from a human to an posthuman condition as individuals. We believe that individual transhumanizing will also allow us to form relationships, cultures, and polities of unprecedented innovation, richness, freedom, and responsibility.

We reserve the right to make further amendments collectively and individually. Rather than seeking a state of final perfection, we will continue to pursue new forms of excellence according to our own values, and as technology allows.

Your ambitious human offspring.

42

Progress and Relinquishment

Ray Kurzweil

Technology has always been a double-edged sword, bringing us longer and healthier lifespans, freedom from physical and mental drudgery, and many new creative possibilities, on the one hand, while introducing new and salient dangers on the other. Technology empowers both our creative and destructive natures. Genetic engineering is in the early stages of enormous strides in reversing disease and aging processes.

Ubiquitous nanotechnology, now about two decades away, will continue an exponential expansion of these benefits. These technologies will create extraordinary wealth, thereby overcoming poverty, and enabling us to provide for all of our material needs by transforming inexpensive raw materials and information into virtually any type of product. Lingering problems from our waning industrial age will be overcome. We will be able to reverse remaining environmental destruction.

Nanoengineered fuel cells and solar cells will provide clean energy. Nanobots in our physical bodies will destroy pathogens, remove debris such as misformed proteins and protofibrils, repair DNA, and reverse aging. We will be able to redesign all of the systems in our bodies and brains to be far more capable and durable. And that's only the beginning.

There are also salient dangers. The means and knowledge exist in a routine college bioengineering lab to create unfriendly pathogens more dangerous than nuclear weapons. Unrestrained nanobot replication ("unrestrained" being the operative word here) would endanger all physical entities, biological or otherwise. As for "unfriendly" AI, that's the most daunting challenge of all because intelligence is inherently the most powerful force in the Universe.

Awareness of these dangers has resulted in calls for broad relinquishment. Bill McKibben, the environmentalist who was one of the first to warn against global warming, takes the position that we have sufficient technology and that further progress should end. In his

Statement for Extropy Institute Vital Progress Summit February 18, 2004.

The Transhumanist Reader: Classical and Contemporary Essays on the Science, Technology, and Philosophy of the Human Future, First Edition. Edited by Max More and Natasha Vita-More.

latest book, titled *Enough: Staying Human in an Engineered Age*, he metaphorically compares technology to beer and writes that "one beer is good, two beers may be better; eight beers, you're almost certainly going to regret." McKibben's metaphor comparing continued engineering to gluttony misses the point, and ignores the extensive suffering that remains in the human world, which we will be in a position to alleviate through sustained technological progress.

Another level of relinquishment, one recommended in Bill Joy's *Wired* magazine cover story, "Why the Future Doesn't Need Us" (*Wired* 8.04, April 2000), would be to forgo certain fields – nanotechnology, for example – that might be regarded as too dangerous. But such sweeping strokes of relinquishment are equally untenable. Nanotechnology is simply the inevitable end result of the persistent trend towards miniaturization that pervades all of technology. It is far from a single centralized effort, but is being pursued by a myriad of projects with many diverse goals.

Abandonment of broad areas of technology will only push them underground, where development would continue unimpeded by ethics and regulation. In such a situation, it would be the less stable, less responsible practitioners (e.g., terrorists) who would have all the expertise.

The siren calls for broad relinquishment are effective because they paint a picture of future dangers as if they were released on today's unprepared world. The reality is that the sophistication and power of our defensive technologies and knowledge will grow along with the dangers. When we have "gray goo" (unrestrained nanobot replication), we will also have "blue goo" ("police" nanobots that combat the "bad" nanobots). The story of the twenty-first century has not yet been written, so we cannot say with assurance that we will successfully avoid all misuse. But the surest way to prevent the development of the defensive technologies would be to relinquish the pursuit of knowledge in broad areas. This was the primary moral of the novel Brave New World.

Consider software viruses. We have been able to largely control harmful software virus replication because the requisite knowledge is widely available to responsible practitioners. Attempts to restrict this knowledge would have created a far less stable situation. Responses to new challenges would have been far slower, and it is likely that the balance would have shifted towards the more destructive applications (that is, the software pathogens). Stopping the "GNR" technologies is not feasible, at least not without adopting a totalitarian system, and pursuit of such broad forms of relinquishment will only distract us from the vital task in front of us. In terms of public policy, the task at hand is to rapidly develop the defensive steps needed, which include ethical standards, legal standards, and defensive technologies. It is quite clearly a race. There is simply no alternative. We cannot relinquish our way out of this challenge.

There have been useful proposals for protective strategies, such as Ralph Merkle's "broadcast" architecture, in which replicating entities need to obtain replication codes from a secure server. We need to realize, of course, that each level of protection will only work to a certain level of sophistication.

The "meta" lesson here is that we will need to place society's highest priority during the twenty-first century on continuing to advance the defensive technologies and to keep them one or more steps ahead of destructive misuse. In this way, we can realize the profound promise of these accelerating technologies, while managing the peril.

Note

Responding to the report of the President's Council on Bioethics, *Beyond Therapy: Biotechnology and the Pursuit of Happiness* (2003), Ray Kurzweil authored a keynote statement for Extropy Institute's Vital Progress Summit, an Internet virtual discussion and debate. Published on Extropy Institute Vital Progress Summit website and KurzweilAI.net, February 18, 2004.

The Vital Progress Summit countered the growing number of groups that attempt to halt scientific advancement and their growing political influence over governments and legislation. It did this by arguing for a more informed and balanced discussion the topic of human enhancement. A major outcome of the Summit was the Proactionary Principle (version 1.0: http://www.extropy.org/proactionaryprinciple.htm and http://strategicphilosophy.blogspot.com/2008/03/proactionary-principle-march-2008.html; version 1.2 : http://www.maxmore.com/proactionary.htm; the most recent version in this volume) as an alternative to the unbalanced strictures of the Precautionary Principle.

Summit keynotes included, in alphabetical order: Ronald Bailey, Aubrey de Grey, Robert A. Freitas, Raymond Kurzweil, Marvin Minsky, Max More, Christine Peterson, Michael D. Shapiro, Lee Silver, Gregory Stock, Natasha Vita-More, Roy Walford, and Michael West. See http://www.extropy.org/summitkeynotes.htm.

Index

*The Transhumanist Reader: Classical and Contemporary Essays on the Science, Technology,
and Philosophy of the Human Future*, First Edition. Edited by Max More and Natasha Vita-More.
© 2013 John Wiley & Sons, Inc. Published 2013 by John Wiley & Sons, Inc.